Tumors of the Sacrum

Pietro Ruggieri • Andrea Angelini
Daniel Vanel • Piero Picci
Editors

Tumors of the Sacrum

Diagnosis and Treatment of Benign and Malignant Tumors

Springer

Editors
Pietro Ruggieri
Department of Orthopedics and
Orthopedic Oncology
University of Padova
PD, Italy

Andrea Angelini
Department of Orthopedics and
Orthopedic Oncology
University of Padova
PD, Italy

Daniel Vanel
Department of Pathology
Istituto Ortopedico Rizzoli
Bologna, Italy

Piero Picci
Laboratory of Experimental Oncology,
Musculoskeletal Oncology,
Istituto Ortopedico Rizzoli
Bologna, Italy

ISBN 978-3-319-51200-6 ISBN 978-3-319-51202-0 (eBook)
DOI 10.1007/978-3-319-51202-0

Library of Congress Control Number: 2017940037

Printed on acid-free paper

This Springer imprint is published by Springer Nature
The registered company is Springer International Publishing AG
The registered company address is: Gewerbestrasse 11, 6330 Cham, Switzerland

Contents

List of Contributors and Author Bios

List of Contributors

Sean Accardo, M.D. Department of Sarcoma, H. Lee Moffitt Cancer Center, Tampa, FL, USA

Andrea Angelini, M.D., Ph.D. Department of Orthopedics and Orthopedic Oncology, University of Padova, Padova, Italy

Alessandra Bartoloni, M.D. Diagnostic and Interventional Radiology, Istituto Ortopedico Rizzoli, Bologna, Italy

Alberto Bazzocchi, M.D. Diagnostic and Interventional Radiology, Istituto Ortopedico Rizzoli, Bologna, Italy

Marilyn M. Bui, M.D., Ph.D. Department of Anatomic Pathology, H. Lee Moffitt Cancer Center, Tampa, FL, USA

Department of Sarcoma, H. Lee Moffitt Cancer Center, Tampa, FL, USA

Angelo Paolo Dei Tos, M.D. Department of Anatomic Pathology, General Hospital of Treviso, Treviso, Italy

Yi Ding, M.D. Department of Pathology, Beijing Jishuitan Hospital, Beijing, China

Stefano Ferrari, M.D. Department of Chemotherapy, Istituto Ortopedico Rizzoli, Bologna, Italy

Alexandra Gangi, M.D. Department of Surgical Oncology, H. Lee Moffitt Cancer Center, Tampa, FL, USA

Ricardo Gonzalez, M.D. Department of Surgical Oncology, H. Lee Moffitt Cancer Center, Tampa, FL, USA

Evita Henderson-Jackson, M.D. Department of Anatomic Pathology, H. Lee Moffitt Cancer Center, Tampa, FL, USA

Department of Sarcoma, H. Lee Moffitt Cancer Center, Tampa, FL, USA

Francis J. Hornicek, M.D., Ph.D. Section of Orthopaedic Oncology, Department of Orthopaedic Surgery, Massachusetts General Hospital, Boston, MA, USA

Matthew T. Houdek, M.D. Department of Orthopedic Surgery, Mayo Clinic, Rochester, MN, USA

Vasilios Igoumenou, M.D. First Department of Orthopaedics, National and Kapodistrian University of Athens, Athens, Greece

David M. Joyce, M.D. Department of Sarcoma, H. Lee Moffitt Cancer Center, Tampa, FL, USA

Douglas G. Letson, M.D. Department of Surgery, University of South Florida, H. Lee Moffitt Cancer Center, Tampa, FL, USA

Laurel A. Littrell, M.D. Department of Radiology, Mayo Clinic, Rochester, MN, USA

Andreas F. Mavrogenis, M.D., Ph.D. First Department of Orthopaedics, National and Kapodistrian University of Athens, Athens, Greece

Steven L. Moran, M.D. Division of Plastic and Reconstructive Surgery, Mayo Clinic, Rochester, MN, USA

John E. Mullinax, M.D. Department of Surgical Oncology, H. Lee Moffitt Cancer Center, Tampa, FL, USA

Erik T. Newman, M.D. Section of Orthopaedic Oncology, Department of Orthopaedic Surgery, Massachusetts General Hospital, Boston, MA, USA

Georgios N. Panagopoulos, M.D. First Department of Orthopaedics, National and Kapodistrian University of Athens, Athens, Greece

Piero Picci, M.D. Laboratory of Experimental Oncology, Musculoskeletal Oncology, Istituto Ortopedico Rizzoli, Bologna, Italy

Peter S. Rose, M.D. Department of Orthopedic Surgery, Mayo Clinic, Rochester, MN, USA

Pietro Ruggieri, M.D., Ph.D. Department of Orthopedics and Orthopedic Oncology, University of Padova, Padova, Italy

Joseph H. Schwab, M.D., M.S. Section of Orthopaedic Oncology, Department of Orthopaedic Surgery, Massachusetts General Hospital, Boston, MA, USA

Franklin H. Sim, M.D. Department of Orthopedic Surgery, Mayo Clinic, Rochester, MN, USA

Daniel Vanel, M.D. Department of Pathology, Istituto Ortopedico Rizzoli, Bologna, Italy

Doris E. Wenger, M.D. Department of Radiology, Mayo Clinic, Rochester, MN, USA

Michael J. Yaszemski, M.D., Ph.D. Department of Orthopedic Surgery and Biomedical Engineering, Mayo Clinic, Rochester, MN, USA

Pier Luigi Zinzani, M.D., Ph.D. Institute of Hematology "L. e A. Seràgnoli," University of Bologna, Bologna, Italy

Author Bios

Andrea Angelini is an orthopedic surgeon at the Department of Orthopedics and Orthopedic Oncology, University of Padova.

Born in Savignano sul Rubicone, Italy, in 1983, he obtained his medical degree (cum laude) from the University of Bologna in 2008. He obtained board certification in orthopedic surgery at the University of Bologna and Istituto Ortopedico Rizzoli in 2014, followed by a Ph.D. in oncology and experimental pathology from the University of Bologna in 2016. His main field of interest is surgery for musculoskeletal tumors: he collaborated for a book (editor of one book), chapters (contributor of four published book chapters), and numerous scientific papers (62 published papers available on PubMed, about 600 citations, H-index 13, IF 85). He has held courses and talks at international meetings (n. 60 presentations), and he is coauthor of more than 200 meeting abstracts. He was awarded for his scientific activity by EFORT, SIOT, EMSOS, and ISOLS. He lives in Bologna and is married with one child.

Piero Picci is director of the Laboratory of Experimental Oncology of Istituto Ortopedico Rizzoli in Bologna, Italy. He obtained his degree in medicine and surgery from the University of Bologna (1979) and completed his board certification in oncology at the same university (1983).

He is coordinator of the EU project PROTHETS (Prognostic and Therapeutic Targets in Ewing Family of Tumors) and research line leader (Ewing sarcoma) in the EU project EUROBONET. He is a participant in four other EU projects.

He is author or coauthor of 446 papers on international journals (433 on Medline, H-index 70), 56 papers on national journals, 71 book chapters, 518 abstracts from international congresses, and 99 abstracts from national congresses.

His memberships include being founder and chairman of the Italian Sarcoma Group (1997); founder, board member, treasurer, vice-president, and president of EMSOS; board member of CTOS; and member of ISS, ASCO, and AIOM.

Pietro Ruggieri is chairman of the Department of Orthopedics and Orthopedic Oncology at the University of Padova, and Director of the Scientific Center for Research of Musculoskeletal Tumors "Mario Mercuri".

Born in Taranto (Italy) in 1958, he graduated in medicine at the University of Bologna in 1982, completed board of orthopedics in 1987 and obtained his Ph.D. in oncology from the University of Bologna in 1989. He was a fellow at the University of Florida, Gainesville, under the direction of Dr. Enneking and Dr. Springfield in

1987 and was a fellow of Dr. Frank Sim at Mayo Clinic in 1991. He is author of more than 800 scientific papers on national/international journals (over 290 of these on PubMed), with an impact factor of over 533 and a citation H-index of 41. He has been a speaker or lecturer in more than 500 international congresses. He has been president of ISOLS. He is board member of EMSOS, co-director of the subspecialty of tumors for SICOT, and scientific coordinator for EFORT. Since October 2016, he is a member of the MSTS Membership Committee. His main fields of research are musculoskeletal oncology, reconstructive surgery, and prostheses in musculoskeletal oncology.

Daniel Vanel is in charge of research and teaching in musculoskeletal tumors at Istituto Ortopedico Rizzoli, Bologna, Italy.

He is former chairman of radiology of Institut Gustave Roussy, France.

He is former president of the European Society of Musculoskeletal Radiology and International Cancer Imaging Society.

He was awarded the Gold Medal of the International Skeletal Society.

He authored 276 articles in Medline.

Part I

General Aspects

Epidemiology of Bone Lesions of the Sacrum

1

Piero Picci

These data come from the Archives of musculoskeletal tumor and pseudotumoral lesions of the Istituto Ortopedico Rizzoli in Bologna. We do not report incidence data, but frequency data registered at a referral center for musculoskeletal lesions. From September 1900 to December 2014, the archive comprises 28,477 cases, of which 790 (2.77%) were lesion of the sacrum. To better understand the specificity of sacrum lesions, data will be compared to the figures of bone lesions affecting the whole skeleton.

1.1 Diagnosis

Conventional bone lesion classification usually subdivides these in "pseudotumoral," "benign," and "malignant," considering the last separately between primary and part of a systemic disease (i.e., carcinoma metastasis, lymphoma, myeloma).

Distribution between these macro-entities differs between the sacrum and all other bone sites. In the sacrum, about three fourths of the cases are malignant, while in the other sites, only one half are malignant. Primary malignant tumors are more frequent in the sacrum (341 cases, 43.2%) followed by systemic lesions (238 cases, 30.1%), benign lesions (195 cases, 24.7%), and pseudotumoral lesions (16 cases, 2.0%). In the whole skeleton, benign lesions are more frequent (11,386 cases, 40.0%), followed by primary tumors (8145 cases, 28.6%), systemic lesions (6149 cases, 21.6%), and pseudotumoral lesions (2797 cases, 9.8%) (Fig. 1.1). Table 1.1 reports all sacrum lesions.

P. Picci, M.D.
Laboratory of Experimental Oncology, Musculoskeletal Oncology, Istituto Ortopedico Rizzoli, Bologna, Italy
e-mail: piero.picci@ior.it

P. Ruggieri et al. (eds.), *Tumors of the Sacrum*,
DOI 10.1007/978-3-319-51202-0_1

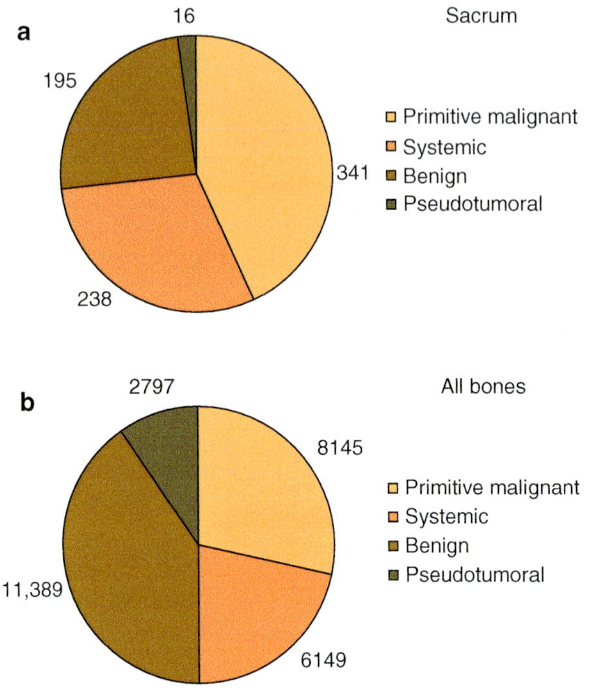

Fig. 1.1 Distribution of bone lesions affecting (**a**) the sacrum and (**b**) the entire skeleton, in the Rizzoli experience. Lesions have been classified as pseudotumoral, benign, primitive malignant and malignant as part of a systemic disease

Frequency of the different entities is totally different from the general distribution in the whole skeleton. From this comparison many important differences are evident, apart from the obvious high frequency of chordomas and intraosseous schwannoma, the latter originating from the sacral roots. There is an important increase in the percentage of systemic lesions as bone metastasis from carcinoma (+25%), lymphoma (+64%), and myeloma (+130%). Among primary malignant tumors, there is an increase of Ewing sarcoma (+54%) and angiosarcoma (+50%), but there is an important decrease in the frequency of osteosarcomas (−54%) and chondrosarcomas (−43%). Within the benign tumors, there is an increase in frequency of giant cell tumor (+40%) and osteoblastoma (+145%), the latter compensated by a decrease in the frequency of osteoid osteoma (−56%).

The frequency of aneurysmal bone cyst and angioma of the bone is not dissimilar from other sites. To be noted is the higher frequency (+120%) of Paget disease in the sacrum. It is important to report that three of the eight secondary osteosarcomas in the sacrum developed on Paget disease. Table 1.2 reports the incidence of the 15 most frequent entities in the sacrum compared to the frequency in the whole skeleton.

Table 1.1 Lesions of the sacrum

Pseudotumoral lesions	*16*
Paget disease	9
Histiocytosis X	6
Solitary bone cyst	1
Benign lesions	*195*
Giant cell tumor	58
Aneurysmal bone cyst	27
Osteoid osteoma	25
Intraosseous schwannoma	25
Osteoblastoma	21
Angioma of bone	9
Fibrous dysplasia	5
Notochordal benign tumor	5
Benign not otherwise specified	5
Solitary osteochondroma	4
Ependymoma	4
Teratoma	4
Chondroblastoma	1
Chondromyxoid fibroma	1
Intraosseous lipoma	1
Primary malignant tumors	*341*
Chordoma	167
Ewing sarcoma	63
Osteosarcomas	46
Classic	35
Secondary	8
Low-grade central	2
Telangiectatic	1
Chondrosarcomas	29
Central	14
Peripheral	6
Clear cell	3
Mesenchymal	3
Dedifferentiated	3
Sarcoma not otherwise specified	10
Angiosarcoma	7
Intraosseous solitary fibrous tumor	6
Undifferentiated pleomorphic sarcoma (UPS)	4
Intraosseous malignant schwannoma	3
Intraosseous leiomyosarcoma	3
Intraosseous synovial sarcoma	2
Intraosseous myoepithelioma	1
Systemic tumors	*238*
Carcinoma metastasis	153
Myeloma	49
Lymphoma	36

Table 1.2 Comparison of frequency in the sacrum and in the whole skeleton for the 15 most frequent entities

	Sacrum		Whole skeleton		Delta
	N°	%	N°	%	%
Chordoma	167	21.1	123	0.4	5175
Metastasis from carcinoma	153	19.4	4305	15.5	25
Ewing sarcoma	63	8.0	1437	5.2	54
Giant cell tumor	58	7.3	1451	5.2	40
Myeloma	49	6.2	745	2.7	130
Osteosarcomas	46	5.8	3507	12.7	−54
Lymphomas	36	4.6	767	2.8	64
Chondrosarcomas	29	3.7	1813	6.5	−43
Aneurysmal bone cyst	27	3.4	1093	3.9	−13
Osteoid osteoma	25	3.2	1992	7.2	−56
Intraosseous schwannoma	25	3.2	17	0.1	3100
Osteoblastoma	21	2.7	311	1.1	145
Paget disease	9	1.1	140	0.5	120
Angioma of bone	9	1.1	279	1.0	10
Angiosarcoma	7	0.9	180	0.6	50

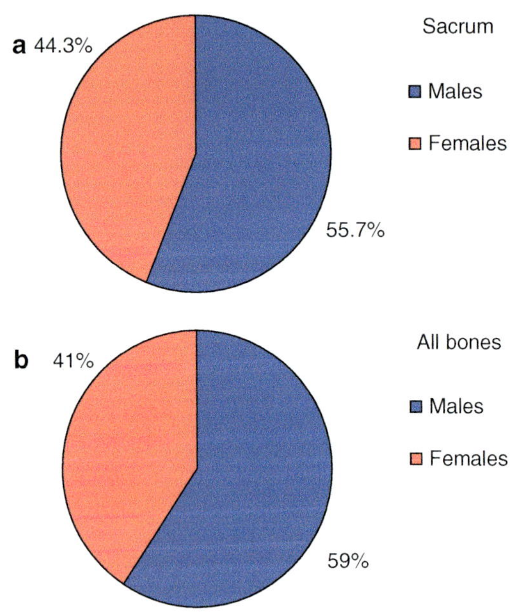

Fig. 1.2 Gender distribution of patients with lesions affecting (**a**) the sacrum and (**b**) the entire skeleton, in the Rizzoli experience

1.2 Gender

A slight prevalence is evident in females with sacral lesions (44.3%) in comparison to other sites (41.0%) (Fig. 1.2).

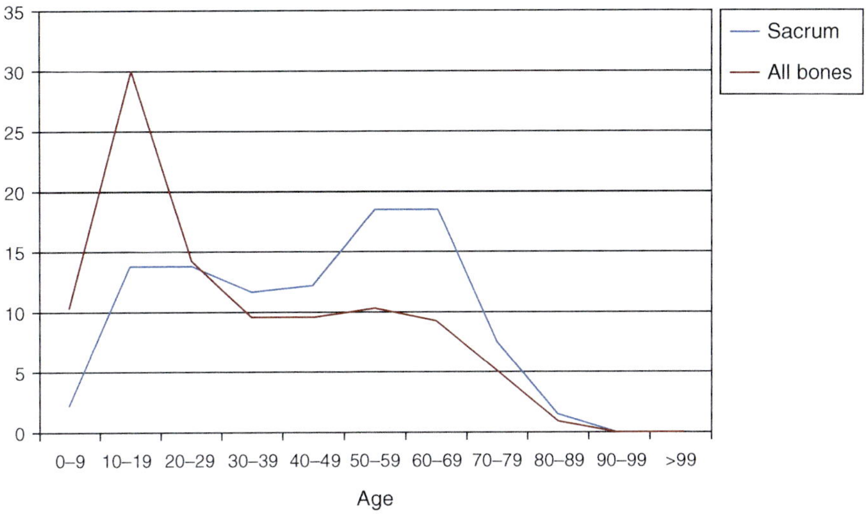

Fig. 1.3 Incidence by age

1.3 Age

The analysis of age shows major differences in the sacrum, compared to other bone sites.

In the sacrum, with a range of 0–89 years, the mean is 44 and the median 47, while in all other sites with a similar age range (from 0 to 103), the mean is 32 and the median is 25.

It is evident that sacral lesions develop in much older patients compared to the other bone sites. Figure 1.3 reports the incidence by decades of the two groups.

Conflict-of-Interest Statement No benefits have been or will be received from a commercial party related directly or indirectly to the subject matter of this article.

Overview on Bone Sacral Tumors

2

Alexandra Gangi and Ricardo Gonzalez

2.1 Introduction

Primary sacral tumors are rare, accounting for approximately 5–7% of all spinal tumors [1]. Metastases are the most common malignant tumors of the sacrum and can be derived from lung, breast, kidney, prostate, head and neck, gastrointestinal, or skin (melanoma) cancers [2, 3, 62]. Primary benign and malignant tumors of the sacrum may arise from bone or neural elements or the bone marrow in cases of hematological malignancies. Approximately 10% of all benign tumors or pseudotumors have been known to involve the sacrum. These can include giant cell tumors (60% of cases), aneurysmal bone cysts (4%), and osteoblastomas. Of malignant bone tumors, 6–8% involve the sacrum and include chordoma (50%), lymphoma (9%) and multiple myeloma (9%), Ewing's sarcoma in children (8%), chondrosarcoma in adults, and osteosarcoma [4].

2.2 Clinical Presentation

Sacral tumors are generally diagnosed late, and the clinical pattern depends on the anatomic location of the lesion within the sacrum and involvement of specific anatomic structures [5–13]. The topic will be discussed in greater detail in the specific chapter.

A. Gangi, M.D. • R. Gonzalez, M.D. (✉)
Sarcoma Department, H. Lee Moffitt Cancer Center,
12902 Magnolia Drive, Tampa, FL 33602, USA
e-mail: Alexandra.Gangi@moffitt.org; Ricardo.Gonzalez@moffitt.org

P. Ruggieri et al. (eds.), *Tumors of the Sacrum*,
DOI 10.1007/978-3-319-51202-0_2

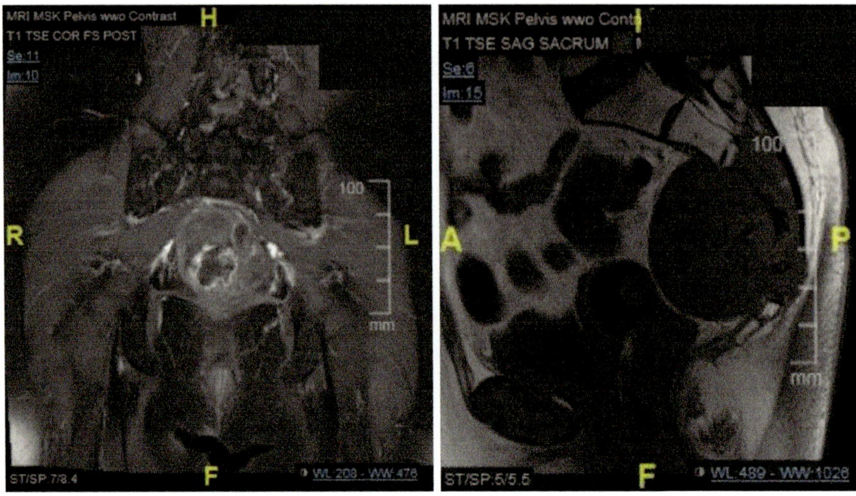

Fig. 2.1 Coronal and sagittal views of 8.5 × 6.5 cm sacral chordoma involving S3-C1

2.3 Imaging

Imaging is a useful adjunct in the diagnosis of sacral tumors. Although the sacrum can be frequently obscured by overlying stool or bowel gas, plain radiographs can be helpful with initial diagnosis. Nonetheless, for more thorough evaluation and better defined spatial understanding, additional imaging such as computed tomography (CT) scan or magnetic resonance imaging (MRI) are required [14, 15, 59].

In general, computed tomography is superior in showing bony details and calcifications and allows for better visualization of adjacent viscera. Lumbar CT scans usually ordered for sciatica of cruralgia must include S1 and S2 in the examination so that sacral lesions are not missed. CT-guided biopsy is particularly useful in the sacrum. If CT is substituted for MRI and there is a presacral soft tissue mass, administration of both rectal and intravenous contrast should be considered to better evaluate involvement of the pelvic structures (Fig. 2.1). When possible, however, MRI is the imaging modality of choice to specify the diagnosis, tumor extent into the sacral canal, neurovascular involvement, and aid in preoperative planning [14, 15]. In some lesions that are hypervascular, such as renal cell carcinoma, leiomyosarcoma, giant cell tumors, and hemangiopericytomas, preoperative angiography and embolization should be considered [15, 16]. This allows for reduced tumor vascularity and safer resection in select patients [15–17].

2.4 Biopsy

Given that the differential diagnosis of sacral tumors is extensive, a biopsy should be performed in almost all cases. A transrectal or transvaginal biopsy should generally not be performed because it violates the containing membranes of presacral fascia and periosteum and could lead to seeding of the rectum or vagina with tumor cells. The preferred biopsy method is image-guided core biopsy, if it can be performed safely.

2.5 Benign Sacral Tumors

Most lesions of the sacrum are benign. Common benign sacral tumors in children are sacrococcygeal teratomas (the most common), lipomas, dermoids, epidermoid cysts, and bone islands or enostoses [18, 19]. Congenital abnormalities such as spina bifida occulta, tethered cord, hairy nevi, dermal sinus tracts, and dimples are associated with tumors of the sacrum in children [6, 20].

Sacrococcygeal teratomas are rare congenital tumors that arise from pluripotent cells. Although approximately 70% are benign, there is a tendency toward malignant transformation [18]. Approximately 20% of sacrococcygeal teratomas are identified prenatally; 70% are identified at birth, and the remaining 10% are identified within the first year of life. In adults, sacrococcygeal teratomas are rare and more commonly benign. On radiographs, the tumors are seen as protruding soft tissue masses with amorphous, punctuate, or spiculated calcifications. CT and MRI usually show a heterogeneous mixture of solid and cystic components [23]. Most sacrococcygeal teratoma resections are performed via a posterior approach, but occasionally a combined abdominal-sacral approach is required. In some patients, extent of resection warrants a temporary and rarely permanent colostomy [24].

While, in children, most sacral tumors tend to be benign, the frequency of benign lesions in adults is significantly lower. The most common benign sacral tumors in adults are giant cell tumors (13% of all sacral tumors), aneurysmal bone cysts, osteoblastomas, schwannomas, osteoid osteomas, skeletal osteochondromas, chondromyxoid fibromas, nerve sheath, and meningeal tumors of the sacrum [24–28, 58, 63].

The sacrum is the third most common location for giant cell tumors which tend to affect patients in their second and fourth decades of life. Giant cell tumors also tend to be more common in females [23, 28, 29]. Sacral giant cell tumors usually develop in an eccentric position, but commonly extend to involve both sides of the midline. Additionally, they tend to have the propensity to cross the sacroiliac joints and intervertebral disks, which is unusual for many other spinal lesions and is a useful distinguishing feature of giant cell tumors [23]. Although generally classified as a benign tumor, 5–10% of giant cell tumors have been reported to be malignant. Malignancy can be characterized based on mitotic activity, $1/mm^2$ or less is highly unlikely to be malignant, and histology and sarcomatous features within the primary specimen can indicate an increased likelihood of malignant degeneration. Additionally, patients may develop lung metastases and recurrence which demonstrate malignancy initially missed in primary tumor pathology evaluation. For these patients prognosis is poor and 5-year tumor-free survival is <50% [30]. The standard treatment for giant cell tumors is wide excision or aggressive curettage followed by adjuvant phenol, hydrogen peroxide, liquid nitrogen or argon beam therapy, embolization, and bone grafting or cementation. Cryosurgery and radiation therapy are also possible options [11, 30–34, 64]. It is important to attempt complete resection, as recurrence rates have been noted to be as high as 50% if complete resection is not achieved [10, 21, 35]. In appropriately selected patients, sacrectomy is an optional procedure which can render the patient free of disease and improve risk of recurrence [31, 32].

The second most common benign tumor in adults is an osteoblastoma. Typically, osteoblastomas affect young adults, with a male/female ratio of 2:1. Approximately 40% of these lesions occur in the spine with approximately 17% arising in the sacrum specifically [3]. Osteoblastomas should be excised. The lesions recur in 10–15% of cases, but the rate approaches 50% in the more aggressive pattern. Malignant transformation of osteoblastoma to osteosarcoma with metastases has also been reported [14].

There are additionally a handful of rarely occurring tumors of the sacrum, osteoid osteomas, cavernous hemangiomas, and chondromyxoid fibromas. Osteoid osteomas of the sacrum represent <2% of sacral tumors [4, 22, 58]. En bloc resection and radiofrequency ablation are both viable options and render low rates of recurrence [2, 33, 34]. Cavernous hemangiomas are the most common benign tumors of the spine, but only exceptionally involve the sacrum [36]. Chondromyxoid fibroma is a rare benign tumor of the sacrum [36]. Differential diagnosis should include chondrosarcoma, chordoma, and giant cell tumor. Surgical excision of the affected area or curettage and bone grafting are the treatments of choice for chondromyxoid fibroma. Radiation therapy should only be considered for the rare surgically inaccessible tumor [36]. Nonetheless, all of these lesions should be considered on the differential diagnosis when considering tumor subtypes.

Nerve sheath tumors may arise from the sacral nerve roots and include schwannomas and neurofibromas (Fig. 2.2). The most common nerve sheath benign sacral tumors are the giant sacral schwannomas; the mean diameter of these tumors is approximately 10.5 cm. Cyst formation, hemorrhage, and necrosis are relatively common in giant sacral schwannomas; unlike neurofibromas, schwannomas tend to be encapsulated. En bloc resection is the treatment of choice. Although difficult because of their size and the presence of critical sacral nerve roots, most can be resected completely, and recurrence is rare [37, 38].

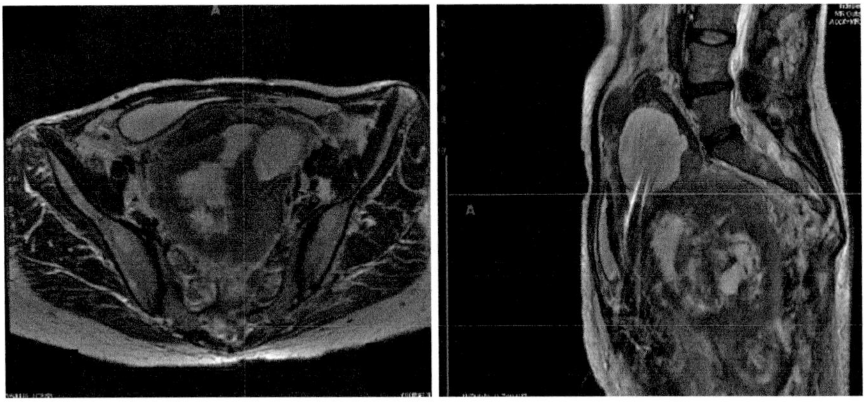

Fig. 2.2 Plexiform neurofibroma involving the sacrum in a patient with history of neurofibromatosis type 1

2.6 Malignant Sacral Tumors

The most common malignant tumors of the sacrum include chordomas, multiple myelomas, Ewing's sarcomas, and primitive neuroectodermal tumors (PNET). Primary lymphomas, osteosarcomas, chondrosarcomas, angiosarcomas, fibrosarcomas, carcinoid, and amyloid tumors of the sacrum are also malignant, but are quite rare.

Chordomas are the most common primary malignant tumor of the sacrum and the most common tumor of any type involving the sacrum [29, 38]. The majority of sacral chordomas occur in the sacrococcygeal region in patients who are 40 years of age or older and occur almost twice as frequently in men compared to women [39]. Chordomas are slow growing and often displace but generally do not invade the rectum and/or the bladder (Figs. 2.3 and 2.4). Metastases are not common, and if

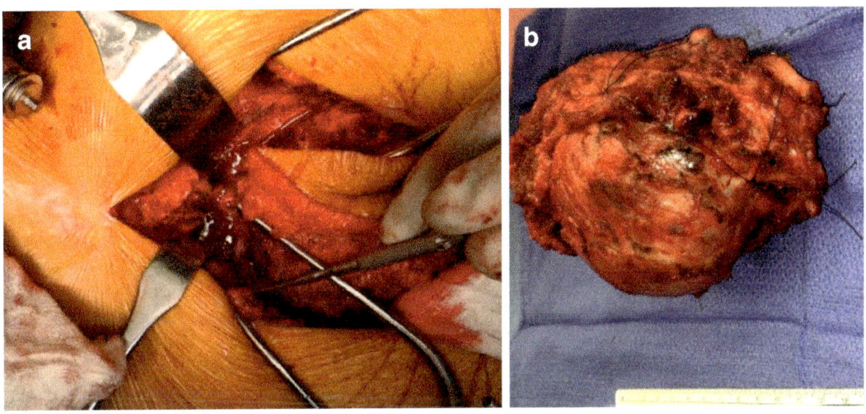

Fig. 2.3 (**a**) Prone approach to resection of sacral chordoma with attempted preservation of nerve roots. (**b**) Resected specimen

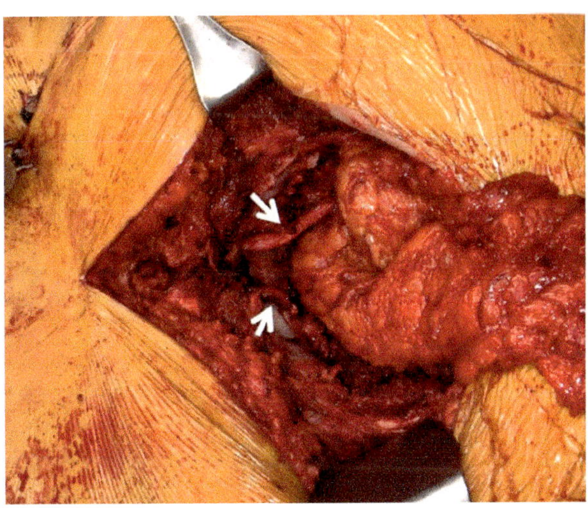

Fig. 2.4 Post-resection of chordoma with intact nerve roots (*arrows*)

metastatic disease is encountered, it is usually a late event [39]. On imaging, there is frequently a well-circumscribed osteolysis without an osteosclerotic rim, and a solid tumor with cystic areas is seen in approximately 50% of cases [3, 14, 15, 23]. Dedifferentiated chordoma is a rare variant that is clinicopathologically analogous to dedifferentiated chondrosarcoma. The sarcomatous component of dedifferentiated chordomas generally demonstrates more aggressive biological behavior and has a higher propensity to metastasize [40]. Primary treatment for chordomas is wide resection, and patient prognosis is dependent upon the completeness of resection and the violation of the tumor margins at the initial surgery. It is imperative to obtain an R0 resection to prevent recurrence; therefore, sacrifice of sacral nerve roots at the time of initial surgery may be necessary and is not uncommon. Total sacrectomy for chordomas involving the S1 nerve root have been reported [32, 41–43]. Local recurrence is the most important predictor of mortality in patients with chordomas and is related to the extent of initial resection. Local recurrence of sacral chordomas results in high morbidity rates and is associated with an approximately 20-fold increased risk of tumor-related death [8, 9, 11, 13, 39]. If the lesion is incompletely resected, adjuvant radiation therapy is another option; however, its efficacy is debatable [7, 11, 13, 44]. Results with brachytherapy techniques for recurrent sacral chordoma have been reported in small numbers of patients with varying success rates [45]. Chemotherapy has been of little value in the management of chordomas [11, 46]. Metastases, which can be found in the liver, lung, and regional lymph nodes, eventually develop in 5–43% of patients [44, 47].

Multiple myeloma is the second most common primary malignant neoplasm of the sacrum. Its incidence peaks in the sixth and seventh decade of life and is more common in males. The earlier solitary form, plasmacytoma, affects younger patients when compared with multiple myeloma. Lesions tend to be larger than those of multiple myeloma and tend to be osteolytic and expansile. These lesions also have poorly defined margins and are frequently associated with a soft tissue mass. Plasmacytomas generally progress to multiple myeloma in 10–15 years [14, 23, 48].

Lymphomas are the third most common primary malignant tumors of the sacrum but represent less than 5% of malignant bone tumors [30]. They predominantly affect men in their fifth to sixth decades of life. Lymphomas can cause aggressive bony destruction, although they tend to extend to the soft tissue leaving the underlying bones intact [14, 23, 49]. Three imaging signs, although nonspecific, are suggestive of lymphomas. These include the intensity and extent of uptake on bone scan (reveals a hot spot), the massive bone marrow invasion on MRI (poorly defined margins with a wide zone of transition) despite normal radiographic findings, and the large soft tissue mass with no visible cortical lesion on CT [50]. This highlights the importance of pursuing investigations (particularly bone scintigraphy and MRI) in patients with persistent pain despite their having no detectable abnormality on conventional radiography [15].

Ewing's sarcoma and PNET represent the fourth most common primary malignant tumors of the spine [26, 61]. Within the spine, the sacrum is the most common site of involvement. The age range for Ewing's sarcoma is 5–30 years, with 75% occurring in the first two decades of life. The male/female ratio is 3:1. Imaging findings tend to show paraspinal soft tissue masses and extradural space involvement [22, 51]. Some cases of sacral Ewing's sarcomas may present as a predominant soft tissue mass, extending to pelvic structures or to the spinal canal, with limited osteolysis [15]. Immunohistochemical studies are needed to distinguish Ewing's sarcoma from PNET, with the latter being characterized by neural differentiation [22, 23, 51, 60]. Primary treatment for Ewing's sarcoma and PNET is chemotherapy and radiation therapy; however, many patients require decompressive surgery and stabilization secondary to symptomatology. Unfortunately, these lesions are associated with the worst prognosis when they occur in the sacrococcygeal region, with low likelihood of local control (60%) and poor long-term survival [19].

There are a number of more rare malignant sacral tumors. Osteosarcomas account for 4% of primary malignant tumors of the sacrum. Many of the osteosarcomas of the sacrum are secondary to Paget's disease [30]. Sacral chondrosarcomas, fibrosarcomas, and angiosarcomas are unusual [52]. A 2% incidence of primary and secondary chondrosarcomas of the sacrum has been reported [4]. Most of sacral fibrosarcomas arise from a pre-existing lesion, usually previously irradiated bone, Paget's disease, or fibrous dysplasia [3].

Another rare malignant lesion is a malignant peripheral nerve sheath tumors (MPNST) (neurofibrosarcomas or malignant schwannomas). These tumors are associated with neurofibromatosis type 1 as they usually arise from pre-existing neurofibromas. Additionally, they have a tendency to recur locally and spread hematogenously, and despite aggressive surgery and adjuvant therapy, the prognosis for patients with MPNST is poor [23].

2.7 Surgical Treatment of Sacral Tumors

For a majority of the aforementioned benign and malignant tumors, complete tumor resection with negative resection is the mainstay of therapy. The surgical goals should be to remove the tumor completely with clear margins while maximizing postoperative function. For malignant lesions, a radical surgical approach such as partial or total sacrectomy, with sacrifice of sacral roots, is often warranted to achieve total resection with clear margins [8]. Various sacrectomies have been described depending on the tumor location, extent, and histology, and decision regarding partial or total sacrectomy for en bloc resection can be made after radiological evaluation and appropriate tissue diagnosis.

Total sacrectomy is indicated when a malignant or aggressive benign lesion involves the proximal sacrum [41, 42]. Partial sacrectomy which includes transverse, sagittal, or a combination of both can be considered for sacral tumors that lie entirely to one side of the sacrum. According to the transverse axis and sacroiliac joint involvement, sacral tumors are considered to be either high midline lesions (above S3 without lateral invasion of a sacroiliac joint), high lateral lesions (above S3 with sacroiliac joint invasion), and low midline lesions (below S3). Lateral lesions with sacroiliac joint involvement should be treated by sagittal sacrectomy, while high or low midline tumors without sacroiliac joint involvement should be treated by transverse sacrectomy [15]. These technically demanding procedures require multidisciplinary (neurosurgery, surgical and orthopedic oncology, and plastic surgery) involvement and should only be undertaken at institutions with experience in treating such patients.

2.8 Radiation Therapy

In those cases where primary complete resection of sacral tumors is difficult because of proximity to neural and vascular structures, radiation therapy may be useful. For sacral metastases, radiation therapy may be the initial treatment of choice, whereas in some cases of primary sacral tumors, conventional radiation therapy may be used in conjunction with surgery as adjuvant treatment (for palliation, prevention of pathological fractures, or to slow progression of or reverse neurologic compromise) [53]. When considering radiation therapy for such patients, it is important to remain cognizant of surrounding structures and to limit radiation doses as appropriate.

2.9 Embolization

Embolization is a useful adjuvant therapy in the management of sacral tumors. Typically, Gelfoam, alcohol embolizing emulsions, coils, ethanol, and microfibrillar collagen are used for embolization [49, 50, 54–57]. If a vascular sacral lesion is suspected based on presentation and imaging, then preoperative angiography should be performed to characterize the vascular anatomy and to determine if the lesion would be amenable to embolization. Of note, sacral tumors may have significant collateral circulation, and tumor neovascular recruitment may result in the formation of an extensive collateral vascular network [55]. It is recommended that embolization should be performed as close as possible to the time of surgery. Typically, timing of embolization is critical and should be planned carefully in conjunction with surgical resection [55–57]. Also, it is important to note that ischemic neuropathy is a potential complication of any pelvic embolization that can result in motor and sensory deficits in the pelvis and lower extremities. Therefore, care must be taken to identify and avoid embolization of the neurovascular anatomy. Rectal ischemia can result from superior hemorrhoidal artery embolization. Any embolization of sacral tumors may result in injury to nontargeted tissue including muscle infarction, injury to the skin, or injury to the colon or other organs [53].

Conclusion

Primary benign and malignant tumors of the sacrum are rare lesions that account for fewer than 7% of all intraspinal primary tumors. Metastatic lesions, multiple myeloma, and lymphoma are far more common than primary sacral tumors. Patients with sacral tumors present with nonspecific symptoms, including pain, palpable mass, and neurologic deficits. Additionally, the management of tumors of the sacrum is challenging. Radical resection through partial or complete sacrectomy can prolong the overall survival of patients with primary malignant or aggressive benign tumors; however, it is necessary to establish immediate stability through spinopelvic reconstruction for early ambulation and preservation of the quality of life. While modern radiation therapy and stereotactic radiosurgery have the potential to reduce complications and embolization can be used as an adjunct to surgery, thorough operative planning by a multidisciplinary team is critical to the success of treatment of such lesions.

Conflict-of-Interest Statement No benefits have been or will be received from a commercial party related directed or indirectly to the subject matter of this article.

References

1. Feldenzer JA, McGauley JL, McGillicudy JE. Sacral and presacral tumors: problems in diagnosis and management. Neurosurgery. 1989;25:884–91.
2. Diel J, Ortiz O, Losada RA, Price DB, Hayt MW, Katz DS. The sacrum: pathologic spectrum, multimodality imaging, and subspecialty approach. Radiographics. 2001;21(1):83–104.
3. Llauger J, Palmer J, Amores S, Bague S, Camins A. Primary tumors of the sacrum: diagnostic imaging. AJR Am J Roentgenol. 2000;174(2):417–24.
4. Unni KK. Dahlin's bone tumors: general aspects and data on 11,087 cases. 5th ed. Philadelphia: Lippincott-Raven; 1997.
5. Payer M. Neurological manifestation of sacral tumors. Neurosurg Focus. 2003;15(2):E1.
6. Deutsch H, Mummaneni PV, Haid RW, Rodts GE, Ondra SL. Benign sacral tumors. Neurosurg Focus. 2003;15(2):E14.
7. Chandawarkar RY. Sacrococcygeal chordoma: review of 50 consecutive patients. World J Surg. 1996;20(6):717–9.
8. Cheng EY, Ozerdemoglu RA, Transfeldt EE, Thompson Jr RC. Lumbosacral chordoma. Prognostic factors and treatment. Spine. 1999;24(16):1639–45.
9. Yonemoto T, Tatezaki S, Takenouchi T, Ishii T, Satoh T, Moriya H. The surgical management of sacrococcygeal chordoma. Cancer. 1999;85(4):878–83.
10. Lin PP, Guzel VB, Moura MF, et al. Long-term follow-up of patients with giant cell tumor of the sacrum treated with selective arterial embolization. Cancer. 2002;95(6):1317–25.
11. York JE, Kaczaraj A, Abi-Said D, et al. Sacral chordoma: 40-year experience at a major cancer center. Neurosurgery. 1999;44(1):74–80.
12. Althausen PL, Schneider PD, Bold RJ, Gupta MC, Goodnight Jr JE, Khatri VP. Multimodality management of a giant cell tumor arising in the proximal sacrum: case report. Spine. 2002;27(15):E361–5.
13. Bergh P, Kindblom LG, Gunterberg B, et al. Prognostic factors in chordoma of the sacrum and mobile spine: a study of 39 patients. Cancer. 2000;88(9):2122–34.
14. Manaster BJ, Graham T. Imaging of sacral tumors. Neurosurg Focus. 2003;15(2):E2.
15. Nair S, Gobin YP, Leng LZ, Marcus JD, Blisky M, Laufer I, Patsalides A. Preoperative embolization of hypervascular thoracic, lumbar, and sacral spinal column tumors: technique and outcomes from a single center. Interv Neuroradiol. 2013;19(3):377–85.
16. Pikis S, Itshayek E, Barzilay Y, Hasharoni A, Kaplan L, Gomori M, Cohen JE. Preoperative embolization of hypervascular spinal tumors: current practice and center experience. Neurol Res. 2014;36(6):502–9.
17. Gerber S, Ollivier L, Leclère J, et al. Imaging of sacral tumours. Skelet Radiol. 2008; 37(4):277–89.

18. Ng EW, Porcu P, Loehrer Sr PJ. Sacrococcygeal teratoma in adults: case reports and a review of the literature. Cancer. 1999;86(7):1198–202.
19. Lam CH, Nagib MG. Nonteratomatous tumors in the pediatric sacral region. Spine. 2002;27(11):E284–7.
20. O'Neill OR, Piatt Jr JH, Mitchell P, Roman-Goldstein S. Agenesis and dysgenesis of the sacrum: neurosurgical implications. Pediatr Neurosurg. 1995;22(1):20–8.
21. Turcotte RE, Sim FH, Unni KK. Giant cell tumor of the sacrum. Clin Orthop Relat Res. 1993;291:215–21.
22. Papagelopoulos PJ, Choudhury SN, Frassica FJ, Bond JR, Unni KK, Sim FH. Treatment of aneurysmal bone cysts of the pelvis and sacrum. J Bone Joint Surg Am. 2001;83(11):1674–81.
23. Peh WC, Koh WL, Kwek JW, Htoo MM, Tan PH. Imaging of painful solitary lesions of the sacrum. Australas Radiol. 2007;51(6):507–15.
24. Wakhlu A, Misra S, Tandon RK, Wakhlu AK. Sacrococcygeal teratoma. Pediatr Surg Int. 2002;18(5–6):384–7.
25. Boretz RS, Lonner BS. Atypical presentation of an osteoid osteoma in a child. Am J Orthop. 2002;31(6):347–8.
26. Popuri R, Davies AM. MR imaging features of giant presacral schwannomas: a report of four cases. Eur Radiol. 2002;12(9):2365–9.
27. Pogoda P, Linhart W, Priemel M, Rueger JM, Amling M. Aneurysmal bone cysts of the sacrum. Clinical report and review of the literature. Arch Orthop Trauma Surg. 2003;123(5):247–51.
28. Campanacci M, Baldini N, Boriani S, Sudanese A. Giant-cell tumor of bone. J Bone Joint Surg Am. 1987;69(1):106–14.
29. Disler DG, Miklic D. Imaging findings in tumors of the sacrum. AJR Am J Roentgenol. 1999;173(6):1699–706.
30. Gong L, Liu W, Sun X, Sajdik C, Tian X, Niu X, Huang X. Histological and clinical characteristics of malignant giant cell tumor of the bone. Virchows Arch. 2012;460(3):327–34.
31. Ozaki T, Liljenqvist U, Halm H, Hillmann A, Gosheger G, Winkelmann W. Giant cell tumor of the spine. Clin Orthop Relat Res. 2002;401:194–201.
32. Sar C, Eralp L. Surgical treatment of primary tumors of the sacrum. Arch Orthop Trauma Surg. 2002;122(3):148–55.
33. Wuisman P, Lieshout O, Sugihara S, van Dijk M. Total sacrectomy and reconstruction: oncologic and functional outcome. Clin Orthop Relat Res. 2000;381:192–203.
34. Lackman RD, Khoury LD, Esmail A, Donthineni-Rao R. The treatment of sacral giant-cell tumours by serial arterial embolisation. J Bone Joint Surg Br. 2002;84(6):873–7.
35. Randall RL. Giant cell tumor of the sacrum. Neurosurg Focus. 2003;15(2):E13.
36. Lath R, Rajshekhar V, Chacko G. Sacral haemangioma as a cause of coccydynia. Neuroradiology. 1998;40(8):524–6.
37. Klimo Jr P, Schmidt RH, Schmidt MH. Nerve sheath tumors involving the sacrum. Case report and classification scheme. Neurosurg Focus. 2003;15(2):E12.
38. Abernathey CD, Onofrio BM, Scheithauer B, Pairolero PC, Shives TC. Surgical management of giant sacral schwannomas. J Neurosurg. 1986;65(3):286–95.
39. Fourney DR, Gokaslan ZL. Current management of sacral chordoma. Neurosurg Focus. 2003;15(2):E9.
40. Fleming GF, Heimann PS, Stephens JK, et al. Dedifferentiated chordoma. Response to aggressive chemotherapy in two cases. Cancer. 1993;72(3):714–8.
41. Guo Y, Yadav R. Improving function after total sacrectomy by using a lumbar-sacral corset. Am J Phys Med Rehabil. 2002;81(1):72–6.
42. Jackson RJ, Gokaslan ZL. Spinal-pelvic fixation in patients with lumbosacral neoplasms. J Neurosurg. 2000;92(1 Suppl):61–70.
43. Tomita K, Tsuchiya H. Total sacrectomy and reconstruction for huge sacral tumors. Spine. 1990;15(11):1223–7.
44. Bjornsson J, Wold LE, Ebersold MJ, Laws ER. Chordoma of the mobile spine. A clinicopathologic analysis of 40 patients. Cancer. 1993;71(3):735–40.

45. Kumar PP, Good RR, Skultety FM, Leibrock LG. Local control of recurrent clival and sacral chordoma after interstitial irradiation with iodine-125: new techniques for treatment of recurrent or unresectable chordomas. Neurosurgery. 1988;22(3):479–83.
46. Azzarelli A, Quagliuolo V, Cerasoli S, et al. Chordoma: natural history and treatment results in 33 cases. J Surg Oncol. 1988;37(3):185–91.
47. Papagelopoulos PJ, Mavrogenis AF, Galanis EC, Savvidou OD, Boscainos PJ, Katonis PG, Sim FH. Chordoma of the spine: clinicopathological features, diagnosis, and treatment. Orthopedics. 2004;27(12):1256–63.
48. Lanzieri CF, Sacher M, Solodnik P, Hermann G, Cohen BA, Rabinowitz JG. Unusual patterns of solitary sacral plasmacytoma. AJNR Am J Neuroradiol. 1987;8(3):566–7.
49. Chiras J, Cognard C, Rose M, et al. Percutaneous injection of an alcoholic embolizing emulsion as an alternative preoperative embolization for spine tumor. AJNR Am J Neuroradiol. 1993;14(5):1113–7.
50. Shimada A, Sugimoto KJ, Wakabayashi M, Imai H, Seikguchi Y, Nakamura N, Sawada T, Ota Y, Komatsu N, Noguchi M. Primary sacral non-germinal center type diffuse large B-cell lymphoma with MYC translocation: a case report and review of the literature. Int J Clin Exp Pathol. 2013;6(9):1919–28.
51. Grubb MR, Currier BL, Pritchard DJ, Ebersold MJ. Primary Ewing's sarcoma of the spine. Spine. 1994;19(3):309–13.
52. Shives TC, McLeod RA, Unni KK, Schray MF. Chondrosarcoma of the spine. J Bone Joint Surg Am. 1989;71(8):1158–65.
53. Gibbs IC, Chang SD. Radiosurgery and radiotherapy for sacral tumors. Neurosurg Focus. 2003;15(2):E8.
54. Gottfried ON, Schmidt MH, Stevens EA. Embolization of sacral tumors. Neurosurg Focus. 2003;15(2):E4.
55. Yakes WFJ, Carrasco CH, Luethke JM. Embolization of lumbosacral lesions. In: Doty JR, Rengachary SS, editors. Surgical disorders of the sacrum. New York: Thieme; 1994. p. 294–308.
56. Hess T, Kramann B, Schmidt E, Rupp S. Use of preoperative vascular embolisation in spinal metastasis resection. Arch Orthop Trauma Surg. 1997;116(5):279–82.
57. Smith TP, Gray L, Weinstein JN, Richardson WJ, Payne CS. Preoperative transarterial embolization of spinal column neoplasms. J Vasc Interv Radiol. 1995;6(6):863–9.
58. Biagini R, Orsini U, Demitri S, et al. Osteoid osteoma and osteoblastoma of the sacrum. Orthopedics. 2001;24(11):1061–4.
59. Knoeller SM, Uhl M, Gahr N, Adler CP, Herget GW. Differential diagnosis of primary malignant bone tumors in the spine and sacrum. The radiological and clinical spectrum: minireview. Neoplasma. 2008;55(1):16–22.
60. Fiandaca MS, Ross WK, Pearl GS, Bakay RA. Carcinoid tumor in a presacral teratoma associated with an anterior sacral meningocele: case report and review of the literature. Neurosurgery. 1988;22(3):581–8.
61. Schnee CL, Hurst RW, Curtis MT, Friedman ED. Carcinoid tumor of the sacrum: case report. Neurosurgery. 1994;35(6):1163–7.
62. Capanna R, Briccoli A, Campanacci L. Benign and malignant tumors of the sacrum. In: Frymore J, editor. The adult spine: principles and practice. Philadelphia: Lippincott-Raven; 1997. p. 2367–405.
63. Papagelopoulos PJ, Currier BL, Shaughnessy WJ, et al. Aneurysmal bone cyst of the spine. Management and outcome. Spine. 1998;23(5):621–8.
64. Feigenberg SJ, Marcus Jr RB, Zlotecki RA, Scarborough MT, Berrey BH, Enneking WF. Radiation therapy for giant cell tumors of bone. Clin Orthop Relat Res. 2003;411:207–16.

Clinical and Neurological Manifestations of Sacral Tumors

3

Alexandra Gangi and Ricardo Gonzalez

3.1 Clinical Presentation

Sacral tumors are generally diagnosed late and can present as large, advanced neoplastic masses because of mild initial symptoms. The clinical pattern depends on the anatomic location of the lesion within the sacrum, its extension, and whether it compresses or invades neighboring structures [1]. The pain may initially be nonspecific and as clinical examination is usually poor, these tumors may remain clinically silent for long periods of time. The most common initial symptom of a sacral tumor is local pain due to its mass effect and compression. Occasionally smaller lesions could become symptomatic secondary to involvement of critical structures, such as nerves or ureters, or because of pathologic fractures. Generally, however, these tumors remain asymptomatic until they are quite large, and lower sacral tumors can grow large enough for their anterior portion to be palpated during a rectal examination [1–3]. While lateral extension of sacral tumors across the sacroiliac joints causes local pain at the joint, invasion of the origin of the gluteus maximus and piri formis muscles leads to local pain and subsequently decreases hip extension and external rotation strength [3–7].

Subsequently, as nerve roots become increasingly compressed or infiltrated by tumor, multiradicular sensory deficits develop and can include radicular pain radiating uni- or bilaterally into the buttocks, posterior thigh or leg, external genitalia, and/or perineum (Fig. 3.1).

As this continues to progress, motor deficits, and eventually, bladder, bowel, and/or sexual dysfunction from anterior extension of the tumor into the presacral space can be noted [1].

A. Gangi, M.D. • R. Gonzalez, M.D. (✉)
Sarcoma Department, H. Lee Moffitt Cancer Center, 12902 Magnolia Drive, Tampa, FL 33602, USA
e-mail: Alexandra.Gangi@moffitt.org; Ricardo.Gonzalez@moffitt.org

P. Ruggieri et al. (eds.), *Tumors of the Sacrum*,
DOI 10.1007/978-3-319-51202-0_3

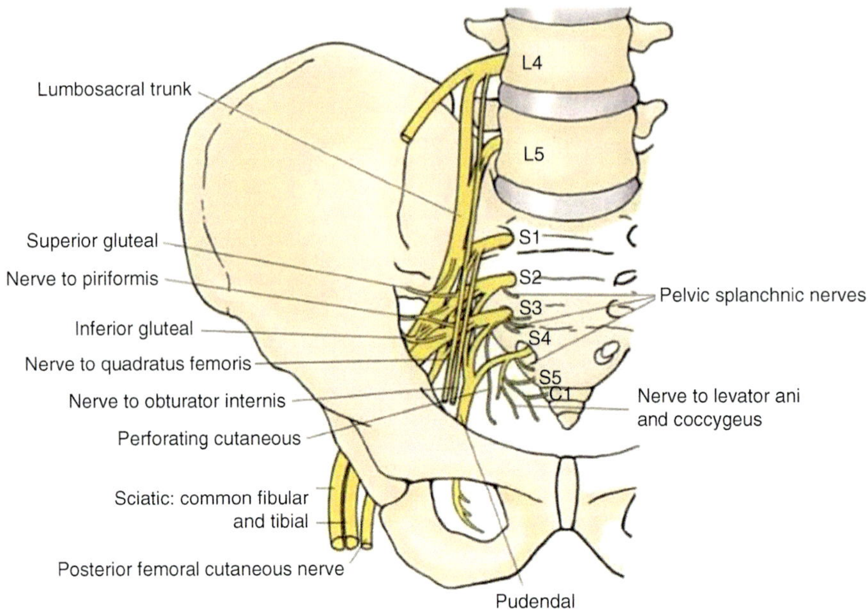

Fig. 3.1 Sacral nerve roots (2016, June). Retrieved July, 2016, from http://wiki.ahuman.org/index.php/HumanNervesSpinalRoots

Involvement of lumbosacral nerve roots in sacral lesions leads to certain specific deficits. A lesion involving the L-5 nerve root, commonly in its L5-S1 foraminal or extraforaminal course, may cause radicular pain and hypesthesias in the lateral thigh and calf as well as dorsum of the foot to the great toe [1, 2, 4]. Motor weakness of the L-5 nerve root may result in weakened ankle dorsiflexion, great toe extension, knee flexion, and hip abduction. The straight-leg raise test, or Lasegue's sign, which involves raising the patients leg with a straight knee while the patient is supine, would result in sciatic pain and render a positive result. A lesion involving the S-1 nerve root, in its canalicular, S1-2 foraminal or extraforaminal course, typically causes radicular pain and hypesthesias in the posterior thigh and calf as well as at the lateral and plantar face of the foot and the small toe. A motor deficit due to an S-1 lesion may result in weakened ankle plantar flexion, knee flexion, and hip extension. A unilateral lesion to the S2 or S3 nerve root usually leads to mild or moderate bladder, bowel, and/or sexual dysfunction [8, 9]. A bilateral lesion of the S2 or S3 roots almost always results in complete bladder, bowel, and sexual dysfunction, and although a unilateral lesion at the same nerve root may cause symptoms, they are generally more nonspecific. However, unilateral or even bilateral lesions of the S4 and/or S5 roots do not result in autonomic dysfunction, although anatomical work has shown some S4 and S5 root contribution to bladder and bowel function [10]. Performance of a thorough physical exam in such patients is critical and can significantly aid in diagnosis and ancillary testing.

Conflict-of-Interest Statement No benefits have been or will be received from a commercial party related directed or indirectly to the subject matter of this article.

References

1. Payer M. Neurological manifestation of sacral tumors. Neurosurg Focus. 2003;15(2):E1.
2. Deutsch H, Mummaneni PV, Haid RW, Rodts GE, Ondra SL. Benign sacral tumors. Neurosurg Focus. 2003;15(2):E14.
3. Chandawarkar RY. Sacrococcygeal chordoma: review of 50 consecutive patients. World J Surg. 1996;20(6):717–9.
4. Cheng EY, Ozerdemoglu RA, Transfeldt EE, Thompson Jr RC. Lumbosacral chordoma. Prognostic factors and treatment. Spine. 1999;24(16):1639–45.
5. Yonemoto T, Tatezaki S, Takenouchi T, Ishii T, Satoh T, Moriya H. The surgical management of sacrococcygeal chordoma. Cancer. 1999;85(4):878–83.
6. Lin PP, Guzel VB, Moura MF, et al. Long-term follow-up of patients with giant cell tumor of the sacrum treated with selective arterial embolization. Cancer. 2002;95(6):1317–25.
7. York JE, Kaczaraj A, Abi-Said D, et al. Sacral chordoma: 40-year experience at a major cancer center. Neurosurgery. 1999;44(1):74–80.
8. Althausen PL, Schneider PD, Bold RJ, Gupta MC, Goodnight Jr JE, Khatri VP. Multimodality management of a giant cell tumor arising in the proximal sacrum: case report. Spine. 2002;27(15):E361–5.
9. Unni KK. Dahlin's bone tumors: general aspects and data on 11,087 cases. 5th ed. Philadelphia: Lippincott-Raven; 1997.
10. Bergh P, Kindblom LG, Gunterberg B, et al. Prognostic factors in chordoma of the sacrum and mobile spine: a study of 39 patients. Cancer. 2000;88(9):2122–34.

Imaging of Sacral Tumors and Tumor Simulators: Experience of the Mayo Clinic

4

Laurel A. Littrell and Doris E. Wenger

4.1 Introduction

Imaging of the sacrum can be a challenging task. On conventional radiographs, the sacrum is difficult to evaluate due to its complex anatomy as a flat and irregular bone with the posteriorly angled and slightly curved shape of the sacrum combined with the complex ring-shaped geometry of the pelvis. These features result in overlap with additional bones of the pelvis, as well as overlying stool, bowel gas, and soft tissues that can significantly limit the ability to detect pathology involving the sacrum [1]. Nevertheless, radiographs are recommended as the modality of choice to begin the imaging workup of a patient with known or suspected sacral pathology. Although careful scrutiny may allow detection and initial characterization of a lytic, expansile, sclerotic, or mineralized tumor, sacral tumors and other abnormalities can easily escape detection on conventional radiographs.

When an abnormality is detected in the sacrum on conventional radiographs or clinical suspicion warrants, cross-sectional imaging with CT and/or MRI allows for improved detection, characterization, and staging of sacral masses and other abnormalities [2]. CT provides an advantage over MRI in its ability to evaluate the integrity of the cortex, to assess and characterize periosteal new bone formation, and to detect and characterize matrix mineralization. With these features, CT provides the ability to evaluate the imaging features of a lesion that are helpful in distinguishing between benign and malignant bone tumors. The advantages of MRI include its superior soft tissue contrast resolution, which provides the ability to sensitively detect lesions, characterize tissue types, and accurately stage tumors locally for their anatomic extent in the bone and soft tissues. In many cases, the information from CT and MRI are complimentary and interpreted in conjunction to provide

L.A. Littrell, M.D. (✉) • D.E. Wenger, M.D.
Department of Radiology, Mayo Clinic, Rochester, MN, USA
e-mail: littrell.laurel@mayo.edu; wenger.doris@mayo.edu

P. Ruggieri et al. (eds.), *Tumors of the Sacrum*,
DOI 10.1007/978-3-319-51202-0_4

optimal tumor characterization. It is also important to determine the size and number of lesions, since the differential diagnosis varies significantly for solitary versus multiple lesions.

4.2 General Imaging Features

When a solitary mass is detected in the sacrum, it is important to evaluate it using the same features that are used to characterize a tumor in a long bone. The imaging features that can be utilized to determine if a lesion is benign or malignant include the lesion margination, zone of transition, pattern of destruction (osteolytic, osteosclerotic, or mixed), presence and character of periosteal new bone formation, and matrix mineralization as well as the integrity of the cortex and evidence of soft tissue extension. In long bones, these features are often accurately evaluated on conventional radiographs. However, in the sacrum, these features are often difficult to discern for the reasons previously mentioned. When information regarding these features cannot be determined on conventional radiographs, then CT is the next best imaging modality to establish these criteria.

4.3 Cross-Sectional Imaging with Computed Tomography (CT) and Magnetic Resonance Imaging (MRI)

CT exams are typically performed with axial image acquisition and multiplanar 2D image reconstruction in coronal oblique and sagittal planes. Conversely, if a lesion is detected on MRI, then it is important to compare the MRI with either a CT or radiographs to fulfill the assessment of these criteria. MRI is advantageous for local tumor staging, detecting the presence of a soft tissue mass and evaluating its relationship with the traversing neural elements and adjacent pelvic organs. For example, dedicated imaging of the sacrum allows for visualization of individual nerve roots as they course through and exit the neural foramen and can reveal evidence of nerve encasement or perineural spread of tumor that may not be visible on CT. In addition, MRI is more accurate for evaluating the extent of lesions in the bone marrow and may show evidence of marrow infiltration that is not apparent on CT. Additionally, MRI is more sensitive for the detection of additional lesions that would impact the appropriate differential diagnosis of a sacral tumor. For example, diffusely abnormal marrow throughout the pelvis or multiple discrete lesions would suggest the possibility of a marrow-infiltrating process such as metastases, multiple myeloma, or lymphoma.

For MR imaging of tumors, T1-weighted sequences, fluid-sensitive sequences with fat suppression, and post gadolinium contrast T1-weighted sequences provide a useful combination of imaging sequences to optimally detect and characterize pathology in the sacrum. True T1-weighted imaging is invaluable and should always be performed in the evaluation of a tumor or other indeterminate lesion in the sacrum. In general, complete replacement of the internal fat within the bone marrow is one of the most important features for distinguishing normal red marrow or edema from a marrow-replacing tumor.

In addition to T1-weighted imaging, an abnormality in the sacrum should be carefully examined for signal characteristics on a fluid-sensitive sequence as well as fat-saturated T2-weighted fast spin-echo (FSE) sequences or inversion recovery (IR) sequences [3, 4]. In general, FSE T2-weighted images with fat saturation provide improved spatial resolution and signal to noise compared with inversion recovery imaging. However, inversion recovery images can provide improved fat saturation in the setting of metallic hardware. Bone marrow rich in "yellow marrow" should be dark on a fat-saturated fluid-sensitive sequence. Red marrow usually demonstrates minimal T2 signal abnormality, usually only minimally brighter than the adjacent fatty bone marrow. On T2-weighted or IR images, many benign and malignant neoplastic processes are hyperintense and brighter than either yellow or red marrow. However, bone lesions that are diffusely sclerotic and heavily mineralized or contain significant blood products can demonstrate intermediate or dark signal intensity on T2-weighted imaging. The intermediate or dark components are often intermixed within areas of bright signal intensity. However, in the case of a purely sclerotic lesion such as a sclerotic metastasis, the lesion may be homogeneously dark and may be missed on T2-weighted imaging alone making careful correlation with T1-weighted images critical. Although most pathologic processes involving bone are bright on fluid-sensitive sequences, focal increased T2 signal within the sacrum is a nonspecific finding alone and can be seen in a wide range of benign and malignant diseases including stress fracture, infection, metastases, and primary bone tumors, both malignant and benign. Careful correlation with the morphology of the signal abnormality, the T1-weighted imaging findings, as well as conventional radiographic and/or CT findings is crucial.

Gadolinium contrast-enhanced images are usually performed in the evaluation of a suspected tumor within the sacrum. However, gadolinium enhancement is a nonspecific feature that can be seen in a broad spectrum of benign/reactive and neoplastic processes, including reactive edema, osteomyelitis, vascular red marrow, and a variety of malignant and benign bone tumors. The enhancement pattern may help distinguish benign from malignant diseases in some cases [3]. For example, gadolinium enhancement can help distinguish solid from cystic masses. It can also be utilized to evaluate for areas of necrosis, either in the primary tumor or in response to chemoradiation therapy. It can also provide guidance for biopsy planning in order to target a solid enhancing portion rather than a non-enhancing necrotic portion to improve diagnostic yield [5].

4.4 Differential Diagnosis of Sacral Masses

When a mass is detected in the sacrum, the differential diagnosis is broad and includes a wide range of both benign and malignant disease processes. However, the differential diagnosis for a specific tumor can be narrowed based on factors such as

Table 4.1 Pneumonic for the differential diagnosis of a sacral mass, "**N**o **G**ood **C**omes **O**f **A** **S**acral **M**ass"

No	Neurogenic tumors
	Benign neurofibromas schwannomas
	Malignant peripheral nerve sheath tumor
Good	Giant cell tumor
Comes	Chordoma
	Benign notochord cell tumor (BNCT)
Of	Osteoblastoma
A	Aneurysmal bone cyst (ABC)
Sacral	Sarcomas
	Ewing's sarcoma
	Osteosarcoma
	Chondrosarcoma
	"Simulators"
	Red marrow
	Paget disease
	Stress fractures
Mass	Mets, myeloma, lymphoma
	Meningocele and Tarlov cysts

patient's age, sex, and specific imaging findings including those listed above such as the presence of matrix mineralization, margination, periosteal reaction, and precise location within the sacrum. A helpful pneumonic for remembering the multitude of diagnostic possibilities when a sacral tumor is encountered is "**N**o **G**ood **C**omes **O**f **A** **S**acral **M**ass," where "N" stands for neurogenic tumors and includes both benign neurofibromas and schwannomas and malignant peripheral nerve sheath tumors (MPNST), "G" for giant cell tumor, "C" for chordoma (and benign notochord cell tumors or BNCT), "O" for osteoblastoma and osteoid osteoma, "A" for aneurysmal bone cyst (ABC), "S" for sarcoma (including Ewing's sarcoma, osteosarcoma, and chondrosarcoma) as well as simulators of tumor (including red marrow, Paget disease, and stress fracture), and "M" for metastases and the marrow-infiltrating lesions (including myeloma and lymphoma) and also for meningocele (and Tarlov cysts) (Table 4.1).

The diagnoses on the differential diagnosis can be subdivided into general categories based on the patient's age. For example, ABC, osteoblastoma, Ewing's sarcoma, and osteosarcoma tend to occur in patients less than 20 years old. Since osteosarcomas in the spine tend to occur in older patients than osteosarcoma in other locations, osteosarcoma should also be included in the differential for a malignant-appearing destructive solitary mass in the sacrum of a patient between the ages of 20 and 40 years. Neurogenic tumors and giant cell tumors tend to occur in patients between the ages of 20 and 40 years. Chordomas, metastases, myeloma, lymphoma, chondrosarcoma, and secondary osteosarcomas as well as the tumor simulators tend to occur in patients over the age of 40 (Table 4.2) [1, 2, 5–9].

Table 4.2 General guidelines for formulating an appropriate differential diagnosis for sacral tumors based on age

Age in years	Less than 20	20–40	Greater than 40
Benign	ABC	Giant cell tumor	Tarlov cysts
	Osteoblastoma	Schwannoma	Tumor simulators
		Neurofibroma	Stress fracture
			Paget disease
			Red marrow
Malignant	Ewing's sarcoma	MPNST	MPNST, usually <50
	Osteosarcoma	Osteosarcoma	Chordoma
			Mets
			Myeloma
			Lymphoma
			Chondrosarcoma
			Osteosarcoma (secondary to radiation and Paget disease)

4.5 Imaging Findings of the Most Common Benign and Malignant Neoplasms in the Sacrum and Tumor Simulators

4.5.1 Neurogenic/Peripheral Nerve Sheath Tumors

Peripheral nerve sheath tumors (PNSTs) are divided into benign and malignant categories. Benign PNSTs include neurofibromas and schwannomas and most commonly occur in patients between the ages of 20 and 40 years of age. The malignant categories, formerly referred to as neurofibrosarcomas, malignant schwannomas, and neurogenic sarcomas, are currently termed malignant peripheral nerve sheath tumors (MPNST) by the World Health Organization and are most commonly seen in patients between the ages of 20 and 50 years [7–9]. Any of these categories can be associated with neurofibromatosis type 1, and the risk of malignant degeneration is higher in these patients due to the multiplicity and long-standing nature of these tumors. In the general population, the lifetime risk of malignant transformation of a benign neurogenic tumor is 3–5%. In patients with neurofibromatosis type 1, the risk is as high as 15–20% [10]. Although neurogenic tumors can arise in any location, they most commonly occur near the trunk. The sacral plexus is one of the most common sites, along with the sciatic nerve and brachial plexus. These are typically intradural extramedullary lesions and are not true primary tumors of the sacrum but take their origin within the sacral spinal canal and/or within the sacral neural foramen, with resultant expansion or infiltration of the surrounding bone. Subsequently, they may present as a mass involving the sacrum with a significant presacral soft tissue mass. They may also present as a predominantly presacral soft tissue mass with or without direct anatomic extension into adjacent sacral neural foramina.

Pathologically, neurofibromas and schwannomas have distinctly different relationships to the parent nerve. Neurofibromas show more intimate involvement of the nerve with the parent nerve entering and exiting the fusiform mass, whereas schwannomas show more eccentric involvement of the nerve. It is often impossible to differentiate schwannomas from neurofibromas based on imaging features. This is especially true in the sacrum where the entering nerve segment is much shorter and, therefore, more difficult to characterize the relation of the mass to the parent nerve [2, 7, 11]. The majority of neurofibromas and schwannomas are solitary. However, the presence of multiple nerve sheath tumors suggests a diagnosis of neurofibromatosis.

Benign peripheral nerve sheath tumors grow along nerve segments and often cause chronic indolent remodeling of the cortical surfaces of the sacrum. This growth pattern manifests as expansion of the spinal canal and/or neural foramina and sclerosis along the margins of the expanded bone (Fig. 4.1). The chronic indolent character of the bone remodeling is best evaluated on CT (Fig. 4.1). Most benign peripheral nerve sheath tumors in or around the sacrum will present as a soft tissue mass filling and expanding the associated neural foramen and/or spinal canal with frequent extension into the presacral soft tissue spaces. They often present with a dominant presacral component. Long-standing benign schwannomas may reach huge sizes in the pelvis and often contain areas of cystic degeneration and

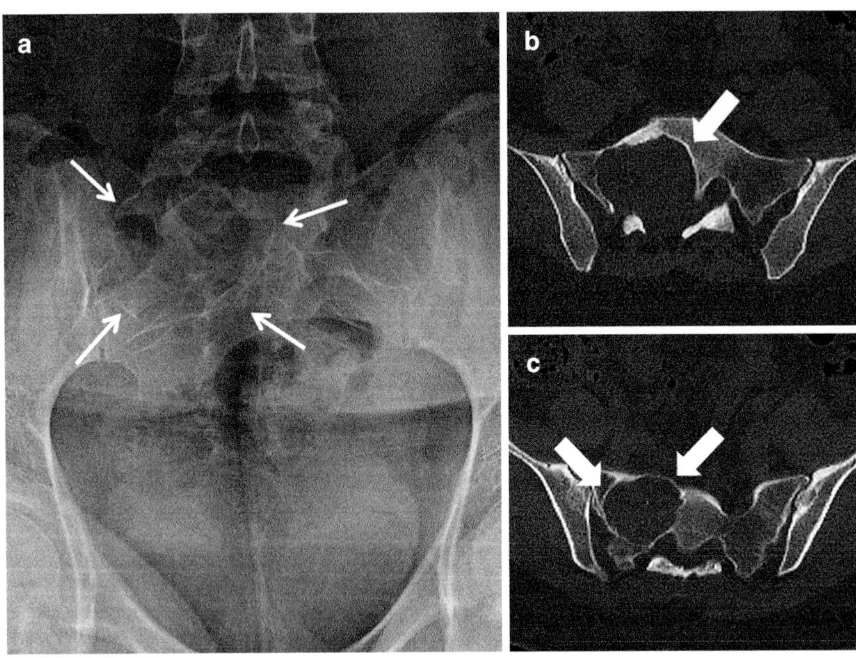

Fig. 4.1 AP radiograph (**a**) and axial CT images (**b** and **c**) of the sacrum in a 33-year-old female with a *schwannoma* demonstrate a lytic expansile lesion centered upon the right S1 neural foramen. Although the lesion is detected on the radiograph (*thin arrows*), it could easily be confused with overlying bowel gas. The CT shows the lesion to better advantage and characterizes the benign nature of the growth pattern with expansion of the bone and a thin peripheral rim of sclerosis (*thick arrows*)

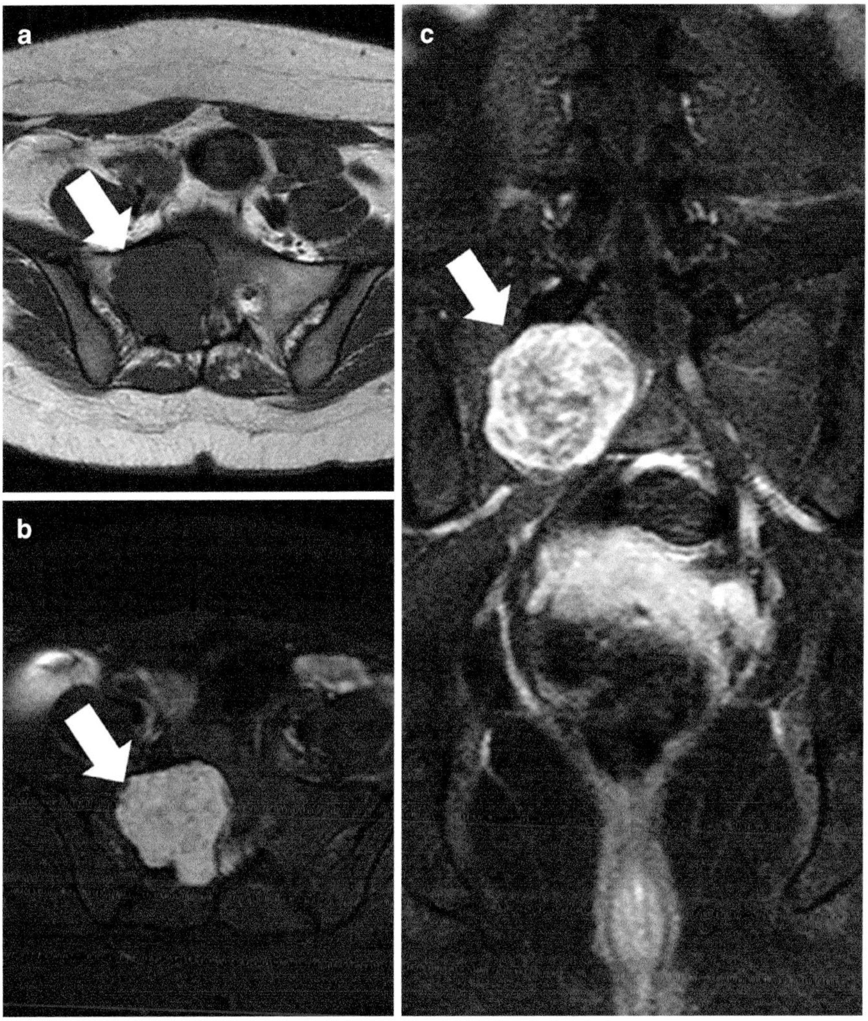

Fig. 4.2 Axial T1 (**a**), T2 with fat suppression, (**b**) and gadolinium-enhanced SPGR (**c**) MR images from the patient illustrated in Fig. 4.1 show typical signal characteristics of a *schwannoma* with intermediate signal on T1, heterogeneous predominantly hyperintense signal on T2, and avid heterogeneous enhancement

calcifications (sometimes referred to as "ancient schwannomas"). On MRI (Fig. 4.2), most benign peripheral nerve sheath tumors are intermediate (similar or isointense to skeletal muscle) on T1 and either homogeneously or heterogeneously hyperintense on T2, sometimes showing a "target sign" with a central hypointense area within the T2 hyperintense mass [7, 8]. Up to 70% of benign peripheral nerve sheath tumors will show some degree of heterogeneity on T2 [8]. On post gadolinium images, these lesions usually enhance avidly, usually homogeneously or with mild heterogeneity. However, large long-standing schwannomas may show more heterogeneity with areas of non-enhancing cystic degeneration.

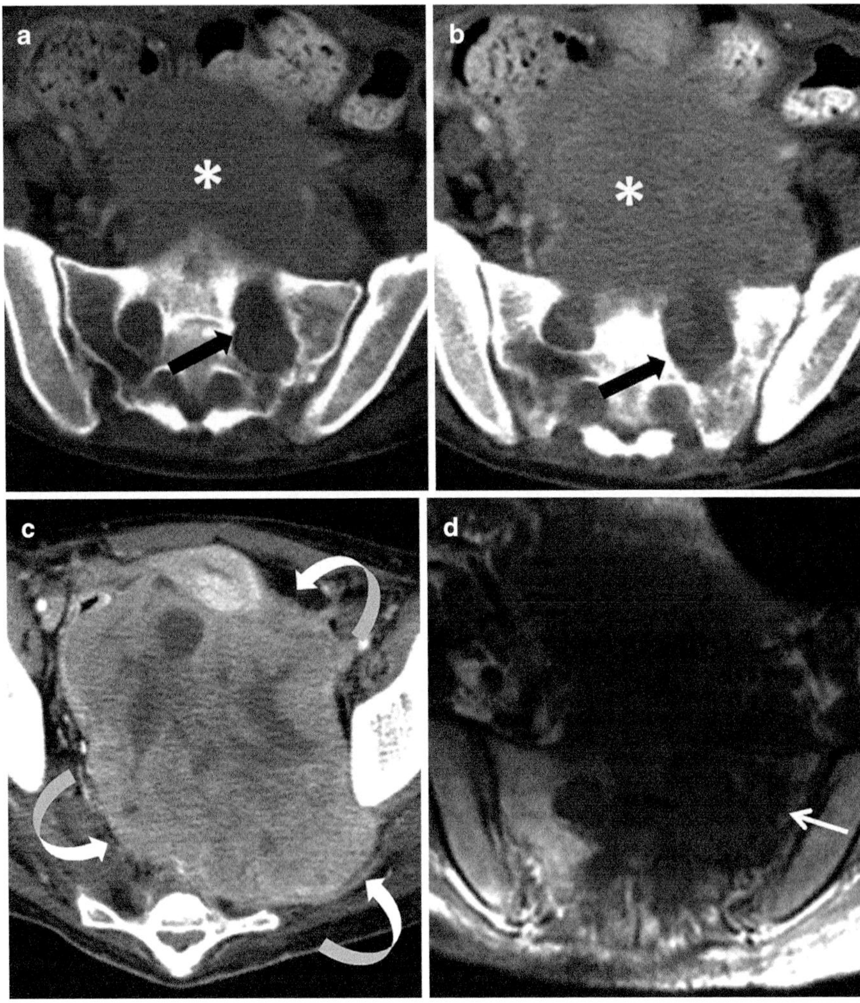

Fig. 4.3 Axial CT images of the upper pelvis (**a** and **b**) of a 16-year-old female with a *malignant peripheral nerve sheath tumor* demonstrate a mass involving the left S1 nerve root with associated chronic-appearing expansion of the neural foramen (*black arrows*). The mass is in anatomic continuity with a large solid heterogeneous presacral soft tissue mass (*asterisks*). Axial CT of the lower pelvis (**c**) shows that the soft tissue mass extends inferiorly where it fills nearly the entire pelvis and courses toward the left sciatic notch (*curved arrows*). Axial T1-weighted MRI (**d**) shows that despite the chronic-appearing expansion of the left S1 neural foramen, there is evidence of permeation of the tumor into the adjacent sacral ala (*thin arrow*)

There is significant overlap in the imaging appearance of benign and malignant peripheral nerve sheath tumors. Although size alone cannot be used to differentiate benignity from malignancy, MPNSTs are generally larger than their benign counterparts, with average measurements reported at 10 cm, whereas the average size of a benign neurofibroma has been reported to be 5 cm [8] (Figs. 4.3 and 4.4). On CT imaging of MPNSTs, bony involvement may be more infiltrative with

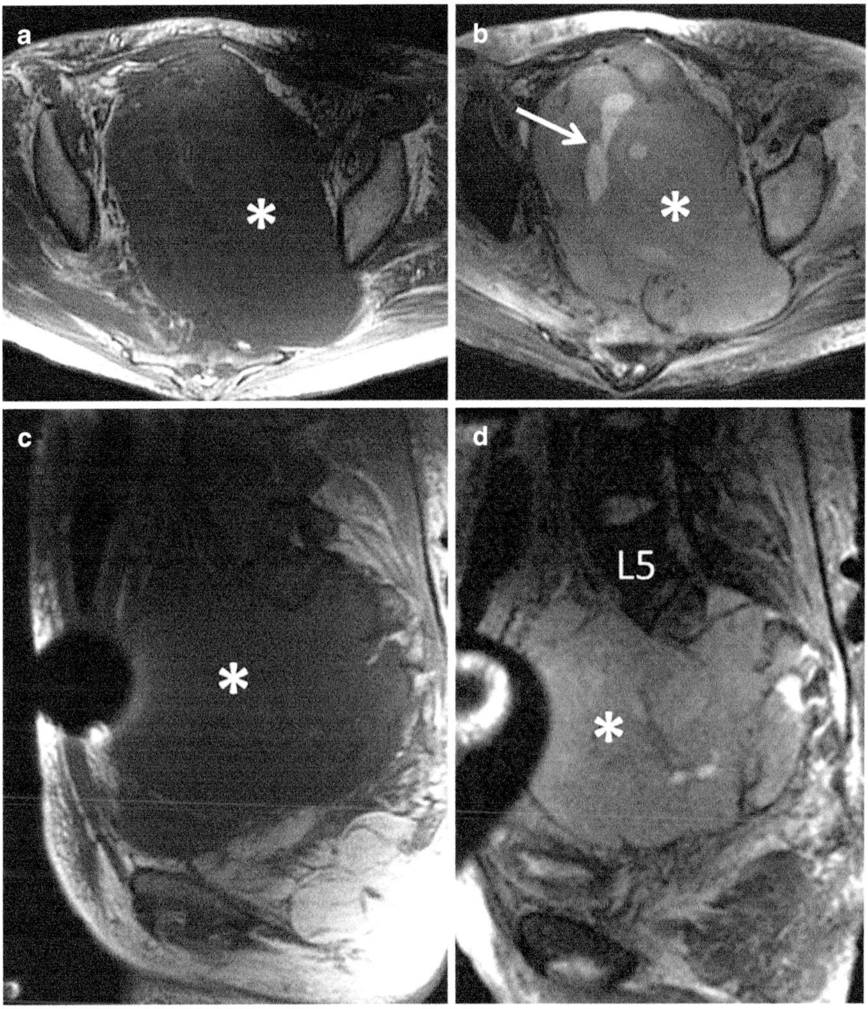

Fig. 4.4 Axial (**a**) and sagittal (**c**) T1-weighted and axial (**b**) and sagittal (**d**) T2-weighted MR images of the patient in Fig. 4.3 with a *malignant peripheral nerve sheath tumor* illustrate the massive size of the tumor which fills the entire pelvis (*asterisks*) and is in anatomic continuity with the mass involving the S1 nerve root. The mass is markedly heterogeneous with focal areas of internal necrosis (*arrow*) and is associated with perilesional edema on the T2-weighted images

irregular margins between the mass and the adjacent bone (Fig. 4.3). However, more chronic benign-appearing foraminal expansion and cortical remodeling are often seen in MPNTs. The presence of chronic bone remodeling and the absence of infiltration into adjacent bone should not be used to assume benignity. On MRI, MPNSTs often demonstrate more heterogeneity on all imaging sequences. Although benign neurogenic tumors may have cystic change and heterogeneity, dominant areas of intratumoral cystic change and necrosis and a peripheral enhancement pattern with or without intratumoral cystic change should raise the level of suspicion that a neurogenic tumor may be malignant (Fig. 4.4). In addition, the presence of perilesional edema with feathery areas of increased T2-weighted signal adjacent to the mass should also raise suspicion of a malignant mass in the setting of a suspected nerve sheath tumor [7–9]. Pain and rapid growth are also concerning features.

Benign peripheral nerve sheath tumors are at risk for malignant degeneration, especially plexiform neurofibromas in patients with neurofibromatosis type 1. These patients typically have innumerable complex plexiform masses of varying sizes, and determining which lesions are suspicious for malignant degeneration can be extremely challenging. Recently, ^{18}FDG PET–CT has been shown to be a promising imaging tool for identifying tumors that are suspicious for malignant degeneration [10, 12]. Full-body imaging can be performed which is particularly advantageous in patients with neurofibromatosis and multiple masses. Lesions with higher FDG uptake are considered worrisome for malignant transformation. Although different threshold standard uptake values (SUV) have been described, in general, masses with an SUV less than 4 are at low risk for malignancy. Lesions with an SUV between 4 and 7 are intermediate risk, and an SUV greater than 7 is highly suspicious for malignant degeneration [10]. In addition, these plexiform masses are often huge, and PET–CT can be useful for identifying a specific area within a large mass to target for preoperative image-guided biopsy, decreasing the chance of sampling error.

4.5.2 Giant Cell Tumors

The majority of giant cell tumors (GCT) of the bone are benign and composed of a spindle cell stroma with intermixed ovoid mononuclear giant cells that have osteoclastic activity [5, 13, 14]. Although usually benign, they can be locally aggressive and may recur after resection. Approximately 5–10% are malignant, either primary malignant giant cell tumor of the bone or dedifferentiation within a recurrence [2, 15]. Metastases to the lungs, although rare, may occur with benign tumors [2, 13]. These tumors generally occur in patients in the second through fourth decades of life, more commonly in females [5]. Giant cell tumor (GCT) of the bone is most commonly found in the ends of long bones of skeletally mature patients, manifesting as a well-defined eccentrically located lytic lesion, usually without a sclerotic margin, extending to the subchondral bone of the articular surface. However, 15% of GCT involve flat bones and up to 7% of cases of GCT have been reported in the spine. Of the cases occurring in the spine, 90% occur in the sacrum [1, 2, 5, 13, 14]. GCT is the second most common primary bone tumor of the sacrum after chordoma. When GCT involves the sacrum, they most commonly occur in the upper sacrum and often involve both sides of midline but are usually eccentrically located, lateralizing to one of the sacral alae [1].

In the sacrum, radiographic and CT findings are also of a lytic lesion but may be more destructive than typically seen in long bones, often destroying the cortex of

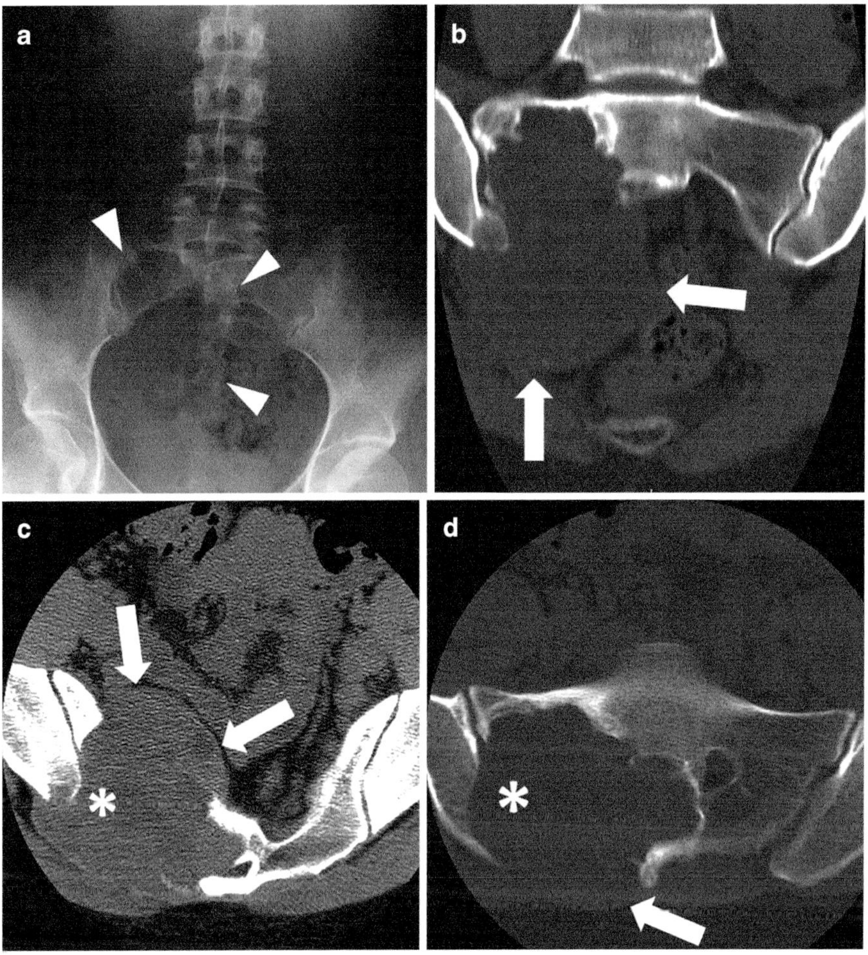

Fig. 4.5 AP radiograph (**a**), coronal (**b**) and axial (**d**) unenhanced bone window, and axial soft tissue window (**c**) CT images show typical imaging features of a *giant cell tumor* of the sacrum in a 29-year-old female. The lesion demonstrates a purely lytic pattern of destruction with a peripheral rim of sclerosis and a large associated soft tissue mass anteriorly and posteriorly (*arrows*). The lesion also crosses the SI joint (*asterisk*) and involves the adjacent ilium

the sacral neural foramina and frequently extending across the sacroiliac joint (Fig. 4.5). On CT, these masses are soft tissue attenuation and appear expansile or purely lytic without any evidence of mineralization. Although there is usually a narrow zone of transition *without* a sclerotic rim as in GCT of the long bones, in the sacrum, and in the spine, a thin rim of sclerosis may occasionally be seen [13]. Large soft tissue masses may also be present (Fig. 4.5).

On MRI (Fig. 4.6), GCT of the bone usually demonstrate low to intermediate signal on T1 but may have areas of increased T1 signal associated with intralesional hemorrhage. On T2-weighted or fluid-sensitive sequences, there may be significant

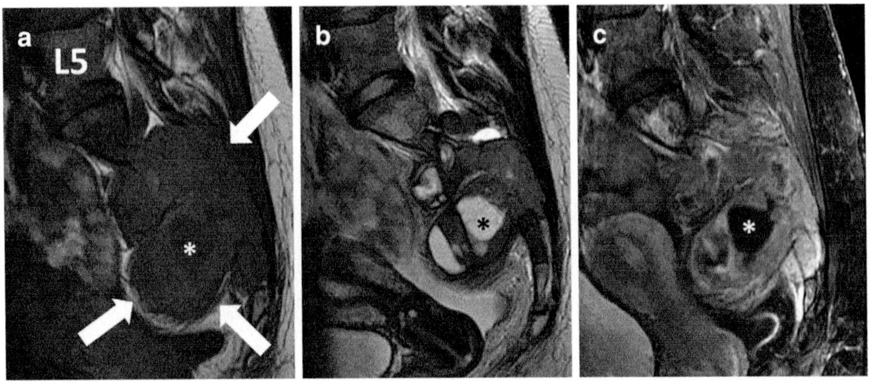

Fig. 4.6 Sagittal T1 (**a**), sagittal T2 (**b**), and sagittal gadolinium-enhanced SPGR (**c**) MR images of the *giant cell tumor* from patient illustrated in Fig. 4.5 show a large destructive heterogeneous mass extending from S1 to S4 with a large associated soft tissue mass extending both anteriorly and posteriorly. The mass is markedly heterogeneous on all of the image sequences with areas of solid heterogeneous enhancement and scattered foci of fluid signal intensity (*asterisk*) that could be due to cystic change or necrosis. Of interest, there are significant areas of low to intermediate signal on the T2-weighted image in the bone and soft tissue component of the tumor which can be seen in GCT due to the presence of fibrous tissue and hemosiderin

heterogeneity due to hemorrhage or necrosis, but these tumors frequently have predominantly low to intermediate T2 signal due to the presence of fibrous components and hemosiderin. The low T2 signal may aid in differentiating GCT from malignant and other benign masses in the sacrum that usually show predominantly bright T2 signal [13]. However, areas of increased T2 signal are often present as well due to fluid and cystic changes. Secondary aneurysmal bone cyst formation occurs in up to 14% of GCT of the bone which may result in prominent areas of cystic change and extensive fluid–fluid levels [14]. On post contrast CT and MR imaging, these tumors usually show significant enhancement of the non-cystic components.

4.5.3 Chordoma and Benign Notochordal Cell Tumors

Chordoma: Chordomas are rare tumors, accounting for 2–4% of all primary malignant bone tumors. However, excluding lymphoproliferative malignancies, it is the most common primary tumor of the sacrum, accounting for 40% of all primary sacral neoplasms, including both benign and malignant tumors [1, 13, 16]. Chordomas are malignant neoplasms that develop from remnants of the primitive notochord. During development, the notochordal tissue is relegated to the intervertebral regions to become the nucleus pulposus as the cylinder of notochord tissue is replaced by cartilage-producing sclerotomes. Vestiges of nonneoplastic notochord tissue are found in up to 2% of cadavers, usually in the midline near the spheno-occipital synchondrosis and in the sacrococcygeal regions, paralleling the

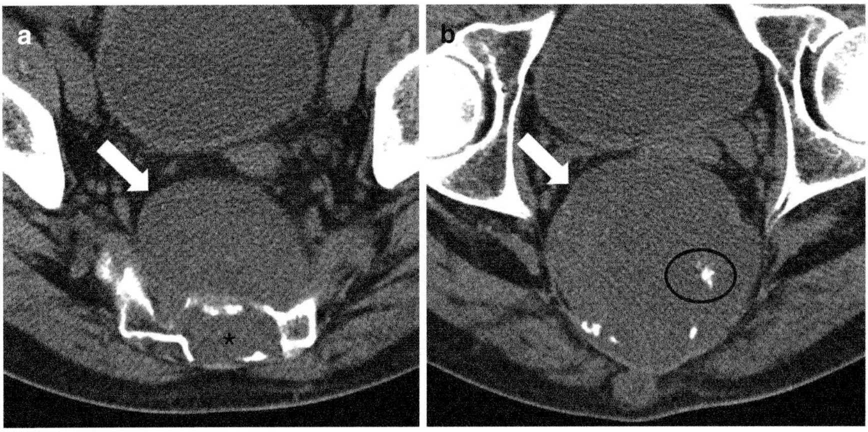

Fig. 4.7 Axial soft tissue window CT images of the lower sacrum of a 61-year-old male show typical imaging features of a *chordoma* with a lytic destructive lesion in the lower sacrum (*asterisk*) that is centered on the midline, has a large associated exophytic presacral soft tissue mass (*arrows*), and contains scattered punctate calcifications (*circle*)

most common locations for chordomas with 30–35% occurring in the spheno-occipital region and 50–60% in the sacrococcygeal region. In the sacrum, chordomas are more common in the fourth and fifth sacral segments [1, 2, 13, 16, 17]. Chordomas occur in all age groups but occur most commonly in the fourth to seventh decades of life and are more common in males, with a 2:1 male to female ratio [2, 17].

Radiographs may reveal a lytic lesion in the sacrum with a soft tissue mass containing calcifications. CT will show a destructive lytic lesion, typically in the midline or paramidline, extending into the sacral spinal with a large lobulated midline exophytic presacral soft tissue mass (Fig. 4.7) [1, 2, 5, 11, 13]. Internal calcifications are frequently seen, occurring in approximately 50–70% of cases, with some series reporting detectable calcifications within the mass in up to 90% of cases on CT [13, 18–21]. The calcifications can be related to chronic areas of hemorrhage and necrosis as well as chondroid matrix [1]. The resulting calcifications may be amorphous, predominantly peripheral or punctate and chondroid in nature, with a similar appearance to the matrix seen in chondrosarcomas. Chondrosarcomas are much less common in the sacrum and, in contrast to chordoma, tend to occur eccentrically within the sacrum [16].

On MRI, chordomas typically present as a solid mass centered within the midline or paramidline lower sacrum with heterogeneous T1 and T2 signal and variable heterogeneous enhancement [1, 2, 5, 11, 13, 16, 18] (Fig. 4.8). Chordomas often have evidence of internal hemorrhage which may show areas of high T1 signal within a heterogeneously T1 low and intermediate signal intensity mass. They often demonstrate prominent lobulated regions of T2 hyperintensity within the lobulated sacral and presacral soft tissue mass, again with significant

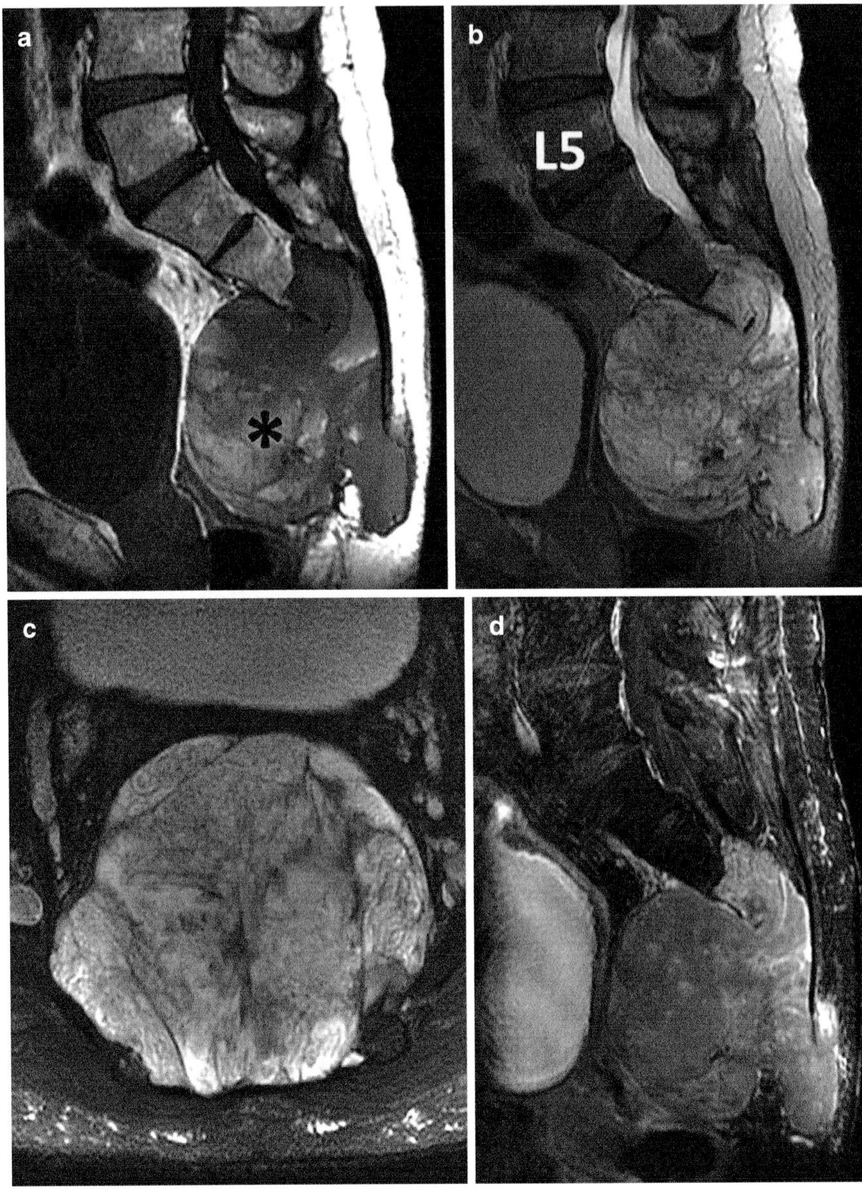

Fig. 4.8 Sagittal T1 (**a**), sagittal T2 (**b**), axial T2 (**c**), and sagittal gadolinium-enhanced (**d**) MR images show a large heterogeneous solid destructive mass involving the majority of the sacrum and coccyx typical of *chordoma* (same patient illustrated in Fig. 4.7). The MRI nicely demonstrates both the intraosseous and extra-osseous extent of the tumor. There are areas of increased signal within the mass on T1 indicative of intralesional hemorrhage (*asterisk*), and the mass shows minimal patchy enhancement that reflects the myxoid component of the tumor

heterogeneity and foci of lower T2 signal related to intralesional hemorrhage and/or calcifications. Chordomas often cross disk spaces or sacral segments, a characteristic that is more unique and distinctive in the tumors involving the mobile spine (the spine above the sacrum). When large, chordomas may also cross the sacroiliac joint [16].

Benign Notochordal Cell Tumors: Benign notochordal cell tumors (BNCTs), previously referred to as benign chordoma, giant notochord rest, and giant notochord hamartoma, are benign intraosseous lesions of notochord cell origin, initially described in 1999. These represent a distinct entity from remnant notochord rests [22–24]. On radiographs, BNCTs are usually occult. Although they may also be occult on CT, BNCTs typically present as a small midline focus of subtle hazy sclerosis without evidence of a destructive osteolytic component (Fig. 4.9). BNCTs are often discovered incidentally on MRI, where they typically present as a small

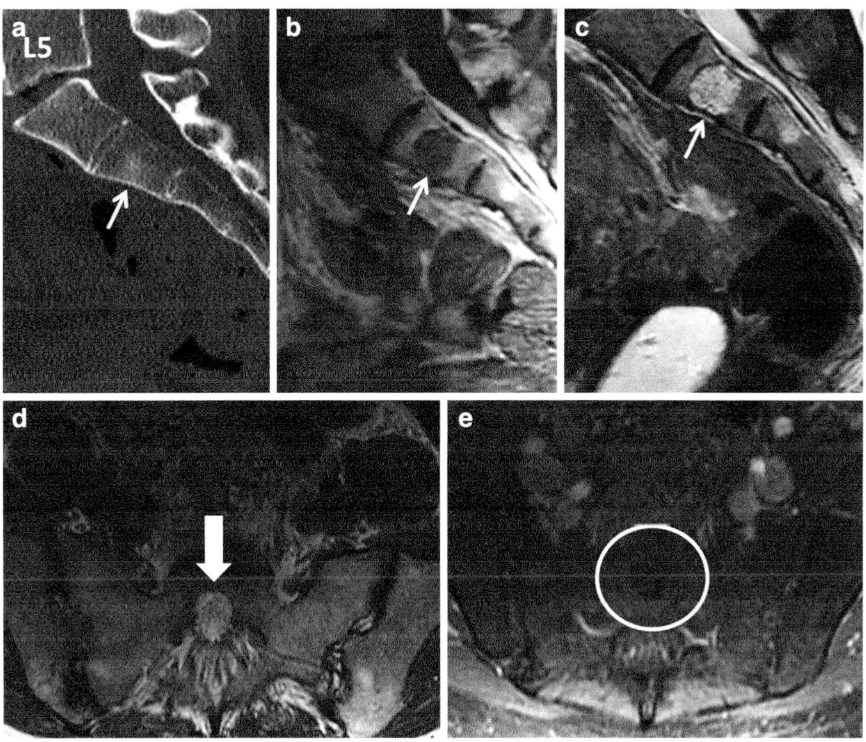

Fig. 4.9 Sagittal CT (**a**) shows a subtle region of hazy sclerosis in the S2 segment. This corresponds with a small nodular mass with predominantly intermediate signal intensity on sagittal T1-weighted (**b**) and hyperintense signal intensity on T2-weighted (**c**) MR images. Axial T2-weighted MRI (**d**) shows that the mass is centered on the midline (*thick arrow*) and axial gadolinium-enhanced SPGR MRI (**e**) shows that there is no enhancement in the mass (*circle*). There is subtle stippling of the signal pattern on the MR images that correlates with tiny foci of intralesional fat. The constellation of imaging findings is typical of a *benign notochordal cell tumor*

intraosseous midline mass with nonspecific intermediate T1 signal, predominantly hyperintense T2 signal, and no significant enhancement on post gadolinium contrast-enhanced images (Fig. 4.9). The margins of the mass are often slightly lobulated. In addition, they may contain tiny foci of bright intralesional fat that can be identified with careful scrutiny of the T1-weighted and corresponding fat-suppressed T2-weighted images. This finding is crucial in differentiating BNCT from chordoma as chordomas should not contain intralesional fat [25]. There have been reported cases of BNCT with atypical features including a small area of cortical permeation and a tiny associated soft tissue mass. In these cases, there was absence of lytic destruction in the bone and there were tiny amounts of intralesional fat suggesting the diagnosis of BNCT. In atypical or equivocal cases as described above, CT-guided biopsy can be performed to make the diagnosis of a BNCT and avoid unnecessary surgical resection [25].

4.5.4 Osteoblastoma and Osteoid Osteoma

Osteoblastoma and osteoid osteoma are similar but distinct lesions with different imaging features and clinical courses [13]. Osteoid osteoma and osteoblastoma are rare in the sacrum [2, 11].

Osteoblastoma is a rare benign but locally aggressive bone producing primary bone tumor that constitutes only 1–2% of all primary bone tumors, usually presenting in the second decade of life. This tumor has a predilection for the spine with 30–40% of cases occurring in the spine [26, 27]. Of osteoblastomas occurring in the spine, 7–17% occur in the sacrum [26, 27]. Osteoblastomas in the sacrum usually occur in the posterior elements of the upper sacrum and can have a varied CT and radiographic appearance. They range from a round well-defined radiolucent lesion greater than 1.5 cm with surrounding sclerosis to an expansile lesion with a sclerotic rim that contains multiple small internal calcifications [13]. They may also present with more aggressive features as an expansile destructive mass with infiltrative margins [13]. The calcifications in osteoblastoma are often punctate with chondroid-like features (Fig. 4.10). The MRI findings are varied and generally nonspecific with intermediate to low signal on T1-weighted images, heterogeneously hyperintense T2 signal with varying amounts of intermediate and low T2 signal depending on the amount of calcified osteoid matrix (Fig. 4.11). However, the hallmark of these tumors is extensive peritumoral edema, which can make evaluation of margins and tumor extent difficult. Due to the ability of MRI to exaggerate the overall size of the process on fluid-sensitive sequences and the nonspecific MR signal characteristics of the lesion, correlation with CT is imperative to avoid the misdiagnosis of an osteosarcoma.

Although 10% of osteoid osteomas occur in the spine, only 2% of spinal osteoid osteomas occur in the sacrum [2, 11, 13]. They most commonly occur in males between 10 and 20 years of age. Osteoid osteomas most commonly arise in the posterior elements of the spine and, when in the sacrum, are most commonly located in the articular process of S1. On radiographs, they may be occult or

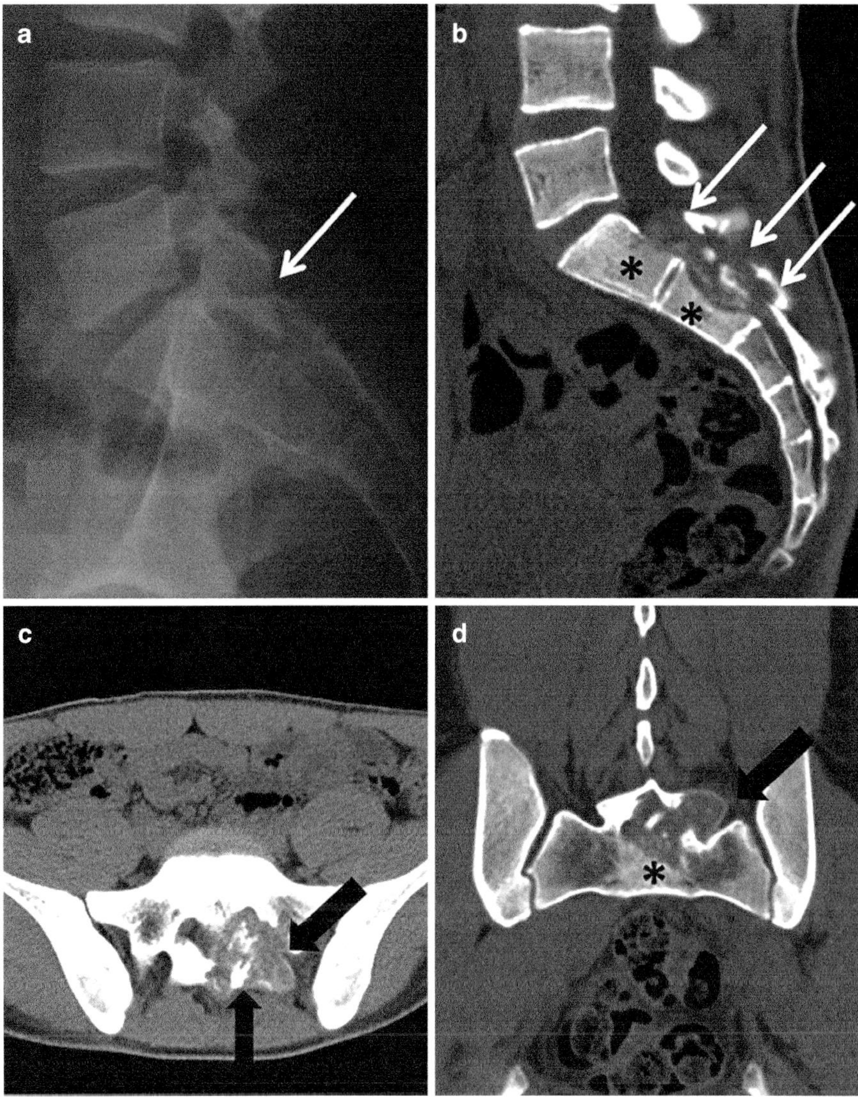

Fig. 4.10 Lateral radiograph of the upper sacrum (**a**) and sagittal (**b**), axial (**c**), and coronal (**d**) CT images of a 17-year-old male with an *osteoblastoma* show a solid mass with internal calcifications involving the posterior elements of S1 and S2 (*thin arrows*) that is associated with expansion of the bone (*thick black arrows*) as well as surrounding medullary sclerosis (*asterisks*)

present as a sclerotic lesion. The lucent nidus is often obscured by the complex anatomy and overlap that occurs with spinal radiographs. CT is the imaging modality of choice when the diagnosis of osteoid osteoma is suspected. On CT, osteoid osteomas usually present as a small radiolucent lesion that by definition is less than 1.5 cm in diameter. They may contain a central focus of calcification and

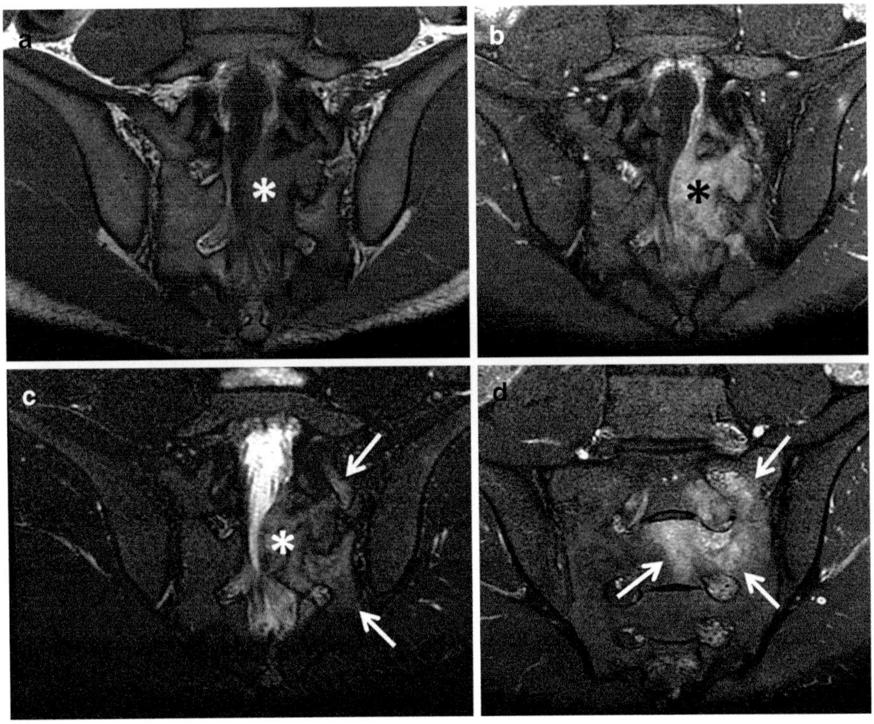

Fig. 4.11 Coronal T1 (**a**), T2 (**c**), and gadolinium-enhanced SPGR (**b** and **d**) MR images of the patient in Fig. 4.10 show typical MR imaging features of an *osteoblastoma*. The mass has intermediate signal intensity on T1-weighted and heterogeneous intermediate and high signal intensity on T2-weighted images and shows avid enhancement with gadolinium (*asterisks*). Of interest, the mass is associated with extensive surrounding bone marrow edema (*thin arrows*) with is typical of osteoblastoma

are notorious for inciting exuberant surrounding sclerosis and cortical thickening. On MRI, detection of the nidus is often difficult due to the extensive surrounding increased T2 signal in the bone and soft tissues due to edema and inflammatory change that results in exaggeration of the overall size of the process. When identified, the tumor is typically low to intermediate on T1 and intermediate to high on T2-weighted images. The tiny focus of central calcification demonstrates low signal on all pulse sequences.

4.5.5 Aneurysmal Bone Cyst

Aneurysmal bone cysts (ABCs) are relatively rare benign expansile bone lesions with blood-filled cystic spaces which, until relatively recently, were thought to represent a reactive process. However, a neoplastic origin in primary ABC has been demonstrated with evidence of USP6 gene rearrangement in primary tumors

[28]. The majority of ABCs are considered primary lesions with no underlying neoplasm found. When associated with an underlying tumor, as secondary ABC, giant cell tumor of the bone and chondroblastoma are the most common lesions on the differential diagnosis. However, they can be associated with other benign and malignant tumors. Most aneurysmal bone cysts are diagnosed by the age of 20 years with a slightly higher prevalence in females. The spine is involved in 12–30% of cases of ABC. Of spinal cases, 13% occur in the sacrum [5, 13]. Although, usually, the lesion is comprised of blood-filled cystic cavities with thin vascular septations between the cysts, a "solid variant" has been described and is more common in the spine. Spinal ABCs may cross the disk space or SI joint, similar to chordoma and GCT.

On radiographs and CT, ABCs typically present as a well-defined lytic lesion with varying degrees of expansion and a thin peripheral rim of sclerosis (Figs. 4.12 and 4.13). CT and MRI imaging generally show multiple cystic spaces with intervening septations and the distinguishing fluid–fluid levels. The fluid–fluid levels are a hallmark of ABCs and can be seen with CT or MRI but are typically more conspicuous on MRI (Fig. 4.13). Significant heterogeneity due to blood products of varying ages is usually seen with increased T1 signal due to methemoglobin within either the dependent or nondependent portions. On T2, there are usually hyperintense areas as well as dark areas, again due to fluid and blood products. On post contrast CT and MR imaging, there is usually thin smooth enhancement of the periphery and internal septations. Solid areas of enhancement may be due to a solid variant of ABC but should raise the possibility of an underlying neoplasm with secondary ABC. Secondary ABC most commonly occurs with benign tumors such as giant cell tumor and chondroblastoma. Fluid–fluid levels can also be seen in malignant tumors such as telangiectatic osteosarcoma due to intralesional hemorrhage. Since radiographs provide limited detail in the sacrum, CT is helpful for distinguishing ABC from GCT or telangiectatic osteosarcoma, since ABC shows benign expansion of the bone with preservation of a peripheral shell of the bone, whereas GCT may be associated with cortical destruction and a soft tissue mass. Telangiectatic osteosarcomas almost universally present as an aggressive osteolytic lesion with significant cortical destruction and soft tissue mass.

4.5.6 Primary Sarcomas of Bone

Chondrosarcoma: Chondrosarcoma of the spine is relatively rare with approximately 7% occurring in the mobile spine and 5% in the sacrum. The most common location in the mobile spine is the thoracic region [29–31]. However, excluding lymphoproliferative malignancies, chondrosarcoma is the second most common primary malignant bone tumor in the spine and sacrum after chordoma [11]. Men are affected two to four times more often than women and the mean age at diagnosis is 45 years [29]. Sacral chondrosarcomas are most commonly located eccentrically in the upper sacrum.

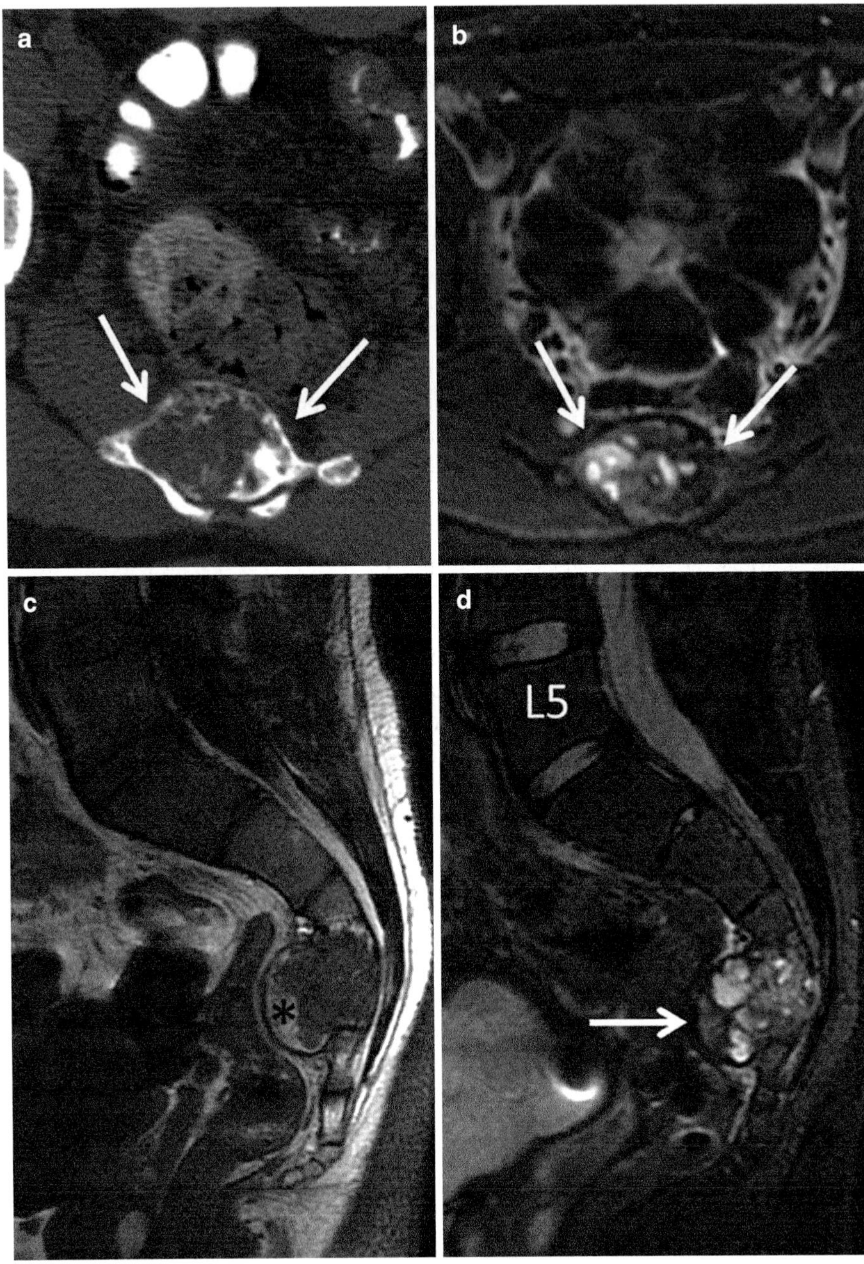

Fig. 4.12 Axial CT (**a**) and sagittal T1-weighted (**c**) and axial (**b**) and sagittal (**d**) T2-weighted MR images of the sacrum show an *aneurysmal bone cyst* involving S3 in an 18-year-old male. The lesion is predominantly lytic and is associated with marked expansion of the anterior cortex, which is otherwise intact (*arrows* on CT). The lesion is markedly heterogeneous and contains multiple rounded areas of varying signal intensity, some of which have fluid signal intensity and others low signal intensity due to hemosiderin. One of the spaces along the anterior aspect of the mass contains increased T1 signal indicative of subacute hemorrhage (*asterisk*)

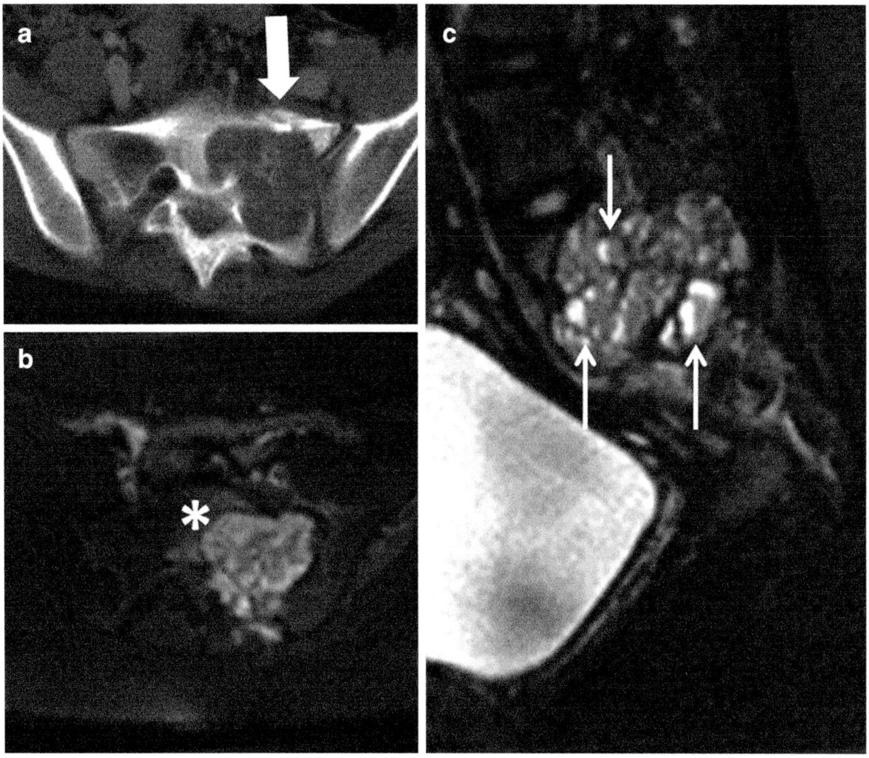

Fig. 4.13 Axial CT (**a**), axial T2-weighted (**b**), and sagittal T2-weighted (**c**) MR images of a 13-year-old female show a lytic destructive lesion of the upper sacrum on the left with associated expansion and an incomplete pathologic fracture in the anterior cortex (*thick arrow*). The sagittal T2-weighted MRI shows that the lesion is comprised of multiple small round spaces with scattered fluid–fluid levels indicative of intralesional hemorrhage (*thin arrows*). Findings are typical of an *aneurysmal bone cyst*

Radiographs and CT typically show a destructive lytic mass with varying amounts of chondroid matrix (Fig. 4.14). In the spine, the presence of chondroid matrix can be detected on radiographs in 70% of cases [29]. However, the rate of detection may be lower in the sacrum where the significant soft tissue overlap and complex anatomy make it difficult to detect the matrix. CT is the most sensitive modality for detecting and characterizing the matrix, which demonstrates the typical punctate or ring and arc pattern of chondroid matrix [5, 29]. Although chordomas are the most common primary malignant tumor in the sacrum and often contain calcifications with chondroid-type features, they have several distinguishing features from chondrosarcoma. Chordomas are typically in the midline and often in the lower sacrum, whereas chondrosarcomas are typically eccentrically located and more often in the upper sacrum. Given the eccentric location in the upper sacrum, they are often in close proximity to the sacroiliac joint and may cross the joint. Chondrosarcomas in the sacrum and spine are usually low grade

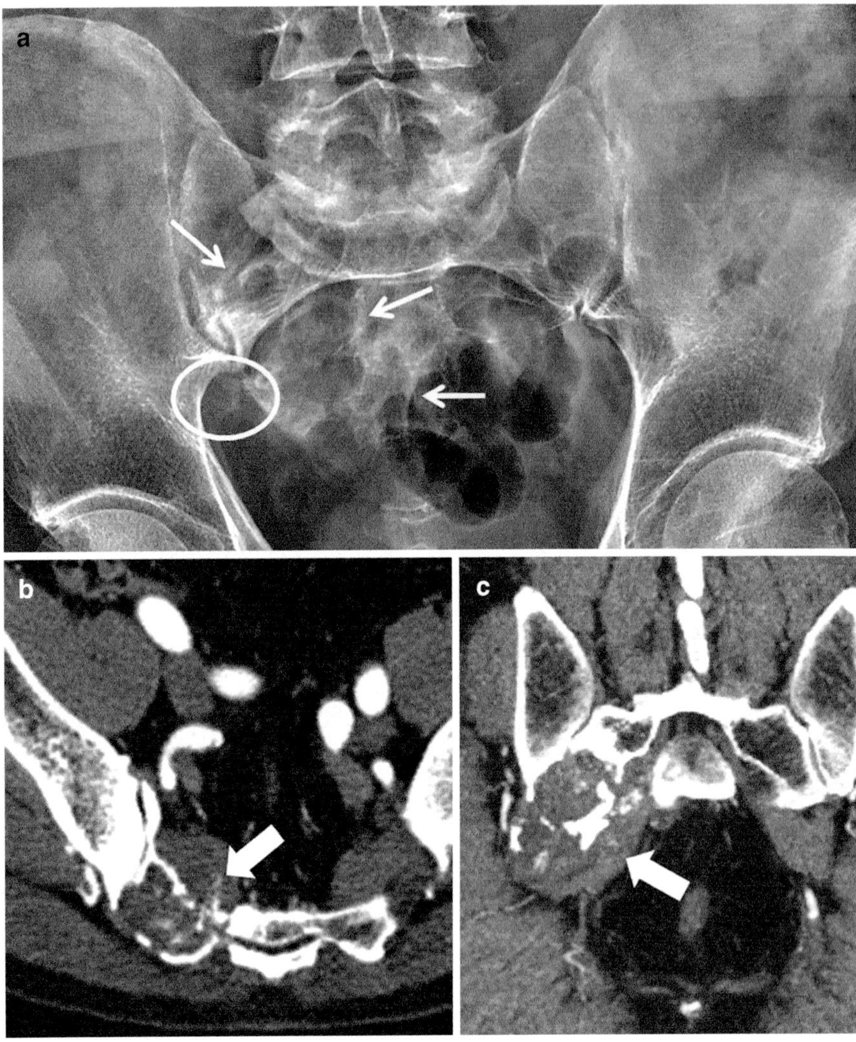

Fig. 4.14 AP radiograph (**a**), axial CT (**b**), and coronal CT (**c**) of a 58-year-old male with a *chondrosarcoma* of the sacrum show a large lytic destructive mass involving the lower sacrum that is associated with expansion of the bone and a thick peripheral rim of sclerosis. Although the chondroid matrix is evident on the radiograph (*circle*), it is more apparent and better characterized on the CT. The CT shows that the lesion involves the right SI joint and is associated with soft tissue extension anteriorly (*thick arrows*)

and often show some evidence of their indolent nature. There may be some element of expansion and/or surrounding reactive sclerosis (Fig. 4.14). A mineralized lobulated soft tissue mass is often present with chondrosarcomas as well as chordomas, but, again, the location within the sacrum and pelvis may help differentiate the two. If there is a large soft tissue mass associated with a cartilage tumor of the sacrum without any detectable mineralized matrix, the question of dedifferentiated chondrosarcoma should be raised [32].

On MRI, sacral chondrosarcomas tend to show imaging characteristics typical of cartilage neoplasms elsewhere in the skeleton with intermediate to low T1 signal and lobulated markedly T2 hyperintense signal within both the destructive sacral mass and associated soft tissue mass (Fig. 4.15). There are usually foci of hypointense T1- and T2-weighted signal corresponding to the punctate chondroid calcifications [32, 33]. The pattern of enhancement on post gadolinium images can be

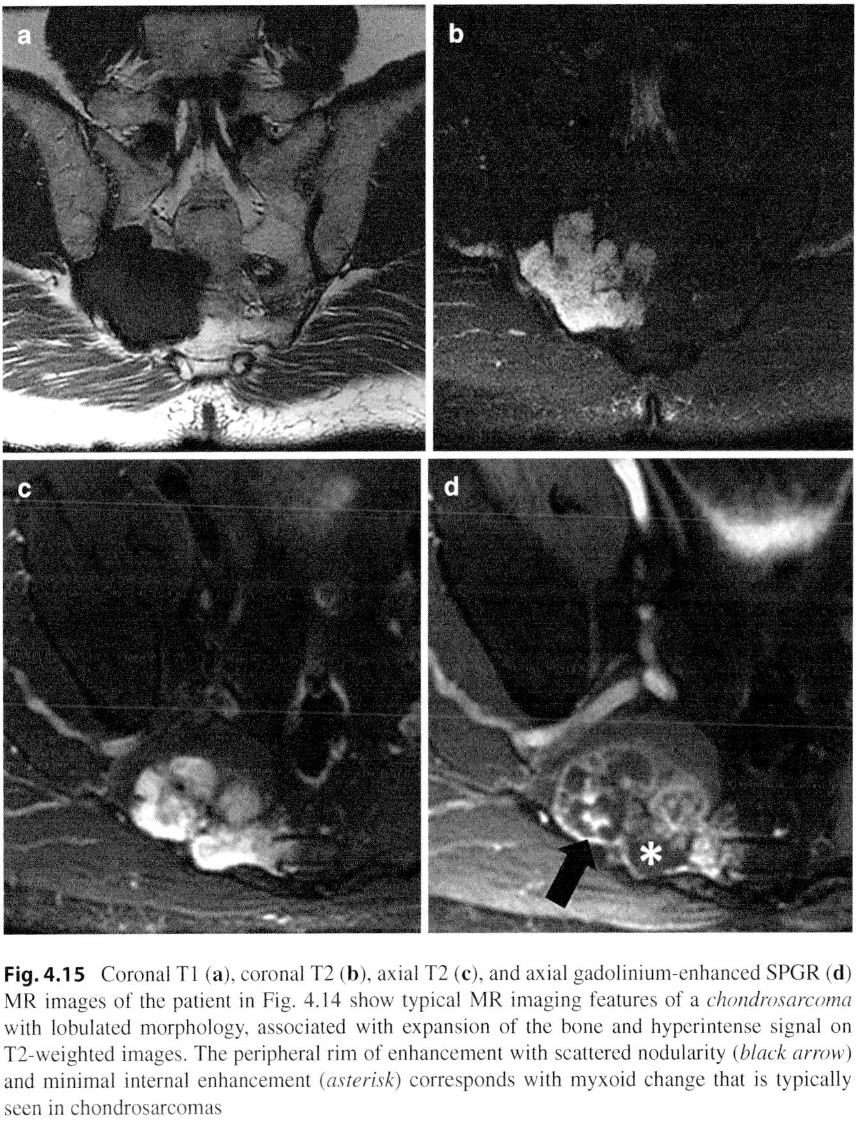

Fig. 4.15 Coronal T1 (**a**), coronal T2 (**b**), axial T2 (**c**), and axial gadolinium-enhanced SPGR (**d**) MR images of the patient in Fig. 4.14 show typical MR imaging features of a *chondrosarcoma* with lobulated morphology, associated with expansion of the bone and hyperintense signal on T2-weighted images. The peripheral rim of enhancement with scattered nodularity (*black arrow*) and minimal internal enhancement (*asterisk*) corresponds with myxoid change that is typically seen in chondrosarcomas

instrumental in making the diagnosis of chondrosarcoma. They typically show areas of peripheral or peripheral nodular enhancement, scattered foci of punctate enhancement, and central areas of non-enhancement due to myxoid change (Fig. 4.15). More dominant solid areas of enhancement may also be seen [32, 33].

Osteosarcoma: Of 4887 cases of primary osteosarcoma (not occurring secondary to radiation or Paget disease) seen at the Mayo Clinic between 1915 and 2001, 4% occurred in the spine. Of these spinal cases, 21% occurred in the sacrum. Although rare, osteosarcoma is the fifth most common malignant primary bone tumor of the sacrum [1]. Although osteosarcoma can occur in all age groups, compared to osteosarcoma in the appendicular skeleton, the average age of patients with spinal osteosarcomas is slightly higher with an average age of 35 years [1, 34]. Secondary osteosarcomas typically occur in older patients and are related to malignant transformation of Paget disease of the bone or are radiation-induced sarcomas occurring 5–20 years following pelvic radiation [5, 35]. In the case of Paget disease, the average patient's age is 66 years but has been reported in patients in their fourth through ninth decades of life. Virtually all osteosarcomas of the sacrum involve the sacral ala and body. Osteoblastic osteosarcoma is by the far the most common subtype with chondroblastic osteosarcoma being the second most common subtype.

Approximately 80% of cases show matrix mineralization on radiographs and/or CT, often marked or dense with an amorphous pattern typical of osteoid matrix production (Fig. 4.16). Although these typically present as a destructive lesion with associated soft tissue mass and mineralized matrix, they are occasionally confined to the bone. When they are located within the posterior elements of the upper

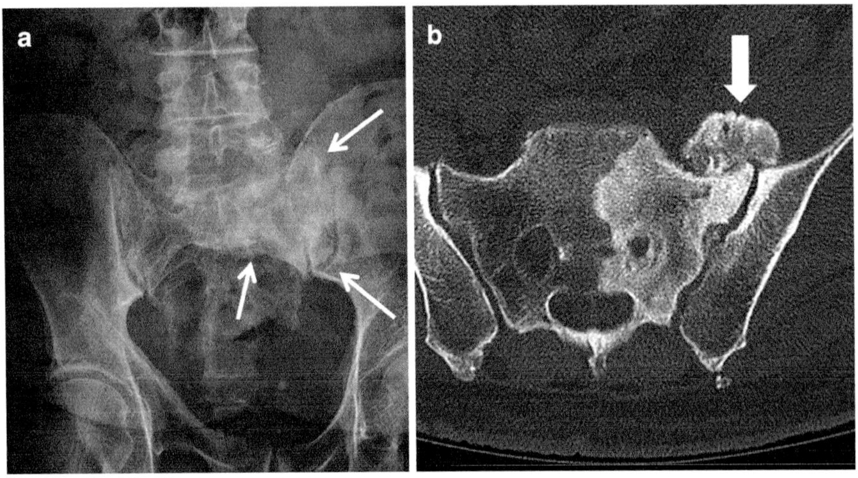

Fig. 4.16 AP radiograph (**a**) and axial CT (**b**) of a 68-year-old male show a densely sclerotic lesion in the upper sacrum on the left that has an associated mineralized soft tissue mass anteriorly (*thick arrow*). Although the mass is evident of the radiograph as an area of increased density (*thin arrows*), it is better defined and characterized as a mineralized mass with osteoid matrix on the CT where the imaging features are typical of an *osteosarcoma*

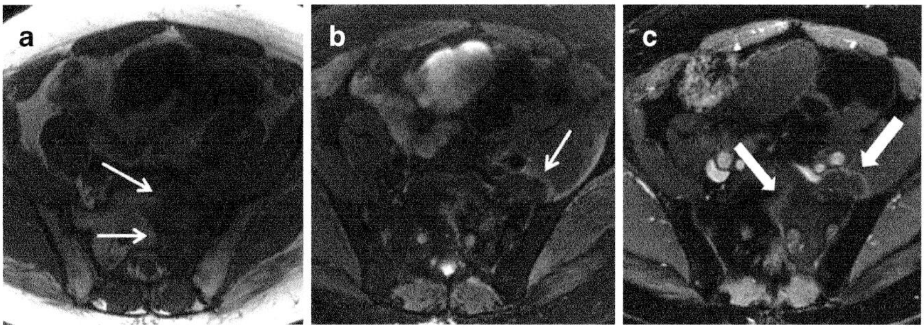

Fig. 4.17 Axial T1 (**a**), axial T2 (**b**), and axial gadolinium-enhanced SPGR (**c**) MR images of the patient in Fig. 4.16 show that both the intra- and extra-osseous portions of the *osteosarcoma* demonstrate predominantly low signal intensity on T1- and T2-weighted images (*thin arrows*) and show minimal internal enhancement with a margin of peripheral enhancement (*thick arrows*) typical of a heavily mineralized osteosarcoma

sacrum, they may mimic an osteoblastoma. In some cases, they can also mimic an osteoblastic metastasis. It has been reported that up to 20% of cases occurring in the spine will show a purely lytic pattern. A lytic pattern may occur with any subtype but occurs in the majority of telangiectatic and fibroblastic subtypes [1, 5, 13, 34]. Although the chondroblastic subtype may mimic a chondrosarcoma, usually at least a component of osteoid matrix can be identified within the tumor to suggest the correct diagnosis [36].

On MRI, lesions with large amounts of dense amorphous osteoid matrix will be predominantly dark on all imaging sequences (Fig. 4.17). Consequently, they may be relatively inconspicuous on T2-weighted images compared to other bone tumors in the sacrum, which are typically hyperintense on T2-weighted images. These cases may only show mild to moderate enhancement, usually greatest along the periphery of the densely mineralized areas of the tumor (Fig. 4.17). The purely lytic or less densely mineralized masses will show more typical nonspecific signal patterns with intermediate or a combination of intermediate and dark signal on T1 and bright or a combination of bright and dark signal on T2, with the areas of lower T1 and T2 signal correlating with the areas of heavy mineralization.

Ewing's Sarcoma: Ewing's sarcoma is an aggressive malignant round cell tumor. Only 3–10% of primary Ewing's sarcomas occur in the spine. However, Ewing's sarcoma is the most common primary malignant tumor of the spine in children, most commonly occurring in the sacrococcygeal region and usually in the first two decades of life [1, 13]. Like osteosarcoma, Ewing's sarcoma should be included on the differential diagnosis for a malignant-appearing destructive mass in the sacrum in younger patients. Ewing's sarcoma typically occurs in younger patients than osteosarcoma since osteosarcoma in the spine tends to occur in a slightly older population than primary osteosarcoma elsewhere in the skeleton.

The imaging features of Ewing's sarcoma are generally nonspecific with bony destruction and lucency on radiographs and CT, often showing a large enhancing nonmineralized soft tissue mass on cross-sectional imaging studies. However, up to 38%

of all cases of Ewing's sarcoma may show prominent sclerosis, usually intermixed with lytic areas. This bony sclerosis correlates with osteonecrosis pathologically. In the spine, sclerosis is even more common, reported in up to 69% of spinal lesions [37]. On MRI, the lytic destructive portions of the mass and any soft tissue mass are usually hyperintense on T2 and intermediate on T1. Areas of sclerosis on radiographs or CT will often correlate with areas of dark signal on both T1- and T2-weighted images.

4.5.7 Metastases, Myeloma, and Lymphoma

Metastases: Metastases are the most common sacral neoplasm. Lung, breast, kidney, and prostate cancer are the most frequent metastases encountered. Lytic metastases are the most common and may be caused by lung, breast, thyroid, kidney, or colon cancer in adults or neuroblastoma in children. Breast and prostate metastases are the most common causes of osteoblastic metastases and may be sclerotic or mixed lytic and sclerotic. However, lymphoma, carcinoid tumors, mucinous adenocarcinomas of the gastrointestinal tract, pancreatic adenocarcinoma, and bladder carcinoma may cause sclerotic skeletal metastases in adults. Neuroblastoma and medulloblastoma are the most common causes of sclerotic metastases in children. The presence of multiple lesions in the sacrum and throughout the remainder of the pelvis should suggest the diagnosis of metastases (or myeloma) (Fig. 4.18), but occasionally, a metastatic lesion may be solitary, mimicking a primary bone tumor (Fig. 4.19). In addition to hematogenous spread of disease, direct anatomic extension from adjacent pelvic tumors into the sacrum can occur with carcinomas of the rectum, uterus, prostate, and bladder [2, 5].

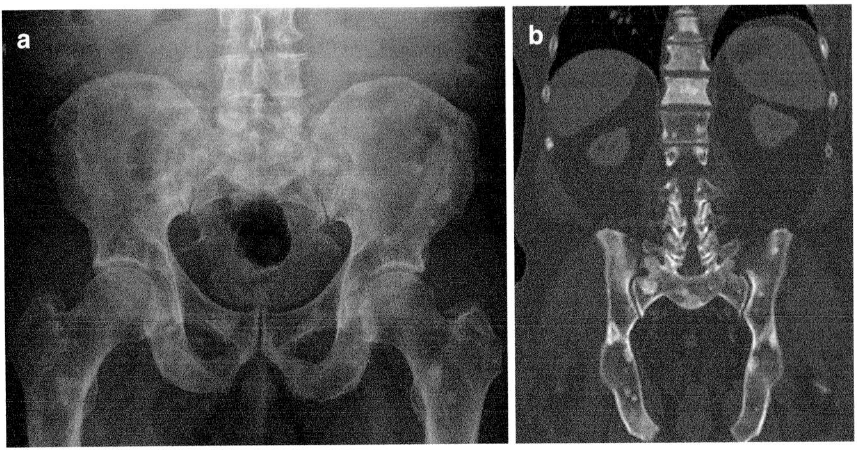

Fig. 4.18 AP radiograph of the pelvis (**a**) and coronal CT of the abdomen and pelvis (**b**) of a 71-year-old male with metastatic adenocarcinoma of the prostate reveal innumerable osteoblastic lesions involving nearly all of the visualized bones, including the sacrum, typical of *skeletal metastases*

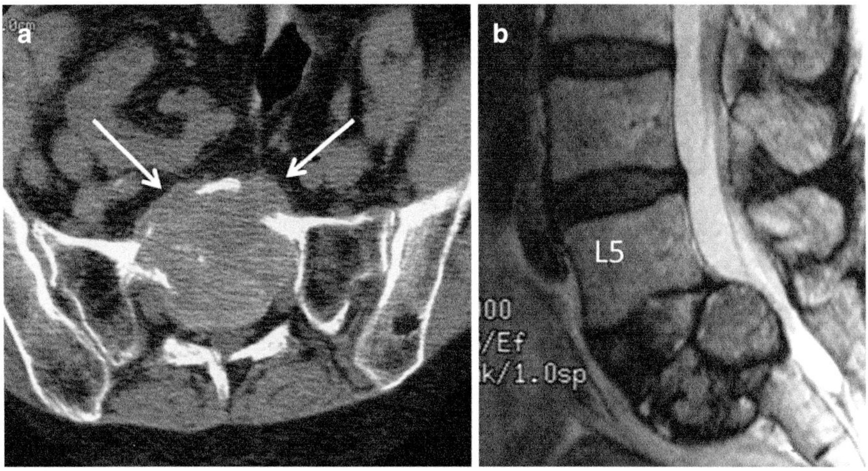

Fig. 4.19 Axial CT (**a**) and sagittal T2-weighted MRI (**b**) of a 65-year-old female show a solid heterogeneous destructive lesion involving S1. The mass has nonspecific imaging features with differential diagnostic possibilities including a metastasis, chordoma, multiple myeloma, or primary sarcoma. The biopsy revealed a solitary *skeletal metastasis* due to metastatic adenocarcinoma of the breast

Multiple Myeloma: Multiple myeloma is due to a neoplastic clonal proliferation of plasma cells and is the second most common primary malignant neoplasm of the sacrum. Multiple myeloma peaks in the sixth and seventh decades of life and lesions are most common in areas that produce hematopoietic marrow in adults [1]. Solitary plasmacytomas are due to focal proliferation of malignant plasma cells without the diffuse involvement present in multiple myeloma. Plasmacytoma, an uncommon tumor occurring in 3–7% of patients with plasma cell neoplasms, is typically considered to represent an early stage of multiple myeloma. It often presents a decade or two earlier than the diffuse form of the disease.

Plasmacytoma and multiple myeloma most commonly produce lytic, destructive lesions that may have an expansile component (Fig. 4.20). Multiple myeloma typically presents with multiple small round lytic lesions in the cancellous bone, without sclerotic margins, which results in a so-called "punched-out" appearance. Plasmacytomas also preferentially replace cancellous bone and present as lytic lesions with relative preservation of the cortex but are often associated with some degree of expansion of the bone. In about one-third of cases, plasmacytomas present as multilobulated lesions with a bubbly lytic appearance with coarsened intervening septations or trabeculae and may simulate a hemangioma. On MRI, the signal characteristics are usually nonspecific with intermediate T1 signal, hyperintense T2 signal, and homogeneous enhancement on post gadolinium images (Fig. 4.20) [1, 2, 5].

Lymphoma: The majority of osseous lymphoma is secondary and due to late hematogenous metastatic dissemination of nodal lymphoma, usually non-Hodgkin lymphoma or, less commonly, osseous invasion from adjacent lymph nodes. Primary lymphoma of the bone, however, is a rare round cell tumor that represents an

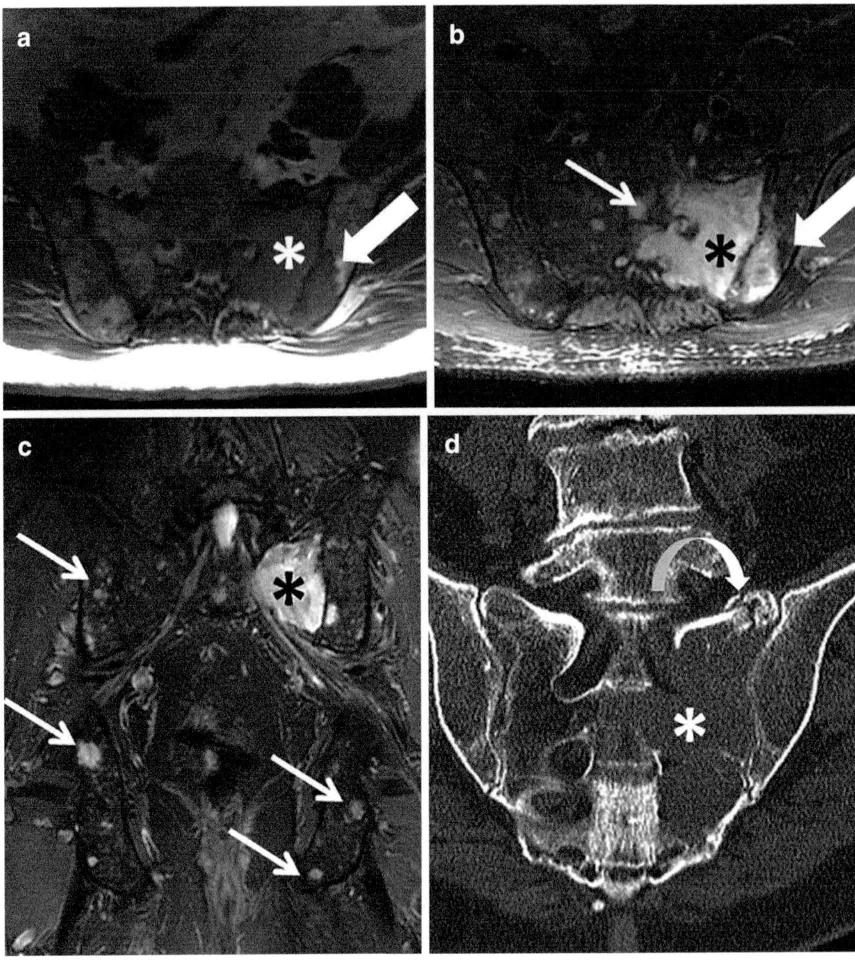

Fig. 4.20 Axial T1 (**a**), axial T2 (**b**), coronal T2 (**c**) MR images and coronal CT (**d**) of a 74-year-old male show a purely lytic destructive lesion involving the mid and upper sacrum on the left (*asterisk*) that crosses the SI joint to involve the adjacent ilium (*thick arrows*) and is associated with a pathologic fracture (*curved arrow*). Although the lesion has nonspecific signal characteristics on the MRI, there are innumerable additional small lesions scattered throughout all of the visualized bones (*thin arrows*). Findings are typical of *multiple myeloma*

extranodal manifestation of the lymph node counterpart of non-Hodgkin lymphoma. It accounts for only 1–3% of all lymphomas. Primary lymphoma of the bone is most common in the fifth to seventh decades of life with a strong 6:1 male to female predilection [5, 38]. Primary lymphoma of the bone has a better prognosis than secondary osseous involvement [38].

The pattern of destruction of primary lymphoma of the bone is variable. The lytic destructive pattern is most common, reported in 70% of cases. The lytic pattern may be permeative (or moth eaten) with multiple elongated ill-defined lucencies or may manifest as an area of either poorly marginated or well-defined osteolysis. The mixed lytic and sclerotic pattern is the next most common appearance. Although possible, purely sclerotic lesions are the least common pattern of bone destruction in primary lymphoma of the bone [38]. Lymphomatous lesions are typically readily detected with cross-sectional imaging. However, radiographic findings and, in some cases, CT findings are often quite subtle. Although a destructive lesion may be seen on conventional radiographs or CT, one of the unique features of lymphoma is that the degree of bone marrow replacement on MR imaging is often markedly out of proportion to the radiographic and/or CT findings and this may be a key feature for suggesting the diagnosis and distinguishing lymphoma from other bone tumors (Fig. 4.21). In addition, this tumor has a propensity for extending into soft tissues

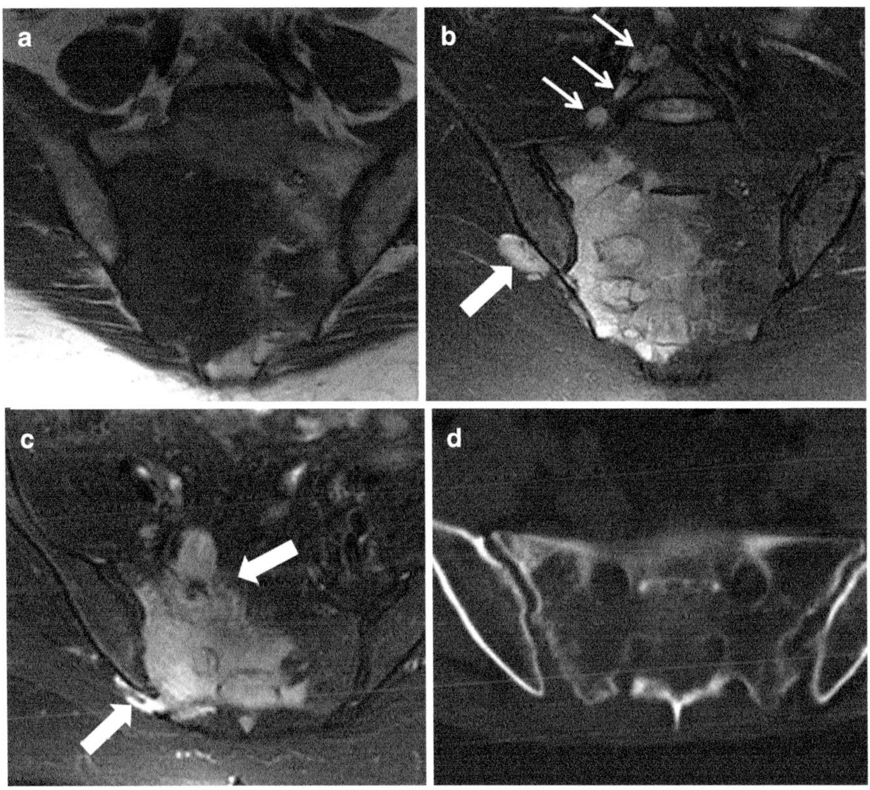

Fig. 4.21 Coronal T1 (**a**), coronal T2 (**b**), and axial T2 (**c**) MR images and axial CT (**d**) of a 57-year-old female with *non-Hodgkin lymphoma* show a large infiltrative mass involving nearly the entire right hemisacrum with an associated soft tissue mass anteriorly and posteriorly (*thick arrows*). The mass encases all of the right sacral nerve roots in their foramina. Of interest, the destructive findings are not as great as expected for the extent of involvement on the MRI with relative preservation of the definition of the foramina, sacral struts, and spinal canal. The discrepancy of MRI findings out of proportion to findings on radiographs or CT is typical of lymphoma. Additionally, there are a multiple small but numerous lymph nodes that could provide an additional clue to the diagnosis (*thin arrows*)

often while leaving the intervening cortex intact [1]. The imaging findings are otherwise nonspecific with lytic destruction on radiographs and CT. MR signal characteristics are nonspecific with intermediate T1 signal, bright T2 signal, and homogeneous enhancement on post contrast images (Fig. 4.21).

4.5.8 Meningocele and Tarlov Cyst

Sacral Meningoceles: Sacral meningoceles should be included on the differential for an expansile sacral and presacral soft tissue mass. Meningoceles are due to an anterior or posterior defect in the vertebral column with herniation of the CSF-filled meninges through the defect. Posterior meningoceles are more common, and the spectrum of disease includes myeloceles, myelomeningoceles, and lipomyelomeningoceles. Posterior meningoceles are often associated with a tethered cord. These are typically clinically apparent in the early postnatal period or may be detected on prenatal ultrasound. Anterior meningoceles may be asymptomatic and may be found incidentally on imaging studies performed from other reasons. However, 80% of anterior meningoceles are present in childhood with symptoms related to pressure on pelvic contents, such as chronic constipation or urinary problems. Neurologic deficits are rare [39, 40].

Anterior sacral meningoceles may be associated with congenital sacral abnormalities. On conventional radiographs, sacral agenesis may be seen or a chronic crescentic-shaped defect of one side of the sacrum related to hemisacral agenesis [2, 39]. On CT, the chronic underlying sacral abnormality should be apparent with a low-density soft tissue mass related to the CSF-filled herniated meninges. Chronic extrinsic erosive changes are commonly seen in the area of the sacral defect related to pressure changes and may be mistaken for a destructive sacral mass. However, careful evaluation of the CT and radiographic findings and correlation with MRI should demonstrate the underlying sacral abnormality and the purely cystic nature of the mass with a connection to the dural sac.

Tarlov Cysts: Tarlov cysts, also known as perineural cysts, meningeal cysts, and arachnoid cysts, are common and very often seen on cross-sectional imaging studies of the lumbar spine, sacrum, and pelvis. They have been reported to be present in 5% of patients undergoing MRI of the lumbar spine [2]. These cysts are related to dilatations of the meninges within the sacral canal or neural foramen and communicate freely with the subarachnoid space. These cysts are frequently associated with chronic expansion and remodeling of the sacral spinal canal and/or involved sacral neural foramen. CT shows chronic widening of the sacral spinal canal or neural foramen with low-density fluid within the cyst. MRI is helpful for confirming the relationship of the cyst to the sacral nerve roots. On MRI, they present as a well-circumscribed homogeneous mass with signal intensity isointense with CSF on all pulse sequences and a variable degree of expansion of the spinal canal or neural foramen (Fig. 4.22).

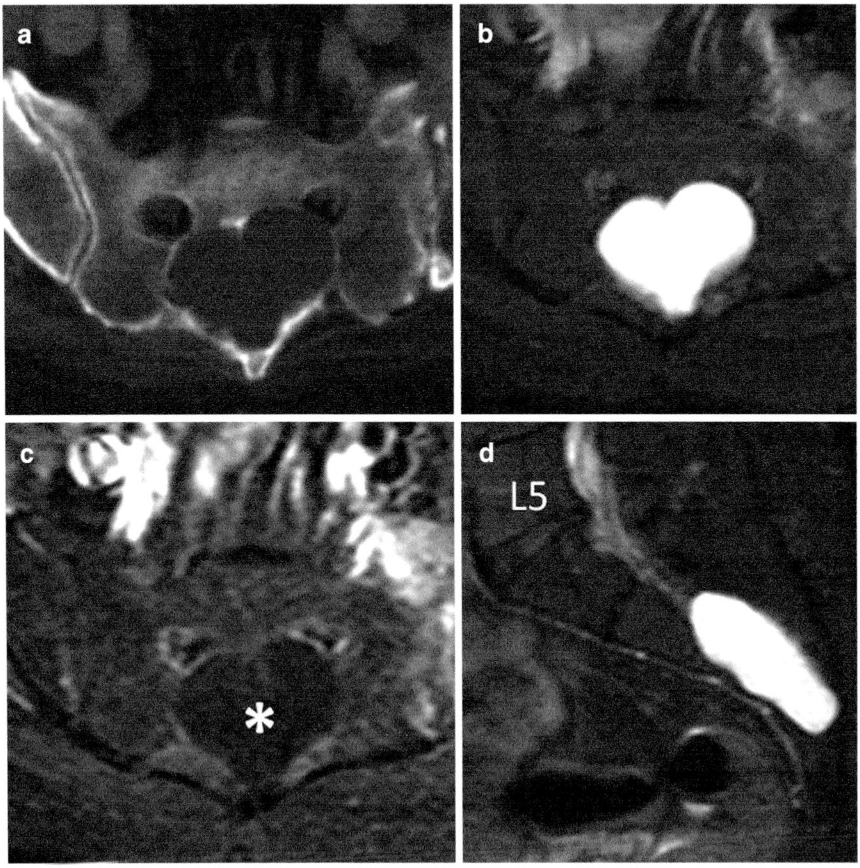

Fig. 4.22 Axial CT (**a**) and axial T2 (**b**) and axial gadolinium-enhanced (**c**) and sagittal T2 (**d**) MR images of the sacrum show typical imaging features of a *Tarlov cyst* presenting as a lesion with fluid signal intensity and associated expansion of the spinal canal. The mass is hypodense on CT and shows homogeneous high signal intensity on T2 and no central enhancement with gadolinium (*asterisk*). These findings are characteristic of a cyst with signal intensity isointense with CSF on all pulse sequences

4.5.9 Tumor Simulators

Some benign nonneoplastic processes have imaging features that simulate tumors in the sacrum. The more common tumor simulators in the sacrum include red marrow hyperplasia, insufficiency-type stress fractures, and Paget disease. It is important to be familiar with the imaging findings in these benign processes in order to avoid unnecessary biopsy and patient anxiety.

Paget Disease: Paget disease is a chronic metabolic disorder of abnormal bone remodeling in adults, usually in patients greater than 40 years of age. Paget disease may involve the sacrum, but when it does, it usually occurs in the setting of polyostotic disease [2]. However, monostotic cases involving the sacrum have been reported [41, 42]. Paget disease may simulate a lytic and/or sclerotic primary bone tumor or metastasis. However, Paget disease has characteristic imaging findings that should enable an accurate diagnosis to be made based upon imaging, obviating the need for biopsy.

On radiographs and CT, the imaging findings vary according to the stage of disease. In the early phase, lytic changes are observed related to osteoclastic activity and intense bone resorption [43]. This is followed by a mixed lytic and sclerotic phase reflecting mixed osteoclastic and osteoblastic activity that results in abnormal bone remodeling. Finally, the last phase is the late inactive or osteoblastic phase, where there are diffuse sclerotic changes.

The lytic and mixed lytic and sclerotic phases have a very characteristic appearance in the long bones with a well-circumscribed area of lucency along the advancing edge of the process described as having a "blade-of-grass" appearance. This finding is seen in association with the typical features of Paget disease, including thickening of the cortex, coarsening of the trabecular pattern, and enlargement of the bone. In the sacrum, these characteristic features can be more difficult to discern, but similar changes in the innominate bone or proximal femur may be helpful for making the diagnosis [43].

During the late or sclerotic phase, radiographs and CT will show progression of diffuse enlargement of the entire sacrum and any other affected pelvic bones as well as progression of cortical thickening and trabecular coarsening (Figs. 4.23 and 4.24). In the sacrum, the cortical thickening may preferentially affect the neural foramina and the lateral cortices adjacent to the sacroiliac joints [2]. Because of the previously noted limitations of radiographs in evaluating the pelvis and sacrum, CT is advantageous and considered as the modality of choice for visualizing and characterizing the pathognomonic changes of Paget disease (Fig. 4.23). In addition to the previously described features, CT is also helpful for demonstrating preservation of the marrow fat with Paget disease. The latter finding is more apparent on the soft tissue window settings and is a helpful feature for distinguishing Paget disease from tumor on CT.

On MRI, findings in Paget disease may be easily confused with a variety of benign and malignant bone tumors, especially in the lytic and mixed lytic and sclerotic phases when there may be nonspecific increased T2 signal and mild diffuse enhancement on post gadolinium images (Fig. 4.24). The sclerotic phase may have a more characteristic appearance with low T1 and T2 signal changes in the areas of cortical thickening and trabecular coarsening. The hallmark for distinguishing between Paget disease and all tumors is the relative preservation of the marrow fat signal on the T1-weighted images in Paget disease. The MRI findings should also be correlated with conventional radiographs and/or CT to confirm the diagnosis [2, 5, 43].

Sarcomatous transformation is one of the known complications of Paget disease of the bone. The rate of malignant transformation is dependent on the extent of skeletal involvement with Paget disease. In patients with widespread Paget disease, the rate of sarcoma has been reported in up to 5–10% of cases. In patients with less extensive or monostotic involvement, the rate is less than 1% [43, 44]. Osteosarcoma

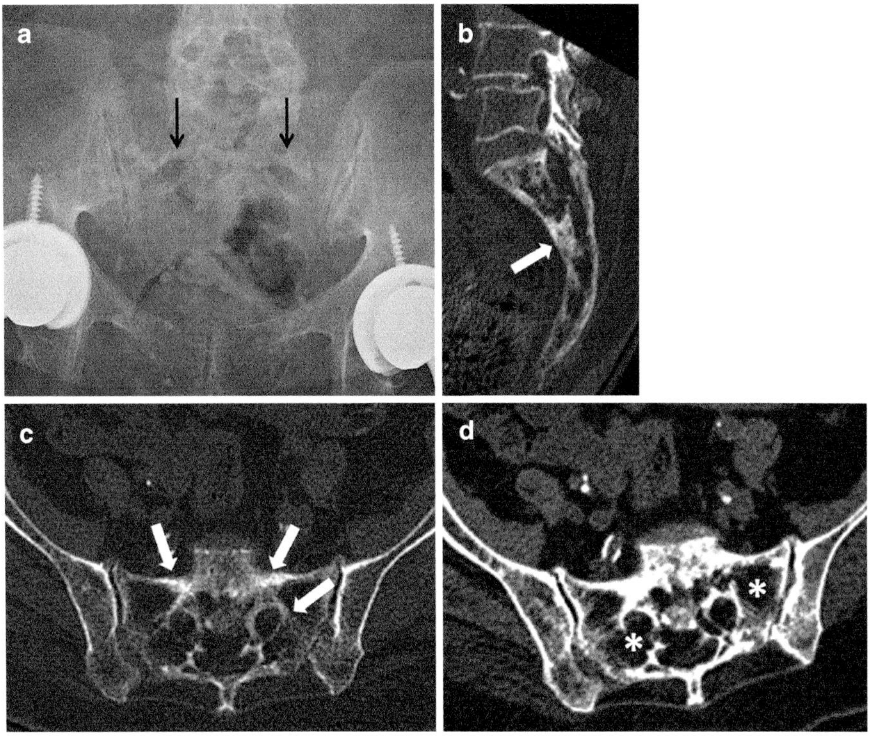

Fig. 4.23 AP radiograph of the pelvis (**a**), and sagittal bone window (**b**), axial bone window (**c**), and axial soft tissue window (**d**) CT images of an 85-year-old female with Paget disease of the sacrum. The findings are subtle on the radiographs but there is evidence of cortical thickening of the sacral struts (*thin arrows*). The CT images show typical findings of *Paget disease* with cortical thickening (*thick arrows*), coarsening of the trabecular pattern, enlargement of the bone, and preservation of the marrow fat density throughout the sacrum (*asterisks*)

is the most common tumor that arises, comprising 50–70% of cases. These tumors typically present as malignant-appearing destructive lesions within the pagetic bone, often with associated cortical destruction and a soft tissue mass [44]. In the case of degeneration to osteosarcoma, osteoid matrix may be identified within the destructive lesion to suggest the diagnosis.

Sacral Insufficiency-Type Stress Fractures: Sacral insufficiency-type stress fractures may occur secondary to osteoporosis or sequela of radiation therapy and have been increasingly recognized over the last several decades [2, 45, 46]. The findings may be very subtle or occult on radiographs but may show a linear vertical lucency or band of sclerosis involving the sacral ala on radiographs and/or CT. However, occasionally the sclerosis and reactive changes may simulate a sclerotic tumor, either primary or metastatic. Findings may be more difficult to interpret in the setting of radiation osteitis. However, CT is sensitive for the detection of the fracture demonstrating the characteristic linear sclerosis or lucent fracture line that parallels the SI joint (Fig. 4.25). The fractures are associated with a variable degree of surrounding sclerosis depending upon the age of the fracture. Additional insufficiency-type stress

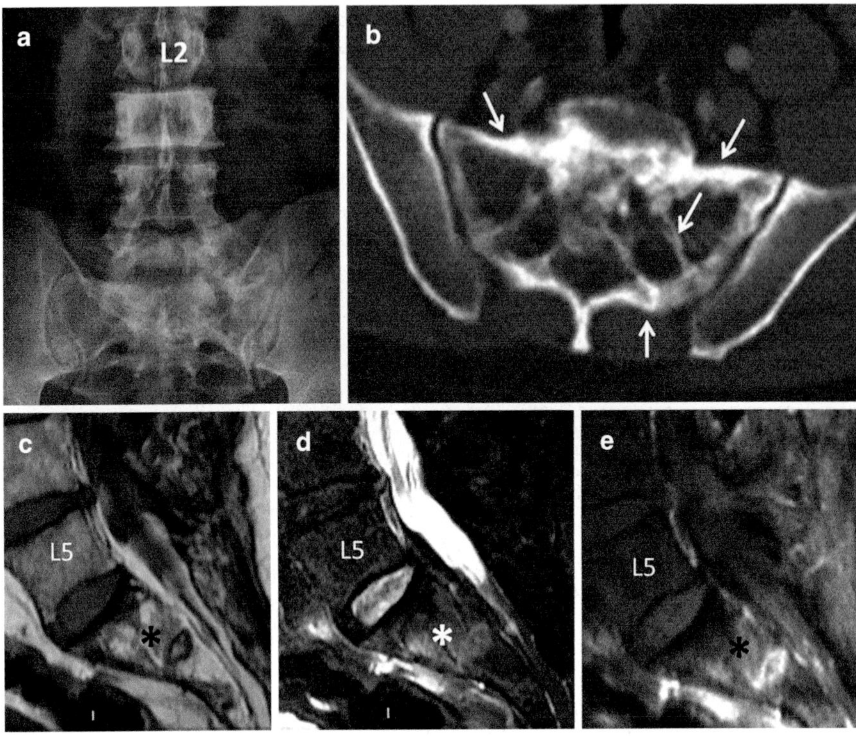

Fig. 4.24 AP radiograph of the lumbar spine and sacrum (**a**), axial CT (**b**) and sagittal T1 (**c**), fat-suppressed T2 (**d**), and gadolinium-enhanced SPGR (**e**) MR images of L5 and upper sacrum of a 71-year-old male with typical findings of *Paget disease* of L3, L5, and the sacrum. The radiographs and CT show enlargement of the bone with cortical thickening and coarsening of the trabecular pattern. The MRI shows patchy increased T2 signal and enhancement in the visualized portion of the sacrum (*asterisks*). The T1-weighted images show complete preservation of the marrow fat signal (*asterisk*), which is typical of Paget disease and aids in distinguishing it from neoplasm

fractures are often identified in the bones of the pelvis, most often in the contralateral sacral ala or the pubic bone. Unilateral and bilateral sacral insufficiency fractures have been reported at equal frequency in the literature. When bilateral in the sacral ala, there may be a horizontal component through the sacral body, resulting in an H-shape pattern [45–47]. Insufficiency-type stress fractures can also occur in the iliac bones and are more common when there is a history of prior pelvic radiation [45]. With insufficiency-type stress fractures, there should not be evidence of an underlying destructive bone lesion or soft tissue mass.

On MRI, insufficiency-type stress fractures present with extensive bone marrow edema in the sacral ala, with a poorly marginated region of increased T2 signal (Fig. 4.25). The T2 signal abnormality may have a band-like morphology but is usually out of proportion to the degree of abnormal signal on T1-weighted images. The decreased T1 signal is typically patchy and poorly defined without evidence of focal geographic marrow replacement (Fig. 4.25). The discrepancy between the findings on T1- and T2-weighted images is typical of bone marrow

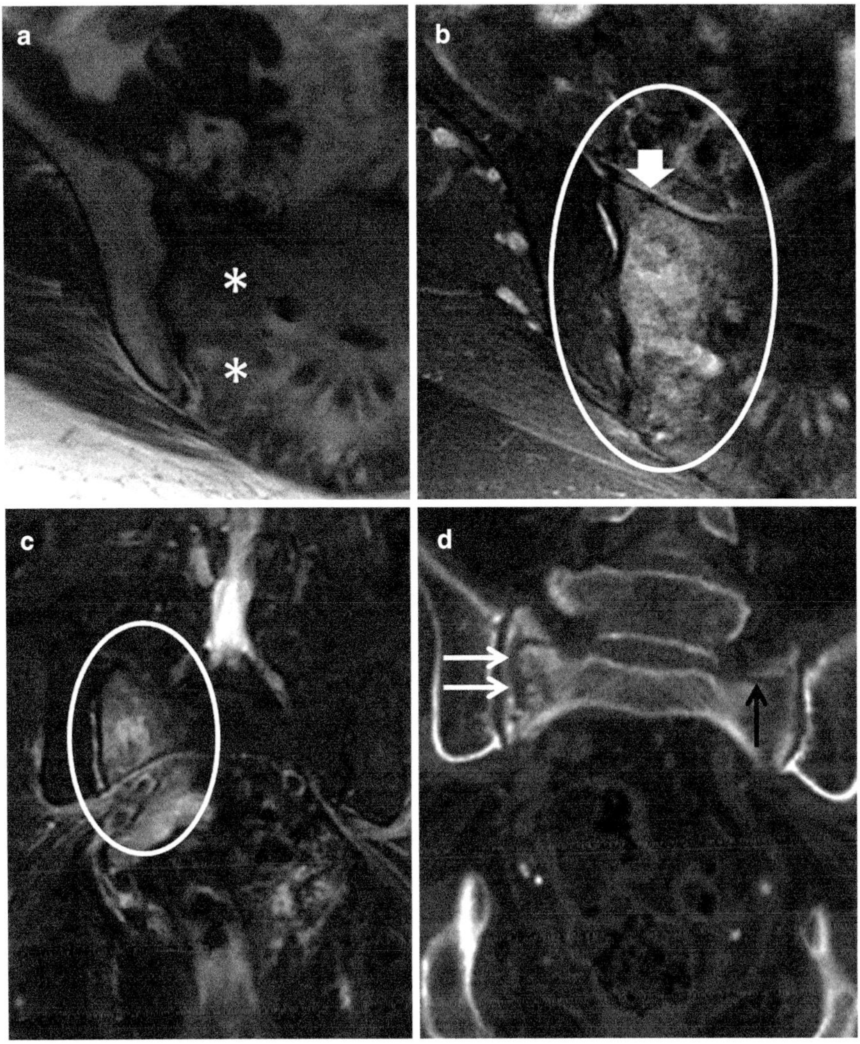

Fig. 4.25 Axial T1 (**a**), axial T2 (**b**), and coronal T2 (**c**) MR images of the mid and upper sacrum of an 80-year-old female with history of breast cancer show a large region of abnormal increased T2 signal in the right sacral ala (*circle*). The corresponding T1-weighted image shows hazy diffuse decreased signal but does not show areas of confluent focal marrow fat replacement. This pattern is indicative of bone marrow edema and should suggest an *insufficiency-type stress fracture*. Although the vertically oriented fracture that parallels the SI joint is more evident on the coronal CT (**d**, *white arrows*), there was evidence of a fracture involving the anterior cortex on the MRI (*thick arrow*). The CT (**d**) was obtained 5 days following the MRI and also showed a new stress fracture of the left sacral ala (*black arrow*)

edema and should provide a clue to suggesting the diagnosis of fracture rather than tumor. The hypointense linear fracture line may be identified as on either the T1- or T2-weighted images [2, 48]. When MR images are carefully scrutinized, the fracture line is identified in 94% of cases. Although MRI is more sensitive for the detection of sacral insufficiency fractures, if the fracture line is not identified on MRI and the diagnosis remains in question, CT may be helpful for demonstrating the fracture line as demonstrated by the arrows in the coronal CT (d). Hematomas are only rarely associated with insufficiency fractures [48]. If a soft tissue mass is present in conjunction with the sacral fracture, it should not be assumed to be a hematoma, and suspicion for a pathologic fracture should increase.

Red Marrow Hyperplasia: At birth, nearly all bone marrow is comprised of hematopoietically active red marrow. Conversion to hematopoietically inactive yellow marrow occurs in a predictable pattern with conversion usually completed by age 25. However, red marrow remains relatively concentrated in the axial and proximal appendicular skeleton throughout adulthood, including within the pelvis and sacrum [49]. The imaging appearance of bone marrow in the pelvis and sacrum of adult patients is variable. It may be comprised entirely of fatty yellow marrow or entirely of red marrow or have a heterogeneous appearance with patchy areas of red and yellow marrow scattered throughout the pelvis and sacrum. In general, the amount of yellow marrow involving the bones of the pelvis progresses with age, with elderly patients frequently demonstrating only fat signal intensity in their bone marrow.

A focal area of red marrow within the sacrum or the patchy heterogeneous pattern may be confused with a focal mass or masses (in the case of patchy red marrow). Although extensive red marrow reconversion in an elderly patient may be a sign of an underlying chronic illness such as anemia, the red marrow itself is benign, and biopsy should be unnecessary in most cases.

Bone marrow patterns are not visible on conventional radiographs and, therefore, only appreciated on CT or MRI. On CT, red marrow presents as hazy areas of mildly increased density compared to adjacent hypodense fatty yellow marrow and should not be associated with bone destruction. However, on MRI, focal or multifocal patchy red marrow is readily identified and more often a diagnostic dilemma than on other modalities.

Because yellow marrow is composed predominantly of fat, it has signal intensity isointense with fat on all imaging sequences [4, 49]. Although red marrow contains fat, it also contains hematopoietic elements responsible for the production of red blood cells, white blood cells and platelets that affect its signal intensity. Red marrow tends to have intermediate signal intensity on T1-weighted images (darker than fat but usually brighter than intervertebral disk or skeletal muscle), resulting in a hazy decrease in marrow fat signal on T1-weighted images [4]. On fluid-sensitive sequences, red marrow usually demonstrates minimal T2 signal abnormality, usually only minimally brighter than the adjacent fatty bone marrow [50]. Red marrow typically shows mild enhancement with gadolinium.

It is usually possible to distinguish the hazy decrease in T1 signal related to red marrow involving the bones of the pelvis in adult patients from benign and malignant tumors. The red marrow results in a hazy gray pattern on T1-weighted images, in contrast to tumors that show confluent areas of focal replacement that have low to intermediate signal intensity (dark or darker than skeletal muscle). However, in challenging cases, chemical shift imaging can be helpful for distinguishing red marrow from neoplasm [3].

Chemical shift imaging, commonly referred to as "in-phase and opposed-phase" imaging, is useful for detecting microscopic fat as is the case with decreased T1 signal due to either red marrow or edema. When both fat and water are present within the same imaging voxel, the signal will be lower or darker on the opposed-phase images compared to the in-phase images. This finding is helpful for confirming the presence of microscopic fat and suggesting benign red marrow rather than a marrow-replacing tumor [51]. This sequence can be performed for problem solving when red marrow is suspected but cannot be confirmed definitively with conventional T1-weighted imaging. The diagnosis of focal or diffuse red marrow can be made and unnecessary biopsy avoided for a T2 isointense or mildly hyperintense enhancing focus within the bone marrow of the sacrum that shows signal dropout on the opposed-phase images (compared to in-phase images) (Fig. 4.26).

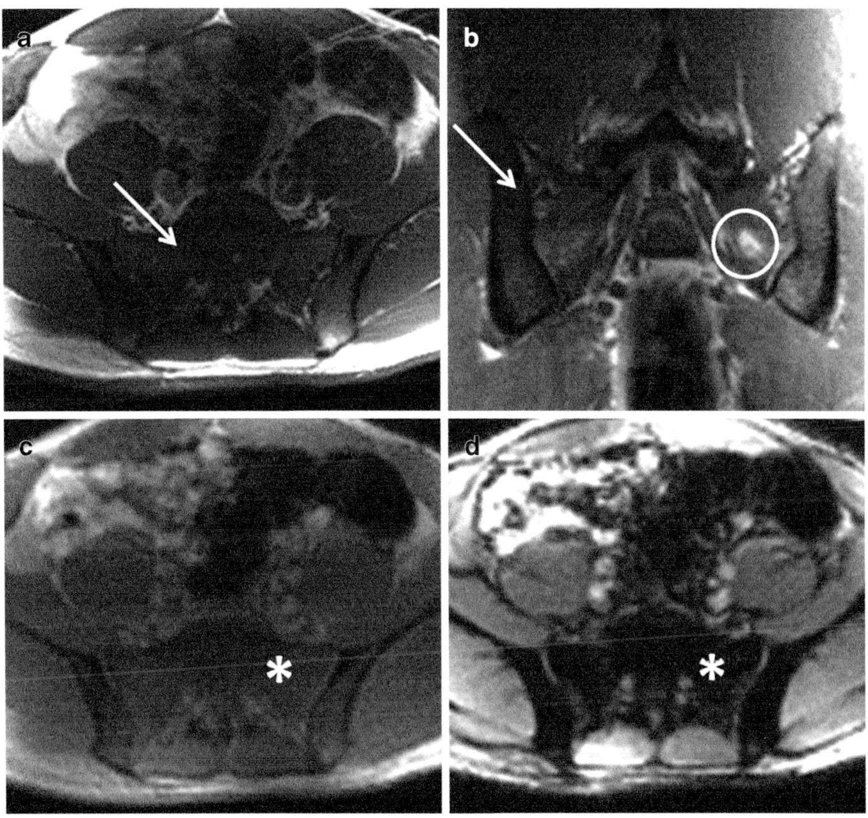

Fig. 4.26 Axial (**a**) and coronal (**b**) T1-weighted MR images of the pelvis in a 31-year-old male with back and pelvic pain demonstrate diffuse decrease in signal intensity in the sacrum and innominate bones (*arrows*) with marked decrease in the expected quantity of yellow marrow fat signal for a patient of this age. There was a small focus of preserved fat signal in the left sacral ala (*circle*). Axial dual gradient echo in-phase (**c**) and opposed-phase (**d**) MR images show marked diffuse signal dropout (*asterisks*) indicative of significant intravoxel fat. The confirmation of the presence of fat confirms the diagnosis of *red marrow hyperplasia* and excludes the possibility of marrow-infiltrating neoplasm such as leukemia, lymphoma, or diffuse metastatic disease

Conclusion

In conclusion, there is a broad spectrum of pathology involving the sacrum ranging from benign and malignant processes to tumor simulators. The imaging workup for a patient with a known or suspected tumor or abnormality involving the sacrum is variable but should always begin with a conventional radiograph. In some cases, the radiographs are diagnostic. However, given the complexity of the anatomy of the bones of the pelvis, further imaging with CT and/or MRI is often required for optimal characterization. In some cases, the constellation of imaging findings are diagnostic, and unnecessary patient anxiety and biopsy can be avoided. In other cases, the lesions have indeterminate imaging features and biopsy is required for definitive diagnosis. The information provided in this chapter will serve as a helpful guide for either making the diagnosis or formulating an appropriate differential diagnosis for tumors involving the sacrum, based on a combination of the imaging findings along with pertinent clinical information, including the patient's age, gender, and any known syndromes. Being familiar with the advantages and disadvantages of the available imaging tools along with the expected findings associated with the spectrum of pathology plays a critical role in guiding management of these patients and ultimately in providing optimal patient care.

Conflict-of-Interest Statement No benefits have been or will be received from a commercial party related directly or indirectly to the subject matter of this article.

References

1. Disler DG, Miklic D. Imaging findings in tumors of the sacrum. AJR. 1999;173:1699–706.
2. Diel J, Ortiz O, Losada RA, Price DB, Hayt MW, Katz DS. The sacrum: pathologic spectrum, multimodality imaging, and subspecialty approach. Radiographics. 2001;21:83–104.
3. Howe BM, Johnson GB, Wenger DE. Current concepts in MRI of focal and diffuse malignancy of bone marrow. Semin Musculoskelet Radiol. 2013;17:137–44.
4. Shah LM, Hanrahan CJ. MRI of spinal bone marrow: part I, techniques and normal age-related appearances. AJR. 2011;197:1298–308.
5. Rodallec MH, Feydy A, Larousserie F, Anract P, Campagna R, Babinet A, Zins M, Drape J. Diagnostic imaging of solitary tumors of the spine: what to do and say. Radiographics. 2008;28:1019–41.
6. Miller T. Bone tumors and tumorlike conditions: analysis with conventional radiography. Radiology. 2008;246:662–74.
7. Lin J, Martel W. Cross-sectional imaging of peripheral nerve sheath tumors: characteristic signs on CT, MR imaging and sonography. AJR. 2001;176:75–82.
8. Wasa J, Nishida Y, Tsukushi S, Shido Y, Sugiura H, Nakashima H, Ishiguro N. MRI features in the differentiation of malignant peripheral nerve sheath tumors and neurofibromas. AJR. 2010;194:1568–74.
9. Hrehorovich PA, Hubert FR, Maximin S, Caracta P. Malignant peripheral nerve sheath tumor. Radiographics. 2003;23:790–4.
10. Karabatsou K, Kiehl TR, Wilson DM, Hendler A, Guha AM. Potential role of 18fluorodeoxyglucose-positron emission tomography/computed tomography in differentiating benign neurofibroma from malignant peripheral nerve sheath tumor associated with neurofibromatosis 1. Neurosurgery. 2009;65(4 Suppl):A160–70.

11. Llauger J, Palmer J, Amores S, Bague S, Camins A. Primary tumors of the sacrum: diagnostic imaging. AJR. 2000;174:417–24.
12. Combemale P, Valeyrie-Allanore L, Giammarile F, Pinson S, Guillot B, Goulart DM, Wolkenstein P, Blay JY, Mognetti T. Utility of 18F-FDG PET with a semi-quantitative index in the detection of sarcomatous transformation in patients with neurofibromatosis type 1. PLoS One. 2014;9(2):e85954.
13. Murphey MD, Andrews CL, Flemming DJ, Temple HT, Smith WS, Smirniotopoulos JG. Primary tumors of the spine: radiologic-pathologic correlation. Radiographics. 1996;16:1131–58.
14. Chakarun CF, Forrester DM, Gottsegen CF, Patel DB, White EA, Matcuk GR. Giant cell tumor of bone: review, mimics, and new developments in treatment. Radiographics. 2013;33: 197–211.
15. Gong L, Liu W, Sun X, Sajdik C, Tian X, Niu X, Huang XY. Histologic and clinical characteristics of malignant giant cell tumor of bone. Virchows Arch. 2012;460:327–34.
16. Farsad K, Kattapuram SV, Sackoff R, Ono J, Nielsen GP. Best cases from the AFIP: sacral chordoma. Radiographics. 2009;29:1525–30.
17. Bjornsson J, Wold LE, Ebersold MJ, Laws ER. Chordoma of the mobile spine: a clinicopathologic analysis of 40 patients. Cancer. 1993;71:735–40.
18. Rosenthal DI, Scott JA, Mankin HJ, Wismer GL, Brady TJ. Sacrococcygeal chordoma: magnetic resonance imaging and computed tomography. AJR. 1985;145:143–7.
19. De Bruine FT, Kroon HM. Spinal chordoma: radiologic features in 14 cases. AJR. 1988;150:861–3.
20. Firoonzia H, Pinto RS, Lin JP, Baruch HH, Zausner J. Chordoma: radiologic evaluation of 20 cases. AJR. 1976;127:797–805.
21. Firoonzia H, Golimbo C, Rafii M, Reede DL, Kricheff II, Bjorkengren A. Computed tomography of spinal chordomas. J Comput Assist Tomogr. 1986;10:45–50.
22. Yamaguchi T, Iwata J, Sugihara S, McCarthy EF, Karita M, Murakami H, Kawahara N, Tsuchiya H, Tomita K. Distinguishing benign notochordal cell tumors from vertebral chordoma. Skelet Radiol. 2008;37:291–9.
23. Nishiguchi T, Mochizuki K, Ohsawa M, Inoue T, Kageyama K, Suzuki A, Takami T, Miki Y. Differentiating benign notochordal cell tumors from chordomas: radiographic features on MRI, CT, and tomography. AJR. 2011;196:644–50.
24. Yamaguchi T, Yamato M, Saotome K. First histologically confirmed case of a classic chordoma arising in a precursor benign notochordal lesion: differential diagnosis of benign and malignant notochordal lesions. Skelet Radiol. 2001;31:413–8.
25. Pasalic D, Luetmer PH, Hunt CH, Rose PS, Diehn FE, Folpe AL, Wenger DE. Benign notochordal cell tumor of the sacrum with atypical imaging features: the value of CT guided biopsy for diagnosis. Open Neuroimaging J. 2013;7:36–40.
26. Ruggieri P, Huch K, Mavrogenis AF, Merlina B, Angelini A. Osteoblastoma of the sacrum: report of 18 cases and analysis of the literature. Spine. 2014;39:E97–E103.
27. Unni KK. Benign osteoblastoma (giant osteoid osteoma). In: Unni KK, editor. Dahlin's bone tumors: general aspects and data on 11087 cases. 5th ed. Philadelphia: Lippincott-Raven; 1996. p. 131–42.
28. Oliveira AM, Perez-Atayde AR, Inwards CY, Medeiros F, Derr V, Hsi BL, Gebhardt MC, Rosenberg AE, Fletcher JA. USP6 and CDH11 oncogenes identify the neoplastic cell in primary aneurysmal bone cysts and are absent in so-called secondary aneurysmal bone cysts. Am J Pathol. 2004;165(5):1773–80.
29. Shives TC, McLeod RA, Unni KK, Schray MF. Chondrosarcoma of the spine. JBJS. 1989;71:1158–65.
30. Stuckey RM, Marco RAW. Chondrosarcoma of the mobile spine and sacrum. Sarcoma. 2011;2011:4. doi:10.1155/2011/274281.
31. Gitelis S, Bertoni F, Picci P, Campanacci M. Chondrosarcoma of bone. The experience at the Istituto Ortopedico Rizzoli. J Bone Joint Surg Am. 1981;63(8):1248–57.
32. Littrell LA, Wenger DE, Wold LE, Bertoni F, Unni KK, White LM, Kandel R, Sundaram M. Radiographic, CT, and MR imaging features of dedifferentiated chondrosarcomas: a retrospective review of 174 de novo cases. Radiographics. 2004;24:1397–409.

33. Murphey MD, Walker EA, Wilson AF, Kransdorf MF, Temple T, Gannon FH. Imaging of primary chondrosarcoma: radiologic-pathologic correlation. Radiographics. 2003;23:1245–78.
34. Ilaslan H, Sundaram M, Unni KK, Shives TC. Primary vertebral osteosarcoma: imaging findings. Radiology. 2004;23:697–702.
35. Deyrup AT, Montag AG, Inwards CY, Xu Z, Swee RG, Unni KK. Sarcomas arising in Paget disease of bone: a clinicopathologic analysis of 70 cases. Arch Pathol Lab Med. 2007;131:942–6.
36. Shives TC, Dahlin DC, Sim FH, Pritchard DJ, Earle JD. Osteosarcoma of the spine. JBJS. 1986;68A(5):660–8.
37. Shirley SK, Gilula LA, Siegal GP, Foulkes MA, Kissane JM, Askin FB. Roentgenographic-pathologic correlation of diffuse sclerosis in Ewing sarcoma of bone. Skelet Radiol. 1984; 12(2):69–78.
38. Krishnan A, Shirkhoda A, Tehranzadeh J, Armin AR, Irwin R, Les K. Primary bone lymphoma: radiographic-MR imaging correlation. Radiographics. 2003;23:1371–87.
39. Mohta A, Das S, Jindal R. Anterior sacral meningocele presenting as constipation. J Pediatr Neurosci. 2011;6(1):40–3.
40. Hain KS, Pickhardt PJ, Lubner MG, Menias CO, Bhalla S. Presacral masses: multimodality imaging of a multidisciplinary space. Radiographics. 2013;33:1145–67.
41. Yorulmaz G, Akalin A, Serbetci BS. Paget's disease of sacrum: a case report. Endocr Abstr. 2009;20:275.
42. Singh AK, Murray SA. Paget disease of the sacrum: a case report. Orthop Proc. 2006. ISSN:1358–992X.
43. Theodorou DJ, Theodorou SJ, Kakitsubata Y. Imaging of Paget disease of bone and its musculoskeletal complications: review. AJR. 2011;196:S64–75.
44. Moore TE, King AR, Kathol MH, el-Khoury GY, Palmer R, Downey PR. Sarcoma in Paget disease of bone: clinical, radiologic, and pathologic features in 22 cases. AJR. 1991;156: 1199–203.
45. Cooper KL, Beabout JW, Swee RG. Insufficiency fractures of the sacrum. Radiology. 1985; 156:15–20.
46. Peh WCG, Khong PL, Yin Y, Ho WY, Evans NS, Gilula LA, Yeung HWD, Davies AM. Imaging of pelvis insufficiency fractures. Radiographics. 1996;16:335–48.
47. Lyders EM, Whitlow CT, Baker MD, Morris PP. Imaging and treatment of sacral insufficiency fractures. Am J Neuroradiol. 2010;31:201–10.
48. Carrabus MC, Ambekar A, Lu Y, Link TM. MRI and CT of insufficiency fractures of the pelvis and the proximal femur. AJR. 2008;191:995–1001.
49. Vogler III JB, Murphy WA. Bone marrow imaging. Radiology. 1988;168(3):679–93.
50. Shah LM, Hanrahan CJ. MRI of spinal bone marrow: part 2, techniques and normal age-related appearances. AJR. 2011;197:1298–308.
51. Merkle EM, Nelson RC. Dual gradient-echo in-phase and opposed-phase hepatic MR imaging: a useful tool for evaluating more than fatty infiltration or fatty sparing. Radiographics. 2006;26:1409–18.

Imaging of Sacral Tumors: Experience of the Rizzoli Institute

5

Alessandra Bartoloni, Alberto Bazzocchi, and Daniel Vanel

5.1 Introduction

The sacrum is composed of bone, cartilage, and bone marrow as well as notochord remnants. Malignant bone tumors can arise from any of these components.

The sacrum, which contains hematopoietic bone marrow, is a common site of metastases and hematological malignancies such as myeloma, lymphoma, or plasmacytoma. Metastases are the most common malignancies of this region.

Chordoma is the most common primary malignant bone tumor of the sacrum. Primary sarcomas of the sacrum are rare and include chondrosarcoma, Ewing Sarcoma, and osteosarcoma, in order of decreasing incidence [1].

Benign sacral bone tumors include giant cell tumors (GCT), aneurysmal bone cyst, osteoid osteoma, osteoblastoma.

5.2 Primary and Secondary Malignant Bone Tumors

5.2.1 Metastases

Metastases from lung, breast, kidney, prostate, head and neck, gastrointestinal, or skin (melanoma) cancers are the most common malignancies of the sacrum. Metastases are usually osteolytic, or more rarely osteoblastic (prostate, breast). In the case of multiple sacral and spinal lesions, a diagnosis of metastatic disease or multiple myeloma is first suggested.

A. Bartoloni, M.D. • A. Bazzocchi, M.D.
Diagnostic and Interventional Radiology, Istituto Ortopedico Rizzoli, Bologna, Italy
e-mail: abazzo@inwind.it

D. Vanel, M.D. (✉)
Department of Pathology, Istituto Ortopedico Rizzoli, Bologna, Italy
e-mail: vanel.daniel@yahoo.fr

P. Ruggieri et al. (eds.), *Tumors of the Sacrum*,
DOI 10.1007/978-3-319-51202-0_5

5.2.2 Sacral Involvement of Multiple Myeloma and Plasmacytoma

Patients with multiple myeloma are usually >60 years at presentation. CT usually shows an osteolytic lesion without a peripheral rim of sclerosis with a "soap bubble" appearance sometimes associated with a space-occupying lesion [2]. Plasmacytoma [3] is a focal, isolated, proliferation of malignant plasma cells and is considered to be often an early stage of multiple myeloma. It appears as an osteolytic, space-occupying lesion, generally larger than multiple myeloma lesions. The remaining bone trabeculae are thick. On MRI, a Plasmacytoma is hypointense on T1-w images, hyperintense on T2-w images, and enhances avidly post-contrast. PET/CT or whole body MRI can help in the diagnosis of multiple myeloma.

5.2.3 Bone Lymphoma

Bone lymphoma can be either primary or associated with lymph node and visceral involvement. It usually manifests after the age of 10 years, but can occur at any age with a male predominance.

Bone lymphoma is an aggressive lesion associated with extensive moth-eaten osteolysis, inconstant reactive sclerosis, and soft tissues invasion.

Radiographic and CT findings are often absent or a permeative lesion without cortical disruption can be present. At MRI, bone marrow involvement appears as a well-delineated T1-w hypointense and T2-w hyperintense area with intense contrast enhancement [4, 5].

Discrepancy between massive bone marrow invasion at MRI and normal radiography, a large soft tissue mass with no visible cortical lesion at CT and an increased uptake on scintigraphy, are all suggestive signs of bone lymphoma, although nonspecific [6].

5.2.4 Chordoma

Chordoma is the most common primary tumor of the sacrum, representing 40% of all sacral tumors and one half of all malignant bone tumors.

It is more common in individuals aged 40–70 with a peak in the fifth decade and a strong male predominance [7]. Chordomas derive from notochordal remnants, and they involve the sacrococcygeal region in 50–60% of cases and the clivus or spheno-occipital region in 30–35% of cases [8]. It is a malignant tumor essentially due to local invasion. Metastatic disease is uncommon, but secondary sites may be observed.

Sacral chordoma usually arises from the third, fourth, or fifth vertebra as a large osteolytic lesion in the midline or in a paramedian location associated with a soft tissue mass, usually anterior [9].

CT shows a well-defined osteolytic lesion without any sclerotic rim, but sometimes associated with bulging of the cortex. Internal calcifications are demonstrated in 50–60% of sacral chordomas. In >50% of cases, there are areas of low attenuation within the mass reflecting the myxoid matrix of the tissue. A fibrous pseudocapsula may be present [10].

When there is an extra-osseous involvement, sacral chordomas can extend upward into the sacral canal or anteriorly in the presacral space, ("dumbbell shape" appearance).

An extension to the sacro-iliac joint or intervertebral disc may be present although this is not typical for sacral chordoma.

At MRI, the classical feature of sacral chordoma is the high signal intensity on T2-weighted images, reflecting the abundant mucoid matrix of the tumor, similar to that of the nucleus pulposus. On T1-w images, chordomas show an iso-hypointense signal with moderate contrast enhancement (Fig. 5.1). Hyperintense foci can be seen on T1-w images representing areas of hemorrhage or mucoid material.

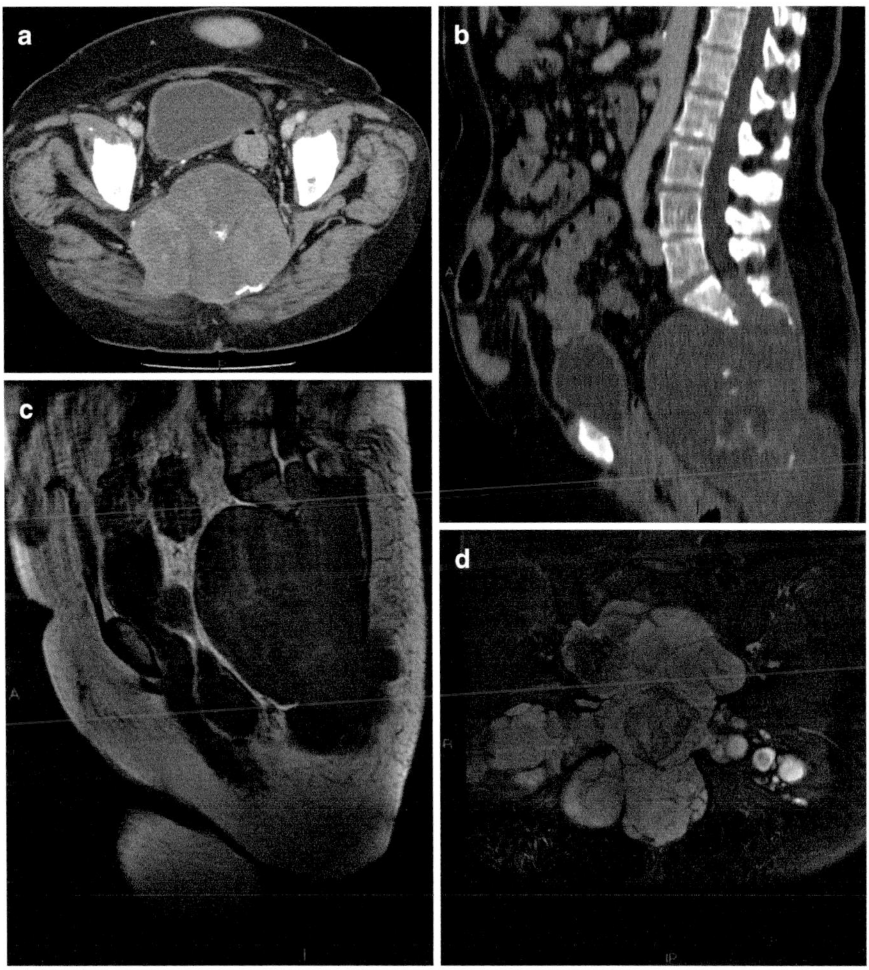

Fig. 5.1 Sacral chordoma in a 55-year-old woman. (**a**, **b**) Axial and sagittal CT scan. Large osteolytic lesion arising in the midline from the lower sacrum. The mass shows low attenuation and some internal calcifications. (**c**) Sagittal T1-w MRI, (**d**) oblique coronal T-2 weighted MRI: the lesion has a low signal intensity on T1-w images and a high signal intensity on T2-w images; it extends in the spinal canal and in the presacral space

Septations can be present and appear as hypointense on T2-w images. Small foci of low signal intensity on T2-w images can represent hemosiderin deposits from previous hemorrhage [11].

The main differential diagnosis of sacral chordoma include chondrosarcoma, benign notochordal cell tumor (BNCT), giant cell tumor, Plasmacytoma, myxopapillary ependymoma, and metastases.

The characteristic signs in favor of chordoma are its usually midline position, situated very low in the sacrum (S3 to S5) and extended upward in the sacral canal.

Chondrosarcoma constitutes the major differential diagnosis, especially in the presence of tumor calcifications, often observed in chondroid chordomas. The location (chondrosarcoma arise off midline, from the sacro-iliac cartilage), a heterogeneous signal intensity on T2-w images, the lack of areas of hemorrhage within the tumor, and septations contrast enhancement may help in the diagnosis of chondrosacroma [12]. Diffusion weighted-MRI can be useful in differential diagnosis since ADC values seem to be higher in chondrosarcoma than in chordoma [13].

Chordoma should also be distinguished from Benign Notochordal Cell Tumor (BNCT), a benign lesion arising from notochord remnants (previously called giant "notochordal rests" or "notochordal hamartomas") and believed to be rarely a precursor of chordoma. It is very frequent on autopsies (20% of the population) but rare on imaging exams (probably because not enough large to be detected) [14]. On radiographs, BNCT are often invisible or can show a vague sclerosis. CT shows a sclerotic lesion without cortical disruption or expansion. On MRI, BNCT are hyperintense on T2-w images and hypointense on T1-weighted images without any contrast enhancement (Fig. 5.2). Unlike chordoma, no soft tissue component is present [15–17]. If radiological characteristics are typical of BNCT, biopsy is not necessary unless the lesion changes; follow-up is recommended.

Giant cell tumors usually affect younger patients, have an eccentric and upper-sacral location, polycystic areas, fluid–fluid level, and frequently involve the sacro-iliac joint.

Myxopapillary ependymomas may show very similar characteristics to those of chondroma but they arise in the spinal canal rather than in the bone and usually demonstrate a more intense Gadolinium contrast enhancement.

After surgery, MRI follow-up of chordomas should be performed every 6 months for the first year after diagnosis to detect local recurrence or progression. The whole spine must be studied on MRI to detect leptomeningeal recurrences. Thereafter, if there is no progression, MRI is recommended yearly for at least 15 years [18].

5.2.5 Chondrosarcoma

Chondrosarcomas accounts for 7–12% of malignant primary tumor of the spine and are more common in the thoracic spine, while they are rare in the sacrum.

Primary chondrosarcoma of the sacrum predominantly affects patients between 30 and 70 years, with a male predominance (2-4:1) [19].

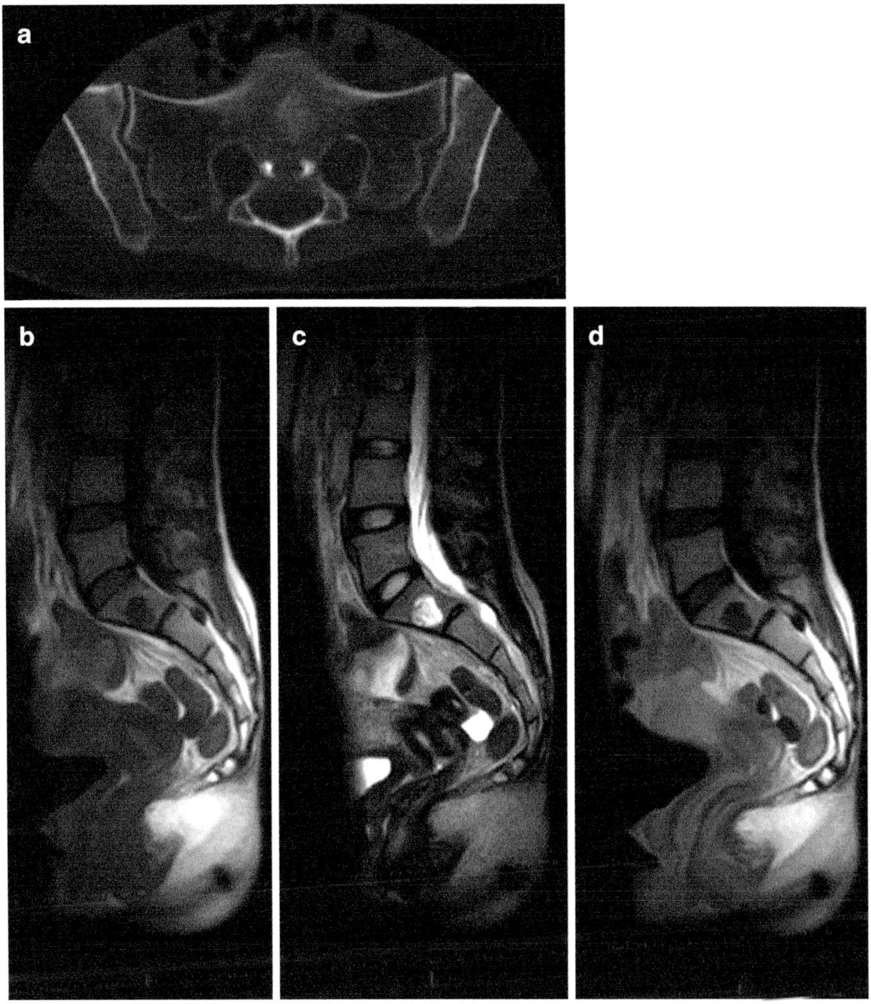

Fig. 5.2 Benign notochordal cell tumor (*BNCT*) in a 31-year-old woman: (**a**) axial CT scan shows a sclerotic lesion in S1. (**b**) Sagittal T1-w MRI, (**c**) sagittal T2-w MRI, (**d**) sagittal T1-w MRI after Gd: the lesion has a low signal intensity on T1-w images, is hyperintense on T2-w images, and shows no contrast enhancement

On radiographs and CT, chondrosarcoma appears as a destructive lytic lesion, usually eccentric in location, with a lobulated contour and endosteal scalloping. The lesion can be associated with a soft tissue mass [10].

On CT, the non-mineralized, cartilaginous portion of the tumor has a low density while the mineralized portion can show typical "ring and arc" calcifications.

On MRI, cartilaginous nodules are iso-hypointense on T1-w images and show lobular high intensity on T2-w images; calcifications are seen as areas of signal void on all MRI sequences (Fig. 5.3). Contrast enhancement is usually mild and can be

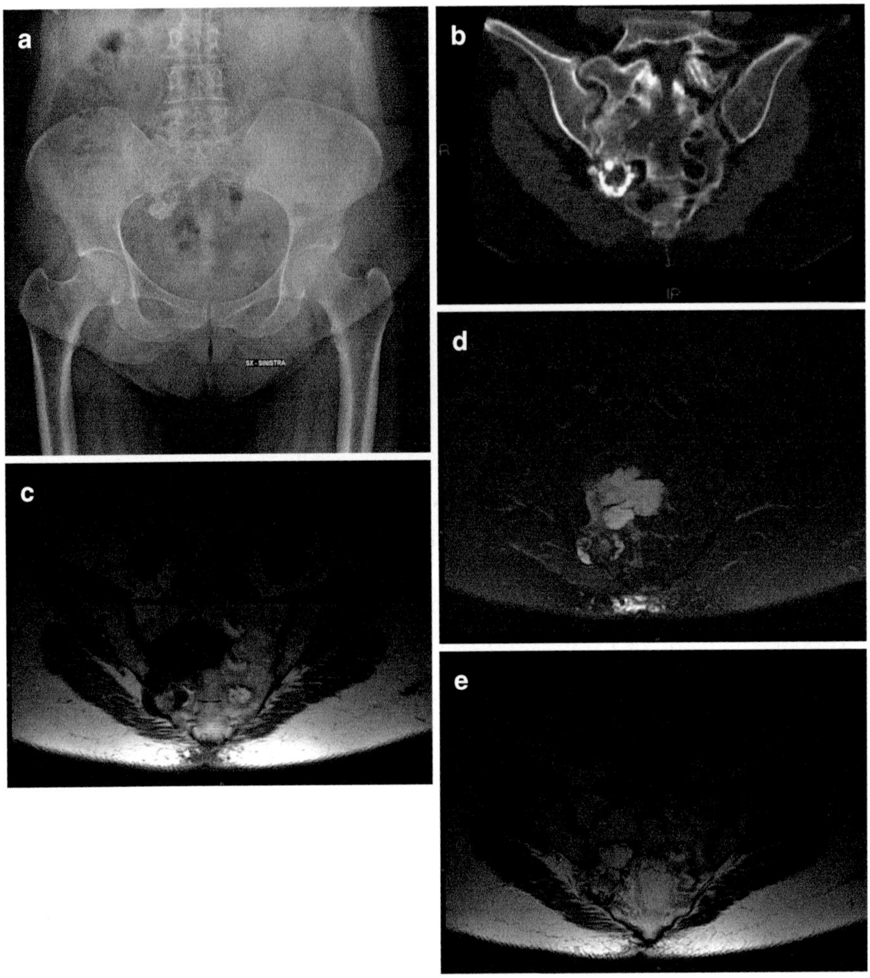

Fig. 5.3 Chondrosarcoma of the right sacral wing in a 60-year-old woman. (**a**) X-ray, (**b**) oblique coronal CT scan. "Ring and arc" calcifications in the osteolytic lesion (**c**) oblique coronal T1-w MRI image, (**d**) oblique coronal T2-w Fat Sat MRI, (**e**) oblique coronal T1-w MRI after Gd. The lesion is iso-hypointense on T1-w images and has a lobular high intensity on T2-w images

either nodular, septal, or diffuse [1]. Dedifferentiation can be detected on CT or MRI in a part of the tumor taking up contrast medium strongly. The biopsy must include this suspicious location.

5.2.6 Ewing Sarcoma

Ewing sarcoma usually affects patients between the age of 10 and 30 years with a male predominance. More than one half of vertebral Ewing sarcoma arise in the sacrum (70% in the sacral wing) [20], but just 0.5% of all Ewing sarcoma involve this region.

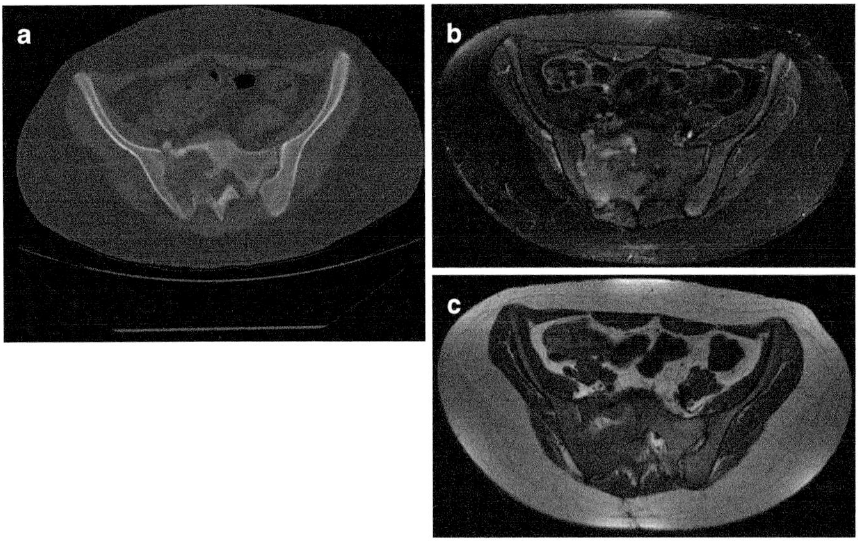

Fig. 5.4 Ewing sarcoma in a 20-year-old woman: (**a**) coronal CT, (**b**) axial T1-w MRI image, (**c**) axial T2-w Fat Sat MRI image. The lesion appears as a destructive osteolysis with a sclerotic reaction and invasion of right sacral foramina and sacro-iliac joint

These tumors typically fill the bone marrow cavity and destroy the cortex. The soft tissue mass associated to the tumor is often larger than the intra-osseous component.

Radiography and CT show a osteolytic destructive lesion, often associated with a sclerotic reaction [21]. CT better depicts the soft tissue involvement and the extension of the bony lesion.

MRI clearly depicts both intra- and extra-osseous components of the tumor, including paraspinal, extradural, and presacral involvement. MRI features are nonspecific; the lesion is iso-hypointense on T1-w and iso-hyperintense on T2-w images with variable contrast enhancement. Both CT and MRI are useful for staging of the tumor but are nonspecific because the osteolysis and the soft tissue mass can be limited and the lesion can be located either anterior or posterior to the spinal canal (Fig. 5.4).

5.2.7 Osteosarcoma

Sacral osteosarcoma is rare with only 1% of osteosarcoma involving the sacrum with a peak of incidence in the fourth decade [22].

Most sacral osteosarcomas are secondary, occurring after radiotherapy or Paget's disease. The tumor has an aggressive, permeative osteolytic pattern with cortical disruption and soft tissue involvement. Tumor extension across the sacro-iliac joint and into the spinal canal is common [23]. On CT, most sacral osteosarcomas contain "cloud-like" osteoid mineralization [24]. MRI shows no specific features.

5.2.8 Other Malignant Bone Tumors

Fibrosarcomas of the sacrum are rare; they arise from a preexisting lesion in about ¼ of cases, usually previously irradiated bone, Paget's disease, bone infarct or giant cell tumour, fibrous dysplasia, or ameloblastic fibroma.

Clear cell sarcoma (CCS) is a very rare tumor (1% of soft tissue sarcomas) that usually arises from tendons or aponeuroses of the extremities. It usually affects young patients (25–40 years), presenting with a slowly growing, painless mass [25, 26].

Few cases of clear cell sarcoma of the sacrum are reported. MR is the gold standard imaging method for the diagnosis of the CCS.

The lesion usually is hyperintense on T1-weighted images and hypointense on T2-weighted images due to the melanin content of sarcomatous cells [27].

Angiosarcoma, *hemangiopericytoma*, and *pleomorphic sarcoma* in the sacrum are exceptional.

5.3 Benign Bone Tumors

Ten percent of all benign tumors (pseudotumors) involve the sacrum. The most common are giant cell tumours (60% of cases) followed by aneurysmal cysts (4%) and osteoblastoma.

5.3.1 Giant Cell Tumour

Giant cell tumour (GCT) is the second most frequent primary tumor of the sacrum after chordoma; the peak of frequency is between 20 and 30 years with a female predominance (2/1).

Although usually benign, GCT are locally aggressive and 5–10% can undergo malignant transformation [28].

GCT usually involves the upper sacrum and has an eccentric location.

On CT, GCT appears as a well-demarcated polycyclic expansile lesion, inducing usually circumscribed osteolysis and rarely associated with a rim of sclerosis, classically with no calcifications.

The tumor is locally invasive, disrupting the cortex, and invading soft tissues. Crossing of the sacro-iliac joint is frequent (Figs. 5.5 and 5.6).

MRI shows anterior and posterior extension of the mass with a heterogeneous signal both on T1 and T2-w images. Generally, the tumor has a low-to-intermediate signal intensity on T1-w images. On T2-w images, GCT is iso-hypointense to the normal spinal cord in 63–96% of cases [29]. This seems to be related to the relative collagen content of fibrous components and hemosiderin within the tumor. Although this feature is not unique to GCT, it can help in the differential diagnosis because most other spinal neoplasms (metastases, myeloma, lymphoma, and chordoma) show high signal intensity on T2-w images.

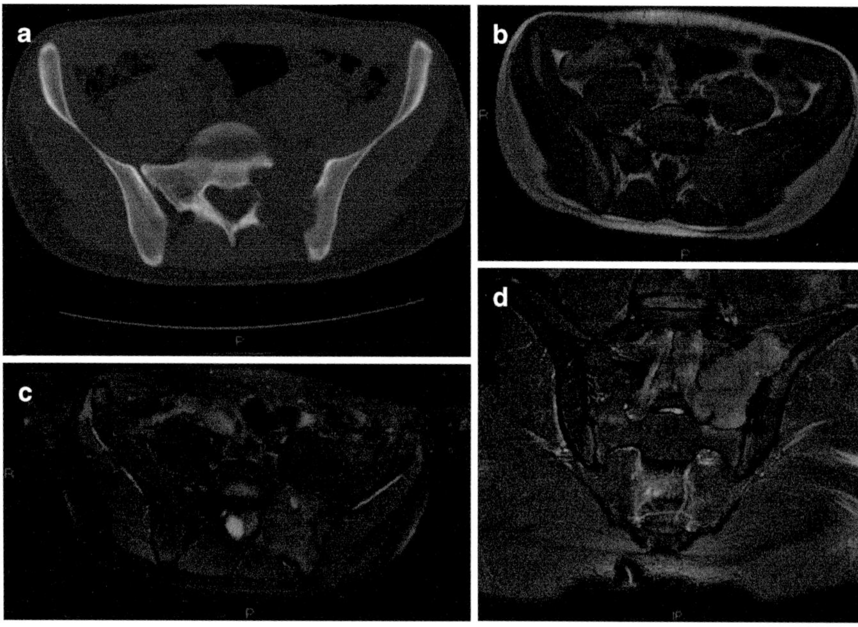

Fig. 5.5 Giant cell tumor (*GCT*) in a 30-year-old man: (**a**) axial CT scan shows an eccentric osteolytic lesion in the upper sacrum crossing the left sacro-iliac joint, (**b**) axial T1-w MRI, (**c**) axial T2-w FS image, (**d**) coronal T2-w FS image. On MRI, the lesion has a heterogeneous low to intermediate signal intensity on T1-w and on T2-w images

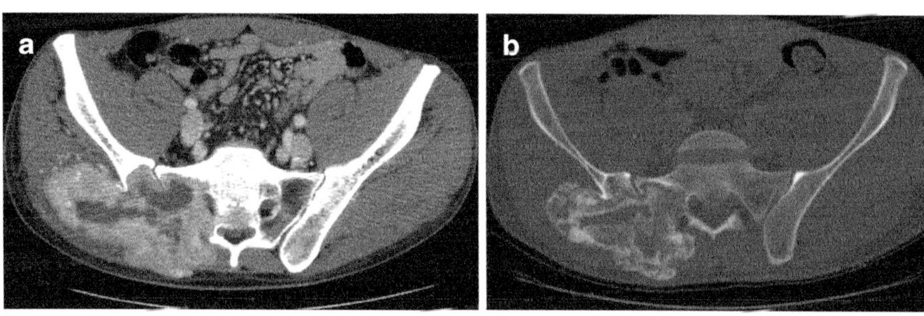

Fig. 5.6 Giant cell tumor in a 25-year-old man. Axial CT scan before (**a**) and after (**b**) treatment with Denosumab. The lesion is massively ossified. That indicates an efficient treatment, and must not be misdiagnosed as malignant transformation

Evidence of hemorrhage (with high signal intensity on T1-w and T2-w sequences or T2-w hypointense foci for hemosiderin deposits) and necrosis in the center of the tumor, with fluid–fluid levels, are characteristic [30]. Secondary aneurismal bone cyst with fluid–fluid levels can be detected.

5.3.2 Aneurysmal Cyst

Aneurysmal cyst is a space-occupying lesion comprising blood-filled cysts and is rare in the sacrum (<5%). About 80% of aneurysmal cysts are discovered before the age of 20, with a slight female predominance (56%) [10].

On CT, it appears as a purely lytic lesion without solid components, surrounded by a thin calcified border. MRI shows a well-limited multiloculated lesion with a high signal intensity on T2-w images, associated with fluid–fluid levels and surrounded by a hypointense rim (Fig. 5.7). The lesion presents a strong contrast enhancement because it is highly vascularized.

No solid tissue component, and a T2-w hypointense rim, regularly hyperdense on CT in an expansile sacral lesion with fluid–fluid level in a young patient are typical features that suggest the diagnosis of aneurismal cyst. However, biopsy remains necessary especially for the differential diagnosis with GCT or rarely with telangiectatic osteosarcoma that may both present fluid–fluid levels [6].

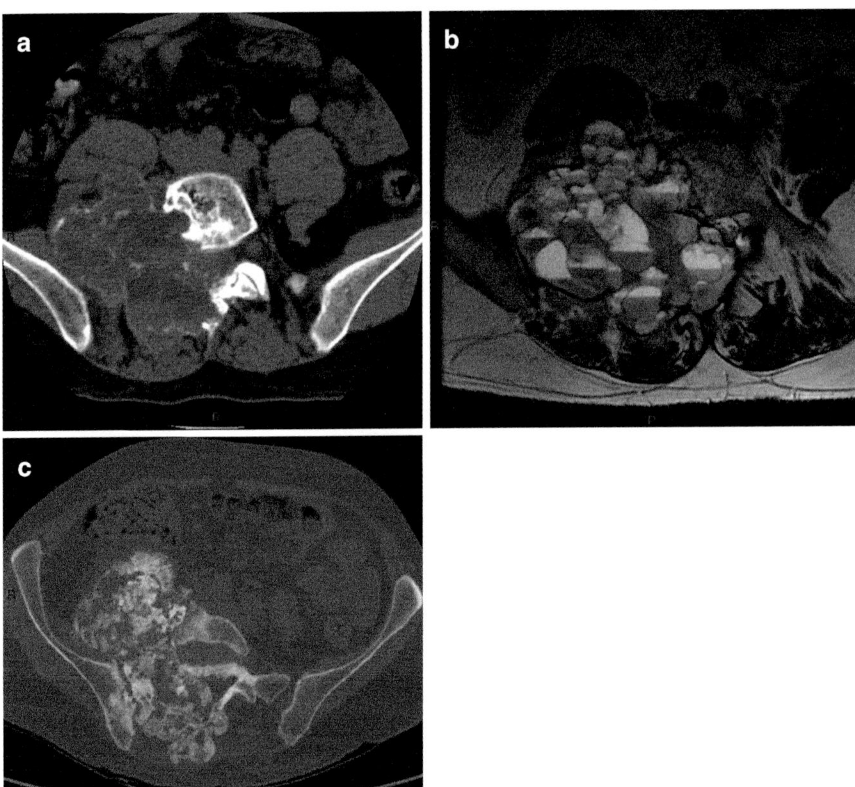

Fig. 5.7 Aneurismal bone cyst in an 18-year-old boy. (**a**) Axial CT scan (soft tissues window) depicts an osteolytic lesion in the right sacral wing surrounded by a thin sclerotic border. (**b**) Axial T2-w MRI: the lesion is multiloculated with fluid–fluid levels, (**c**) axial CT scan post-embolization (bone window) shows a sclerotic ossification within the cyst

5.3.3 Osteoid Osteoma

Osteoid osteoma rarely involves the sacrum (2%) but it represents 9% of all benign sacral tumors. Seventy-five percent of osteoma osteoid occur in patients before the age of 25 with a male predominance [21]. The classical symptom is dull pain, worse at night, and relieved by aspirin.

Sacro-iliac joint is a common location for osteoid osteoma.

CT shows the typical feature of osteoid osteoma: a round low-density area (less than 2 cm in diameter) with a central mineralized area in the center (the nidus); CT also demonstrates the surrounding osteoblastic response as a peripheral rim of sclerosis [31].

On MRI, often an extensive bone marrow edema and inflammatory changes can obscure the lesion that usually appears hypointense on T1-w images and iso-hypointense on T2-w images.

Bone scintigraphy is accurate in the detection of osteoid osteoma revealing the "double density sign": the central area of the nidus has an intense radionuclide uptake compared to the surrounding zone of bone sclerosis.

5.3.4 Osteoblastoma [32–34]

Osteoblastoma is a rare, benign, bone-forming tumor that may occur in any skeletal segment with a predilection for the spine. Sacrum is rarely affected. Ninety percent of osteoblastoma are discovered before the age of 30, with a peak of incidence at 20 and a male predominance. Even if osteoblastoma and osteoid osteoma share some histological features, osteoblastoma differs by its more expansile nature, a larger dimension (>2 cm) and therefore a more common clinical presentation with neurological symptoms.

On CT (and X-ray), osteoblastoma can present as a well-delimited osteolytic expansile lesion with multifocal calcifications and a sclerotic rim.

CT scanning is the best modality to identify the lesion and characterize the tumor matrix; it also assesses the degree of sclerosis and the extent of bone involvement.

MRI shows the inflammatory reaction around the lesion and in surrounding soft tissues as a hyperintense area on T2-w images (Fig. 5.8).

The differential diagnosis essentially include osteosarcoma. Aggressive forms of osteoblastoma have been described, probably corresponding to osteosarcoma rather than malignant transformation of osteoblastoma.

5.3.5 Other Benign Sacral Bone Tumors

Chondroma, *osteochondroma*, *chondromyxoid fibroma*, *lipoma*, *fibrous histiocytoma*, and *cavernous hemangioma* are extremely rare in the sacrum.

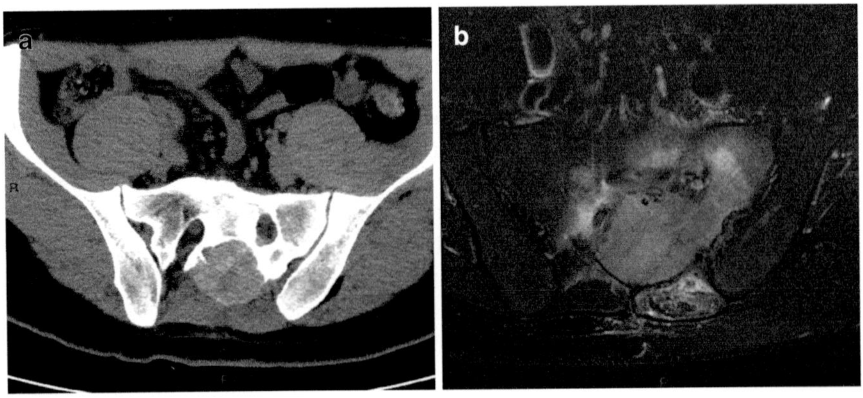

Fig. 5.8 Osteoblastoma in a 20-year-old boy. (**a**) Axial CT scan shows a well-delimited expansile osteolytic lesion with a mineralized matrix and a very thin sclerotic rim. (**b**) Axial T2-w FS MRI: the inflammatory reaction around the lesion and in surrounding soft tissues appears hyperintense on T2-w FS images

5.4 Non-osseous Tumors or Pseudotumors

5.4.1 Sacrococcygeal Germ Cell Tumors

Germ cell tumors arise from totipotent primitive neural cells during embryogenesis and are usually located on the midline of the body, 19% of them occurring in the sacrococcygeal region. Sacrococcygeal teratoma is the most common presacral germ cell tumor in children and the most common solid tumor in neonates with a female predominance (3-4:1) and is benign in 60% of cases [35]. In adults, sacrococcygeal teratoma is rare and generally benign. More than 90% of teratomas are diagnosed in children under 2 years of age and are usually predominantly external. Most of yolk sac tumors are diagnosed between the third and the seventh year of life.

Sacrococcygeal teratomas usually present a heterogeneous appearance on imaging, depending on their components. Benign teratomas contain only mature tissues and are predominantly cystic, with fluid attenuation at CT [36]. Areas of bone, fat, and calcifications may be seen.

At MRI, signal intensity depends on fat and calcifications content and fluid–fluid levels may be present. MRI also shows intra-sacral and extra-sacral extent of the tumor.

Malignant teratomas and yolk sac tumors have a more solid component, with areas of hemorrhage and necrosis. Yolk sac tumors have aggressive features with heterogeneous contrast enhancement and invasion of adjacent organs.

5.4.2 Meningeal Tumors

Meningoceles are herniations of the dural sac through a defect in the anterior surface of the sacrum and are most commonly congenital.

5.4.3 Perineural Cysts

Also known as Tarlov cysts, perineural cysts are congenital meningeal dilatations of the posterior nerve rootlets and most commonly originate at the level of the second or third sacral root. They are usually asymptomatic but large cysts can cause low back and/or leg pain as well as urinary, gastrointestinal, or neurological symptoms. At radiographs and CT, a bone remodelling or an asymmetrical enlargement of a sacral foramina may be seen. At CT, they appear as a cystic mass isoattenuating relative to cerebrospinal fluid [37], causing regular bone erosion and surrounded by a thin peripheral rim. No contrast enhancement, calcifications, or soft tissue masses are seen. MRI best demonstrates the relationship between the cyst and the nerve roots; their signal intensity is the same as cerebrospinal fluid on all sequences [38].

Lumbosacral meningiomas are exceptional in the sacrum.

5.5 Nerve Tumors

5.5.1 Neurofibromas and Schwannomas [35, 36, 39, 40]

These are intra-dural extra-medullary masses arising from sacral nerve roots sheath and present a slow growth and a benign appearance on imaging.

Neurofibromas are benign neural tumors that consist of fibroblasts, Schwann cells, and neural elements that expand and diffusely infiltrate a nerve. They can be multiple in patients with neurofibromatosis type 1 (NF1).

Typically, neurofibroma is a well-delimited rounded lesion causing enlargement of a sacral foramen. At CT, it has a lower attenuation compared to that of adjacent soft tissues.

At MRI, they are iso-hypointense on T1-w sequences, with a homogeneous contrast enhancement. On T2-w imaging, neurofibromas have a classical target appearance that consists of a central zone of low signal intensity related to their fibrous content and a hyperintense rim due to the myxoid component.

Intraosseous schwannoma (neurilemmoma) is rare, but 1–5% of spinal schwannomas originate in the sacrum that is the most frequent site after the mandible.

It is a benign slowly growing tumor that usually manifests as a large mass.

Radiographs and CT show a well-limited osteolysis, surrounded by a thin sclerotic rim. Calcifications can be present. When they are large, they tend to remodel or erode the bone and cause foramina enlargement. At MRI, large schwannomas present soft tissues involvement and are heterogeneous, with low signal intensity on T1-weighted images and high signal intensity on T2-weighted images, and can present small cystic areas, a thin pseudocapsule and fluid–fluid level (Fig. 5.9).

Neuroblastomas, *ganglioneuroblastomas*, and *ganglioneuromas* are pediatric neurogenic masses possibly located in the sacrum, especially at its anterior aspect.

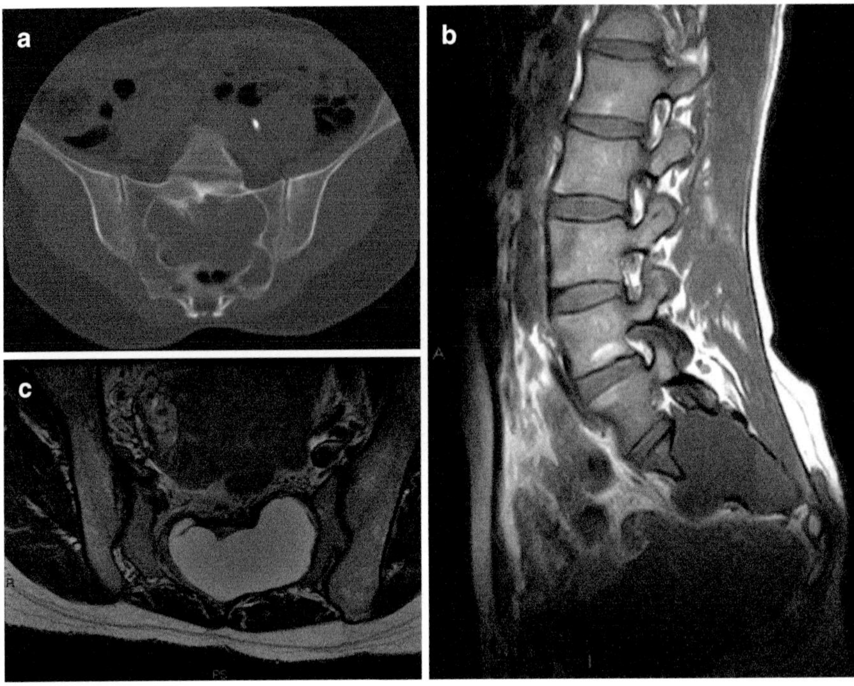

Fig. 5.9 Schwannoma in a 45-year-old woman. (**a**) Oblique coronal CT scan. Well-limited osteolytic lesion that enlarges sacral foramina. (**b**) Sagittal T1-w MRI, (**c**) axial T2-w MRI. The lesion has a low signal intensity on T1-weighted images and a high signal intensity on T2-weighted images

5.5.2 Ependymoma

Ependymomas is a malignant tumor that occasionally occurs outside the central nervous system and can involve sacrococcygeal region in childhood. It can be either primary, arising from ependymal cells of the conus medullaris or a metastasis from a primary tumor of the central nervous system [41, 42].

5.5.3 Metastases

Metastases from primary central nervous system tumors can involve the spinal canal of the sacrum (PNET, germ cell tumors, choroid plexus tumors, glioblastomas).

5.5.4 Carcinoid Tumors

Primary and secondary carcinoid tumors of the sacral dural sac have been reported [43, 44].

5.5.5 Sacral Involvement of Pelvic Lesions

Sacrum invasion from a pelvic mass must be differentiated from primary sacral bone tumors.

5.5.6 Imaging in Postoperative Follow-Up

The aim of postoperative follow-up is to assess any residual tumor and to detect local recurrence; furthermore, it can monitor adjuvant therapy efficacy. It is usually performed by contrast-enhanced MRI although artifacts may be produced by prosthetic material.

MRI examination has to distinguish inflammatory and fibrotic changes of the scar from a residual tumor in case of incomplete surgical resection; a local recurrence should be detected at the site of the initial tumor in case of complete resection.

If the tumor is inoperable, MRI can monitor changes of the lesion size and signal intensity after radiotherapy and chemotherapy.

In hematogenous malignancies and primary bone sarcoma, PET/CT has a role in evaluating tumor response after adjuvant therapy.

Conflict-of-Interest Statement No benefits have been or will be received from a commercial party related directly or indirectly to the subject matter of this chapter.

References

1. Thornton E, Krajewski KM, O'Regan KN, Giardino AA, Jagannathan JP, Ramaiya N. Imaging features of primary and secondary malignant tumours of the sacrum. Br J Radiol. 2012; 85:279–86.
2. Rodallec MH, Feydy A, LaRousserie F, Anract P, Campagna R, Babinet A, et al. Diagnostic imaging of solitary tumors of the spine: what to do and say. Radiographics. 2008; 28:1019–41.
3. Lanzieri CF, Sacher M, Solodnik P, Hermann G, Cohen B, Rabinowitz JG. Unusual patterns of solitary sacral plasmocytoma. AJNR Am J Neuroradiol. 1978;8:566–7.
4. Nayil K, Makhdoomi R, Ramzan A, Malik R, Alam S, Wani A, Chhiber S. Primary sacral lymphoma: a case report and review of the literature. Turk Neurosurg. 2011;21(4):659–62.
5. Mulligan ME, McRae GA, Murphey MD. Imaging features of primary lymphoma of bone. AJR Am J Roentgenol. 1999;173:1691–7.
6. Gerber S, Ollivier L, Leclère J, Vanel D, Missenard G, Brisse H, De Pinieux G, Neuenschwander S. Imaging of sacral tumours. Skelet Radiol. 2008;37:277–89.
7. Llauger J, Palmer J, Amores S, Bagué S, Camins A. Primary tumors of the sacrum: diagnostic imaging. AJR Am J Roentgenol. 2000;174:417–24.
8. Farsad K, Kattapuram SV, Sacknoff R, Ono J, Nielsen GP. Best cases from the AFIP sacral chordoma. Radiographics. 2009;29:1525–30.
9. Yamaguchi T, Yamato M, Saotome K. First histologically confirmed case of a classic chordoma arising in a precursor benign notochordal lesionn: differential diagnosis of benign and malignanat notochordal lesions. Skelet Radiol. 2002;31:413–8.

10. Murphey MD, Andrews CL, Flemming DJ, Temple HT, Smith WS, Smirniotopoulos JG. Primary tumors of the spine: radiologic-pathologic correlation. Radiographics. 1996;16: 1131–58.
11. Sung MS, Lee GK, Kang HS, Kwon ST, Park JG, Suh JS, et al. Sacrococcygeal chordoma: MR imaging in 30 patients. Skelet Radiol. 2005;34:87–94.
12. Si MJ, Wang CS, Ding XY, Yuan F, Du LJ, Lu Y, Zhang WB. Differentiation of primary chordoma, giant cell tumor and schwannoma of the sacrum by CT and MRI. Eur J Radiol. 2013;82:2309–15.
13. Yeom KW, Lober RM, Mobley BC, et al. Diffusion-weighted MRI: distinction of skull base chordoma from chondrosarcoma. Am J Neuroradiol. 2013;34:1056–61.
14. Picci P, Manfrini M, Fabbri N, Gambarotti M, Vanel D. Atlas of musculoskeletal tumors and tumor-like lesions. The Rizzoli case archive. New York: Springer.
15. Yamaguchi T, Iwata J, Sugihara S, EF Jr MC, Karita M, et al. Distinguish benign notochordal cell tumors from vertebral chordoma. Skelet Radiol. 2008;37:291–9.
16. Kyriakos M. Benign notochordal lesions of the axial skeleton: a review and current appraisal. Skelet Radiol. 2011;40:1141–52.
17. Kreshak J, et al. Difficulty distinguishing benign notochordal cell tumor from chordoma further suggests a link between them. Cancer Imaging. 2014;14:4.
18. Stacchiotti S, Sommer J, Chordoma Global Consensus Group. Building a global consensus approach to chordoma: a position paper from the medical and patient community. Lancet Oncol. 2015;16(2):e71–83.
19. Murphey MD, Walker EA, Wilson AJ, Kransdorf MJ, Temple HT, Gannon FH. From the archives of the AFIP: imaging of primary chondrosarcoma: radiologic-pathologic correlation. Radiographics. 2003;23:1245–78.
20. Ilaslan H, Sundaram M, Unni KK, et al. Primary Ewing sarcoma of the vertebral column. Skelet Radiol. 2004;230:697–702.
21. Disler DG, Miklic D. Imaging findings in tumors of the sacrum. AJR Am J Roentgenol. 1999;173:1699–706.
22. Unni KK, Inwards CY. Dahlin's bone tumors. 6th ed. Philadelphia: Lippincott Williams & Wilkins; 2010.
23. Ilaslan H, Sundaram M, Unni KK, et al. Primary vertebral osteosarcoma: imaging findings. Radiology. 2004;230:697–702.
24. Ko O, Ritchie DA. Pictorial essay: tumours and pseudotumours of sacrum. Can Assoc Radiol J. 2014;65:113–20.
25. Kawai A, Hosono A, Nakayama R, et al. Clear cell sarcoma of tendons and aponeuroses: a study of 75 patients. Cancer. 2007;109(1):109–16.
26. Hantschke M, Mentzel T, Rutten A, et al. Cutaneous clear cell sarcoma: a clinicopathologic, immunohistochemical, and molecular analysis of 12 cases emphasizing its distinction from dermal melanoma. Am J Surg Pathol. 2010;34(2):216–22.
27. Zhang W, Shen Y, Wan R, Zhu Y. Primary clear cell sarcoma of the sacrum: a case report. Skelet Radiol. 2011;40:633–9.
28. Ha AS, Chew FS. Imaging of sacral masses: self-assessment module. AJR Am J Roentgenol. 2010;195:S32–6.
29. Resnick D. Diagnosis of bone and joint disorders. 3rd ed. Philadelphia: Saunders; 1995. p. 3785–806.
30. Kwon JW, Chung HW, Cho EY, Hong SH, Choi SH, Yoon YC, Yi SK. MRI findings of giant cell tumors of the spine. AJR Am J Roentgenol. 2007;189:246–50.
31. Abdel Razek AAK, Castillo M. Imaging appearance of primary bony tumors and pseudotumors of the spine. J Neuroradiol. 2010;37:37–50.
32. Gamba JL, Martinez S, Apple J, Harrelson JM, Nunley JA. Computed tomography of axial skeletal osteoid osteomas. AJR Am J Roentgenol. 1984;142:769–72.
33. Kroon H, Schurmans J. Osteoblastoma: clinical and radiologic findings in 98 new cases. Radiology. 1990;175:783–90.

34. Ruggieri P, Huch K, Mavrogenis AF, Merlino B, Angelini A. Osteoblastoma of the sacrum: report of 18 cases and analysis of the literature. Spine (Phila Pa 1976). 2014;39(2):E97–103.
35. Kocaoglu M, Frush DP. Pediatric presacral masses. Radiographics. 2006;26:833–57.
36. Hain KS, Pickhardt PJ, Lubner MG, Menias CO, Bhalla S. Presacral masses: multimodality imaging of a multidisciplinary space. Radiographics. 2013;33:1145–67.
37. Paulsen RD, Call GA, Murtagh FR. Prevalence and percutaneous drainage of cysts of the sacral nerve root sheath (Tarlov cysts). AJNR Am J Neuroradiol. 1994; 15(2): 293–7; discussion 298–9.
38. Davis SW, Levy LM, LeBihan DJ, et al. Sacral meningeal cysts: evaluation with MR imaging. Radiology. 1993;187:445–8.
39. Leeson MC, Hite M. Ganglioneuroma of the sacrum. Clin Orthop Relat Res. 1989;246: 102–5.
40. Ortolan EG, Sola CA, Gruenberg MF, Carballo Vazquez FC. Giant sacral schwannoma. A case report. Spine (Phila Pa 1976). 1996;21(4):522–6.
41. Moelleken SMC, Seeger LL, Eckardt JJ, Batzdork U. Myxopapillary ependymoma with extensive sacral destruction: CT and MR findings. J Comput Assist Tomogr. 1992;16:164–6.
42. Aktug T, Hakguder G, Sarioglu S, Akgur FM, Olguner M, Pabuccuoglu U. Sacrococcygeal extraspinal ependymomas: the role of coccygectomy. J Pediatr Surg. 2000;35:515–8.
43. Schnee CL, Hurst RW, Curtis MT, Friedman ED. Carcinoid tumor of the sacrum: case report. Neurosurgery. 1994;35:1163–7.
44. Dujardin F, Beaussart P, de Mure A, Rosset P, Waynberger E, Mulleman D, de Pinieux G. Primary neuroendocrine tumor of the sacrum: case report and review of the literature. Skelet Radiol. 2009;38:819–23.

6 Biopsy and Staging of Sacral Tumors

John E. Mullinax and Ricardo J. Gonzalez

6.1 Introduction

Tumors arising within the sacrum are rare and often present a diagnostic challenge. The etiology of the tumor is the primary consideration at the time of presentation so as to direct therapy appropriately. Initial imaging such as plain radiographs or computed tomography (CT) often suggests a primary sacral neoplasm (Fig. 6.1).

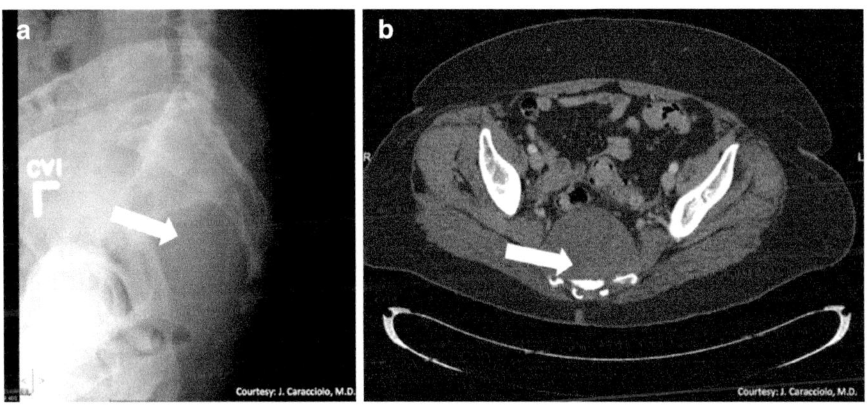

Fig. 6.1 Initial imaging of sacral mass. (**a**) Sagittal radiograph demonstrating hypodense lesion immediately anterior to sacrum. (**b**) Computed tomography scan confirms a primary sacral mass with bony destruction

J.E. Mullinax, M.D. (✉)
Department of Surgical Oncology, H. Lee Moffitt Cancer Center, 12902 Magnolia Drive, Tampa, FL 33602, USA
e-mail: john.mullinax@moffitt.org

R.J. Gonzalez, M.D.
Sarcoma Department, H. Lee Moffitt Cancer Center, FOB-1, 12902 Magnolia Drive, Tampa, FL 33612, USA

P. Ruggieri et al. (eds.), *Tumors of the Sacrum*,
DOI 10.1007/978-3-319-51202-0_6

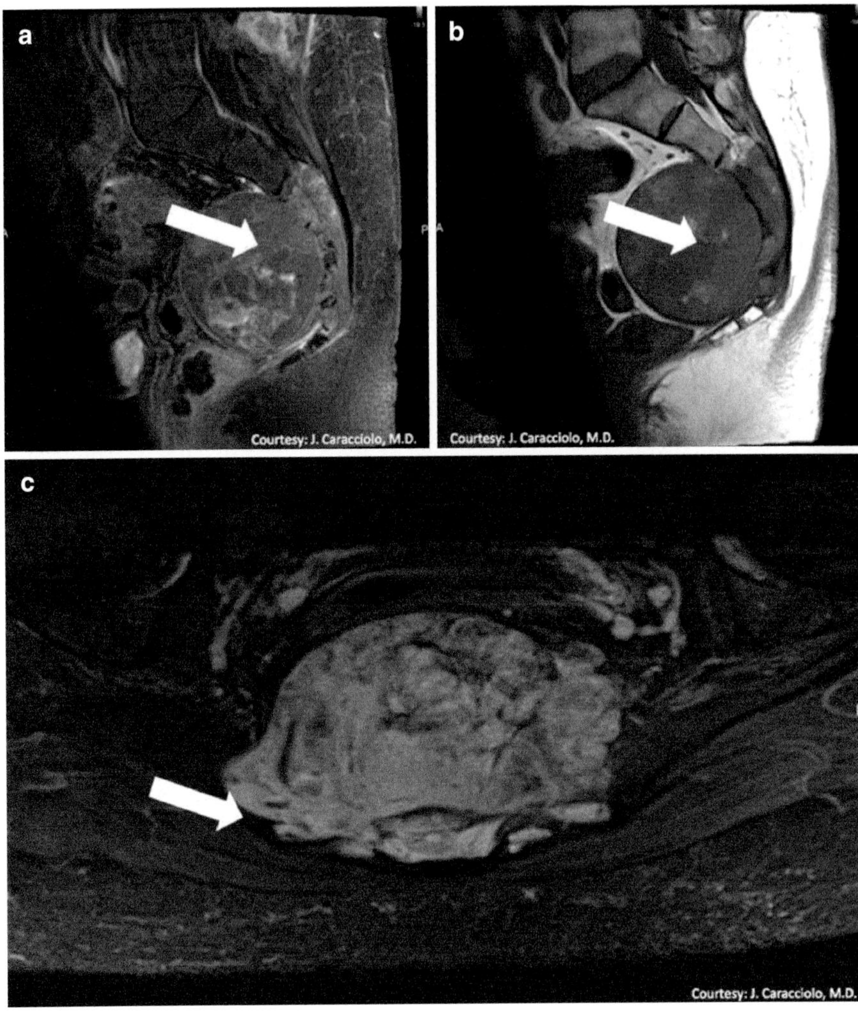

Fig. 6.2 Magnetic resonance imaging of sacral mass. Subsequent imaging modality revealed an encapsulated, heterogeneous mass emanating from the sacrum. (**a**) T1 phase and (**b**) T2 phase confirm heterogeneous density. (**c**) Axial view demonstrates clear plane between mass and gluteus maximus mm

Magnetic resonance imaging (MRI) can be used to stratify the lesion as benign or malignant (Fig. 6.2). In the latter category, a history of previous malignancy will help to delineate between a primary or metastatic lesion. Since metastatic lesions are far more common in the sacrum than primary malignancies, a thorough history is a critical component of the diagnostic decision-making. Following this thorough history, a biopsy is indicated to confirm diagnostic suspicion from the initial imaging. Once a diagnosis is confirmed on biopsy, staging studies are required to complete the management plan and define optimal modes of therapy. This chapter will review the differential diagnosis, the optimal biopsy method, and the staging studies required for optimal management of sacral tumors.

6.2 Method of Biopsy

The need for biopsy is clear and absolute due to the multiple underlying histologies of neoplasm, both benign and malignant, within the sacrum. The method of biopsy, however, is less clear and the source of much controversy. Historical descriptions of biopsy technique have included open (incisional) biopsy, excisional biopsy, core needle biopsy, and fine needle aspiration with the last two performed by either image guidance or direct palpation. Recent experience has clarified the role of each with some significant pitfalls now recognized.

Incisional biopsy should only rarely be undertaken for the diagnosis of a sacral tumor. With modern image guidance and large bore core biopsy needles, there is no need for tumor disruption to obtain diagnosis. Incisional biopsy is fraught with complications, most severely the spread of tumor across planes of tissue not otherwise invaded by the malignant process. Local bleeding of the tumor and biopsy site allows for the diffuse spread of tumor cells and negatively impacts the outcome. Many times, a complete oncologic resection is not possible simply due to biopsy technique. This unfortunate outcome can be avoided with proper planning.

Small (<3 cm) tumors which have clear benign features on imaging can be biopsied by complete excision [1]. Using this method, adherence to oncologic principles is required in the event a high-grade neoplasm is identified on final pathologic analysis. Great care should be taken to not disrupt uninvolved tissue planes and ensure adequate hemostasis during dissection. The primary benefit of this technique is an adequate tissue sample for analysis by the pathologist. Architecture of the tumor is preserved maximally which allows for description of tumor heterogeneity and identification of poorly differentiated areas within the larger specimen.

Percutaneous biopsy can be performed by either fine needle aspiration (FNA) or core needle biopsy (Fig. 6.3). Prior to selection of technique, imaging should be reviewed directly between the treating physician and diagnostic radiologist focusing on two components. First, the *a priori* probability of metastatic disease should be determined. For those patients with a high probability of metastatic tumor, FNA is appropriate to confirm the suspicion. Second, the heterogeneity of the tumor should be discussed to ensure proper sampling of the biopsy. There should be a focus on any high-grade components, as these foci within the primary lesion can contain characteristic genetic alterations used to guide therapy.

Use of FNA for the diagnosis of soft tissue sarcoma is appropriate when performed in the setting of a multidisciplinary team. As mentioned above, the sampling of the tumor should be planned from the initial imaging and the biopsy should be performed under image guidance for tumors with significant heterogeneity. The pathologist should immediately assess adequacy of the specimen so that a core biopsy can be performed, if needed. Using this method, FNA is adequate for diagnosis in 77% of cases and 78% of the time the diagnosis correlates with malignant radiographic findings. For those lesions with benign features on imaging, FNA is not as helpful as the final diagnosis is in agreement in only 44% of cases. In the case of indeterminate image characteristics, FNA can differentiate benign from malignant lesions in 63% of cases [2]. FNA utility is increasing as subtypes are

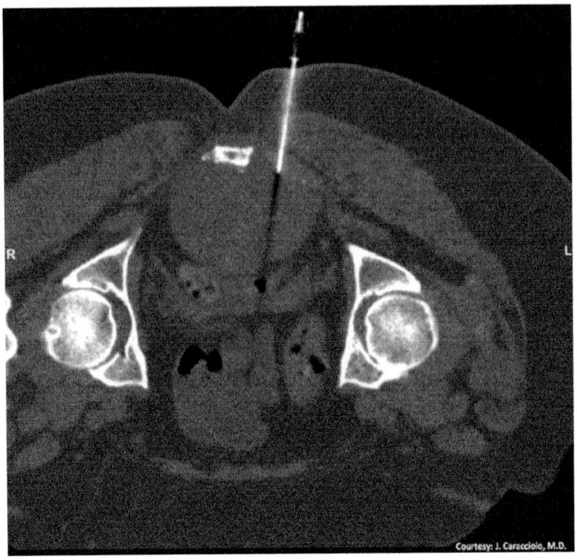

Fig. 6.3 Computed tomography-guided biopsy. A posterior approach was used to biopsy the lesion and confirm the histology as chordoma

increasingly diagnosed by cytogenetic techniques since a relatively small number of cells is needed for analysis.

If resection of the tumor is considered in the treatment algorithm, then the surgeon should direct the biopsy plan after discussion with the diagnostic radiologist. Many times the biopsy tract can be placed within the planned incision, making excision at the time of tumor extirpation possible. At times, there are limitations of biopsy approach due to anatomic constraints and in those cases, placement of the biopsy tract outside the planned surgical incision cannot be avoided. It is not mandatory to excise a core biopsy tract if it will yield an unacceptable increase in morbidity but the biopsy cavity from an incisional biopsy should always be excised. Local recurrence (9%) following core biopsy without excision of the biopsy tract is rare compared to distant recurrence risk (25%) in the same patients [3].

6.3 Differential Diagnosis

6.3.1 Primary Benign Sacral Tumors

The primary consideration on biopsy of sacral tumors is whether a malignant process is responsible for the lesion identified on imaging. Not all lesions identified are malignant and several benign primary lesions occur within the sacrum. The most common benign tumor of the sacrum is a giant cell tumor (GCT), which is responsible for approximately 60% of benign lesions within the sacrum and 13% of all sacral tumors [4]. While only 7% of GCT involve the spine, the sacrum is the most common site of involvement within the spine [5]. The histologic hallmark of these lesions is the presence of large, osteoclast-like multinucleated cells (giant cells) scattered within spindle cell stroma. There are often hemorrhagic and fibrotic areas found within the tumor [6, 7]. Genetic hallmarks of GCT include telomere fusion, termed telomeric association (tas), which is found in 50% of GCT. Rearrangements of chromosome 17 (described below) have also been reported which hints at the presence of aneurysmal bone cysts within the larger lesion [7].

The second most common benign tumor found in the sacrum is the aneurysmal bone cyst (ABC). The spine is the location of approximately 20% of all ABCs and about 20% of spinal ABCs are located within the sacrum, which means the sacrum is the primary site for 3–4% of all ABCs [4–6, 8]. The histologic findings associated with ABC include large blood filled cystic spaces which are formed by septae of fibroblasts. There is little evidence of atypia within the cellular component of these lesions though mitoses can be common. The osteoclast-like giant cells seen in GCT are seen in ABCs as well but the large cystic areas distinguish these lesions from the former [7]. Cytogenetic rearrangements of the ubiquitin-specific peptidase 6 (USP6) gene on chromosome 17 are seen in 70% of primary ABC [7].

The spine is the primary location of osteoblastoma in 40% of cases and the sacrum is the site of 17% of these spinal lesions, thus the sacrum accounts for only 1% of all osteoblastomas [4, 5]. There are three classically described patterns of osteoblastoma on imaging and the most aggressive pattern of bone destruction with infiltration of adjacent structures carries a local recurrence rate approaching 50% [4]. This aggressive form is termed "epithelioid osteoblastoma" but there is no evidence that it has a worse prognosis compared to other subtypes [7]. Histologic hallmarks include disorganized spicules of woven bone lined with osteoblasts which do not demonstrate any degree of atypia [7]. There have been no genetic alterations described for osteoblastoma.

The final category of benign sacral tumors includes schwannomas and neurofibromas which arise from the neural elements of the sacrum. Schwannomas can be quite large at diagnosis with a mean diameter of 10.5 cm [4, 8]. Neurofibromas are often smaller tumors and can be distinguished by the lack of a capsule as opposed to the schwannomas which often are encapsulated. The malignant form of neurofibroma, called malignant peripheral nerve sheath tumor, can occur in patients with neurofibromatosis type 1. The hallmark schwannomas is the biphasic cellular components, termed Antoni A and B tissue. The former is characterized by spindle cells arranged in a compact group while the latter is more loosely arranged spindle cell foci within the tumor. This characteristic finding is readily identified and, when present with a fibrous capsule, is diagnostic for a schwannoma. The biphasic cellular component of the schwannoma contrasts the more loosely arranged spindle cell infiltrate of nerves found with neurofibroma. Genetic associations between these two entities include mutations in the NF2 gene which lead to schwannoma tumorigenesis and mutations in the NF1 gene which are found commonly within neurofibromas [7].

6.3.2 Primary Malignant Sacral Tumors

Chordoma is the most common tumor found in the sacrum and accounts for 2–4% of malignant bone tumors [5, 9]. These tumors are found along the axial skeleton and equally distributed between the skull base, spine, and sacrococcygeal region [5, 10]. This distribution is indicative of the pathogenesis of this tumor which is derived from the primitive fetal notochord [9–13]. Studies have shown that there are rests of primitive notochord cells within the adult vertebrae which further corroborates the cell of origin for these tumors. Chordomas are slow growing and generally present late with involvement of pelvic viscera and sacral nerve roots. Histologic hallmarks of these tumors include intracellular vacuoles which are termed physaliferous and are pathognomonic for chordoma [7, 9–13].

The differentiation of chordomas from other primary malignant sacral lesions, specifically chondrosarcomas has been historically very challenging. Chordomas are immunoreactive to S-100, a primitive neural crest marker, cytokeratin 8, 18, and 19 while chondroid neoplasms also have immunoreactivity to S-100. Chondroid chondrosarcomas have been particularly difficult to distinguish from chordoma due to the patchy appearance of cytokeratin immunostains, which are not present in the chondroid component of the tumor [12]. This diagnostic dilemma was ameliorated by Vujovic et al, with the report of brachyury as a pathognomonic biomarker for the diagnosis of chordoma [12]. Brachyury is synonymous with the T gene, located on chromosome 6 and is a transcription factor expressed by the notochord of the human embryo [12, 14]. The function of the gene is to direct mesoderm differentiation in embryologic development and as such should not be expressed in adult tissue.

The unique expression of brachyury in chordomas yields significant utility to immunostains and is well documented. There is no expression in other lesions commonly found within the sacrum. In a recent series of 305 cases, there was no expression in clear cell renal cell carcinoma (most common metastatic lesion to sacrum) or germ cell tumors [13]. Other reports have documented the lack of expression in chondrosarcoma, liposarcoma, and mucinous carcinoma [11, 15]. The combination of brachyury and AE1/AE3 immunostains yields 98% sensitivity and 100% specificity for chordoma [15]. The utility of brachyury expression is limited to diagnosis and not prognosis. A recent report of 78 chordoma patients failed to show a correlation between brachyury expression by immunohistochemistry and clinical outcome [16].

Most exciting is the therapeutic potential of this biomarker. Through analysis of 40 chordoma patients with 358 ancestry-matched controls, it was shown that the mutation in the T gene, resulting in overexpression of brachyury, is a single nucleotide polymorphism in exon 4. This unique mutation and expression is being exploited as a target for immunotherapy. *In silico* analysis demonstrated HLA binding regions for brachyury peptides. Follow up *in vitro* experiments with brachyury-peptide pulsed dendritic cells demonstrated CD8+ lymphocyte proliferation and cytotoxic activity as measured by interferon-γ release assay [17]. Thus, a marker with significant diagnostic utility may also be used as an immunotherapy target.

The second most common primary malignant tumor of the sacrum is multiple myeloma (plasma cell myeloma) or the solitary, indolent form; plasmacytoma [4].

These are found due to the rich marrow deposit located within the sacrum. Histologic findings of these tumors demonstrate a plasmacytic proliferation with immunoreactivity to CD138. The features of solitary plasmacytoma and plasma cell myeloma are difficult to distinguish microscopically and the diagnosis is made by laboratory studies where M-protein is found in the blood or urine for plasma cell myeloma. Cytogenetics can be helpful in the diagnosis since there are translocations involving the immunoglobulin heavy chain (IGH) locus found in patients with plasma cell myeloma of the bone [7].

Another primary malignancy associated with the hematopoietic component of the sacrum is primary bone lymphoma. This is the third most common lesion in the sacrum and the imaging characteristics are so unique that thorough imaging is generally diagnostic. On microscopic analysis, the lesions are destructive centrally with normal cortical bone. There is significant pleomorphism among the cells and nuclear atypia is prominent. These lymphomas are B-cell derived and therefore immunostains for CD20 are positive [7].

Rare primary malignant lesions of the sacrum include Ewing's sarcoma and osteosarcoma. Ewing's sarcoma accounts for approximately 8% of primary malignant lesions in the sacrum and there are very specific therapeutic recommendations for this lesion. These tumors have characteristic small, round, blue cells and demonstrate unique cytogenetics with a translocation between the EWSR1 gene and a transcription factor from the ETS family, most commonly FLI1 [7]. There are presently clinical trials targeting these translocations and preoperative therapy is recommended, making an accurate diagnosis on biopsy of paramount importance. Osteosarcoma represents 4% of the primary malignant lesions in the sacrum, and there is no immunophenotype or unique histologic finding associated with this diagnosis. There are multiple subtypes of osteosarcoma but there is currently no relationship between histologic subtype and treatment [7].

6.3.3 Metastatic Disease

Despite the multiple subtypes of primary malignant and benign sacral tumors, the most common lesions found within the sacrum are metastatic deposits from other primary lesions. Common metastatic lesions to the sacrum include clear cell renal cell carcinoma, prostate cancer, and adenocarcinomas from the gastrointestinal tract. Biopsy for these lesions is generally performed as a confirmatory test following conclusions drawn from the history in clinic rather than from imaging.

6.4 Staging

The most important determinant of staging studies for patients with sacral tumors is the history of other primary malignancies. For those patients, all evaluation should be undertaken with the assumption that the sacral tumor is a metastatic lesion until definitive biopsy proves otherwise. Staging studies in these cases should focus on the identification of other metastatic deposits, and for this reason positron emission tomography (PET) scans are recommended.

Other methods of axial imaging should be performed for primary sacral malignancies. In these cases, computed tomography (CT) of the thorax, abdomen, and pelvis are required for adequate assessment of distant metastatic disease. Magnetic resonance imaging (MRI) of the pelvis is helpful in staging because assessment of local invasion is more readily appreciated with this modality. MRI also offers the ability to enhance surgical planning for those patients without distant disease identified on CT. Bone marrow biopsy, skeletal survey, and serum protein electrophoresis are mandatory tests to stage patients with multiple myeloma or plasmacytoma.

6.5 Summary

Primary sacral malignancies are rare and management requires a broad knowledge of the histologic possibilities arising within the sacrum. The most common benign diagnosis is giant cell tumor and the most common primary malignancy is a chordoma. Decisions regarding the technique of biopsy should be discussed with the primary treating surgeon in conjunction with the interpreting pathologist. This is especially true for heterogeneous masses and when there is ambiguity regarding a diagnosis of chordoma or chondroscarcoma. Due to the paucity of cases, the collaborative effort of a multidisciplinary team is recommended to achieve optimal outcomes.

Conflict-of-Interest Statement No benefits have been or will be received from a commercial party related directly or indirectly to the subject matter of this chapter.

References

1. Clarke M, Mendel E, Vrionis F. Primary spine tumors: diagnosis and treatment. Cancer Control. 2014;21(2):114–23.
2. Phadke D, Lucas DR, Madan S. Fine-needle aspiration biopsy of vertebral and intervertebral disc lesions. Arch Pathol Lab Med. 2001;125:1463–8.
3. Binitie O, Tejiram S, Conway S, Cheong D, Temple HT, Letson GD. Adult soft tissue sarcoma local recurrence after adjuvant treatment without resection of core needle biopsy tract. Clin Orthop Relat Res. 2013;471(3):891–8.
4. Mavrogenis A, Patapis P, Kostopanagiotou G, Papagelopoulos P. Tumors of the sacrum. Orthopedics. 2009;32(5):342.
5. Diel J, Ortiz O, Losada R, Price D, Hayt M, Katz D. The sacrum: pathologic spectrum, multimodality imaging, and subspecialty approach. Radiographics. 2001;21:83–104.
6. Llauger J, Palmer J, Amores S, Bague S, Camins A. Primary tumors of the sacrum: diagnostic imaging. Am J Roentgenol. 2000;174:417–24.
7. Fletcher CDM, Bridge J, Hogendoorn PC, Mertens F. WHO classification of tumours of soft tissue and bone. 4th ed. Lyon, France: International Agency for Research on Cancer; 2013.
8. Deutsch H, Mummaneni P, Haid R, Rodts G, Ondra S. Benign sacral tumors. Neurosurg Focus. 2003;15(2):E14.

9. Crapanzano JP, Ali S, Ginsberg MS, Zakowski M. Chordoma: a cytologic study with histologic and radiologic correlation. Cancer Cytopathol. 2001;93:40–51.
10. Walcott BP, Nahed BV, Mohyeldin A, Coumans J-V, Kahle KT, Ferreira MJ. Chordoma: current concepts, management, and future directions. Lancet Oncol. 2012;13(2):e69–76.
11. Barresi V, Ieni A, Branca G, Tuccari G. Brachyury: a diagnostic marker for the differential diagnosis of chordoma and hemangioblastoma versus neoplastic histological mimickers. Dis Markers. 2014;2014:514753.
12. Vujovic S, Henderson SR, Presneau N, et al. Brachyury, a crucial regulator of notochordal development, is a novel biomarker for chordomas. J Pathol. 2006;209:157–65.
13. Sangoi AR, Karamchandani J, Lane B, et al. Specificity of brachyury in the distinction of chordoma from clear cell renal cell carcinoma and germ cell tumors: a study of 305 cases. Mod Pathol. 2011;24(3):425–9.
14. Pillay N, Plagnol V, Tarpey PS, et al. A common single-nucleotide variant in T is strongly associated with chordoma. *Nat Genet*. 2012;44(11):1185–7.
15. Oakley GJ, Fuhrer K, Seethala RR. Brachyury, SOX-9, and podoplanin, new markers in the skull base chordoma vs chondrosarcoma differential: a tissue microarray-based comparative analysis. Mod Pathol. 2008;21(12):1461–9.
16. Zhang L, Guo S, Schwab J, et al. Tissue microarray immunohistochemical detection of brachyury is not a prognostic indicator in chordoma. PLoS One. 2013;8(9):e75851.
17. Palena C, Polev DE, Tsang KY, et al. The human T-box mesodermal transcription factor Brachyury is a candidate target for T-cell-mediated cancer immunotherapy. Clin Cancer Res. 2007;13(8):2471–8.

Histopathology of Sacral Tumors and Pseudotumors

7

Marilyn M. Bui, Yi Ding, Evita Henderson Jackson, and Angelo Paolo Dei Tos

The sacrum is composed of bone, cartilage, soft mesenchymal tissue, bone marrow, and notochordal remnants, which give rise to tumors or pseudotumors. Tumors of the sacrum include primary and metastatic/systemic origin. The primary tumors consist of malignant and benign entities. Systemic diseases include metastases and hematopoietic malignancies such as lymphoma, multiple myeloma, or plasmacytoma. The incidence of sacral tumors and pseudotumors at the Rizzoli institute is described in the epidemiology chapter of this book. Personal communication with Dr. Xiaohui Niu, Professor and Chair of the Department of Orthopedic Oncology Surgery of the Jishuitan (JST) Hospital in Beijing, China, the largest and a premier Orthopedic Oncology hospital in China, also confirms the most frequently occurring sacral tumors (Table 7.1). This data is retrieved from the JST epidemiology website of musculoskeletal tumors (www.sarcoma-jst.net) based on a collection of 18, 419 cases [1]. In this chapter, the histopathology as well as pertinent ancillary diagnostic, prognostic, and predictive information of these common tumors and pseudotumors will be discussed.

M.M. Bui, M.D., Ph.D. (✉) • E.H. Jackson, M.D.
Department of Anatomic Pathology, Moffitt Cancer Center, Tampa, FL, USA

Department of Sarcoma, Moffitt Cancer Center, Tampa, FL, USA
e-mail: Marilyn.Bui@moffitt.org

Y. Ding, M.D.
Department of Pathology, Jishuitan Hospital, Beijing, China

A.P.D. Tos, M.D.
Department of Medicine, University of Padua School of Medicine, Padua, Italy

P. Ruggieri et al. (eds.), *Tumors of the Sacrum*,
DOI 10.1007/978-3-319-51202-0_7

Table 7.1 Frequency of sacral tumor and pseudotumors (JST data)

Diagnosis	Cases
Primary malignant tumors	
Chordoma	172
Undifferentiated high-grade pleomorphic sarcoma	27
Chondrosarcoma	18
Ewing Sarcoma	12
Small blue round cell tumor	9
Osteosarcoma	11
Malignant peripheral nerve sheath tumor	3
Fibrosarcoma of bone	2
Malignancy in giant cell tumor of bone	2
Angiosarcoma	1
Subtotal	*257*
Benign lesions	
Giant cell tumor of bone	124
Schwannoma/neurofibroma	75
Aneurysmal bone cyst	8
Bone cyst	9
Osteoblastoma	5
Paraganglioma	5
Hemangioma	4
Desmoplastic fibroma of bone	2
Fibrous dysplasia	2
Angiomatosis, Langerhans cell histiocytosis, Lipoma, Myopericytoma, Osteochondroma, Osteoid osteoma	6
Subtotal	*240*
Systemic diseases	
Metastatic disease	84
Plasma cell myeloma	13
Primary non-Hodgkin lymphoma of bone	8
Subtotal	*105*
Total	602

7.1 Malignant Tumors

Malignant tumors include primary sarcoma, primary hematopoietic malignancy, and metastatic diseases. Primary sarcoma may derive from bone or soft tissue. The histological type of a primary bone sarcoma is often indicative of the tumor grade. The most common bone sarcomas are of high-grade malignancy. Soft tissue sarcoma occurring in sacrum is rare. Histological type and grade predict tumor behavior. The Federation Nationale des Cenres de Lutte Contre Le (FNCLCC) grading system is well accepted.

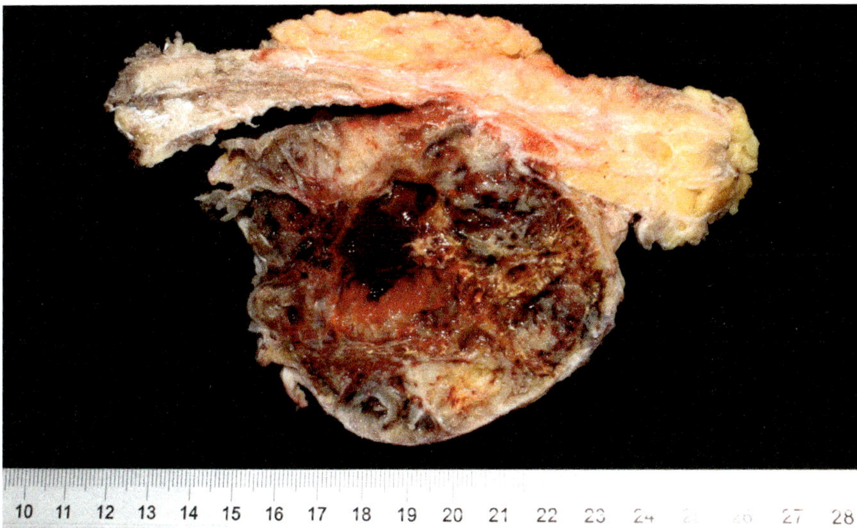

Fig. 7.1 Gross image of a sacral chordoma

7.1.1 Chordoma

Chordoma is the most common primary malignancy occurring in sacrum arising from notochordal rests [2]. Although it is mainly located in the base of the skull, 29.2–60% of chordomas occur in the sacrococcygeal region [3, 4]. It is usually a slow-growing and low-grade tumor, but metastatic disease is seen more frequently in sacral chordomas than in skull base chordomas [5].

Grossly, the tumor has an expansile, lobulated structure with cortical invasion. The cut surface is gelatinous with chondroid texture (Fig. 7.1). By definition, chordoma is a malignant tumor showing notochordal differentiation [3]. Notochordal differentiation is exhibited by epithelioid cells arranged in nests or cords with clear or eosinophilic cytoplasm; some have vacuolated "bubbly" cytoplasm, so called "physaliphorous cells." The tumor cells are separated by fibrous septa, which give rise to the lobulated appearance and are embedded in abundant extracellular myxoid matrix. In a low-grade tumor, the nuclei are small with coarse chromatin. In a high-grade tumor, the nuclei may become larger, pleomorphic and with greater mitotic activity.

Most of the chordomas are designated as chordomas, not otherwise specified (NOS) [3]. Chondroid chordoma is a rare variant which contains hyaline cartilage component. Its behavior is similar to chordoma, NOS, but it may be confused as chondrosarcoma morphologically. Brachyury is a specific immunohistochemical diagnostic marker for chordoma [6]. Nuclear immunoreactivity to Brachyury is seen in chordoma but not in chondrosarcoma, and is therefore extremely helpful in the differential diagnosis. Figure 7.2 shows the histological and immunohistochemical features of a chordoma. In practice, we prefer to use the more specific monoclonal antibody of brachyury than the polyclonal to prevent false positivity; we also

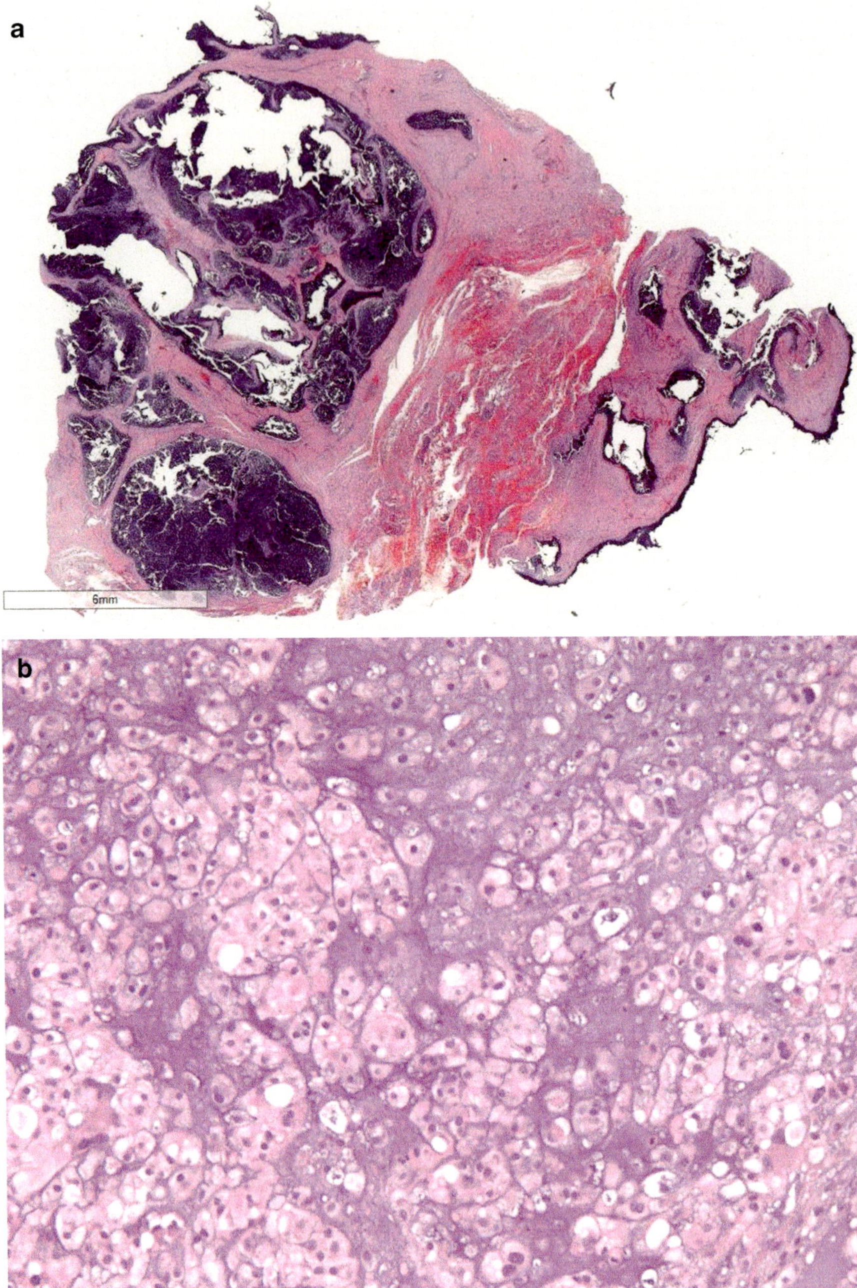

Fig. 7.2 Microscopic images of a chordoma. (**a**) HE digitalized whole slide image. (**b**) HE ×200. (**c**) HE ×600. (**d**) Brachyury stain ×200

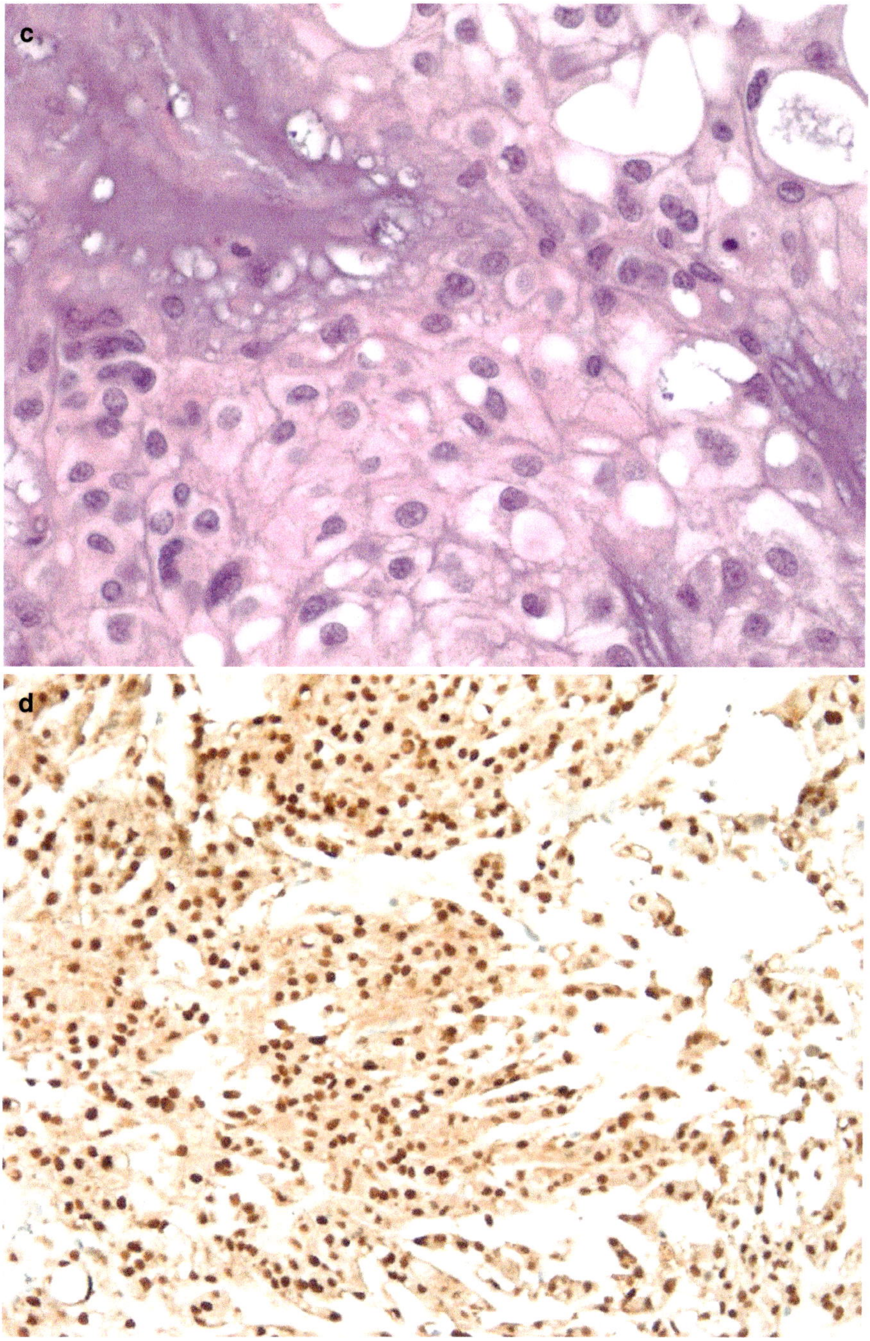

Fig. 7.2 (continued)

prefer to use non-decalcified specimen for brachyury testing to prevent false negativity. Other traditional helpful positive diagnostic immunohistochemical markers for chordoma include keratin, epithelial membrane antigen, and S-100 protein. New markers such as loss of PTEN and loss of INI-1 expression have recently been found in chordoma [7, 8]. Dedifferentiated chordoma is a high-grade and biphasic tumor which consists of a high-grade undifferentiated spindle cell sarcoma or osteosarcoma in association to chordoma, NOS [3]. Recognizing the conventional chordoma component is the key to this diagnosis because the dedifferentiated component does not express the diagnostic markers described here.

7.1.2 Chondrosarcoma

Chondrosarcoma is a locally aggressive malignant tumor that produces cartilaginous matrix [3]. There are four histological variants of chondrosarcoma: conventional, dedifferentiated, mesenchymal, and clear cell (Table 7.2). The histological grade is the single most important prognostic factor of conventional chondrosarcoma. Chondrosarcoma can be classified on the basis of its location in the bone. Central chondrosarcomas are located in the medullary cavity, peripheral chondrosarcomas arise from the surface of the bone, and periosteal (juxtacortical) chondrosarcomas arise from the surface of the bone and the periosteum [3]. According to its origin, a primary chondrosarcoma arises de novo, and secondary chondrosarcoma is a result of malignant transformation of an enchondroma (central) or osteochondroma (peripheral). All types can affect the pelvic bones, including the sacrum; however, peripheral secondary chondrosarcoma is seen more commonly in younger patients than in central primary chondrosarcoma, which predominantly affects patients more than 50 years of age [9]. The majority of the conventional and dedifferentiated chondrosarcomas exhibits somatic mutations of the *isocitrate dehydrogenase genes 1 and 2* (*IDH1 and IDH2*) [10]. However, this finding is absent in mesenchymal and clear cell chondrosarcoma indicating their different pathogenesis. The presence of (*IDH1 and IDH2*) mutation can be used to differentiate a chondroblastic

Table 7.2 Characteristics of histological variants of chondrosarcoma

Tumor type	Component	Prognosis
Conventional	Chondrosarcoma	Depends on grade
	Grade I	
	Grade II	
	Grade III	
Dedifferentiated	Low-grade conventional chondrosarcoma plus high-grade dedifferentiated sarcoma or osteosarcoma	Poor
Mesenchymal	Low-grade conventional chondrosarcoma plus poorly differentiated malignant small round cells	Poor
Clear cell	Clear cells or chondroblastoma-like cells	Depends on grade
	Note: Usually occurs in the ends of long bones; patients younger than conventional	

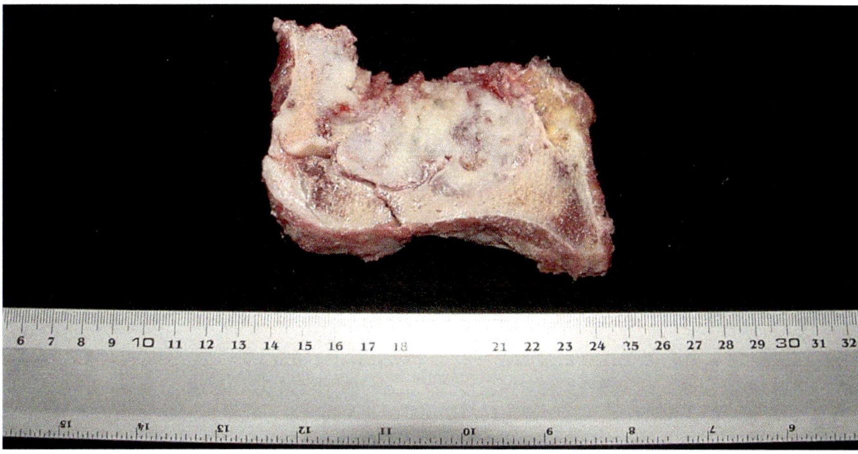

Fig. 7.3 Gross image of a sacral chondrosarcoma

osteosarcoma when it is deemed necessary. These molecular findings also warrant further investigation for their role as potential therapeutic targets [11].

As shown in Fig. 7.3, conventional chondrosarcomas grossly have the cut surface of hyaline cartilage with irregularly lobular appearance. Myxoid, cystic, and calcification changes can be seen. Microscopically, the distinction between enchondroma and grade I chondrosarcoma can be challenging due to overlapping morphological features. A generally accepted minimum diagnostic criteria for chondrosarcoma include hypercellularity, permeation of the host bone, absence of host bone encasement, open chromatin, mucoid matrix, and older patient (age >45 years) [3]. After establishing a diagnosis of chondrosarcoma, the next step is to grade the tumor using the following histological features: cellularity, nuclear size, degree of hyperchromasia, and mitoses. The grade I chondrosarcoma has similar nuclear features of enchondroma, except the architectural changes as described above. Grade III chondrosarcoma exhibits high cellularity, markedly enlarged nuclei, pleomorphic nuclei with nucleoli, and frequent mitoses compared to grade II chondrosarcoma. Tumor grade is the single most important prognostic factor of chondrosarcoma [9, 12]. When a chondrosarcoma has a spectrum of histology from grade I to grade III, it is a good practice to report the percentage of the high-grade component which predicts a worse prognosis. Figure 7.4 is the histological illustration of chondrosarcoma of various grades and dedifferentiated chondrosarcoma.

7.1.3 Ewing Sarcoma

Ewing sarcoma is a high-grade malignancy with small, round tumor cells harboring pathognomonic molecular signatures [3]. Approximately 85% of the Ewing sarcoma harbors a somatic chromosomal translocation t(11;22)(q24;q12) which rearrange *EWSR1* gene to fuse with *FLI1* gene [13]. The fusion protein EWSR1-FLI1 is an oncoprotein and is responsible for the pathogenesis of Ewing sarcoma [14, 15].

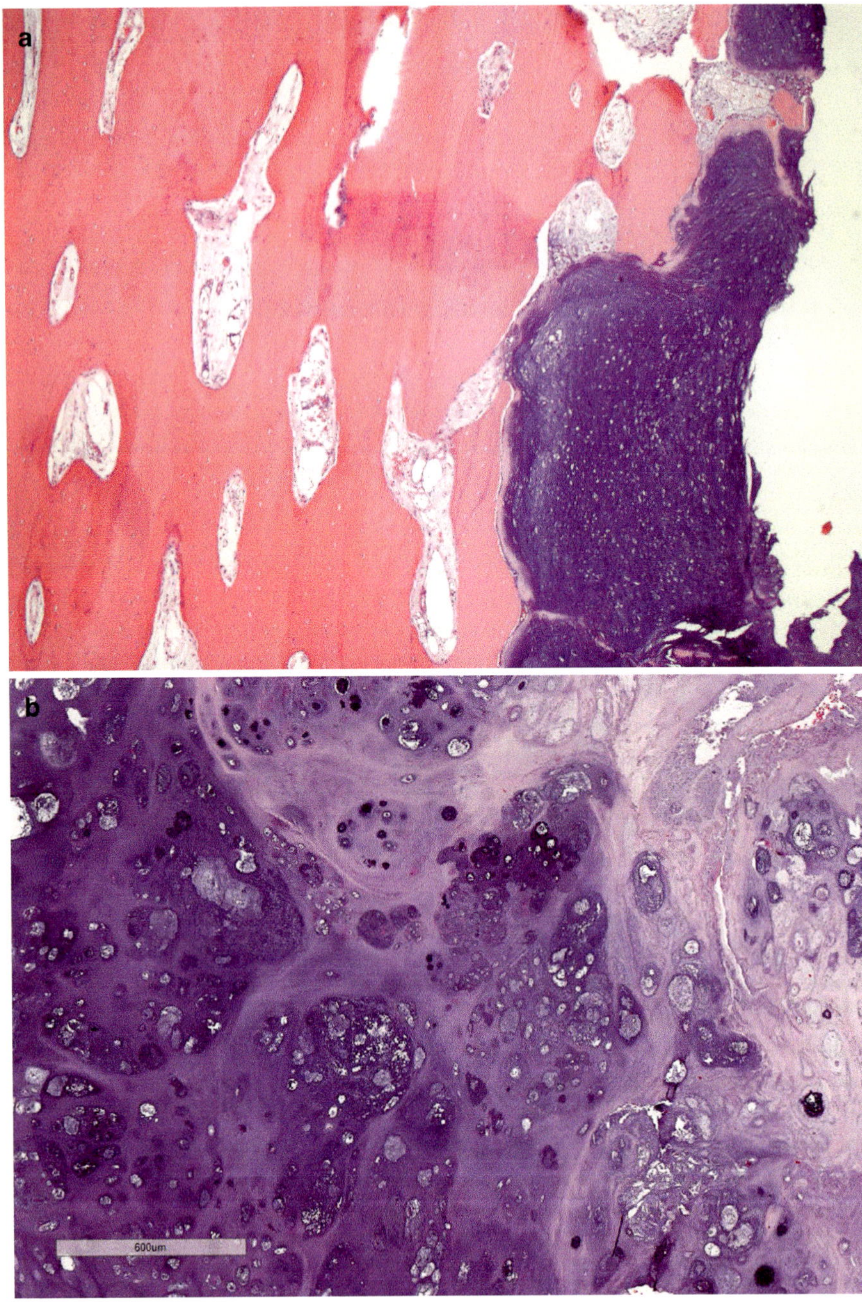

Fig. 7.4 Microscopic images of chondrosarcoma. (**a**) Chondrosarcoma invasion of bone. HE ×40. (**b**) Grade I chondrosarcoma. (**c**) Grade II. HE ×200. (**d**) Grade III. (**e**) Dedifferentiated chondrosarcoma. HE ×400

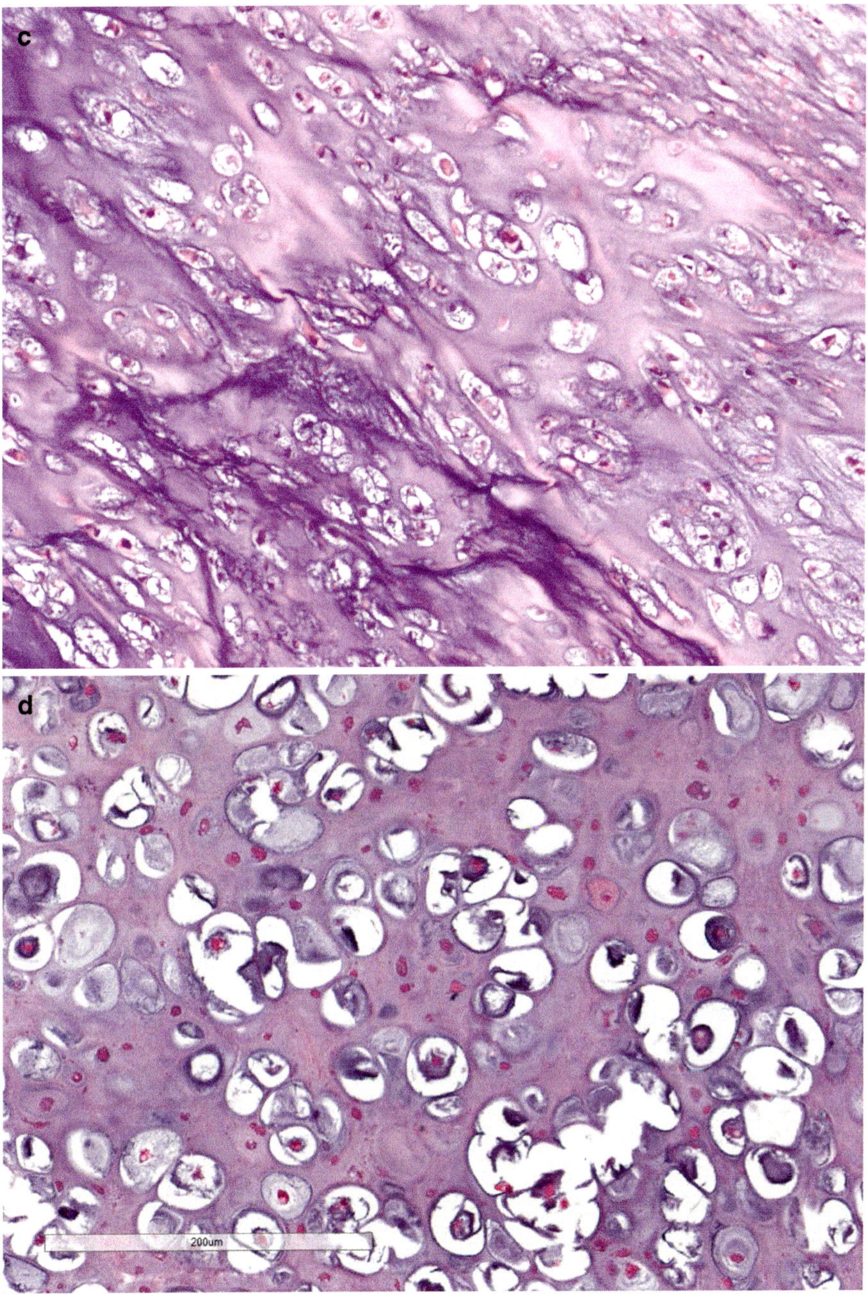

Fig. 7.4 (continued)

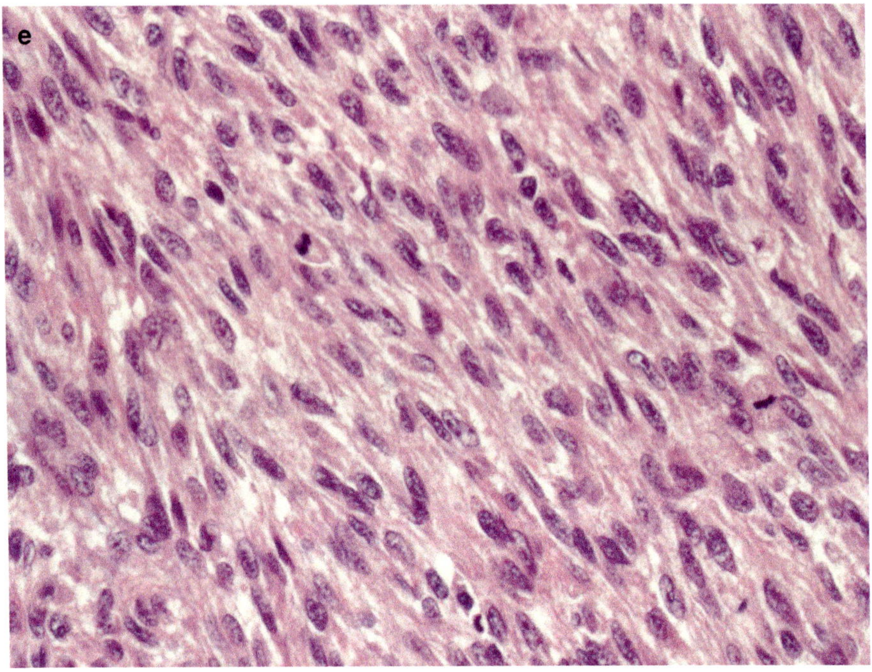

Fig. 7.4 (continued)

The *EWSR1* gene also has many other fusion partners such as the *ERG* gene [13]. Molecular testing for the signature gene and products are useful in confirming the diagnosis [16, 17]. While reverse transcription polymerase chain reaction (RT-PCR) may confirm the presence of *EWSR1-FLI1* or *EWSR1-ERG* fusion products, specific for Ewing sarcoma, the detection of rearrangement of *EWSR1* gene by fluorescence in situ hybridization (FISH) is not specific, because other sarcomas may harbor *EWSR1* gene rearrangements [3].

Primary Ewing sarcoma of the spine including sacrum is uncommon (only 3–10%); while metastatic disease from extraspinal Ewing sarcoma is more frequent. The sacral ala is the most common site for primary Ewing sarcoma of the spine [18, 19]. The prognosis is worse for sacrococcygeal Ewing sarcoma than for extraspinal Ewing sarcoma, usually due to larger tumor size at presentation because of delayed clinical presentation [20].

Grossly, the tumor has tan-grey cut surface with no bone or cartilaginous matrix. Necrosis and hemorrhage can be seen. In a classic Ewing sarcoma, the tumor is composed of small round cells with scant cytoplasm and round nuclei arranged in a vaguely lobular pattern or completely dyscohesive. This latter appearance resembles lymphoma. However, the cytoplasm of Ewing sarcoma appears clear and contains glycogen, which stains positively with periodic acid-Schiff (PAS). Ewing sarcoma also lacks the lymphoglandular bodies which represent cytoplasmic debris of lymphoma cells. In an atypical Ewing sarcoma, the tumor cells are larger with more pleomorphic nuclei and prominent nucleoli [3]. Neuroectodermal differentiation can be seen with tumor cells forming rosette-like structures. Immunohistochemical stain pattern of Ewing sarcoma includes positive vimentin, CD99 (membranous staining pattern), Keratin (aberrantly expressed in 30% cases), neuroendocrine markers, FLI-1 and, rarely, ERG) [13, 21, 22]. A histological, immunohistochemical and molecular illustration of Ewing sarcoma is in Fig. 7.5.

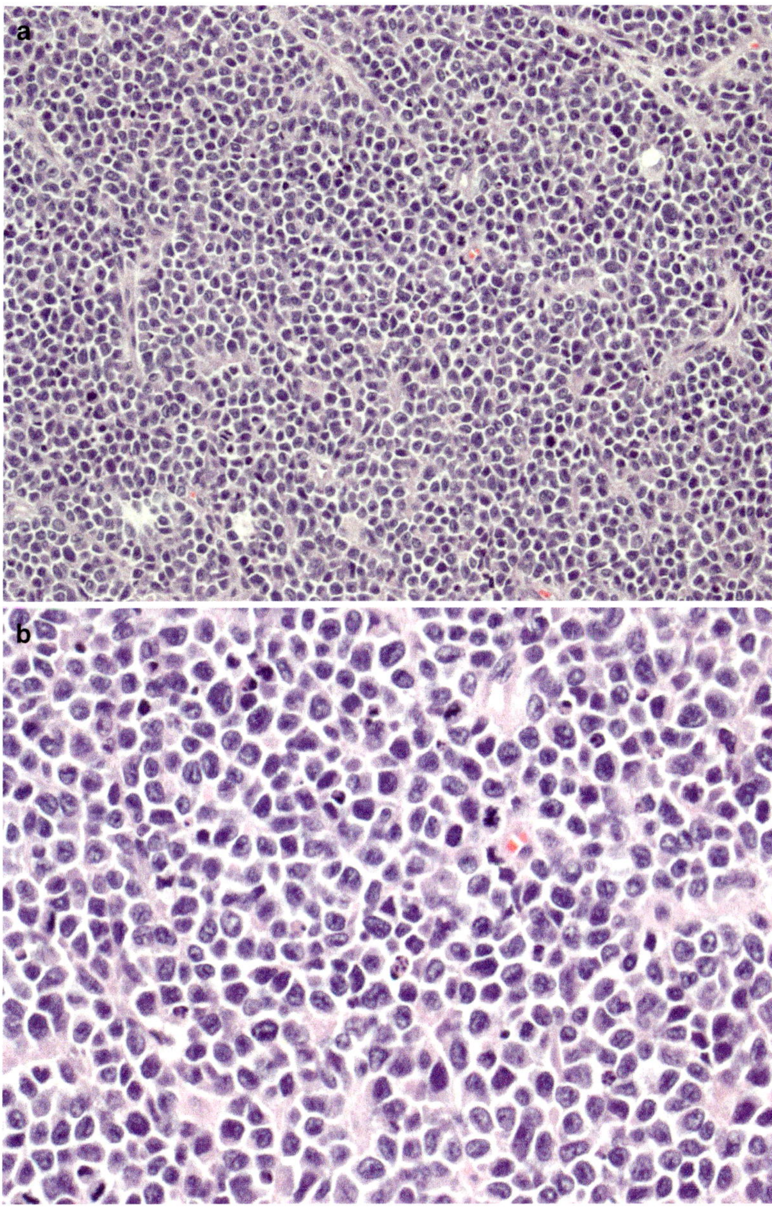

Fig. 7.5 Ewing sarcoma. (**a**) HE ×200. (**b**) HE ×400. (**c**) CD99+ ×400. (**d**) FLI1+ ×400. (**e**) FISH ×1000 showing LSI EWSR1 (22q12) break-apart probe showing EWSR1 rearrangement

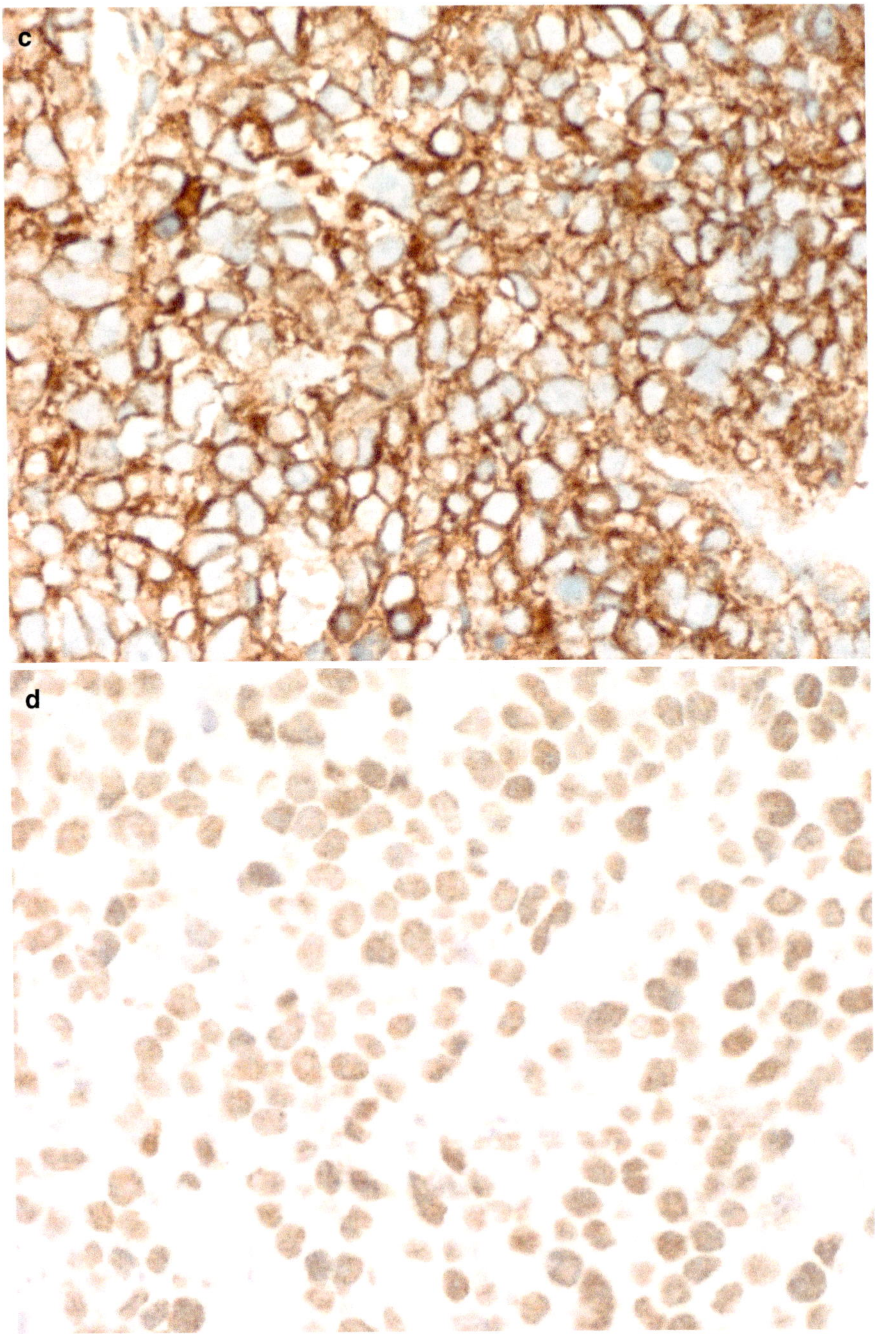

Fig. 7.5 (continued)

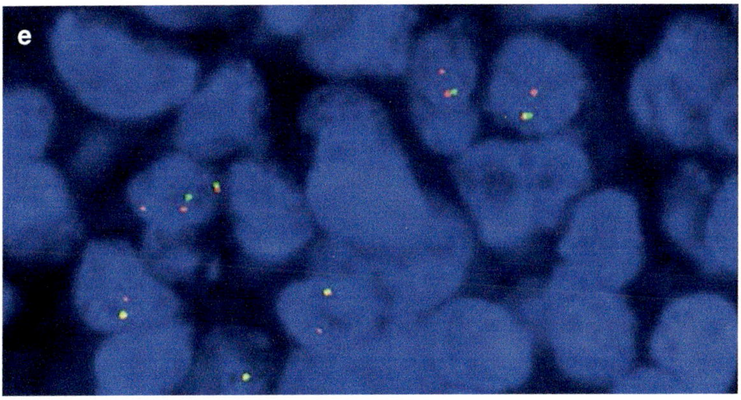

Fig. 7.5 (continued)

Table 7.3 Characteristics of histological variants of primary central osteosarcoma

Tumor type	Component	Prognosis
Conventional	High-grade sarcoma with osteoid formation	High-grade tumor. Subtype does not differ in prognosis and therapy
	Osteoblastic (76–80%) (Fig. 7.6a)	
	Chondroblastic (10–13%) (Fig. 7.6b)	
	Fibroblastic (10%)	
Telangiectatic	High-grade osteosarcoma with characteristic blood lakes and spaces	Similar to conventional type
Giant cell rich	High-grade osteosarcoma with abundant osteoclast-like giant cells (Fig. 7.6c)	Similar to conventional type
Small cell	High-grade osteosarcoma with characteristic small tumor cells (Fig. 7.6d)	Slightly worse prognosis than conventional type
Low-grade central	Low-grade osteosarcoma	Excellent prognosis
	Note: Distinguish from fibrous dysplasia by permeation of the host bone and soft tissue extension; amplification of *MDM2* gene	

7.1.4 Osteosarcoma

Patients with primary lumbosacral osteosarcoma are older at presentation and commonly males [20]. Secondary sacral osteosarcoma occurs in patients with previous radiation treatment or a history of Paget's disease. Elderly patients with polyostotic Paget's disease are most at risk for sarcomatous degeneration [2].

According to its location in the bone, central osteosarcoma is located in the medullary cavity, and peripheral osteosarcoma arises from the surface of the bone [23]. The characteristic of primary central osteosarcoma and surface osteosarcoma are summarized in Tables 7.3 and 7.4. Surface/peripheral osteosarcoma very rarely affects the flat bone.

Table 7.4 Characteristics of histological variants of primary peripheral osteosarcoma

Tumor type	Component	Prognosis
Parosteal (Juxtacortical osteosarcoma)	Low-grade	Excellent
	Spindle cells with mild to moderate atypia, well-formed bone trabeculae arranged in parallel pattern, and associated benign cartilaginous differentiation	
	Note: Amplification of *MDM2* gene	
Periosteal (Juxtacortical chondroblastic osteosarcoma)	Intermediate-grade	Better prognosis than conventional osteosarcoma
	Predominantly atypical cartilage admixed with intermediate-grade osteosarcoma	
High-grade surface osteosarcoma	High-grade osteosarcoma of the surface	Similar to conventional type
	Note: The tumor is predominantly outside the bone; similar variants seen in conventional osteosarcoma	

High-grade osteosarcoma is treated with neoadjuvant chemotherapy. The pathological evaluation of the therapy response is critically important for assessment of prognosis. Osteosarcomas with more than 90% tumor necrosis (less than 10% viable tumor cells) are considered good responders and have better overall and disease-free survival [24]. A generally accepted method of sampling osteosarcoma includes cross-sectioning the central and largest slice of the tumor. The slice is further divided into 1 cm × 1 cm slices and prepared for microscopic examination. Therapy-induced changes include tumor necrosis, pleomorphic changes, cystic changes, fibrosis, etc. However, only the percentage of tumor necrosis characterized by pyknotic, fragmented, or lysed tumor nuclei, which is reversely related to the percentage of viable tumor cells, is accepted as an independent prognostic factor [25].

7.1.5 Undifferentiated Pleomorphic Sarcoma

Undifferentiated pleomorphic sarcoma (UPS) is a group of high-grade tumors that have no identifiable line of differentiation when analyzed by current technologies, and therefore represents a diagnosis of exclusion. Figure 7.7 shows a gross image of a sacral undifferentiated sarcoma. UPS histology is variable and may show several morphologic patterns from storiform areas composed of spindle cells to areas composed of large, pleomorphic neoplastic cells with marked nuclear atypia [3, 26]. Mitotic activity is prominent with atypical mitotic figures.

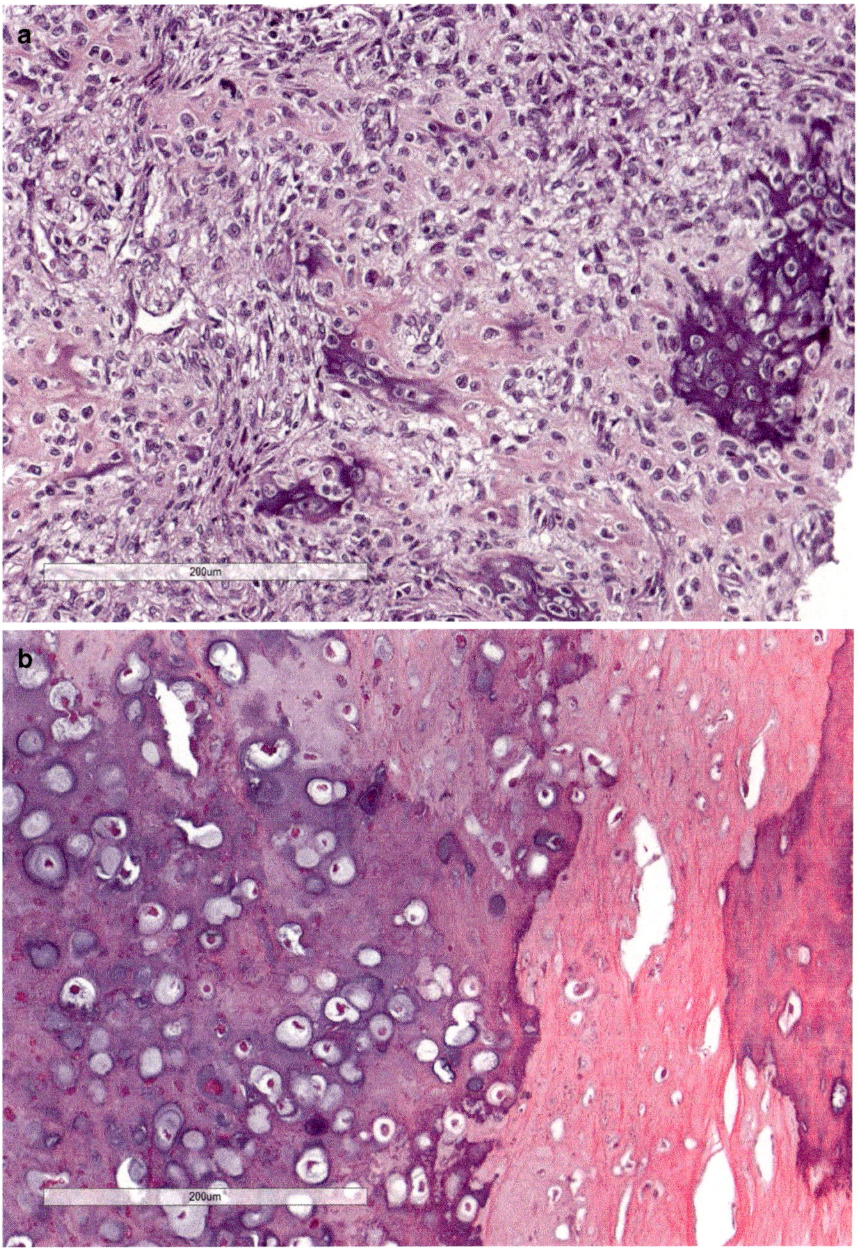

Fig. 7.6 Osteosarcoma. (**a**) Osteoblastic osteosarcoma. (**b**) Chondroblastic osteosarcoma. (**c**) Giant cell rich osteosarcoma. (**d**) Small cell osteosarcoma

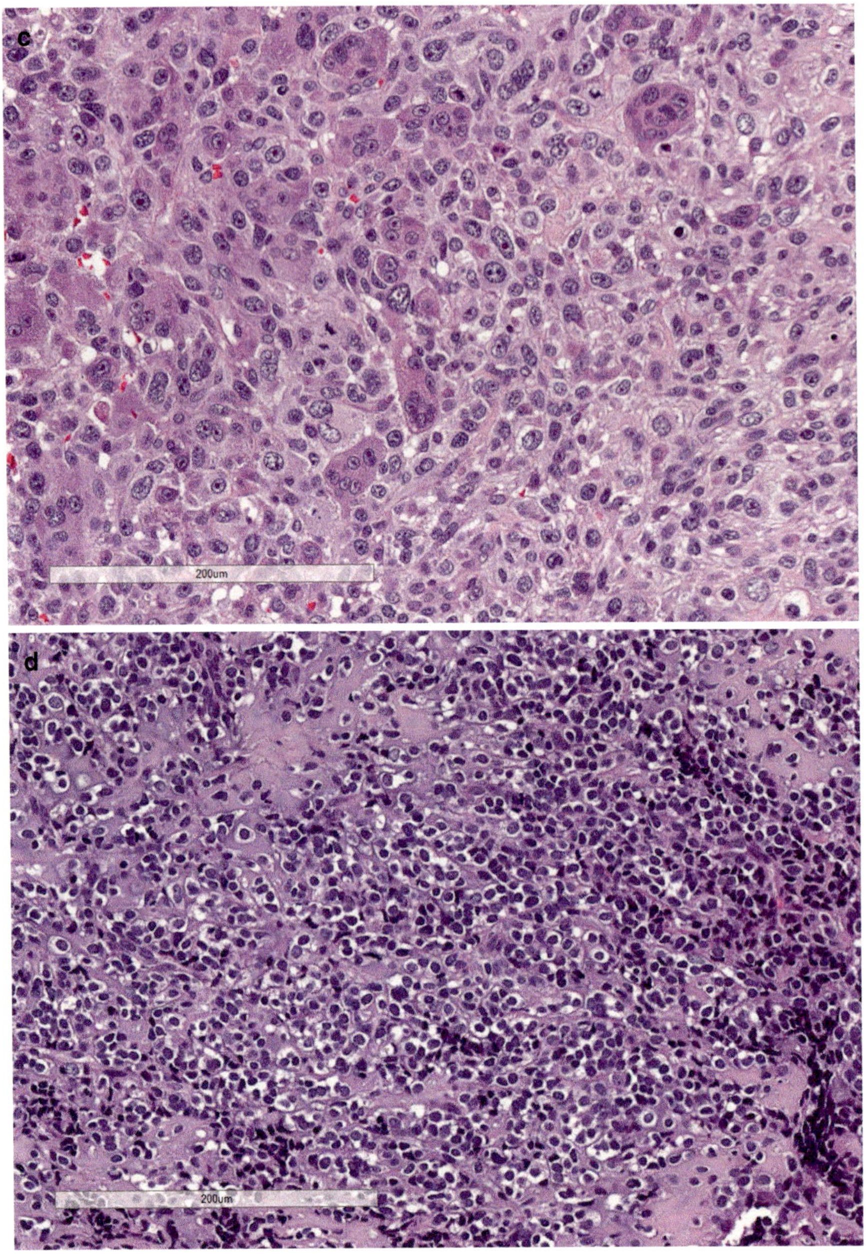

Fig. 7.6 (continued)

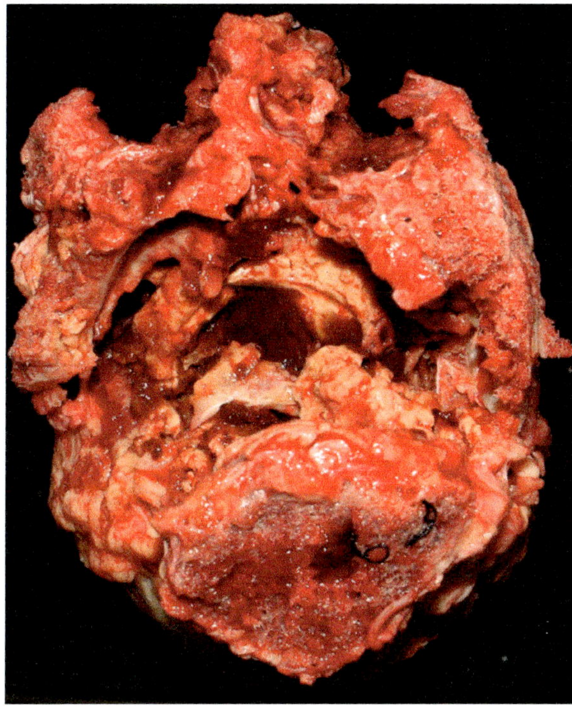

Fig. 7.7 A gross image of undifferentiated sarcoma

7.1.6 Metastatic/Systemic Malignancy

Metastatic disease from epithelial malignancies is the most common secondary malignancy of the sacrum [2]. The primary sites include lung, breast, prostate, kidney, head and neck, and gastrointestinal tract. Melanoma is also a common culprit of metastasis [27]. The most common hematopoietic malignancies of the sacrum are non-Hodgkin lymphoma and multiple myeloma or plasmacytoma These diseases may be either primary of bone or secondary involvement of the bone in disseminated disease. Our institutional review of primary bone lymphoma (PBL) consisted of 70 patients [28, 29]. PBL cases were included in this cohort using the 2013 WHO criteria for bone/soft tissue tumors [3], as disease was restricted to bone and adjacent soft tissue with or without regional nodes at the time of the diagnosis. Bone lymphoma with distant bone marrow involvement as the only other site of extranodal disease was also included. We found that PBL occurs in sacrum less frequently than extremities, but diffuse large B-cell lymphoma is the most common variant of lymphoma.

When a primary tumor is present, the diagnosis of metastatic disease is achieved by comparing the histology of sacral lesion with the primary disease. However, when a primary site unknown histomorphology in conjunction with pertinent ancillary testing including immunohistochemistry, flow cytometry and molecular testing are used to render a definitive diagnosis.

7.1.7 Rare Primary Sacral Sarcomas

The following malignant tumors have occasionally been reported occurring in sacrum [3, 30–32] (see Table 7.5).

7.2 Benign Tumors

7.2.1 Giant Cell Tumor of Bone

Giant cell tumor of bone (GCTB) is a benign but locally aggressive tumor. The tumor is composed of numerous characteristic giant cells which are large and osteoclast-like. These cells are impressive morphologically; however, they are the background cells reactive to the true neoplastic cells which are primitive mesenchymal stromal cells. The neoplastic cells are mononuclear and express receptor activator for NF-κB ligand (RANKL), the master regulator of osteoclast differentiation. Macrophages and osteoclasts express RANK. The interaction between the

Table 7.5 Rare primary sarcomas of sacrum

Tumor type	Definition	Histology and immunophenotype	Prognosis
Undifferentiated/ unclassified sarcoma	High-grade malignancy showing no identifiable specific lineage of differentiation	Pleomorphic, spindle cell, round cell, epithelial cell	Limited data
		No consistent finding	
Angiosarcoma	Aggressive malignancy with endothelial differentiation	Epithelial, spindle	Poor prognosis associated with high grade, presence of macronucleolus, older age, large size, increased mitoses, and high Ki-67 index
		Express vascular markers (CD34, CD31, ERG, and FLI1)	
Fibrosarcoma	Intermediate- to High-grade fibroblastic spindle cell malignancy	Less pleomorphic than undifferentiated pleomorphic sarcoma	Depend on age, tumor site, grade, and stage
		Rare report of slerosing epithelioid fibrosarcoma	
		No consistent finding	
Malignant solitary fibrous tumor	Malignant variant of solitary fibrous tumor	Large tumor size, infiltrative margin, hypercellularity, nuclear pleomorphism, tumor necrosis, and high mitotic activity (>4/10 HPF)	Depend on age, tumor site, grade, and stage
		Express STAT6 (nuclear), CD34, CD99, and Bcl-2	

neoplastic mononuclear stromal cells and macrophages/osteoclasts by a RANKL-dependent mechanism via the stimulation of macrophage-colony stimulation factor (MCSF) results in neoplastic proliferation and induces osteoclast formation. During this process, tumor-associated macrophage-like osteoclast precursors, which are also mononuclear cells, are recruited by tumoral stromal cells to participate in osteoclast differentiation and activation. Because osteoclast formation is the major consequence of GCTB, inhibition of osteoclast formation and activity is the key therapeutic approach. For example, bisphosphonate inhibits osteoclast-mediated resorption of bone/osteolysis and anti-RANKL antibody targets the RANKL-dependent mechanism of GCTB formation.

Osteoprotegerin (OPG) is a soluble decoy receptor that is produced by osteoblasts to inhibit osteoclast differentiation through its binding to RANKL, which prevents RANK binding. OPG expression reflects a protective mechanism of the skeleton to compensate increased bone resorption. Bone remodeling is mainly controlled by the balance of RANKL/OPG. Osteoprotegerin ligand (OPGL), also named receptor activator of RANKL, is also expressed in the stroma-like tumor cells of GCTB. The ratio of OPGL/OPG by tumor cells may contribute to the degree of osteoclastogenesis and bone resorption [33].

Although giant cell tumors of the bone (GCTB) within the vertebrae are rare (2.7–6.5% of all GCTB), the sacrum may be the most common spinal site for this lesion [34–36]. In a collaborative study with Beijing Jishuitan Hospital, we found that GCTB has significant higher incidences than the Mayo Clinic group [37]. JST group also published an article described two GCTBs of sacrum with pulmonary metastasis [38].

Grossly, the tumor is red-brown with hemorrhage (Fig. 7.8). Yellow areas reflect lipid laden macrophage rich areas. Histologically (Fig. 7.9) the tumor is composed of numerous giant cells with multinucleation and scattered mononuclear cells that are round or spindle. Lipid laden or hemosiderin laden macrophages are also

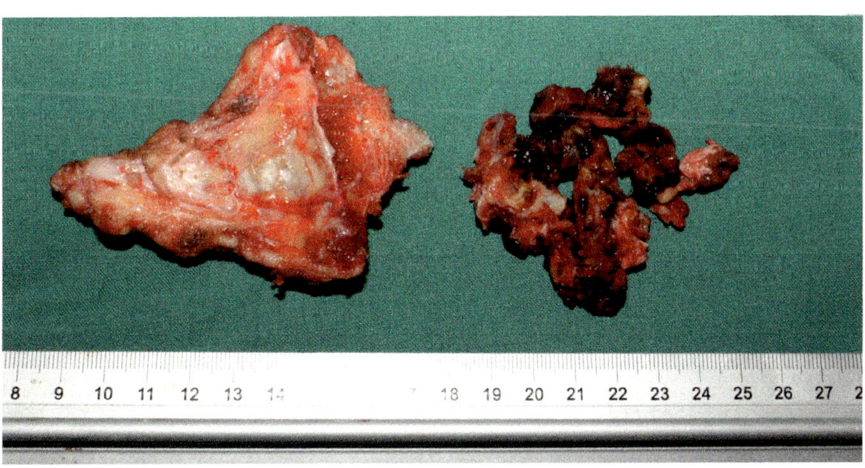

Fig. 7.8 A gross image of a sacral giant cell tumor

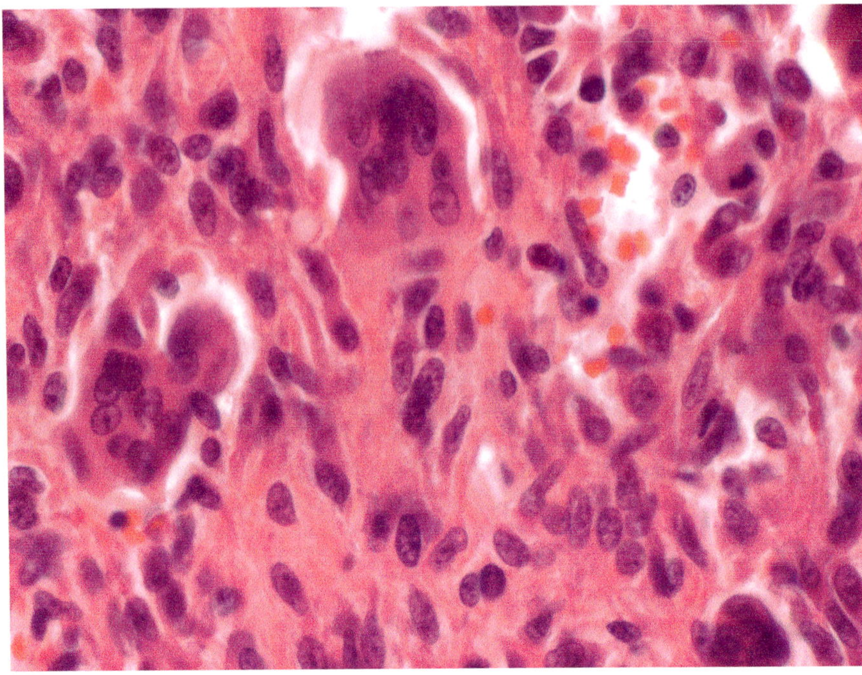

Fig. 7.9 Microscopic images of giant cell tumor

present. The tumor is mainly solid and may contain cystic areas. Secondary aneurysmal bone cyst component is seen in 10% of GCTB. The tumor may be mitotically active; however, a benign giant cell tumor typically does not have atypical mitosis or significant nuclear atypia. The latter is associated with a malignant transformation of GCTB. One diagnostic pitfall is to avoid misdiagnosing an osteosarcoma when a pathological fracture is in association with a malignant giant cell tumor.

7.2.2 Benign Neurogenic Tumor

Benign neurogenic tumors occur in paraspinal or presacral locations. Sacral schwannomas or neurofibromas grow within the sacral canal and only rarely expand through the anterior sacral foramina into the presacral space [39]. Schwannoma (Fig. 7.10) consists of well-differentiated Schwann cells, is usually encapsulated and cut surfaces have a pink, white, or yellow appearance. Classic histology (Fig. 7.11a, b) shows a pattern of alternating Antoni A (cellular areas of spindle cells with occasional palisading) and Antoni B (loose myxoid areas with scattered spindle cells and thick-walled, hyalinized vessels) areas. Degenerative changes such as cyst formation, calcification, hemorrhage, and hyalinization may be present,

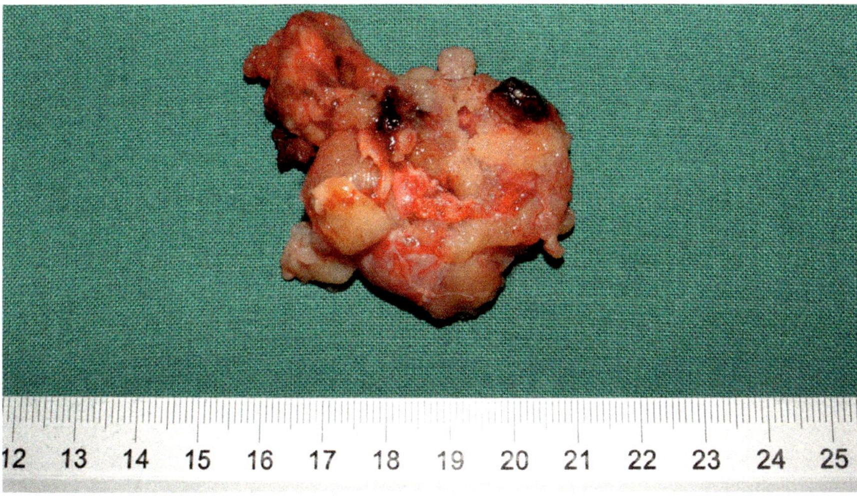

Fig. 7.10 A gross image of a sacral schwannoma

especially if the tumor has been there for a long duration. Ancient schwannoma is characterized by Schwann cells with large and hyperchromatic nuclei, the manifestation of degenerative change. Schwannomas with increased cellularity and occasional mitoses are referred to as cellular schwannomas, a variant of schwannoma. These variants of schwannoma behave similar to conventional schwannomas. Immunohistochemically, schwannomas express strongly and diffusely S-100 protein as well as SOX10, a new marker of neural crest differentiation [40]. Neurofibroma, originating from sacral nerve roots, is composed of Schwann cells, perineurial-like cells, fibroblasts, and axons and are associated with a myxoid or fibrous stroma.

Malignant transformation can occur, often seen in the setting of neurofibromatosis type 1. Differentiation of benign and malignant neoplasms can be difficult, but increased size, rapid growth, infiltrative border, necrosis, increased cellularity, and increased mitotic activity with atypical mitosis favor malignancy. Cellular schwannoma can be misdiagnosed as malignant peripheral nerve sheath tumor (MPNST) (Fig. 7.11c). Morphologic features distinguishing cellular schwannoma from MPNST are the presence of perivascular accentuation of cellularity, tumor herniation into vascular lumens, presence of necrosis, and loss of expression of H3K27me [41].

Other rare neurogenic tumors include sacral ependymomas that arise from ependymal cells of the terminal filum, expand the sacral canal, and are usually of the myxopapillary type. Sacral meningiomas are even more rare than sacral ependymomas and schwannomas and arise within the sacral canal. Neuroblastoma is derived from embryonic neural crest tissue and clinically manifests in infancy. Ganglioneuroma is originated from sympathetic ganglion cells [39]. Ependymomas and meningioma have both benign and malignant variants.

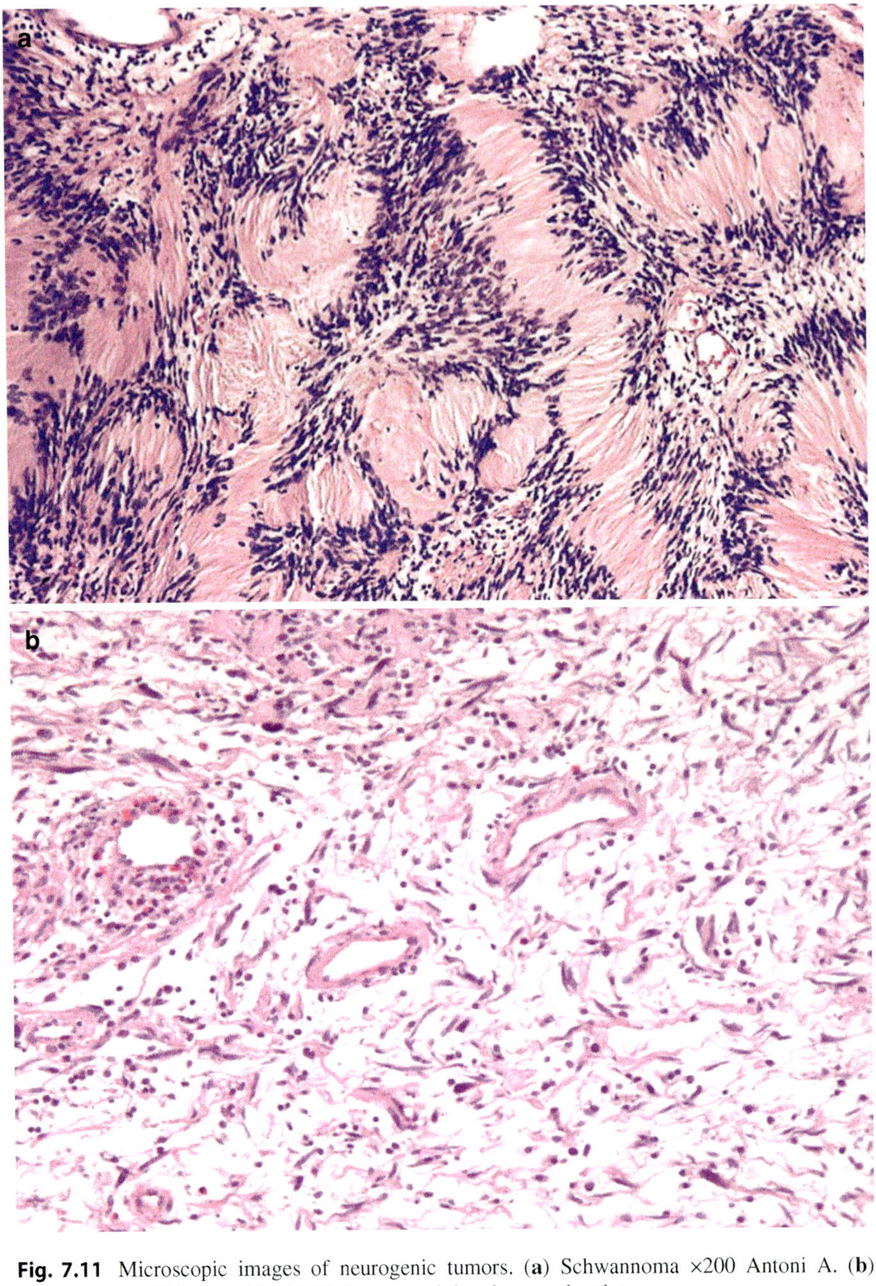

Fig. 7.11 Microscopic images of neurogenic tumors. (**a**) Schwannoma ×200 Antoni A. (**b**) Schwannoma ×200 Antoni B. (**c**) Malignant peripheral nerve sheath tumor

Fig. 7.11 (continued)

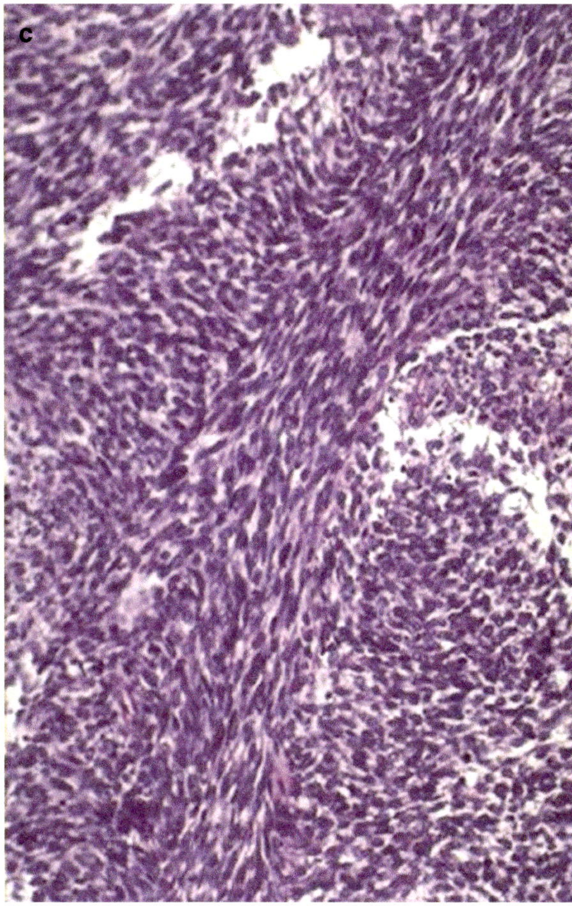

7.2.3 Aneurysmal Bone Cyst

Aneurysmal bone cyst (ABC) is a benign tumor. Grossly it is well defined and composed of blood-filled pseudocystic spaces. The cysts lack specific cell-lining and consist of a wall of spindle cells with scattered osteoclast-type multinucleated giant cells. The neoplastic cells are spindle shaped and indistinguishable from reactive fibroblasts and myofibroblasts. However, the tumor cells show *USP6* rearrangement in 70% of ABC [42]. The spindle cells are bland. Mitoses may be frequent without atypical forms. Reactive woven bone may be seen with osteoblastic rimming.

7.2.4 Other Rare Benign Primary Intraosseous Sacral Lesions

Although the true incidence has not been established, the lesions listed here (Table 7.6) rarely occur in sacrum. The diagnosis is mainly based by histologic examination with clinicoradiological correlations. Ancillary testing is not widely used for diagnosis. The ancillary testing described in Table 7.6 are mostly for academic interest except for fibrous dysplasia and Langerhans cell histiocytosis.

7.2.5 Sacrococcygeal Teratoma

Sacrococcygeal teratoma is a germ cell tumor and the most common sacral tumor in neonates, although it is very rare in adults [39]. These tumors are composed of multiple tissues foreign to the tissue in which they arise, which usually include skin, teeth, central nervous system tissue, and respiratory and alimentary mucosa. Mature teratoma (dermoid cyst) is benign and most common. Struma ovarii is a rare form of mature teratoma that contains mostly benign thyroid tissue. Immature teratoma is

Table 7.6 Rare benign primary intraosseous sacral lesions

Name	Nature	Histology	Ancillary testing for diagnosis
Chondroblastoma	Neoplastic	Round to polygonal chondroblasts with round to ovoid nucleus exhibit longitudinal grooves and well-defined cytoplasmic borders. Well. "Chicken wire" calcifications and multinucleated osteoclast-like giant cells are seen	S-100 protein and SOX9 expression by IHC
Chondromyxoid fibroma	Neoplastic	A lobular pattern with cellular stellate or spindle cells at the periphery and less cellular center with myxoid or chondromyxoid matrix. Multinucleated osteoclast-like giant cells, hyaline cartilage and calcification are seen	S-100 protein and SOX9 expression by IHC
Osteochondroma	Neoplastic	Perichondrium, cartilage, and bone	None
Osteoid osteoma	Neoplastic	Nidus consisting of a combination of osteoid and woven bone surrounded by osteoblasts. The nidus is vascular rich with the appearance of granulation tissue. The nidus is surrounded by sclerotic bone	Runx2 and Osterix
Osteoblastoma	Neoplastic	Similar features as seen in osteoid osteoma	None
Fibrous dysplasia	Neoplastic	Bland spindle fibroblastic cells admixed with irregular bony spicules without osteoblastic rimming	*GNAS* mutation

Table 7.6 (continued)

Name	Nature	Histology	Ancillary testing for diagnosis
Langerhans cell histocytosis/ eosinophilic granuloma	Likely neoplastic	Langerhans cells are specialized histiocytes with nuclear grooves (reniform nuclei), which are admixed with inflammatory cells including prominent eosinophilia	CD1a, CD207/ Langerin, and CD45 expression by IHC
Paget disease	Nonneoplastic metabolic disorder of bone remodeling susceptible to deformities and fractures; increased risk to primary bone malignancy	Increase in osteoclastic resorption and secondary bone formation resulting in a disorganized and fragile lamellar bone mosaic pattern	None
	Monostotic or polyostotic		
Simple bone cyst	Nonneoplastic	Unilocular cysts of bone with a fibrous membrane lining. The cyst contains serous or serosanguineous fluid	None

uncommon which differs from mature teratoma by the presence of immature tissue and exhibits malignant clinical behavior.

7.2.6 Developmental Lesions

Sacral meningocele is a cerebrospinal fluid-filled protrusion of the meninges through a defect in the sacrum [39]. Benign sacral meningeal cysts are frequent coincidental findings in the radiological examination of the sacrum, and their pathogenesis is poorly understood.

7.2.7 Intraoperative Pathologic Evaluation of Bone and Soft Tissue Lesions

Intraoperative pathologic diagnosis of bone and soft tissue lesions is an important yet challenging tool in clinical musculoskeletal oncology practice. Indications for frozen section include making a diagnosis, evaluating margin status, determining tumor extent/spread, and obtaining an adequate sample for permanent section and diagnosis. Frozen section pathological evaluation provides real-time guidance to therapeutic intervention. In our practice, intraoperative cytology is used as an adjunct to frozen section. This approach has proven useful to enhance the accuracy of diagnosing bone and soft tissue lesion [43, 44], including sacral lesions.

References

1. Xu H, Seifert RP, Niu X, Li Y, Bui MM. The establishment and utility of a free online database of primary bone tumors. Pathol Oncol Res. 2016;22(1):129–33. PubMed PMID: 26377426.
2. Thornton E, Krajewski KM, O'Regan KN, Giardino AA, Jagannathan JP, Ramaiya N. Imaging features of primary and secondary malignant tumours of the sacrum. Br J Radiol. 2012;85(1011):279–86. PubMed PMID: 22167504. Pubmed Central PMCID: PMC3473982.
3. Fletcher CDM, World Health Organization, International Agency for Research on Cancer. WHO classification of tumours of soft tissue and bone. 4th ed. Lyon: IARC Press; 2013. p. 468.
4. Diel J, Ortiz O, Losada RA, Price DB, Hayt MW, Katz DS. The sacrum: pathologic spectrum, multimodality imaging, and subspecialty approach. Radiographics. 2001;21(1):83–104. PubMed PMID: 11158646.
5. Ha AS, Chew FS. Imaging of sacral masses: self-assessment module. AJR Am J Roentgenol. 2010;195(3 Suppl):S32–6. PubMed PMID: 20729410.
6. Vujovic S, Henderson S, Presneau N, Odell E, Jacques TS, Tirabosco R, et al. Brachyury, a crucial regulator of notochordal development, is a novel biomarker for chordomas. J Pathol. 2006;209(2):157–65. PubMed PMID: 16538613.
7. Chen K, Mo J, Zhou M, Wang G, Wu G, Chen H, et al. Expression of PTEN and mTOR in sacral chordoma and association with poor prognosis. Med Oncol. 2014;31(4):886. PubMed PMID: 24535608
8. Mobley BC, McKenney JK, Bangs CD, Callahan K, Yeom KW, Schneppenheim R, et al. Loss of SMARCB1/INI1 expression in poorly differentiated chordomas. Acta Neuropathol. 2010;120(6):745–53. PubMed PMID: 21057957.
9. Gelderblom H, Hogendoorn PC, Dijkstra SD, van Rijswijk CS, Krol AD, Taminiau AH, et al. The clinical approach towards chondrosarcoma. Oncologist. 2008;13(3):320–9. PubMed PMID: 18378543.
10. Amary MF, Bacsi K, Maggiani F, Damato S, Halai D, Berisha F, et al. IDH1 and IDH2 mutations are frequent events in central chondrosarcoma and central and periosteal chondromas but not in other mesenchymal tumours. J Pathol. 2011;224(3):334–43. PubMed PMID: 21598255.
11. Taylor BS, Barretina J, Maki RG, Antonescu CR, Singer S, Ladanyi M. Advances in sarcoma genomics and new therapeutic targets. Nat Rev Cancer. 2011;11(8):541–57. PubMed PMID: 21753790. Pubmed Central PMCID: PMC3361898.
12. Evans HL, Ayala AG, Romsdahl MM. Prognostic factors in chondrosarcoma of bone: a clinicopathologic analysis with emphasis on histologic grading. Cancer. 1977;40(2):818–31. PubMed PMID: 890662.
13. Henderson-Jackson EB, Bui MM. Molecular pathology of soft-tissue neoplasms and its role in clinical practice. Cancer Control. 2015;22(2):186–92. PubMed PMID: 26068763.
14. Surdez D, Benetkiewicz M, Perrin V, Han ZY, Pierron G, Ballet S, et al. Targeting the EWSR1-FLI1 oncogene-induced protein kinase PKC-beta abolishes Ewing sarcoma growth. Cancer Res. 2012;72(17):4494–503. PubMed PMID: 22930730.
15. Delattre O, Zucman J, Plougastel B, Desmaze C, Melot T, Peter M, et al. Gene fusion with an ETS DNA-binding domain caused by chromosome translocation in human tumours. Nature. 1992;359(6391):162–5. PubMed PMID: 1522903.
16. Coppola D. Mechanisms of oncogenesis: an update on tumorigenesis. Dordrecht: Springer; 2010. xii, 314p.
17. Coppola D. Molecular pathology and diagnostics of cancer. New York: Springer; 2013.

18. Llauger J, Palmer J, Amores S, Bague S, Camins A. Primary tumors of the sacrum: diagnostic imaging. AJR Am J Roentgenol. 2000;174(2):417–24. PubMed PMID: 10658718.
19. Rodallec MH, Feydy A, Larousserie F, Anract P, Campagna R, Babinet A, et al. Diagnostic imaging of solitary tumors of the spine: what to do and say. Radiographics. 2008;28(4):1019–41. PubMed PMID: 18635627.
20. Murphey MD, Andrews CL, Flemming DJ, Temple HT, Smith WS, Smirniotopoulos JG. From the archives of the AFIP. Primary tumors of the spine: radiologic pathologic correlation. Radiographics. 1996;16(5):1131–58. PubMed PMID: 8888395.
21. Olsen SH, Thomas DG, Lucas DR. Cluster analysis of immunohistochemical profiles in synovial sarcoma, malignant peripheral nerve sheath tumor, and Ewing sarcoma. Mod Pathol. 2006;19(5):659–68. PubMed PMID: 16528378.
22. Rossi S, Orvieto E, Furlanetto A, Laurino L, Ninfo V, Dei Tos AP. Utility of the immunohistochemical detection of FLI-1 expression in round cell and vascular neoplasm using a monoclonal antibody. Mod Pathol. 2004;17(5):547–52. PubMed PMID: 15001993.
23. Dodd L, Bui MM. Atlas of soft tissue and bone pathology: with histologic, cytologic, and radiologic correlations. New York: Demos Medical; 2015. viii, 419p.
24. Anninga JK, Gelderblom H, Fiocco M, Kroep JR, Taminiau AH, Hogendoorn PC, et al. Chemotherapeutic adjuvant treatment for osteosarcoma: where do we stand? Eur J Cancer. 2011;47(16):2431–45. PubMed PMID: 21703851.
25. Czerniak B, Dorfman HD. Dorfman and Czerniak's bone tumors. 2nd ed. Philadelphia: Elsevier; 2016.
26. Goldblum JR, Folpe AL, Weiss SW, Enzinger FM, Weiss SW. Enzinger and Weiss's soft tissue tumors. 6th ed. Philadelphia: Saunders/Elsevier; 2014. xiv, 1155p.
27. Disler DG, Miklic D. Imaging findings in tumors of the sacrum. AJR Am J Roentgenol. 1999;173(6):1699–706. PubMed PMID: 10584822.
28. Wu H, Zhang L, Shao H, Sokol L, Sotomayor E, Letson D, et al. Prognostic significance of soft tissue extension, International Prognostic Index, and multifocality in primary bone lymphoma: a single institutional experience. Br J Haematol. 2014;166(1):60–8. PubMed PMID: 24673481.
29. Wu H, Bui MM, Leston DG, Shao H, Sokol L, Sotomayor EM, et al. Clinical characteristics and prognostic factors of bone lymphomas: focus on the clinical significance of multifocal bone involvement by primary bone large B-cell lymphomas. BMC Cancer. 2014;14:900. PubMed PMID: 25465716. Pubmed Central PMCID: PMC4265495.
30. Nakamura M, Tsushima K, Yasuo M, Yamazaki Y, Honda T, Koizumi T, et al. Angiosarcoma with sacral origin metastasizing to the lung. Intern Med. 2006;45(15):923–6. PubMed PMID: 16946576.
31. Chow LT, Lui YH, Kumta SM, Allen PW. Primary sclerosing epithelioid fibrosarcoma of the sacrum: a case report and review of the literature. J Clin Pathol. 2004;57(1):90–4. PubMed PMID: 14693846. Pubmed Central PMCID: PMC1770169.
32. Dv R, Dm K, Vanel D, Campanacci L, Iv B, Ag T, et al. Malignant solitary fibrous tumor of the sacrum: a case report. J Cancer Res Ther. 2015;3(4):52–5. English.
33. Huang L, Xu J, Wood DJ, Zheng MH. Gene expression of osteoprotegerin ligand, osteoprotegerin, and receptor activator of NF-kappaB in giant cell tumor of bone: possible involvement in tumor cell-induced osteoclast-like cell formation. Am J Pathol. 2000;156(3):761–7. PubMed PMID: 10702390. Pubmed Central PMCID: PMC1876848.
34. Shimada Y, Hongo M, Miyakoshi N, Kasukawa Y, Ando S, Itoi E, et al. Giant cell tumor of fifth lumbar vertebrae: two case reports and review of the literature. Spine J. 2007;7(4):499–505. PubMed PMID: 17630149.
35. Bidwell JK, Young JW, Khalluff E. Giant cell tumor of the spine: computed tomography appearance and review of the literature. J Comput Tomogr. 1987;11(3):307–11. PubMed PMID: 3608560.
36. Randall RL. Giant cell tumor of the sacrum. Neurosurg Focus. 2003;15(2):E13. PubMed PMID: 15350044.

37. Niu X, Xu H, Inwards CY, Li Y, Ding Y, Letson GD, et al. Primary bone tumors: epidemiologic comparison of 9200 patients treated at Beijing Ji Shui Tan Hospital, Beijing, China, with 10 165 patients at Mayo Clinic, Rochester, Minnesota. Arch Pathol Lab Med. 2015;139(9):1149–55. PubMed PMID: 25978765.
38. Muheremu A, Huang Z, Niu X. Treatment for giant cell tumor of the spine metastasizing to the lung: A report of two cases and a literature review. Oncol Lett. 2015;9(3):1321–6. PubMed PMID: PMC4315077.
39. Payer M. Neurological manifestation of sacral tumors. Neurosurg Focus. 2003;15(2):E1. PubMed PMID: 15350032.
40. Nonaka D, Chiriboga L, Rubin BP. Sox10: a pan-schwannian and melanocytic marker. Am J Surg Pathol. 2008;32(9):1291–8. PubMed PMID: 18636017.
41. Pekmezci M, Reuss DE, Hirbe AC, Dahiya S, Gutmann DH, von Deimling A, et al. Morphologic and immunohistochemical features of malignant peripheral nerve sheath tumors and cellular schwannomas. Mod Pathol. 2015;28(2):187–200. PubMed PMID: 25189642.
42. Oliveira AM, Perez-Atayde AR, Inwards CY, Medeiros F, Derr V, Hsi BL, et al. USP6 and CDH11 oncogenes identify the neoplastic cell in primary aneurysmal bone cysts and are absent in so-called secondary aneurysmal bone cysts. Am J Pathol. 2004;165(5):1773–80. PubMed PMID: 15509545. Pubmed Central PMCID: PMC3278819.
43. Bui MM, Smith P, Agresta SV, Cheong D, Letson GD. Practical issues of intraoperative frozen section diagnosis of bone and soft tissue lesions. Cancer Control. 2008;15(1):7–12. PubMed PMID: 18094656.
44. Khalbuss WE, Parwani AV. Cytopathology of soft tissue and bone lesions. New York: Springer; 2011.

Part II

Benign Lesions

Giant Cell Tumor of the Sacrum

8

Andreas F. Mavrogenis, Georgios N. Panagopoulos, Andrea Angelini, and Pietro Ruggieri

8.1 Introduction

Giant cell tumors (GCTs) are relatively common, locally aggressive benign neoplasms of bone that demonstrate a high risk for local recurrence and an occasional propensity for metastatic dissemination [1, 2]. The sacrum is the third most common location of GCTs after the knee and distal radius and the most common location in the axial skeleton [1–4]. Most affected patients are between 20 and 40 years old, with approximately 70% of cases occurring in this age group [1].

Sacral GCT is often initially a silent disease, with the patient frequently remaining symptomless until the tumor reaches an alarming size [5]. The optimal treatment of GCTs of the sacrum is a controversial topic in orthopedic oncology [6]. Although generally considered benign, sacral GCTs and their treatment can be associated with a disproportionately high morbidity. Structures potentially at risk, as a result of both tumor extent and standard treatments, include the lumbosacral nerve roots, iliac vessels, bony integrity of the pelvic ring and hip, bladder, ureters, and rectum [6].

8.2 Epidemiology

GCTs of the bone account for 4–10% of all primary bone tumors and approximately 20% of all benign bone tumors [1, 2, 7–9]. Patients present most often in the third decade of their life, with approximately 80% of lesions occurring between 20 and 55

A.F. Mavrogenis, M.D.,Ph.D. • G.N. Panagopoulos, M.D.
First Department of Orthopaedics, National and Kapodistrian University of Athens, Athens, Greece
e-mail: afm@otenet.gr

A. Angelini, M.D., Ph.D. • P. Ruggieri, M.D., Ph.D. (✉)
Department of Orthopedics and Orthopedic Oncology, University of Padova, Padova, Italy
e-mail: andrea.angelini83@yahoo.it; pietro.ruggieri@unipd.it

P. Ruggieri et al. (eds.), *Tumors of the Sacrum*,
DOI 10.1007/978-3-319-51202-0_8

years of age [1, 7, 10]. It is very unusual for a GCT to occur in patients younger than 20 or older than 55 years [1]. There is a slight predilection for females, with ratios ranging from 1.1:1 to 1.5:1 [11]. Even though GCT affects all races, there is a strangely high prevalence of 20% and 30% in China and Southern India, respectively, that has not quite been explained to date [7, 11]. GCTs of the bone typically affect the meta-epiphyseal region of long bones (75–90%), with approximately 84–99% of lesions extending to within 1 cm of subarticular bone [11–14]. Most of these tumors occur around the knee, with this location accounting for 50–65% of all cases [7, 11–14]. The single most common site is the distal femur (23–30%), followed by the proximal tibia (20–25%), the distal radius (10–12%), the sacrum (4–9%), and the proximal humerus (4–8%) [3, 12, 14]. This makes the sacrum the most common location after the knee and the distal radius as well as the most common location of GCT in the axial skeleton [15–18]. In the sacrum, GCT is the second most common bone tumor (15%), preceded by chordoma (25%) and followed by aneurysmal bone cyst (13%), chondrosarcoma (12%), and osteosarcoma (8%) [19].

8.3 Clinical Presentation and Diagnosis

The onset of symptoms in patients with GCT of the sacrum is generally insidious, with the patient typically complaining of a slowly progressive problem evolving over several months. Alternatively, the tumor might remain silent in its initial stages, being easily misdiagnosed or diagnosed with significant delay when the tumor reaches a critical size. Furthermore, superimposition of bowel gas on radiographs and a frequent lack of clinical awareness may cause for the tumor to be missed, even by otherwise experienced clinicians [5]. Symptoms, when present, usually include localized lower back pain that may radiate to one or both legs, frequently mistaken for sciatica [2, 16]. Neurological symptoms, if at all present, may be subtle [20]; vague abdominal discomfort, early satiety, a progressive change in bowel or bladder habits, and sexual dysfunction have been described [2, 16, 18]. A unilateral lesion to the S2 or S3 nerve root usually leads to mild or moderate bladder, bowel, and/or sexual dysfunction. A bilateral lesion of the S2 or S3 roots always results in complete bladder, bowel, and sexual dysfunction [21, 22]. Thus, the diagnostic workup should be thorough.

A careful patient history should be obtained, and a complete physical exam, including abdominal, neurological, spine, and rectal assessments, should be conducted. As radiographs frequently fail to demonstrate the full extent of the disease, a CT and MR imaging scan should be subsequently obtained for a full anatomic assessment of the tumor and evaluation for a potential invasion of surrounding structures or associated soft tissue masses. Bone scintigraphy, even though likely to reveal nonspecific increased activity, is usually also recommended, to evaluate for noncontiguous disease [23]. A staged biopsy is usually the next necessary step in the clinical assessment of the disease in most cases, as the differential diagnosis of sacral tumors is extensive [2]. The minimally invasive nature of true-cut needle biopsy seems to be the most oncologically sound. A transrectal or transvaginal biopsy should not be performed in any case, since it violates the containing membranes of presacral fascia and periosteum, exponentially increasing the risk for inadvertent tumor seeding [24]. If preoperative core needle biopsy has not been performed, an intraoperative frozen section can also be done [25].

8.4 Imaging

In long bones, the radiographic appearance of GCT is rather characteristic, appearing as an eccentric, lytic lesion with a nonsclerotic and sharply defined geographic border [25–27]. Lesions often demonstrate a prominent trabeculation, sometimes referred to as soap bubble appearance [11]. However, these characteristics may be impossible to appreciate in sacral GCTs. The sacrum is difficult to evaluate fully on radiographs because it is often obscured by overlying stool or bowel gas. Furthermore, the sacrum does not have a distinctive trabecular pattern that can be assessed for disruption. Thus, conventional radiography has a limited sensitivity and may rarely reveal gross calcification or ossification in adjacent soft or an associated contiguous pelvic mass [24]. Therefore, the presence of these signs or, more frequently, a high index of suspicion in absence of concrete findings in radiography should warrant further imaging with CT, MRI, or a bone scan.

CT and MR imaging provide for a superior delineation and staging of GCTs of the sacrum [24–27]. CT is particularly useful for the identification of cortical thinning, pathologic fracture, periosteal reaction, assessing the degree of osseous expansile remodeling, confirming the absence of matrix mineralization [11], and guided biopsy [24]. MRI is superior to CT in delineating tumor soft tissue extension. On MR imaging, GCT typically shows low to intermediate signal intensity on T1-weighted sequences and intermediate to high signal intensity on T2-weighted sequences [25]. A cystic appearance with fluid-fluid levels from secondary cyst formation or aneurysmal bone cyst-like changes is present in 10–14% of GCTs (secondary ABC), especially in the pediatric age group [11, 26, 27]. Therefore, when possible, MR imaging should be the imaging modality of choice to specify the diagnosis, tumor extent into the sacral canal, neurovascular involvement, and preoperative planning [28, 29].

Bone scintigraphy demonstrates increased radionuclide uptake in the vast majority of GCTs [30]. Its main role in GCT of sacrum is for evaluation of the presence of noncontiguous disease. Increased radionuclide uptake peripherally with photopenia centrally (the "donut sign") is another pattern reportedly seen in 57% of cases [31]. Increased uptake in bone across an articulation and in adjacent joints is also common (62%) and should not be mistaken for tumor extension. This phenomenon is termed "contiguous bone activity" and is due to increased blood flow and disuse osteoporosis [30–32]. Finally, angiography in GCTs of the sacrum is typically performed in the context of transcatheter, preoperative, therapeutic arterial embolization, aimed to reduce blood loss during surgical resection, as the majority of these lesions are hypervascular (60–65%) [11, 16, 18]. It can also be done repeatedly as primary treatment [16, 33–35].

8.5 Pathology

In gross examination, GCT of the bone is usually a soft, friable, fleshy, red-brown mass with yellowish areas. The cortex may or may not be involved initially, but it can be ultimately destroyed, with the original bone contour expanded. There may be evidence of hemorrhage, hemosiderin deposition, cyst formation, necrosis, and pathological fracture [1]. A secondary ABC can be seen in 10–14% of GCT of the bone [25]. Microscopically, the basic pattern of giant cell tumor is that of a moderately vascularized stroma with oval or plump, spindle-shaped mononuclear cells uniformly interspersed with multinucleated giant cells [1]. The spindled-shaped mononuclear cells have poorly defined cytoplasm and spindle-shaped nuclei and show variable degrees of mitotic activity. They are thought to represent the proper neoplastic cell population [25]. The multinucleated, osteoclast-like giant cells have eosinophilic cytoplasm and vesicular nuclei and are thought to constitute a reactive cell population in the context of the tumor [25].

From a molecular biology standpoint, RANKL is highly expressed by the neoplastic mononuclear stromal cells. It has been demonstrated that the RANK-RANKL interaction and the macrophage colony-stimulating factor (M-CSF) play an important role in osteoclastogenesis by stimulating recruitment of osteoclastic cells from blood-borne mononuclear osteoclast precursor cells that differentiate into multinucleated osteoclast-like giant cells [36–38]. Cytogenetically, the most common chromosomal aberrations in GCTs (50–70%) are represented by telomeric associations, a chromosomal end-to-end fusion [39, 40]. Telomere length maintenance is thought to be an important key factor in the pathogenesis of GCT [41]. Recently, a driver mutation has also been identified in H3F3A, in 92% of GCTs [42]. Furthermore, allelic losses of 1p, 9q, and 19q are common in primary, recurrent, and metastatic GCTB [39]. Mutations of TP53 and HRAS are seen in secondary malignant GCT, probably playing a role in malignant progression [43, 44].

8.6 Biological Behavior

Approximately 25% of conventional GCTs are considered to be locally aggressive on clinical and radiological grounds [45]. These tumors show extensive bone destruction, cortical expansion, and soft tissue invasion [46]. One of the major issues within GCT of bone is the propensity to local recurrence. After simple curettage, 25–35% of GCTs recur, typically within 2–3 years [4, 46]. Neither local aggressiveness nor recurrence has been associated with any specific histologic findings [1]. GCT has a 2–5% incidence of metastasizing to the lung an average of 3–4 years after primary diagnosis, with the risk being greater in locally recurrent tumors [10, 26]. Pulmonary metastases in GCT (sometimes called benign pulmonary implants) are typically slow growing and usually amenable to surgical resection with a prospect for cure [47, 48]. Even though some patients might succumb as a result of multiple lung lesions, prognosis is favorable in more than 70% of patients, and some metastatic foci may resolve spontaneously [2, 49].

Currently, there are no reliable predictors of recurrence or metastatic disease. A recent array comparative genomic hybridization study of 20 frozen tumors has shown that 20q11.1 is frequently amplified in GCT, and its presence correlates with the occurrence of metastatic disease [50]. True malignant variants of GCT also exist. Kransdorf and Murphey [11] describe a modification of a classification of malignant GCT previously reported by Mirra et al. [51]. They distinguish benign metastasizing GCT, which corresponds to the previously described disease with occasional lung nodules; true malignant GCT, which is defined as a high-grade sarcoma arising in a GCT (primary) or at the site of a previously documented GCT (secondary); and, finally, giant cell-containing sarcoma, most commonly occurring in association with other processes, such as severe polyostotic Paget's disease. Secondary malignant GCT is the most common malignant variant, representing about 87% of such cases [11]. A history of pervious radiation therapy is reported in 76% of the patients with secondary malignant GCT, usually after a delay of 10 or more years [52]. With the decline in the use of therapeutic irradiation for giant cell tumors, radiation-induced sarcoma has become exceedingly rare.

8.7 Treatment

Optimal treatment for GCT of sacrum remains challenging and controversial. Several treatment options have been proposed, but all have disadvantages regarding tumor control, complications, and functional outcome (Fig. 8.1). Additionally, published case series are small and surgical approaches heterogeneous, impeding comparison of results (Table 8.1) [4–6, 15, 16, 18, 33–35, 45, 53–57]. The standard treatment for a giant cell tumor is aggressive curettage followed by adjuvant phenol, hydrogen peroxide, high-speed burring, liquid nitrogen or argon beam therapy, and bone grafting or cementation [6, 35, 55, 58–60], or wide excision [22, 61–64]. Although recurrence rates are lowest after en bloc resection (0–16%), curettage with local adjuvants is preferred because it presents less morbidity and functional impairment, with a recurrence rates ranging from 0 to 33% [25, 65–68]. When local adjuvants are not utilized, the mean recurrence rate is approximately 42% (21–65%) [69, 70].

Surgical management of GCT of the sacrum is more complicated, mostly as a result of late discovery, large size, spinal or pelvic instability, and frequent involvement of nerve roots [15–17]. In case of extended involvement of the proximal part of the sacrum, total sacrectomy has been advocated, as it has been associated with low local recurrence rates (0–8%) [18]. However, as there is a high risk of infection (18–46%), neurological deficits (24–38%), and bladder, rectal, or sexual dysfunction (18–47%), it could be considered overtreatment for an essentially benign tumor [64, 71]. Partial sacrectomy is less mutilating and can be performed for sacral involvement distal to the S2 segment, allowing for preservation of bowel and bladder function without the need for lumbopelvic reconstruction [4]. Marginal resection can be performed for lesions distal to the S3 segment.

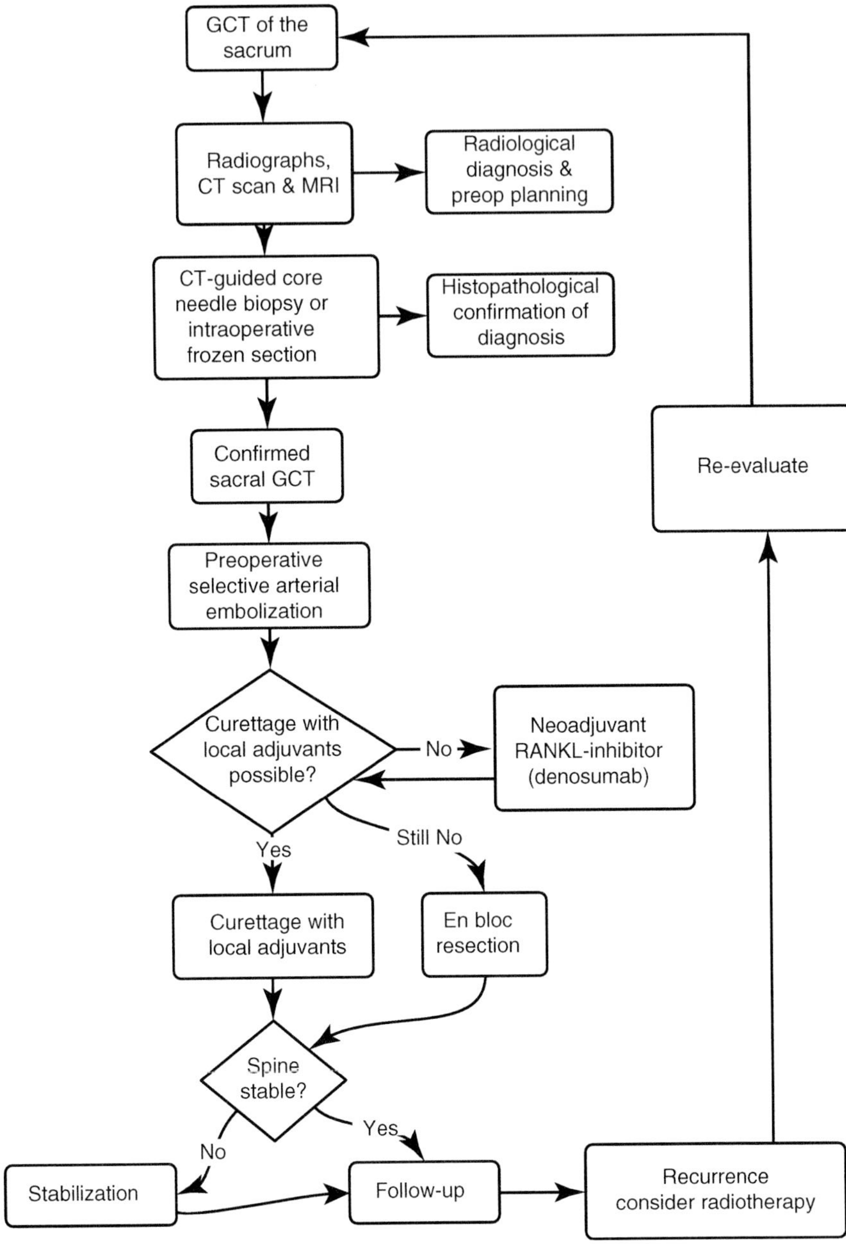

Fig. 8.1 A comprehensive algorithm for the management of GCT of the sacrum

Table 8.1 Summary of the most important published studies on the treatment of GCT of the sacrum

Study	Patients (*n*)	Treatment	Follow-up (months)	Survival to local recurrence (months)
McDonald et al. 1986 [53]	14	Intralesional surgery	Mean, 84; range, 48–312	77% at 84 months
Turcotte et al. 1993 [54]	26	Intralesional surgery, radiation therapy	Mean, 94; range, 84–396	67% at 84 months
Marcove et al. 1994 [55]	7	Cryosurgery and intralesional surgery and/or limited excision	Median, 147; range, 24–170	71.4% at 147 months
Lin et al. 2002 [35]	18	Selective arterial embolization, intra-arterial cisplatin	Median, 105; range, 6–205	69% at 120 months, 57% at 180 and 240 months; no significant effect of cisplatin
Lackman et al. 2002 [34]	5	Serial selective arterial embolization	Mean, 90; range, 48–204	80% at 80.4 months
Leggon et al. 2004 [6]	10	Radiation therapy, intralesional surgery, and chemotherapy	Mean, 96; range, 11–254	80% at 36 months
Hosalkar et al. 2007 [33]	9	Serial selective arterial embolization	Mean, 107; median, 94; range, 46–254	78% at 108 months
Guo et al. 2009 [15]	24	Intralesional surgery, intraoperative occlusion of the abdominal aorta	Mean, 58; median, 50; range, 25–132	69.6% at 60 months
Ruggieri et al. 2010 [4]	31	Intralesional surgery with and without postoperative radiation therapy, selective arterial embolization, phenol, and liquid nitrogen	Mean, 118; median, 108; range, 36–276	90% at 60 and 120 months
Thangaraj et al. 2010 [16]	9	Curettage alone or with embolization ± spinal stabilization ± radiotherapy	Mean, 124; range, 24–256	33% at 19 months
Gaztañaga et al. 2011 [56]	4	Intralesional surgery and radiotherapy	Median, 132; range, 32–144	0% at 32 months
Balke et al. 2011 [45]	10	Curettage and PMMA	Median, 52; range, 15–133	20% at 12 months

(continued)

Table 8.1 (continued)

Study	Patients (n)	Treatment	Follow-up (months)	Survival to local recurrence (months)
Li et al. 2012 [57]	32	Resection (25), curettage (7)	Median, 42; range, 18–115	37.5% at 42 months
Chen et al. 2014 [5]	4	Intralesional curettage and zoledronic acid-loaded cement balls	Mean, 28; range, 25–33	0% at 25 months
Heijden et al. 2014 [18]	26	Intralesional excision with either local adjuvants, radiotherapy, IFN-α, or bisphosphonates	Median, 98; range, 6–229	54% at 13 months

Curettage is less invasive, permitting salvage of nerve roots and visceral structures and maintenance of intrinsic spinal or pelvic support. However, curettage results in relatively high recurrence rates, ranging from 10 to 37% [25]. Caution is warranted with the application of local adjuvants such as phenol or liquid nitrogen in the vicinity of neurovascular structures, as they can induce local necrosis and transient nerve damage [18]. After curettage, spinal or pelvic stability should be assessed and stabilization performed if needed. If at least S1 is preserved after intralesional resection, reconstruction is generally unnecessary. If S1 is partially or completely resected, stabilization with iliolumbar screw fixation is preferred [25].

Selective arterial embolization can be performed serially as primary treatment, or a precursor to surgery to reduce bleeding, as these tumors can be associated with occasional catastrophic intraoperative hemorrhage [16, 33–35]. Systemic therapy alternatives for GCT include bisphosphonates, IFN-a, and denosumab. Denosumab is a human monoclonal antibody and RANKL inhibitor that blocks osteoclast maturation and thus its osteolytic properties. It is currently approved for osteoporosis treatment in postmenopausal women at risk for fracturing, to increase bone mass in patients with prostate or breast cancer who are at risk for fracture due to androgen deprivation therapy or aromatase inhibitor therapy, respectively, and for the prevention of skeletal-related events in patients with bone metastases from solid tumors. It has also been approved by the FDA for the treatment of adults and skeletally mature adolescents with GCTB that is unresectable, or when surgical resection is likely to result in severe morbidity [72]. A recent study has shown clear clinical benefits of denosumab therapy [73]. Finally, another GCT treatment modality is represented by radiotherapy. More used in the near past, it has now gone in misuse, due to concerns for radiation-induced sarcoma. The reported risk of malignant transformation varies between 0 and 5% [74, 75]. Nowadays, radiotherapy should be restricted to those rare cases of unresectable, residual, or recurrent GCTB in which treatment with RANKL inhibitors is not possible or has been proven to be ineffective and when surgery would lead to unacceptable morbidity.

Conclusion

GCT of the sacrum is a benign, but locally aggressive and rarely metastasizing tumor. Aggressive surgery is usually associated with unacceptable morbidity. Treatment decisions should be made by a multidisciplinary team composed of experts in the field of musculoskeletal oncology. Definitive diagnosis should be obtained by accurate imaging, including high-quality radiographs and at least MR imaging. A CT-guided biopsy should complete staging and preoperative planning, for histopathological confirmation of diagnosis. Preoperative selective arterial embolization should be considered in all patients. Preferred treatment is intralesional curettage with local adjuvants. If curettage is not feasible, due to soft tissue extension or neurovascular compromise, neoadjuvant systemic targeted therapy with denosumab should be considered, as it may downsize the lesion and create a calcified rim around the tumor, making excision possible. If curettage is still impossible, en bloc resection may be considered. After surgery, spinopelvic stability should be assessed and reconstruction performed if necessary. Radiotherapy should be restricted to multiple recurrent of refractory GCT, and when denosumab is unavailable, contraindicated or ineffective.

Conflict-of-Interest Statement No benefits have been or will be received from a commercial party related directly or indirectly to the subject matter of this article.

References

1. Dorfman HD, Czerniak B. Bone tumors. St. Louis: Mosby; 1998.
2. Randall RL. Giant cell tumor of the sacrum. Neurosurg Focus. 2003;15(2):E13.
3. Campanacci M, Baldini N, Boriani S, Sudanese A. Giant-cell tumor of bone. J Bone Joint Surg Am. 1987;69(1):106–14.
4. Ruggieri P, Mavrogenis AF, Ussia G, Angelini A, Papagelopoulos PJ, Mercuri M. Recurrence after and complications associated with adjuvant treatments for sacral giant cell tumor. Clin Orthop Relat Res. 2010;468(11):2954–61. doi:10.1007/s11999-010-1448-8.
5. Chen KH, Wu PK, Chen CF, Chen WM. Zoledronic acid-loaded bone cement as a local adjuvant therapy for giant cell tumor of the sacrum after intralesional curettage. Eur Spine J. 2015;24(10):2182–8. doi:10.1007/s00586-015-3978-y.
6. Leggon RE, Zlotecki R, Reith J, Scarborough MT. Giant cell tumor of the pelvis and sacrum: 17 cases and analysis of the literature. Clin Orthop Relat Res. 2004;423:196–207.
7. Turcotte RE. Giant cell tumor of bone. Orthop Clin North Am. 2006;37(1):35–51. doi:10.1016/j.ocl.2005.08.005.
8. Zhang K, Chen K, Zhou M, Chen H, Lu J, Yang H. Extremely large giant-cell tumor of sacrum with successful resection via posterior approach. Spine J. 2015;15(7):1684–5. doi:10.1016/j.spinee.2015.02.007.
9. Feigenberg SJ, Marcus Jr RB, Zlotecki RA, Scarborough MT, Berrey BH, Enneking WF. Radiation therapy for giant cell tumors of bone. Clin Orthop Relat Res. 2003;411:207–16. doi:10.1097/01.blo.0000069890.31220.b4.
10. Reid R, Banerjee S, Sciot R. Giant cell tumour. In: Fletcher D, Unni K, Mertens F, editors. WHO Classification of tumors. Pathology and genetics: tumors of soft tissue and bone. Lyon: IARC Press; 2002. p. 310–2.

11. Kransdorf M, Murphey M. Giant cell tumor. In: Davies M, Sundaram M, James S, editors. Imaging of bone tumors and tumor-like lesions. Berlin: Springer; 2009. p. 321–36.
12. Dahlin DC, Cupps RE, Johnson Jr EW. Giant-cell tumor: a study of 195 cases. Cancer. 1970;25(5):1061–70.
13. Resnick D. Diagnosis of bone and joint disorders. 3rd ed. Philadelphia: Saunders; 1995.
14. Unni KK, Dahlin DC. Dahlin's bone tumors: general aspects and data on 11,087 cases. 5th ed. Philadelphia: Lippincott-Raven; 1996.
15. Guo W, Ji T, Tang X, Yang Y. Outcome of conservative surgery for giant cell tumor of the sacrum. Spine. 2009;34(10):1025–31. doi:10.1097/BRS.0b013e31819d4127.
16. Thangaraj R, Grimer RJ, Carter SR, Stirling AJ, Spilsbury J, Spooner D. Giant cell tumour of the sacrum: a suggested algorithm for treatment. Eur Spine J. 2010;19(7):1189–94. doi:10.1007/s00586-009-1270-8.
17. Martin C, McCarthy EF. Giant cell tumor of the sacrum and spine: series of 23 cases and a review of the literature. Iowa Orthop J. 2010;30:69–75.
18. van der Heijden L, van de Sande MA, van der Geest IC, Schreuder HW, van Royen BJ, Jutte PC, Bramer JA, Oner FC, van Noort-Suijdendorp AP, Kroon HM, Dijkstra PD. Giant cell tumors of the sacrum—a nationwide study on midterm results in 26 patients after intralesional excision. Eur Spine J. 2014;23(9):1949–62. doi:10.1007/s00586-014-3263-5.
19. Bloem JL, Reidsma II. Bone and soft tissue tumors of hip and pelvis. Eur J Radiol. 2012;81(12):3793–801. doi:10.1016/j.ejrad.2011.03.101.
20. Saikia B, Goel A, Gupta SK. Fine-needle aspiration cytologic diagnosis of giant-cell tumor of the sacrum presenting as a rectal mass: a case report. Diagn Cytopathol. 2001;24(1):39–41.
21. Payer M. Neurological manifestation of sacral tumors. Neurosurg Focus. 2003;15(2):E1. doi:10.3171/foc.2003.15.2.1.
22. Althausen PL, Schneider PD, Bold RJ, Gupta MC, Goodnight Jr JE, Khatri VP. Multimodality management of a giant cell tumor arising in the proximal sacrum: case report. Spine. 2002;27(15):E361–5.
23. Higuchi T, Taki J, Sumiya H, Kinuya S, Bunko H, Nonomura A, Tsuchiya H, Tonami N. Intense 201 Tl uptake in giant-cell tumour of bone. Nucl Med Commun. 2002;23(6):595–9.
24. Mavrogenis AF, Patapis P, Kostopanagiotou G, Papagelopoulos PJ. Tumors of the sacrum. Orthopedics. 2009;32(5):342.
25. van der Heijden L, Dijkstra PD, van de Sande MA, Kroep JR, Nout RA, van Rijswijk CS, Bovee JV, Hogendoorn PC, Gelderblom H. The clinical approach toward giant cell tumor of bone. Oncologist. 2014;19(5):550–61. doi:10.1634/theoncologist.2013-0432.
26. Murphey MD, Nomikos GC, Flemming DJ, Gannon FH, Temple HT, Kransdorf MJ. From the archives of AFIP. Imaging of giant cell tumor and giant cell reparative granuloma of bone: radiologic-pathologic correlation. Radiographics. 2001;21(5):1283–309. doi:10.1148/radiographics.21.5.g01se251283.
27. Chakarun CJ, Forrester DM, Gottsegen CJ, Patel DB, White EA, Matcuk Jr GR. Giant cell tumor of bone: review, mimics, and new developments in treatment. Radiographics. 2013;33(1):197–211. doi:10.1148/rg.331125089.
28. Manaster BJ, Graham T. Imaging of sacral tumors. Neurosurg Focus. 2003;15(2):E2.
29. Gerber S, Ollivier L, Leclere J, Vanel D, Missenard G, Brisse H, de Pinieux G, Neuenschwander S. Imaging of sacral tumours. Skeletal Radiol. 2008;37(4):277–89. doi:10.1007/s00256-007-0413-4.
30. Wang K, Allen L, Fung E, Chan CC, Chan JC, Griffith JF. Bone scintigraphy in common tumors with osteolytic components. Clin Nucl Med. 2005;30(10):655–71.
31. Levine E, De Smet AA, Neff JR, Martin NL. Scintigraphic evaluation of giant cell tumor of bone. AJR Am J Roentgenol. 1984;143(2):343–8. doi:10.2214/ajr.143.2.343.
32. Levine E, De Smet AA, Neff JR. Role of radiologic imaging in management planning of giant cell tumor of bone. Skeletal Radiol. 1984;12(2):79–89.
33. Hosalkar HS, Jones KJ, King JJ, Lackman RD. Serial arterial embolization for large sacral giant-cell tumors: mid- to long-term results. Spine. 2007;32(10):1107–15. doi:10.1097/01.brs.0000261558.94247.8d.

34. Lackman RD, Khoury LD, Esmail A, Donthineni-Rao R. The treatment of sacral giant-cell tumours by serial arterial embolisation. J Bone Joint Surg Br. 2002;84(6):873–7.
35. Lin PP, Guzel VB, Moura MF, Wallace S, Benjamin RS, Weber KL, Morello Jr FA, Gokaslan ZL, Yasko AW. Long-term follow-up of patients with giant cell tumor of the sacrum treated with selective arterial embolization. Cancer. 2002;95(6):1317–25. doi:10.1002/cncr.10803.
36. Thomas DM. RANKL, denosumab, and giant cell tumor of bone. Curr Opin Oncol. 2012;24(4):397–403. doi:10.1097/CCO.0b013e328354c129.
37. Roux S, Amazit L, Meduri G, Guiochon-Mantel A, Milgrom E, Mariette X. RANK (receptor activator of nuclear factor kappa B) and RANK ligand are expressed in giant cell tumors of bone. Am J Clin Pathol. 2002;117(2):210–6. doi:10.1309/BPET-F2PE-P2BD-J3P3.
38. Liao TS, Yurgelun MB, Chang SS, Zhang HZ, Murakami K, Blaine TA, Parisien MV, Kim W, Winchester RJ, Lee FY. Recruitment of osteoclast precursors by stromal cell derived factor-1 (SDF-1) in giant cell tumor of bone. J Orthop Res. 2005;23(1):203–9. doi:10.1016/j.orthres.2004.06.018.
39. Rao UN, Goodman M, Chung WW, Swalski P, Pal R, Finkelstein S. Molecular analysis of primary and recurrent giant cell tumors of bone. Cancer Genet Cytogenet. 2005;158(2):126–36. doi:10.1016/j.cancergencyto.2004.09.015.
40. Gorunova L, Vult von Steyern F, Storlazzi CT, Bjerkehagen B, Folleras G, Heim S, Mandahl N, Mertens F. Cytogenetic analysis of 101 giant cell tumors of bone: nonrandom patterns of telomeric associations and other structural aberrations. Genes Chromosomes Cancer. 2009;48(7):583–602. doi:10.1002/gcc.20667.
41. Forsyth RG, De Boeck G, Bekaert S, De Meyer T, Taminiau AH, Uyttendaele D, Roels H, Praet MM, Hogendoorn PC. Telomere biology in giant cell tumour of bone. J Pathol. 2008;214(5):555–63. doi:10.1002/path.2301.
42. Behjati S, Tarpey PS, Presneau N, Scheipl S, Pillay N, Van Loo P, Wedge DC, Cooke SL, Gundem G, Davies H, Nik-Zainal S, Martin S, McLaren S, Goody V, Robinson B, Butler A, Teague JW, Halai D, Khatri B, Myklebost O, Baumhoer D, Jundt G, Hamoudi R, Tirabosco R, Amary MF, Futreal PA, Stratton MR, Campbell PJ, Flanagan AM. Distinct H3F3A and H3F3B driver mutations define chondroblastoma and giant cell tumor of bone. Nat Genet. 2013;45(12):1479–82. doi:10.1038/ng.2814.
43. Oda Y, Sakamoto A, Saito T, Matsuda S, Tanaka K, Iwamoto Y, Tsuneyoshi M. Secondary malignant giant-cell tumour of bone: molecular abnormalities of p53 and H-ras gene correlated with malignant transformation. Histopathology. 2001;39(6):629–37.
44. Saito T, Mitomi H, Izumi H, Suehara Y, Okubo T, Torigoe T, Takagi T, Kaneko K, Sato K, Matsumoto T, Yao T. A case of secondary malignant giant-cell tumor of bone with p53 mutation after long-term follow-up. Hum Pathol. 2011;42(5):727–33. doi:10.1016/j.humpath.2010.08.008.
45. Balke M, Schremper L, Gebert C, Ahrens H, Streitbuerger A, Koehler G, Hardes J, Gosheger G. Giant cell tumor of bone: treatment and outcome of 214 cases. J Cancer Res Clin Oncol. 2008;134(9):969–78. doi:10.1007/s00432-008-0370-x.
46. Sanerkin NG. Malignancy, aggressiveness, and recurrence in giant cell tumor of bone. Cancer. 1980;46(7):1641–9.
47. Dominkus M, Ruggieri P, Bertoni F, Briccoli A, Picci P, Rocca M, Mercuri M. Histologically verified lung metastases in benign giant cell tumours—14 cases from a single institution. Int Orthop. 2006;30(6):499–504. doi:10.1007/s00264-006-0204-x.
48. Donthineni R, Boriani L, Ofluoglu O, Bandiera S. Metastatic behaviour of giant cell tumour of the spine. Int Orthop. 2009;33(2):497–501. doi:10.1007/s00264-008-0560-9.
49. Siebenrock KA, Unni KK, Rock MG. Giant-cell tumour of bone metastasising to the lungs. A long-term follow-up. J Bone Joint Surg Br. 1998;80(1):43–7.
50. Lewis VO. What's new in musculoskeletal oncology. J Bone Joint Surg Am. 2007;89(6):1399–407. doi:10.2106/JBJS.G.00075.
51. Mirra JM, Picci P, Gold RH. Bone tumors: clinical, radiologic, and pathologic correlations. Philadelphia: Lea & Febiger; 1989.

52. Horvai A, Unni KK. Premalignant conditions of bone. J Orthop Sci. 2006;11(4):412–23. doi:10.1007/s00776-006-1037-6.
53. McDonald DJ, Sim FH, McLeod RA, Dahlin DC. Giant-cell tumor of bone. J Bone Joint Surg Am. 1986;68(2):235–42.
54. Turcotte RE, Sim FH, Unni KK. Giant cell tumor of the sacrum. Clin Orthop Relat Res. 1993;291:215–21.
55. Marcove RC, Sheth DS, Brien EW, Huvos AG, Healey JH. Conservative surgery for giant cell tumors of the sacrum. The role of cryosurgery as a supplement to curettage and partial excision. Cancer. 1994;74(4):1253–60.
56. Gaztanaga M, Aristu J, Villas C, San-Julian M. Giant cell tumors of the sacrum treated with intralesional resection and radiotherapy: a case series and review of the literature. Eur Orthop Traumatol. 2011;1:175–9.
57. Li G, Fu D, Chen K, Ma X, Sun M, Sun W, Li J, Cai Z. Surgical strategy for the management of sacral giant cell tumors: a 32-case series. Spine J. 2012;12(6):484–91. doi:10.1016/j.spinee.2012.06.014.
58. Eftekhari F, Wallace S, Chuang VP, Soo CS, Cangir A, Benjamin RS, Murray JA. Intraarterial management of giant-cell tumors of the spine in children. Pediatr Radiol. 1982;12(6):289–93.
59. Gottfried ON, Schmidt MH, Stevens EA. Embolization of sacral tumors. Neurosurg Focus. 2003;15(2):E4.
60. Kollender Y, Meller I, Bickels J, Flusser G, Issakov J, Merimsky O, Marouani N, Nirkin A, Weinbroum AA. Role of adjuvant cryosurgery in intralesional treatment of sacral tumors. Cancer. 2003;97(11):2830–8. doi:10.1002/cncr.11383.
61. Ozaki T, Liljenqvist U, Halm H, Hillmann A, Gosheger G, Winkelmann W. Giant cell tumor of the spine. Clin Orthop Relat Res. 2002;401:194–201.
62. Persson BM, Ekelund L, Lovdahl R, Gunterberg B. Favourable results of acrylic cementation for giant cell tumors. Acta Orthop Scand. 1984;55(2):209–14.
63. Raque Jr GH, Vitaz TW, Shields CB. Treatment of neoplastic diseases of the sacrum. J Surg Oncol. 2001;76(4):301–7.
64. Sar C, Eralp L. Surgical treatment of primary tumors of the sacrum. Arch Orthop Trauma Surg. 2002;122(3):148–55. doi:10.1007/s00402-001-0356-5.
65. Kivioja AH, Blomqvist C, Hietaniemi K, Trovik C, Walloe A, Bauer HC, Jorgensen PH, Bergh P, Folleras G. Cement is recommended in intralesional surgery of giant cell tumors: a Scandinavian Sarcoma Group study of 294 patients followed for a median time of 5 years. Acta Orthop. 2008;79(1):86–93. doi:10.1080/17453670710014815.
66. Algawahmed H, Turcotte R, Farrokhyar F, Ghert M. High-speed burring with and without the use of surgical adjuvants in the intralesional management of giant cell tumor of bone: a systematic review and meta-analysis. Sarcoma. 2010; doi:10.1155/2010/586090.
67. Errani C, Ruggieri P, Asenzio MA, Toscano A, Colangeli S, Rimondi E, Rossi G, Longhi A, Mercuri M. Giant cell tumor of the extremity: a review of 349 cases from a single institution. Cancer Treat Rev. 2010;36(1):1–7. doi:10.1016/j.ctrv.2009.09.002.
68. Klenke FM, Wenger DE, Inwards CY, Rose PS, Sim FH. Giant cell tumor of bone: risk factors for recurrence. Clin Orthop Relat Res. 2011;469(2):591–9. doi:10.1007/s11999-010-1501-7.
69. Trieb K, Bitzan P, Lang S, Dominkus M, Kotz R. Recurrence of curetted and bone-grafted giant-cell tumours with and without adjuvant phenol therapy. Eur J Surg Oncol. 2001;27(2):200–2. doi:10.1053/ejso.2000.1086.
70. Gaston CL, Bhumbra R, Watanuki M, Abudu AT, Carter SR, Jeys LM, Tillman RM, Grimer RJ. Does the addition of cement improve the rate of local recurrence after curettage of giant cell tumours in bone? J Bone Joint Surg Br. 2011;93(12):1665–9. doi:10.1302/0301-620X.93B12.27663.
71. Wuisman P, Lieshout O, Sugihara S, van Dijk M. Total sacrectomy and reconstruction: oncologic and functional outcome. Clin Orthop Relat Res. 2000;381:192–203.

72. Chawla S, Henshaw R, Seeger L, Choy E, Blay JY, Ferrari S, Kroep J, Grimer R, Reichardt P, Rutkowski P, Schuetze S, Skubitz K, Staddon A, Thomas D, Qian Y, Jacobs I. Safety and efficacy of denosumab for adults and skeletally mature adolescents with giant cell tumour of bone: interim analysis of an open-label, parallel-group, phase 2 study. Lancet Oncol. 2013;14(9):901–8. doi:10.1016/S1470-2045(13)70277-8.
73. Thomas D, Henshaw R, Skubitz K, Chawla S, Staddon A, Blay JY, Roudier M, Smith J, Ye Z, Sohn W, Dansey R, Jun S. Denosumab in patients with giant-cell tumour of bone: an open-label, phase 2 study. Lancet Oncol. 2010;11(3):275–80. doi:10.1016/S1470-2045(10)70010-3.
74. Shi W, Indelicato DJ, Reith J, Smith KB, Morris CG, Scarborough MT, Gibbs Jr CP, Mendenhall WM, Zlotecki RA. Radiotherapy in the management of giant cell tumor of bone. Am J Clin Oncol. 2013;36(5):505–8. doi:10.1097/COC.0b013e3182568fb6.
75. Ruka W, Rutkowski P, Morysinski T, Nowecki Z, Zdzienicki M, Makula D, Ptaszynski K, Bylina E, Grzesiakowska U. The megavoltage radiation therapy in treatment of patients with advanced or difficult giant cell tumors of bone. Int J Radiat Oncol Biol Phys. 2010;78(2):494–8. doi:10.1016/j.ijrobp.2009.07.1704.

9 Osteoblastoma of the Sacrum

Andrea Angelini and Pietro Ruggieri

9.1 Introduction

Osteoblastoma is a rare benign bone-forming tumor that accounts for approximately 1% of all bone neoplasm [1–4]. It may occur in any area of the skeleton, but it is more frequently observed in the spine (mainly in the mobile segments whereas sacrum is rarely affected) [1, 5]. Due to the rarity of the tumor and the usual delay in diagnosis, the optimal treatment of sacral osteoblastomas is controversial [1, 5–8]. Although benign, these tumors may occasionally pose a challenge in histopathologic evaluation and differential diagnosis with malignant tumors as well as in the choice of adequate surgical treatment [6, 7].

9.2 Epidemiology, Presentation, and Diagnosis

Sacral osteoblastomas are more rare than those affecting the mobile spine [1, 4], accounting for about 7–17% of all spinal osteoblastomas [1, 5]. The typical presentation is between 10 and 20 years of age [1, 2], with approximately 90% being diagnosed before the age of 30 years [1, 2], and males being affected slightly more frequently [1–5, 9–28]. Most patients with a sacral osteoblastoma remain asymptomatic for a long period of time. Presentation tends to be with pain and neurologic deficits, and there is often a delay of several months between onset of symptoms and surgery due to the wide differential for low back pain seen in routine practice [9, 11]. In a series of 18 patients from a single institution, the mean duration of symptoms was 29 months, ranging from 1 month to 12 years [6]. Pain is the most common presenting symptom and is caused by mass effect and compression, even if

A. Angelini, M.D., Ph.D. • P. Ruggieri, M.D., Ph.D. (✉)
Department of Orthopedics and Orthopedic Oncology, University of Padova, Padova, Italy
e-mail: andrea.angelini83@yahoo.it; pietro.ruggieri@unipd.it

P. Ruggieri et al. (eds.), *Tumors of the Sacrum*,
DOI 10.1007/978-3-319-51202-0_9

osteoblastomas could become symptomatic secondary to involvement of nerves, or because of pathologic fractures. Pain may be either localized, low back, or radicular involving one or more lumbosacral nerve roots, sometimes with sensory defects. Structures including the lumbosacral nerve roots, iliac vessels, the bony support of the pelvic ring, the hip, the ureters, the bladder, and the rectum all can be jeopardized [3, 7, 9, 11, 12, 29].

9.3 Imaging

The most important aspect in the imaging evaluation is the clinical suspect of a sacral lesion. On plain radiographs, the sacrum can be frequently obscured by overlying stool or bowel gas, but sometimes it is possible to identify an osteolytic lesion. Osteoblastoma appears as a well-defined osteolytic lesion typically greater than one cm in diameter that may expand the sacral bone. Minimal perilesional bone sclerosis may be an additional finding. Calcifications, when present, are usually multiple. In some patients, osteoblastomas showing cortical destruction and extension into adjacent soft tissue have an aggressive appearance. Nonetheless, for more thorough evaluation and better defined spatial understanding, additional imaging such as computed tomography (CT) scan or magnetic resonance imaging (MRI) is required. Computed tomography (CT scan) is the preferred imaging modality, since it can identify the lesion, degree of sclerosis, and extent of bony involvement [30]. MRI has a limited role in spinal osteoblastomas because findings can be misleading due to adjacent inflammatory changes [31]. The edema is a nonspecific response of tissue to a stimulus of the tumor inflammation. In addition, visualization of the margin between the osseous and soft tissues is less defined resulting in inaccurate diagnosis of aggressive or malignant lesions [32, 33]. The complementary evaluation of data from both CT scan and MRI is strongly recommended for the preoperative imaging evaluation because while CT scan is essential to properly look at the extent of bony involvement, MRI is complementary and should be obtained when possible to look at the canal, nerve roots, soft tissues, and extraspinal extension.

9.4 Pathology

Osteoblastoma is a benign primary bone tumor composed of well-vascularized connective tissue, in which there is active production of osteoid and primitive woven bone [1–5]. It is defined histologically as a bone-forming neoplasm showing woven bone spicules, which are bordered by prominent osteoblasts without atypia. OBs have a wide spectrum of clinicoradiological and histopathological features. Besides the classic OB, borderline tumors with radiological and histopathological features between OB and osteosarcoma (OS), such as pseudomalignant OB [34, 35], aggressive OB, or malignant OB [8, 36], exist. Moreover, a fraction of OBs may undergo malignant transformation [37, 38]. It is often difficult to distinguish an OB from an OS by routine histopathological procedures alone [3]. Despite similar histologic features, there has not been confirmation of a direct progression from osteoma to osteoblastoma, as well as few reports indicated a malignant degeneration. Osteoblastoma-like osteosarcoma is an entity that can be sometimes misleading and misdiagnosed [3, 8, 29, 39]. Although the exact histopathologic differential diagnosis between osteosarcoma and osteoblastoma may be difficult in some cases [7, 40], it is of clinical importance because the prognosis and the treatment of the two tumor forms differ. OB generally shows an active osteoblastic proliferation with regular alternation of osteoids and woven bone spicules or trabeculae. Scattered foci of osteoclastic bone resorption may appear, but the presence of destructive permeation of preexisting bone tissues is the most helpful criteria in distinguishing OB from osteosarcoma [3, 41]. In some cases of OB, large and plump osteoblasts with a hyperchromatic nucleus and nucleoli, and occasionally mitoses, may be observed. Studies on COX-2 expression in osteoid osteoma and chondroblastoma suggested that COX-2 expression is relatively frequent [42–44]. Hosono et al. confirmed that there was strong and diffused expression of COX-2 in OB, whereas it was only observed in the chondroblastic cells of osteosarcoma, concluding that this is a valuable immunohistochemical marker in the differential diagnosis [41]. Moreover, current molecular genetic examination may help solve this dilemma [29].

9.5 Treatment

Although a slow growing benign neoplasm, osteoblastoma is challenging when it occurs in a difficult location such as mobile spine or the sacrum. While osteoid osteomas are most frequently treated because of the persistent pain associated with them, osteoblastomas are treated both for pain and the increase in size, which leads to destruction of bone and often can become alarming in the pelvis. Although histologically similar to osteoid osteomas, which can be treated with percutaneous ablation techniques and incomplete resections, osteoblastoma tends to be more locally aggressive, of a larger size, and has a higher recurrence rate, as well as a potential for malignant degeneration [8]. Treatment options include radiation therapy, surgery with intralesional margins, surgery with intralesional margins and radiation therapy, surgery with intralesional margins and local adjuvants (phenol or cryosurgical techniques), and resection with wide margins. In the largest review of 306 osteoblastoma cases from the Mayo Clinic, complete treatment and long-term clinic follow-up were available for 75 patients only [3]. In that study, intralesional resection had a significant recurrence rate of 19% (10/52), marginal resection 5.6% (1/18), and wide resection 20% (1/5). Unfortunately, the authors did not explain the type of treatment and outcome of the 13 cases of sacral osteoblastoma, and therefore we cannot get useful information on this specific site [3].

9.5.1 Radiotherapy

The rationale in the use of radiation therapy is the improvement of local control considering that spinal osteoblastoma has the highest recurrence rates of all locations due to the anatomic constraints such as the neurological structures and dura mater [45]. Unfortunately, this has not been shown to prevent recurrence after inadequate excision [45, 46], and disadvantages include local adverse effects and the potential for causing radio-induced sarcomas [39]. Marsh et al. in a review of 197 osteoblastoma cases conclude that "radiotherapy does not alter the course of the disease and appears to be contraindicated" [47]. Through our literature review, we were able to find only one case of sacral osteoblastoma treated with radiotherapy alone: an 18-year-old boy treated to a dose of 45 Gy with regression of the lesion and improvement in pain, motor, and sensory functions at 1 year of follow-up [25]. The insufficient follow-up of this report clearly does not justify to advocate the use of radiotherapy alone.

9.5.2 Intralesional Surgery

Surgery with intralesional margins often can spare nerve roots, pelvic support, and visceral structures depending on the location of the lesion. The disadvantage of intralesional margins for such an aggressive benign tumor implies an increased risk of local recurrence since this procedure leaves behind microscopic disease. Generally, intralesional excision in the form of curettage, with or without addition of local adjuvants, provides a good local control for sacral osteoblastoma [3, 7, 10–13, 21, 22, 27]. Ruggieri et al. reported a high number of intralesional excision treatments in sacral osteoblastoma concluding that it is an effective treatment for osteoblastoma although the recurrence rate was relatively high [6]. Fourteen patients (82%) were successfully treated at first surgery and three patients (18%) after a second time for local recurrence [6]. The other problem associated with intralesional surgery is the robust blood supply, especially in the sacrum. As osteoblastoma is a hypervascular tumor, preoperative embolization can reduce intraoperative bleeding and make surgery more feasible [48–50]. Recently, "ice ball freezing technique" using cryosurgical probe to freeze vascularized neoplastic tissue as an adjunct to surgical excision has been promoted as treatment for highly vascularized bone tumors [51]. Ruggieri et al. reported a case treated with intraoperative cryosurgery with "ice ball" technique in combination with two serial preoperative embolizations, with good control of bleeding during curettage [6] (Fig. 9.1).

9.5.3 Sacral Resection

Resection with wide margins should theoretically minimize the chance of local recurrence but at the cost of increase risk of surgical morbidity, especially for lesion located proximal to S3 [19, 22, 52].

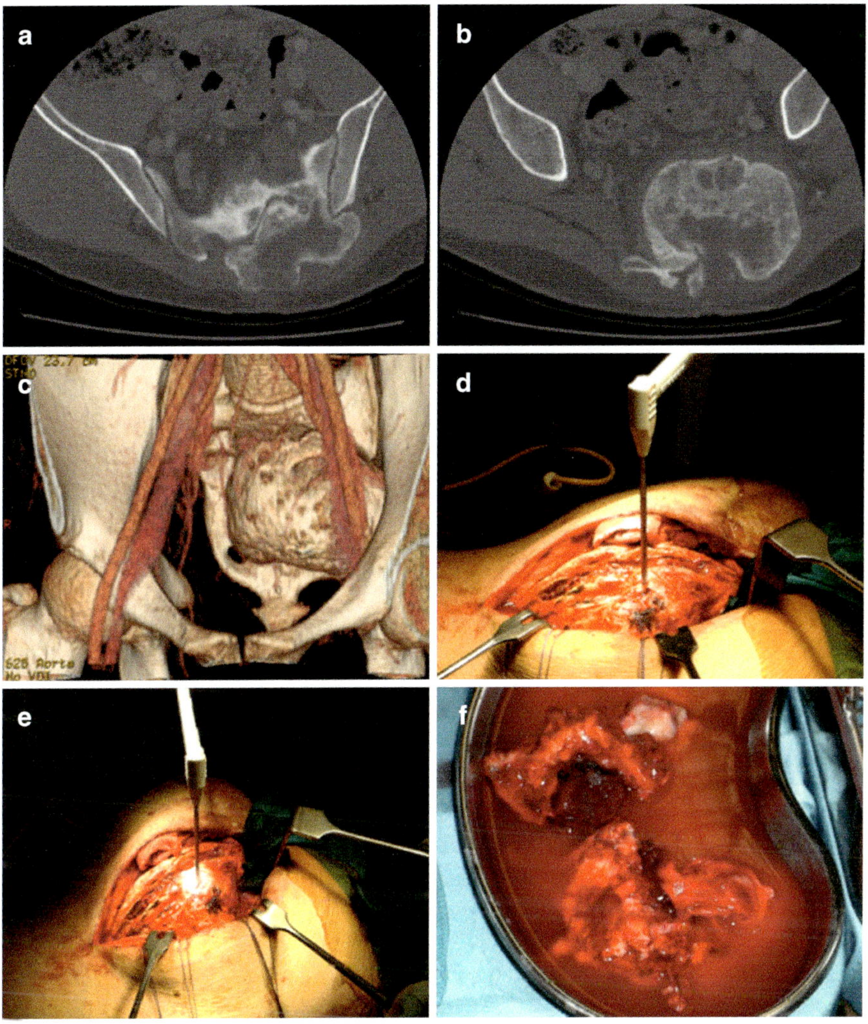

Fig. 9.1 Osteoblastoma of the sacrum in a 19-year-old male. (**a–b**) CT scan axial images show that the lesion is well limited and is surrounded by reactive sclerosis. (**c**) CT-3D reconstruction shows the anatomic relationship with vascular structures. (**d–e**) Intraoperative pictures. A cryosurgery has been performed as local adjuvant. (**f**) Specimen after curettage. Note the "ice balls"

9.5.4 Radio-Frequency Thermal Ablation

Image-guided radio-frequency thermal ablation (RFTA) reduces the pain and improves the function and quality of life of patients with painful bone tumors. It has been used to treat benign bone tumors and tumor-like lesions, and it is the gold-standard procedure for most osteoid osteomas [53]. Even if osteoblastoma is histologically similar to osteoid osteoma, this tumor can exhibit aggressive behavior, and recurrences are not uncommon after classic treatment by surgical excision or curettage [54]. RFTA could be performed in the same way as for osteoid osteomas, using electrodes with a longer active tip or a greater number of ablation sessions or multitip array probes [55].

9.6 Oncologic Outcome

In our literature review, we were able to find only one case of sacral osteoblastoma that died of disease [17]. Dal Cin et al. reported a 35-year-old man with osteoblastoma of the sacroiliac joint treated with partial resection. The pathologic examination revealed an intralesional margin, and the patient was subsequently treated with chemotherapy and radiation therapy (without effect) and died 2 years after diagnosis [17]. The authors explained the aggressive clinical behavior with a possible malignant transformation of the stromal component [17].

The recurrence rates for osteoblastomas of the spine after intralesional excision have been reported between 10 and 19% [3, 56, 57], but the rate approaches 50% in the more aggressive pattern. Some studies reported a correlation between the incidence of recurrence and a previous inadequate treatment in non-referral centers [52, 58]. Boriani et al. [58], in a series of 50 osteoblastomas of the mobile spine, reported an incidence of recurrence among "not intact" patients (cases already treated elsewhere) significantly higher compared to "intact" patients (cases treated in the same institution since the beginning): 50% vs. 5%. Some tumors are more prone to recurrence than others, and some factors relating to surgery may explain this, but the molecular features driving this for osteoblastoma are not known. Also in authors' experience, previous inadequate intralesional surgery was associated with higher rate of local recurrence (40%—two local recurrences in five cases) than patients primarily treated at a specialized tumor center with high levels of surgical and oncologic expertise (7.7%—one local recurrence in 13 cases) [6].

Conflict-of-Interest Statement No benefits have been or will be received from a commercial party related directly or indirectly to the subject matter of this article.

References

1. Unni KK. Benign osteoblastoma (giant osteoid osteoma). In: Unni KK, editor. Dahlin's bone tumours: general aspects and data on 11087 cases. 5th ed. Philadelphia: Lippincott-Raven; 1996. p. 131–42.
2. Greenspan A, Remagen W. Differential diagnosis of tumors and tumor-like lesions of bone and joints. Philadelphia: Lippincott-Raven; 1998. p. 25–366.
3. Lucas DR, Unni KK, McLeod RA, O'Connor MI, Sim FH. Osteoblastoma: clinicopathologic study of 306 cases. Hum Pathol. 1994;25(2):117–34.
4. Campanacci L. Osteoblastoma. In: Picci P, et al., editors. Atlas of musculoskeletal tumors and tumor like lesions. Switzerland: Springer; 2014. p. 81–4.
5. Campanacci M. Bone and soft tissue tumors. New York: Springer; 1993.

6. Ruggieri P, Huch K, Mavrogenis AF, Merlino B, Angelini A. Osteoblastoma of the sacrum: report of 18 cases and analysis of the literature. Spine. 2014;39(2):E97–E103.
7. Bertoni F, Bacchini P, Donati D, Martini A, Picci P, Campanacci M. Osteoblastoma-like osteosarcoma. The Rizzoli Institute experience. Mod Pathol. 1993 Nov;6(6):707–16.
8. Dorfman HD, Weiss SW. Borderline osteoblastic tumors: problems in the differential diagnosis of aggressive osteoblastoma and low-grade osteosarcoma. Semin Diagn Pathol. 1984;1:215–34.
9. Biagini R, Orsini U, Demitri S, et al. Osteoid osteoma and osteoblastoma of the sacrum. Orthopedics. 2001;24(11):1061–4.
10. Bessou P, Lefournier V, Ramoul A, Vasdev A, Boubagra K, Crouzet G. Benign vertebral osteoblastoma. Report of 6 cases. J Neuroradiol. 1998;25(1):21–31.
11. Ozaki T, Liljengvist U, Hillmann A, et al. Osteoid osteoma and osteoblastoma of the spine: experiences with 22 patients. Clin Orthop Relat Res. 2002;397:394–402.
12. Berry M, Mankin H, Gebhardt M, Rosemberg A, Hornicek F. Osteoblastoma: a 30-year study of 99 cases. J Surg Oncol. 2008;98(3):179–83.
13. Poleksic ZR, Lalosevic VJ, Milinkovic ZB. Osteoblastoma of the spine. Acta Chir Iugosl. 2010;57(1):63–8.
14. Chakrapani SD, Grim K, Kaimaktchiev V, Anderson JC. Osteoblastoma of the spine with discordant magnetic resonance imaging and computed tomography imaging features in a child. Spine. 2008;33(25):E968–70.
15. Khan IS, Thakur JD, Chittiboina P, Nanda A. Large sacral osteoblastoma: a case report and review of multi-disciplinary management strategies. J La State Med Soc. 2012;164(5):251–5.
16. Ruggieri P, McLeod RA, Unni KK, Sim FH. Osteoblastoma. Orthopedics. 1996;19(7):621–4.
17. Dal Cin P, Sciot R, Samson I, De Wever I, Van den Berghe H. Osteoid osteoma and osteoblastoma with clonal chromosome changes. Br J Cancer. 1998;78(3):344–8.
18. Della Rocca C, Huvos AG. Osteoblastoma: varied histological presentations with a benign clinical course. An analysis of 55 cases. Am J Surg Pathol. 1996;20(7):841–50.
19. Sar C, Eralp L. Surgical treatment of primary tumors of the sacrum. Arch Orthop Trauma Surg. 2002;122(3):148–55.
20. Jambhekar NA, Desai S, Khapake D. Osteoblastoma: a study of 12 cases. Indian J Pathol Microbiol. 2006;49(4):487–90.
21. Arkader A, Dormans JP. Osteoblastoma in the skeletally immature. J Pediatr Orthop. 2008;28(5):555–60.
22. Puri A, Agarwal MG, Shah M, Puri A, Agarwal MG, Shah M, Srinivas CH, Shukla PJ, Shrikhande SV, Jambhekar NA. Decision making in primary sacral tumors. Spine J. 2009;9(5):396–403.
23. Bouvet R, Vergos M, Chapuis O, André JL, Rochat G. Osteoblastomas of the coccyx. Apropos of a case. Review of the literature. J Chir (Paris). 1994;131(1):40–3.
24. Patel N, Sandeman DR, Cobby M, Nelson IW. Interactive image-guided surgery of the spine—use of the ISG/Elekta Viewing Wand to aid intraoperative localization of a sacral osteoblastoma. Br J Neurosurg. 1997,11(1):60–4.
25. Rajkumar A, Basu R, Datta NR, Dhingra S, Gupta RK. Radiation therapy for sacral osteoblastoma. Clin Oncol (R Coll Radiol). 2003;15(2):85–6.
26. Saghieh S, Rameh C, Birjawi G, Lakkis S. Sacral osteoblastoma presenting as a L5-S1 disc herniation. Int Surg. 2005;90(5):289–92.
27. Witthingham-Jones P, Hughes R, Fajinmi M, Lehovsky J, Saifuddin A. Osteoblastoma crossing the sacro-iliac joint. Skeletal Radiol. 2007;36(3):249–52.
28. Gazzeri R, Tamorri M, Bernardi C, Alfieri A, Gazzeri G. Lumbar spinal osteoblastoma mimicking a dumbbell radicolare schwannoma. Zantralbl Neurochir. 2008;69(4):191–3.
29. Oliveira CR, Mendonca BB, Camargo OP, et al. Classic osteoblastoma, atypical osteoblastoma, and osteosarcoma: a comparative study based on clinical, histological, and biological parameters. Clinics (Sao Paulo). 2007;62(2):167–74.
30. Flemming DJ, Murphey MD, Carmichael BB, et al. Primary tumors of the spine. Semin Musculoskelet Radiol. 2000;4:299–320.

31. Shaikh MI, Saifuddin A, Pringle J, Natali C, Sherazi Z. Spinal osteoblastoma: CT and MR imaging with pathological correlation. Skeletal Radiol. 1999;28:33–40.
32. Hosalkar HS, Garg S, Moroz L, et al. The diagnostic accuracy of MRI versus CT imaging for osteoid osteoma in children. Clin Orthop Relat Res. 2005;433:171–7.
33. Davies M, Cassar-Pullicino VN, Davies AM, et al. The diagnostic accuracy of MR imaging in osteoid osteoma. Skeletal Radiol. 2002;31:559–69.
34. Cheung FM, Wu WC, Lam CK, et al. Diagnostic criteria for pseudomalignant osteoblastoma. Histopathology. 1997;31:196–200.
35. Mirra JM, Kendrick RA, Kendrick RE. Pseudomalignant osteoblastoma versus arrested osteosarcoma: a case report. Cancer. 1976;37:2005–14.
36. Schajowicz F, Lemos C. Malignant osteoblastoma. J Bone Joint Surg Br. 1976;58:202–11.
37. Mayer L. Malignant degeneration of so-called benign osteoblastoma. Bull Hosp Jt Dis. 1967;28:4–13.
38. Seki T, Fukuda H, Ishii Y, Hanaoka H, Yatabe S. Malignant transformation of benign osteoblastoma. A case report. J Bone Joint Surg Am. 1975;57:424–6.
39. Merryweather R, Middlemiss JH, Sanerkin NG. Malignant transformation of osteoblastoma. J Bone Joint Surg Br. 1980;62:381–4.
40. Bertoni F, Unni KK, McLeod RA, Dahlin DC. Osteosarcoma resembling osteoblastoma. Cancer. 1985;55(2):416–26.
41. Hosono A, Yamaguchi U, Makimoto A, Endo M, Watanabe A, Shimoda T, Kaya M, Matsumura T, Sonobe H, Kusumi T, Yamaguchi T, Hasegawa T. Utility of immunohistochemical analysis for cyclo-oxygenase 2 in the differential diagnosis of osteoblastoma and osteosarcoma. J Clin Pathol. 2007;60(4):410–4.
42. Kawaguchi Y, Hasegawa T, Oka S, et al. Mechanism of intramedullary high intensity area on T2 weighted magnetic resonance imaging in osteoid osteoma: a possible role of COX-2 expression. Pathol Int. 2001;51:933–7.
43. Mungo DV, Zhang X, O'Keefe RJ, et al. COX-1 and COX-2 expression in osteoid osteomas. J Orthop Res. 2002;20:159–62.
44. Tsujii M, DuBois RN. Alterations in cellular adhesion and apoptosis in epithelial cells overexpressing prostaglandin endoperoxide synthase 2. Cell. 1995;83:493–501.
45. Harrop JS, Schmidt MH, Boriani S, Shaffrey CI. Aggressive "benign" primary spine neoplasm: osteoblastoma, aneurismal bone cyst, and giant cell tumor. Spine. 2009;34(22 Suppl):S39–47.
46. Berberoglu S, Oguz A, Aribal E, et al. Osteoblastoma response to radiotherapy and chemotherapy. Med Pediatr Oncol. 1997;28:305–9.
47. Marsh BW, Bonfiglio M, Brady LP, et al. Benign osteoblastoma: range of manifestations. J Bone Joint Surg Am. 1975;57:1–9.
48. Mavrogenis AF, Rossi G, Rimondi E, Papagelopoulos PJ, Ruggieri P. Embolization of bone tumors. Orthopedics. 2011;34(4):303–10.
49. Gottfried ON, Schmidt MH, Stevens EA. Embolization of sacral tumors. Neurosurg Focus. 2003;15(2):E4.
50. Kollender Y, Meller I, Bickels J, Flusser G, Issakov J, Merimsky O, Marouani N, Nirkin A, Weinbroum AA. Role of adjuvant cryosurgery in intralesional treatment of sacral tumors. Cancer. 2003;97(11):2830–8. doi:10.1002/cncr.11383.
51. Nader R, Alford BT, Nauta HJ, Crow W, van Sonnenberg E, Hadjepavlou AG. Preoperative embolization and intraoperative cryocoagulation as adjuncts in resection of hypervascular lesions of the thoracolumbar spine. J Neurosurg. 2002;97(3 Suppl):294–300.
52. Ruggieri P, Angelini A, Ussia G, Montalti M, Mercuri M. Surgical margins and local control in resection of sacral chordomas. Clin Orthop Relat Res. 2010;468(11):2939–47.
53. Rosenthal DI, Hornicek FJ, Torriani M, et al. Osteoid osteoma: percutaneous treatment with radiofrequency energy. Radiology. 2003;229:171–5.
54. Frassica FJ, Waltrip RL, Sponseller PD, et al. Clinicopathologic features and treatment of osteoid osteoma and osteoblastoma in children and adolescents. Orthop Clin North Am. 1996;27:559–74.

55. DiCaprio MR, Bellapianta JM. Use of radiofrequency ablation in the treatment of bone tumors. Tech Orthop. 2007;22(2):99–109.
56. Jackson RP. Recurrent osteoblastoma: a review. Clin Orthop Relat Res. 1978;131:229–33.
57. Jackson RP, Reckling FW, Mants FA. Osteoid osteoma and osteoblastoma. Similar histologic lesions with different natural histories. Clin Orthop Relat Res. 1977;128:303–13.
58. Boriani S, Amendola L, Bandiera S, et al. Staging and treatment of osteoblastoma in the mobile spine: a review of 51 cases. Eur Spine J. 2012;21(10):2003–10.

10 Osteoid Osteoma of the Sacrum

Andrea Angelini and Pietro Ruggieri

10.1 Introduction

Osteoid osteoma is a benign bone-forming neoplasm, first described by Jaffe in 1935 [1]. Approximately 10% of all benign bone tumors are osteoid osteomas [2, 3]. It is found most frequently in the second to third decade of life, and there is a pronounced male predominance (2:1 male-to-female predilection). Any portion of the skeleton may be involved, but it is often found (50–60% of cases) in the long bones of the lower extremity [3] and (between 19 and 31% of the cases) upper extremity [4, 5], whereas about 20% occur in the spine [6]. Only 2% of spinal osteoid osteomas are found in the sacrum [2, 7].

10.2 Epidemiology, Presentation, and Diagnosis

Patients with osteoid osteoma typically present with a significant well-localized pain, which is often worse at night and is relieved by nonsteroidal drugs. This lesion is rarely painless, although absence of pain has been reported [8–10]. In some cases pain is not well localized by the patient and can be referred to a nearby joint or in a limb. There are two hypotheses about the source of the pain in osteoid osteoma: (1) abnormally high concentrations of prostaglandins (mainly prostaglandins E2 and I2) have been reported within the nidus, which causes local inflammation and vasodilation [11, 12], as well as strong immunohistochemical staining for cyclooxygenase-2 (COX-2) [13]; (2) pain may be mediated by the nerve fibers located in the reactive bone around the lesion [14–16]. Back pain is a common symptom and this fact may considerably delay the diagnosis of osteoid osteoma of the sacrum

A. Angelini, M.D., Ph.D. • P. Ruggieri, M.D., Ph.D. (✉)
Department of Orthopaedics and Orthopedic Oncology, University of Padova,
Via N. Giustiniani, 3, Padova 35128, Italy
e-mail: andrea.angelini83@yahoo.it; pietro.ruggieri@unipd.it

P. Ruggieri et al. (eds.), *Tumors of the Sacrum*,
DOI 10.1007/978-3-319-51202-0_10

considering a lot of differential diagnosis. Complaints of pain are frequent and mean duration of symptoms is about 12 months [17]. In recent years, however, MRI or CT examination often is used to diagnose patients with back pain, shortening therefore the delay in diagnosis.

10.3 Imaging

Tumors usually present as active, benign stage 2 lesions (Musculoskeletal Tumor Society) and most typically arise from the articular process of S1. Radiographically the majority of the osteoid osteomas were osteosclerotic with or without recognition of a nidus that appear as radiolucent area surrounded by a rim of dense reactive bone. The nidus of an osteoid osteoma is always less than 2 cm in diameter. As "giant osteoid osteomas" were historically defined, the rare cases in which the osteoid osteoma is large (up to 2 cm) retaining the same clinical, imaging, and histological features [2]. Sometimes osteoid osteoma may be obscured by reactive bone and may not be readily visible in a radiograph. In patients with persistent back pain, a bone scan should be obtained to check the existence of this lesion [2, 18]. Bone scintigraphy is constantly positive showing intense focal isotope uptake centered in a less intensely positive and diffused halo (double density sign) [2, 18]. The extent of the isotope uptake is significantly larger than the radiographic dimension of the nidus, encompassing the entire reaction about it. Thin-cut CT scans (1 mm sections) are excellent for diagnosis and precise localization of the nidus. Contrast is usually not needed. Central calcification may be observed within the osteolytic nidus. Sometimes there is a zone of radiolucency between the central area of mineralization and the surrounding reactive bone when ossification of the nidus begins. Some authors reported the use of dynamic contrast-enhanced CT to help differentiate osteoid osteoma from Brodie's abscess, demonstrating vascular flow within the lesion [19]. MR imaging usually shows high signal intensity area in the muscles or bone around the lesion, or both were seen on the T2-weighted image and may be useful for localizing rare intramedullary or periarticular surface osteoid osteomas [20]. However MRI is inferior to CT in depicting the nidus and strongly influenced by the inflammatory reaction of the surrounding tissue.

10.4 Pathology

Grossly, the central nidus of osteoid osteomas appears small and hyperemic, pink to cherry red colored. Histologically, the central portion is composed of abundant, loose, fibrovascular connective tissue between contorted amorphous osteoid and woven trabeculae. Numerous osteoblastic rimming, osteoclasts surrounding the bony trabeculae, and dilated capillaries are observed. The surrounded host bone appears as reactive woven and trabecular bone, more or less mature and sclerotic. Barlow et al., analyzing histologically 10 osteoid osteomas and 20 osteoblastomas (10 spinal and 10 non-spinal), concluded that both tumors are innervated bone-forming lesions which share histomorphological and immunohistochemical features, supporting the view that separate classification is unjustified [21].

10.5 Treatment

In some cases, osteoid osteoma may be self-limiting: rare cases managed by nonsteroidal anti-inflammatory drugs reported pain relief after some years and nidus regression; however, its course is unpredictable and may be protracted. Once the osteoma osteoid has been diagnosed, the physician should discuss nonoperative and operative treatments with the patient. Most patients initially are treated with long-term oral administration of nonsteroidal anti-inflammatory drugs and analgesic drugs [2, 22–25]. If this treatment is ineffective, there are many other alternatives available [26–34].

10.5.1 Radiofrequency Thermal Ablation (RFTA)

Technological advances have allowed for the development of various percutaneous procedures to treat osteoid osteoma. Percutaneous radiofrequency thermal ablation (RFA) has proven to be an effective, reliable, minimally invasive technique in the treatment of osteoid osteoma [32, 35]. The curative approach is operative removal or deactivation of the nidus with RFTA [36], and most of the patients experienced complete disappearance of the pain. If the treatment is not complete, pain persists and additional operative intervention is necessary [37]. RFTA in the spine appears as a safe technique if the lesion is not adjacent to neural structures and the bone cortex is intact [32, 38]. Close proximity of the RFA probe to a neurovascular bun dle is a relative contraindication, but morbidities of other treatment options should be considered.

10.5.2 Surgery

Conventional surgical treatment consists of en bloc resection or curettage of the lesion, which is challenging in certain anatomical locations, such as the acetabulum, femoral neck, spine, and sacrum. Although preoperative radiologic identification of the nidus in osteoid osteoma is not difficult with bone scan, CT, or MRI, localization of the nidus during surgery is difficult [7, 39]. Kirchner et al. [39] reported a probe-guided technique for intraoperative detection of osteoid osteoma and curettage: they injected 99 mTc-methylene diphosphonate 2–3 h before surgery and then identified the point of the maximum count rate during surgery and started curettage of the lesion. They concluded that this method seems to be useful to obtain confirmation of complete removal of the lesion by a continuous check of the count at the same point. If open techniques are preferred, extended intralesional curettage should be performed, and particular care should be taken to remove the entire nidus. Usually no reconstruction may be needed.

10.6 Oncologic Outcome

The recurrence rate after complete nidus excision has been reported to be in the range of 0–25% [4, 7, 23, 37], often in cases in which the nidus was larger than 10 mm. If the tumor has not been excised completely, recurrences are more likely, and it is advisable to carry out further cycles of RFTA to ensure complete removal of the lesion. Specific imaging has proved ineffective to monitor the evolution after treatment, and persistent symptoms appear the most indicative aspect of recurrent/persistent disease.

Conflict of Interest Statement No benefits have been or will be received from a commercial party related directed or indirectly to the subject matter of this article.

References

1. Jaffee HL. "Osteoid osteoma," a benign osteoblastic tumor composed of osteoid and atypical bone. Arch Surg. 1935;31:709.
2. Campanacci M. Osteoid osteoma. In: Campanacci M, editor. Bone and soft tissue tumors. 2nd ed. Padova: Piccin Nuova Libraria; 1999. p. 391–415.
3. Gitelis S, McDonald DJ. Common benign bone tumors and usual treatment. In: Simon MA, Springfield DS, editors. Surgery for bone and soft tissue tumors. Philadelphia: Lippincott-Raven; 1998. p. 181–205.
4. Bednar MS, Weiland AJ, Light TR. Osteoid osteoma of the upper extremity. Hand Clin. 1995;11(2):211–21.
5. Arazi M, Memik R, Yel M, Ogun TC. Osteoid osteoma of the carpal bones. Arch Orthop Trauma Surg. 2001;121(1–2):119–20.
6. Jackson RP, Reckling FW, Mants FA. Osteoid osteoma and osteoblastoma. Similar histologic lesions with different natural histories. Clin Orthop Relat Res. 1977;128:303–13.
7. Capanna R, Ayala A, Bertoni F, Picci P, Calderoni P, Gherlinzoni F, Bettelli G, Campanacci M. Sacral osteoid osteoma and osteoblastoma: a report of 13 cases. Arch Orthop Trauma Surg. 1986;105(4):205–10.
8. Basu S, Basu P, Dowell JK. Painless osteoid osteoma in a metacarpal. J Hand Surg Br. 1999;24(1):133–4.
9. de Smet L, Spaepen D, Zachee B, Fabry G. Painless osteoid osteoma of the finger in a child. Case report. Chir Main. 1998;17(2):143–6.
10. Rex C, Jacobs L, Nur Z. Painless osteoid osteoma of the middle phalanx. J Hand Surg Br. 1997;22(6):798–800.
11. Greco F, Tamburelli F, Ciabattoni G. Prostaglandins in osteoid osteoma. Int Orthop. 1991;15:35–7.
12. Wold LE, Pritchard DJ, Bergert J, Wilson DM. Prostaglandin synthesis by osteoid osteoma and osteoblastoma. Mod Pathol. 1988;1:129–31.
13. Mungo DV, Zhang X, O'Keefe RJ, Rosier RN, Puzas JE, Schwarz EM. COX-1 and COX-2 expression in osteoid osteomas. J Orthop Res. 2002;20(1):159–62.
14. Mahnken AH, Tacke JA, Wildberger JE, Gunther RW. Radiofrequency ablation of osteoid osteoma: initial results with a bipolar ablation device. J Vasc Interv Radiol. 2006;17:1465–70.
15. O'Connell JX, Nanthakumar SS, Nielsen GP, Rosenberg AE. Osteoid osteoma: the uniquely innervated bone tumor. Mod Pathol. 1998;11(2):175–80.
16. Schulman L, Dorfman HD. Nerve fibers in osteoid osteoma. J Bone Joint Surg Am. 1970;52:1351–6.

17. Ozaki T, Liljenqvist U, Hillmann A, Halm H, Lindner N, Gosheger G, Winkelmann W. Osteoid osteoma and osteoblastoma of the spine: experiences with 22 patients. Clin Orthop Relat Res. 2002;397:394–402.
18. Wilson Y, Fogelman I, Evans DM. Detection of an elusive osteoid osteoma using a registration bone scan. J Hand Surg Br. 1997;22(6):801–4.
19. McGrath BE, Bush CH, Nelson TE, Scarborough MT. Evaluation of suspected osteoid osteoma. Clin Orthop Relat Res. 1999;327:247–52.
20. Spouge AR, Thain LM. Osteoid osteoma: MR imaging revisited. Clin Imaging. 2000;24(1):19–27.
21. Barlow E, Davies AM, Cool WP, Barlow D, Mangham DC. Osteoid osteoma and osteoblastoma: novel histological and immunohistochemical observations as evidence for a single entity. J Clin Pathol. 2013;66(9):768–74.
22. Feletar M, Hall S. Osteoid osteoma: a case for conservative management. Rheumatology. 2002;41:585–6.
23. Cohen JD, Harrington TM, Ginsberg WW. Osteoid osteoma: 95 cases and review of the literature. Semin Arthritis Rheum. 1983;12:265–81.
24. Kneisl JS, Simon MA. Medical management compared with operative treatment for osteoid osteoma. J Bone Joint Surg Am. 1992;74:179–85.
25. Golding JSR. The natural history of osteoid osteoma with a report of twenty cases. J Bone Joint Surg Br. 1954;36:218–29.
26. Cantwell CP, Obyrne J, Eustace S. Current trends in treatment of osteoid osteoma with an emphasis on radiofrequency ablation. Eur Radiol. 2004;14:607–17.
27. Skjeldal S, Lilleas F, Folleras G, et al. Real time MRI-guided excision and cryo-treatment of osteoid osteoma in os ischii: a case report. Acta Orthop Scand. 2000;71:637–8.
28. Gangi A, Dietemann JL, Clavert JM, et al. [Treatment of osteoid osteoma using laser photocoagulation: a propos of 28 cases.] (in French). Rev Chir Orthop Reparatrice Appar Mot. 1998;84:676–84.
29. Katz K, Kornreich L, David R, Horev G, Soudry M. Osteoid osteoma: resection with CT guidance. Isr Med Assoc J. 2000;2(2):151–3.
30. Vanderschueren GM, Taminiau AHM, Obermann WR, Bloem JL. Osteoid osteoma: clinical results with thermocoagulation. Radiology. 2002;224:82–6.
31. Campanacci M, Ruggieri P, Gasbarrini A, Ferraro A, Campanacci L. Osteoid osteoma direct visual identification and intralesional excision of the nidus with minimal removal of bone. J Bone Joint Surg Br. 1999;81-B:814–20.
32. Rosenthal DI, Hornicek FJ, Torriani M, Gebhardt MC, Mankin HJ. Osteoid osteoma: percutaneous treatment with radiofrequency energy. Radiology. 2003;229:171–5.
33. Sluga M, Windhager R, Pfeiffer M, Dominkus M, Kotz R. Peripheral osteoid osteoma. Is there still a place for traditional surgery? J Bone Joint Surg Br. 2002;84(2):249–51.
34. Lindner NJ, Ozaki T, Roedl R, Gosheger G, Winkelmann W, Wortler K. Percutaneous radio frequency ablation in osteoid osteoma. J Bone Joint Surg Br. 2001;83-B:391–6.
35. Barei DP, Moreau G, Scarborough MT. Percutaneous radiofrequency thermal ablation of osteoid osteoma. Oper Tech Orthop. 1999;9(2):72–8.
36. Rosenthal DI, Hornicek FJ, Wolfe MW, Jennings LC, Gebhardt MC, Mankin HJ. Percutaneous radiofrequency coagulation of osteoid osteoma compared with operative treatment. J Bone Joint Surg Am. 1998;80(6):815–21.
37. Lee DH, Malawer MM. Staging and treatment of primary and persistent (recurrent) osteoid osteoma. Evaluation of intraoperative nuclear scanning, tetracycline fluorescence, and tomography. Clin Orthop Relat Res. 1992;281:229–38.
38. Osti OL, Sebben R. High-frequency radio-wave ablation of osteoid osteoma in the lumbar spine. Eur Spine J. 1998;7:422–5.
39. Kirchner B, Hillmann A, Lottes G, Sciuk J, Bartenstein P, Winkelmann W, Schober O. Intraoperative, probe-guided curettage of osteoid osteoma. Eur J Nucl Med. 1993;20(7):609–13.

Aneurysmal Bone Cyst of the Sacrum

11

Andrea Angelini, Giuseppe Rossi, Andreas F. Mavrogenis, and Pietro Ruggieri

11.1 Introduction

Aneurysmal bone cyst (ABC) is a benign, reactive, expansile, highly vascular osteolytic tumor-like bone lesion of unknown origin [1, 2]. In about 30% of cases, it is found as secondary lesion to underlying bone diseases (giant cell tumor, osteoblastoma, chondroblastoma, angiosarcoma, and osteosarcoma), while in the other cases it occurs as a primary lesion. Primary ABCs are rare lesions, and their prevalence is about 1% of all primary tumors and about half that prevalence of giant cell tumors [1, 3]. The appearance at imaging evaluation is variable, and sometimes the differential diagnosis with malignant lesions is difficult [1–4]. The behavior of ABC is unpredictable: occasionally it may grow slowly or undergo spontaneous regression [5–7], but usually it grows with aggressive major bone destruction, pathological fracture, and high local recurrence rate [3, 8–10].

A. Angelini, M.D., Ph.D. • P. Ruggieri, M.D., Ph.D. (✉)
Department of Orthopaedics and Orthopedic Oncology, University of Padova, Padova, Italy
e-mail: andrea.angelini83@yahoo.it; pietro.ruggieri@unipd.it

G. Rossi, M.D.
Department of Interventional Angiographic Radiology, Istituto Ortopedico Rizzoli, Bologna, Italy
e-mail: giuseppe.rossi@ior.it

A.F. Mavrogenis, M.D., Ph.D.
First Department of Orthopaedics, National and Kapodistrian University of Athens, Athens, Greece
e-mail: afm@otenet.gr

P. Ruggieri et al. (eds.), *Tumors of the Sacrum*,
DOI 10.1007/978-3-319-51202-0_11

11.2 Epidemiology, Presentation, and Diagnosis

The sacrum is a relatively rare location for ABC, accounting for less than 4% of reported cases [1–4, 9–11], but this histotype represents 15% of all primary sacral tumors. In a series of 289 patients, sacrum was involved in only 4% of the cases [2]. Duration of symptoms prior to diagnosis can reach 2 years. Diagnosis of sacral lesions is difficult due to the nonspecific low-back pain pattern as well as the difficulty in visualization of the lesion on AP radiographs of the pelvis [12]. The most frequently misinterpreted symptoms include radiating pain in the lower extremity that involved the thigh [3]. Moreover, factors associated with delayed diagnosis are inadequate physical examination not including rectal palpation and the use of gonad shields during radiographs of the pelvis. Pain is the main clinical presentation symptom in about all of the reported cases in literature, occasionally associated with localized mass or palpable presacral mass on rectal examination [3]. Neurological signs and symptoms are related to sacral roots involvement, ranging from sphincterial deficiency, leg paresthesias or weakness, up to loss of muscle function. Rarely, a pathologic fracture may occur with acute paraplegia or cauda equina syndrome.

11.3 Imaging

During the early course of the disease, lytic areas may not be recognized on plain radiographs of the pelvis. In larger lesions, direct radiographs show an expansive osteolytic cavity, which swells and sometimes destroys cortical bone. Fluid-fluid levels are visualized most effectively with computed tomography (CT) or magnetic resonance imaging (MRI) [13]. CT imaging reveals multiloculated lytic lesions with multiple internal septations and it is useful for evaluation of bone stock and planning surgery. However, definition and extension of the lesion are better accomplished with weighted MRI than with CT [14]. Multiple fluid levels are best seen on T2-weighted MRI, supporting the diagnosis of ABC although not pathognomonic for this entity. This appearance is also seen in the other bone lesions such as telangiectatic osteosarcoma, giant cell tumor, and chondroblastoma [1, 2]. Although imaging studies are diagnostic methods for many cases, in literature it is noted that biopsy is necessary and cautious for histopathologic confirmation.

11.4 Pathology

At histopathology, the lesion appears as typical spongy pattern. It consists of roundish spaces separated by septa and filled with blood. The septa are characterized by histio-fibroblastic tissue rich in thin blood capillaries and almost always contained benign-appearing multinucleated giant cells. The number of giant cells ranged from sparse to abundant, but present in most of the cases. Bone formation is usually observed, with a typical reactive pattern, quite variable, ranging from small foci with osteoid production to extensive areas of woven bone trabeculae. A peculiar calcified matrix occurred either in the septa or in more solid areas and appeared either as foci of calcification in chondroid-like areas or as filamentous calcification simulating trabeculae of bone. Considered for several years a pseudotumoral lesion of uncertain origin, currently it has been associated with a specific pattern of genetic alterations that result in the activation of the gene USP6 located on 17 p132 [15].

11.5 Treatment

For many years ABC has been treated as a benign bone tumor, and intralesional curettage was widely considered the mainstay of treatment in order to avoid recurrence and future reoperations. The standard of cure was to remove as much of the lesion as possible by curettage, followed by local adjuvant treatments and bone grafting [3, 9, 16–20]. This method of treatment must be individualized in patients with ABC of the sacrum, considering location, extent, and aggressiveness of the lesion and the risk of profuse bleeding during surgery requiring multiple transfusions or CSF leakage. Attempts at removing tumor and sparing nerve roots might have been possible but are technically challenging [21]; in fact, an increasing number of authors have recommended the avoidance of aggressive curettage and instead recommended minimally invasive or noninvasive procedures [20, 22, 23]. Arterial embolization (alone or preoperative in combination with curettage), percutaneous injection of sclerosing agents, drugs (steroid and calcitonin), or bone-inducing substances have all been reported [13, 24–34]. These new therapies are based on an improved understanding of the biology of the tumor and may lead to pain control and ossification of the lesion.

11.5.1 Open Surgical Curettage

ABCs are generally managed by intralesional curettage and bone grafting when long bones of the extremities are involved [9, 16–18]. Avoidance of potentially damaging curettage procedures is particularly important in ABCs of the pelvis and sacrum where special factors need to be considered: relative inaccessibility, significant potential for severe intraoperative bleeding, vulnerability of the sacroiliac joint, proximity to neurovascular structures, and risk of nerve damage [3, 35 37]. Preoperative angiography and selective embolization therapy have been proven to help minimize these complications for lesions larger than 5 cm [1–4, 22, 24, 25, 29, 37–39]. The procedure should be performed by an experienced interventional radiologist to minimize the risk of permanent tissue necrosis. The use of a large bone window [40], a high speed burr [16], and adjuvant therapy with phenol or liquid nitrogen [19, 41–43] has been advocated in order to reduce the risk of local recurrence. On the other hand, some authors suggest to avoid local adjuvants in sacral lesions. Papagelopoulos et al. [3] reported a series including 12 patients treated for their sacral ABC with excision-curettage. They chose a posterior surgical approach avoiding the use of adjunctive chemical cautery, and performed a dissection and preservation of the neural elements whenever possible, with no recurrence within a mean follow-up of 19 years. [3]. Neurological complications in patients with sacral lesions were more likely to be observed comparing to other sites.

11.5.2 Selective Arterial Embolization

Considering the good results reported in literature with selective arterial embolization, it represents the first treatment option for sacral ABC [22] (Fig. 11.1). The technique is a less invasive, more feasible, effective, and repeatable alternative method in cases in which surgery carries significant morbidity, even if the effects can be variable [24, 25]. Some reports suggest that ongoing increase in lesion size or initial unresponsive results can occur, requiring repeated embolization [24, 25]. Exclusion criteria for this modality of treatment include structural instability, pathological or impending fracture, neurological deficits, and technical feasibility.

11.5.3 Sclerosing Agents Injection

The injection of sclerosing agents has been used for ABC in the limb [26], whereas this technique is not recommended in axial lesions (especially in the sacrum) because of possible nerve damage and meningitis [28] caused by the extrusion of the material.

11.5.4 Bone Induction Agents Injection

Recently, the use of bone induction agents to treat ABC is debated. The rational of treatment is to interrupt the destructive osteoclastic process and promote spontaneous bone regeneration. Several materials have been used in clinical setting with conflicting results. Calcium sulfate injections do not appear to be effective [32], whereas demineralized bone matrix seems to be effective, possibly because it induces the bone morphogenic process [44].

Donati et al. reported a case of ABC of the sacrum treated unsuccessfully with arterial embolization. The patient was then treated with percutaneous injection of demineralized bone matrix together with bone marrow concentrate, with evidence of progressive bone production inside the cystic area at 6 and 12 years of follow-up [45]. However, more research on the effectiveness of this technique is needed.

11.5.5 Denosumab

Denosumab is a human monoclonal antibody that inhibits RANKL (receptor activator of nuclear factor kappa-B ligand), reducing bone resorption. The drug has been approved for treatment of osteoporosis and bone metastasis and has been reported

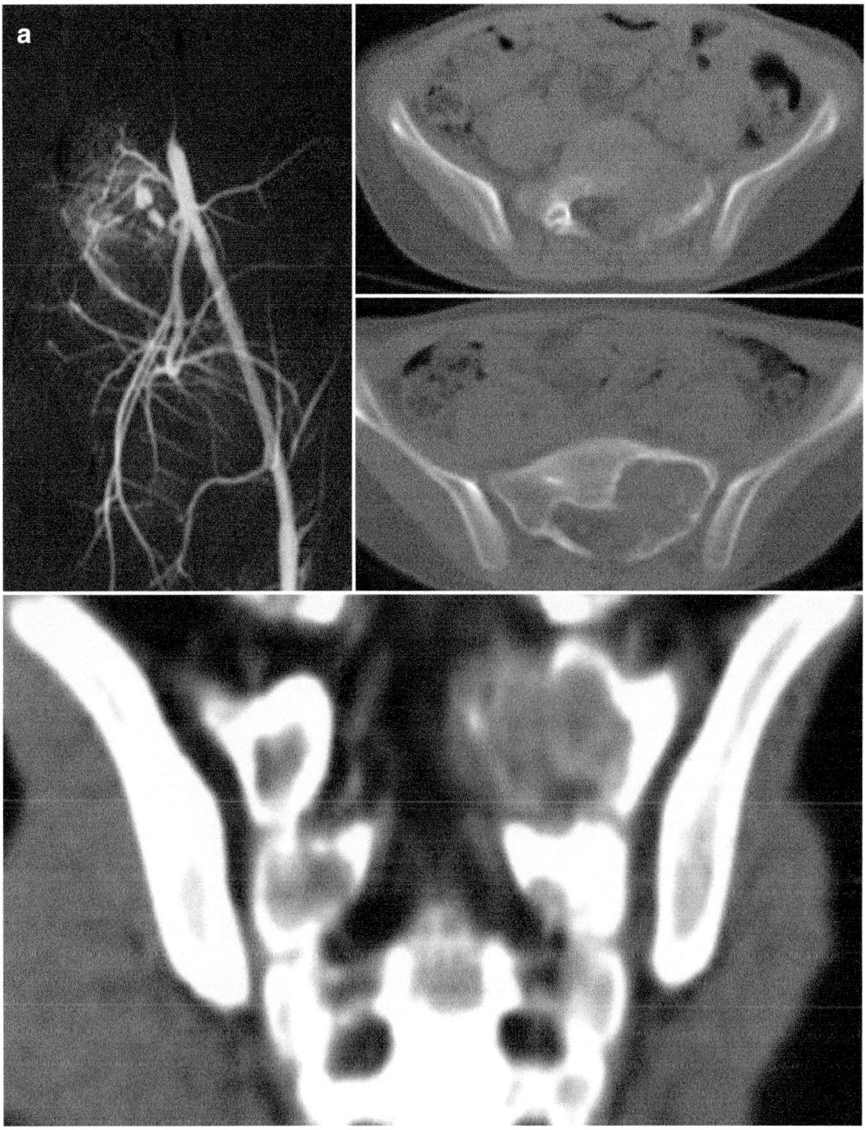

Fig. 11.1 Results after treatment of ABC of the sacrum with selective arterial embolization. (**a**) Digital subtraction angiography (*left corner*) shows the pathological tumor vascularization arising from branches of the internal iliac arteries; axial CT scan (*right corner*) of the pelvis shows an osteolytic lesion extending to the anterior and posterior sacral space; coronal CT scan (*below*) shows the involvement of proximal sacral vertebrae. (**b**) The same imaging studies after embolization show complete occlusion of tumor vascularization and healing of the lesion as evident by ossification and tumor size reduction. The patient is asymptomatic

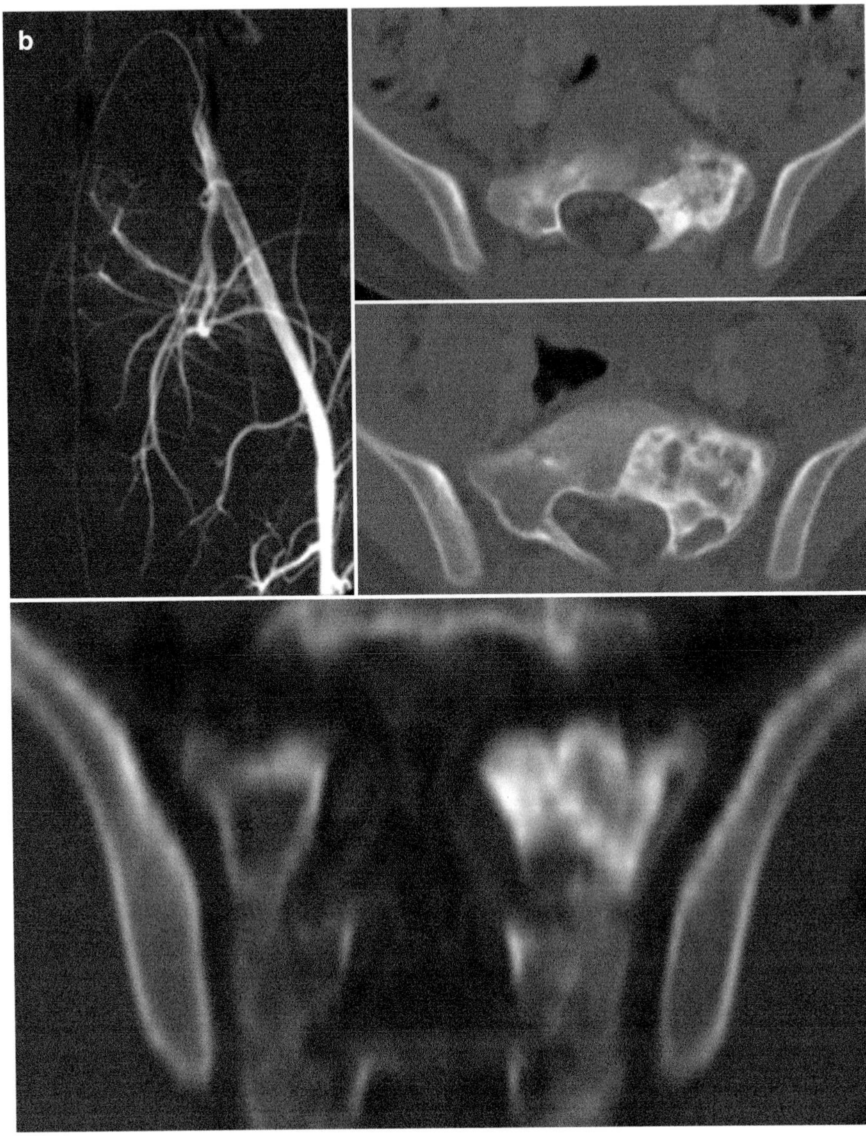

Fig. 11.1 (continued)

active and useful for medical treatment of giant cell tumor of bone. Recently, RANKL has been associated also with ABC growth, justifying use of denosumab as medical treatment [15, 46, 47]. Skubitz et al. reported a gradual pain resolution in a 27 years old male with sacral ABC treated with denosumab administration for 11 months [48]. They confirmed the absence of giant cell and presence of new bone formation at biopsy performed during follow-up. Ghermandi et al. reported good results in term of pain relief and complete ossification of the lesion in two cases unresponsive to selective arterial embolization treated with multiple administration of denosumab [49]. However, many questions remain regarding the use of denosumab in ABC and, awaiting further confirmations from ongoing studies, may be useful in cases not amenable to surgical interventions and unresponsive to selective arterial embolizations.

11.5.6 Radiation Therapy

Radiation therapy as adjuvant treatment or alone has been suggested in the past as possible treatment for ABCs that are difficult to access by surgery, but currently it is not recommended to minimize the risk of postradiation sarcoma and severe complications including osteonecrosis, gonadal damage, and myelopathy [9, 13, 50–53]. Radiation should be reserved only for selected local recurrence cases.

11.6 Oncologic Outcome

Recurrence is reported in 10–44% of the cases [9, 10, 50]. Papagelopoulos et al. reported a recurrence rate of 14% on 35 primary ABCs of the pelvis surgically treated [3], and Capanna et al. reported a similar recurrence rate (13%) on 23 ABCs of the pelvis [54]. Recurrences are associated with incomplete excision [3, 9, 10]. Malignant transformation of ABC is extremely rare [55].

Conflict of Interest Statement No benefits have been or will be received from a commercial party related directly or indirectly to the subject matter of this article.

References

1. Campanacci M. Aneurysmal bone cyst. In: Campanacci M, editor. Bone and soft tissue tumors. 2nd ed. Padova: Piccin Nuova Libraria; 1999. p. 813–40.
2. Unni KK. Dahlin's bone tumors: general aspects and data on 11,087 cases. 5th ed. Philadelphia: Lippincott-Raven; 1996. p. 382–90.
3. Papagelopoulos PJ, Choudhury SN, Frassica FJ, Bond JR, Unni KK, Sim FH. Treatment of aneurysmal bone cysts of the pelvis and sacrum. J Bone Joint Surg Am. 2001;83:1674–81.
4. Cottalorda J, Bourelle S. Modern concepts of primary aneurysmal bone cyst. Arch Orthop Trauma Surg. 2007;127(2):105–14.
5. McQueen MM, Chaimers J, Smith GD. Spontaneous healing of aneurysmal bone cysts. A report of two cases. J Bone Joint Surg Br. 1985;67:310–2.
6. Saglik Y, Kapicioglu MI, Guzel B. Spontaneous regression of aneurysmal bone cyst. A case report. Arch Orthop Trauma Surg. 1993;112:203–4.
7. Malghem J, Maldague B, Esselinckx NH, De Nayer P, Vincent A. Spontaneous healing of aneurysmal bone cysts: a report of three cases. J Bone Joint Surg Br. 1989;71B:645–50.
8. Capanna R, Bertoni F, Bettelli G, Present D, Biagini R, Ruggieri P, Mancini I, Campanacci M. Aneurysmal bone cyst of the pelvis. Arch Orthop Trauma Surg. 1986;105:279–84.

9. Vergel De Dios AM, Bond JR, Shives TC, McLeod RA, Unni KK. Aneurysmal bone cyst. A clinicopathologic study of 238 cases. Cancer. 1992;69:2921–31.
10. Ruiter DJ, van Rijssel TG, van der Veide EA. Aneurysmal bone cysts: a clinicopathological study of 105 cases. Cancer. 1977;39:2231–9.
11. Mirra JM. Aneurysmal bone cyst. In: Mirra JM, Picci P, Gold RH, editors. Bone tumors. Clinical, radiologic, and pathologic correlations. Philadelphia: Lea & Febiger; 1989. p. 1267–311.
12. Honl M, Westphal F, Carrero V, et al. Pelvic girdle reconstruction based on spinal fusion and ischial screw fixation in a case of aneurysmal bone cyst. Sarcoma. 2003;7(3–4):177–82.
13. Tsai JC, Dalinka MK, Fallon MD, Zlatkin MB, Kressel HY. Fluid–fluid level: a nonspecific finding in tumors of bone and soft tissue. Radiology. 1990;175(3):779–82.
14. Davies AM, Cassar-Pullicino VN, Grimer RJ. The incidence and significance of fluid-fluid levels on computed tomography of osseous lesions. Br J Radiol. 1992;65:193–6.
15. Pauli C, Fuchs B, Pfirmann C, Bridge JA, Hofer S, Bode B. Response of an aggressive periosteal aneurismal bone cyst (ABC) of the radius to denosumab therapy. World J Surg Oncol. 2014;12:17.
16. Gibbs CP, Hefele MC, Peabody TD, Montag AG, Aithal V, Simon MA. Aneurysmal bone cyst of the extremities. Factors related to local recurrence after curettage with a high-speed burr. J Bone Joint Surg Am. 1999;81(12):1671–8.
17. Mankin HJ, Hornicek FJ, Ortiz-Cruz E, Villafuerte J, Gebhardt MC. Aneurysmal bone cyst: a review of 150 patients. J Clin Oncol. 2005;23(27):6756–62.
18. Campanacci M, Capanna R, Picci P. Unicameral and aneurysmal bone cysts. Clin Orthop Relat Res. 1986;204:25–36.
19. Peeters SP, Van der Geest IC, de Rooy JW, Veth RP, Schreuder HW. Aneurysmal bone cyst: the role of cryosurgery as local adjuvant treatment. J Surg Oncol. 2009;100(8):719–24.
20. Lin PP, Brown C, Raymond AK, Deavers MT, Yasko AW. Aneurysmal bone cysts recur at juxtaphyseal locations in skeletally immature patients. Clin Orthop Relat Res. 2008;466(3):722–8.
21. Sar C, Eralp L. Surgical treatment of primary tumors of the sacrum. Arch Orthop Trauma Surg. 2002;122(3):148–55.
22. De Cristofaro R, Biagini R, Boriani S, et al. Selective arterial embolization in the treatment of aneurysmal bone cysts and angioma. Skeletal Radiol. 1992;21(8):523–7.
23. Docquier PL, Delloye C. Treatment of aneurysmal bone cysts by introduction of demineralized bone and autogenous bone marrow. J Bone Joint Surg Am. 2005;87:2253–8.
24. Rossi G, Mavrogenis AF, Rimondi E, Ciccarese F, Tranfaglia C, Angelelli B, Fiorentini G, Bartalena T, Errani C, Ruggieri P, Mercuri M. Selective arterial embolisation for bone tumours: experience of 454 cases. Radiol Med. 2011;116(5):793–808.
25. Rossi G, Mavrogenis AF, Papagelopoulos PJ, et al. Successful treatment of aggressive aneurysmal bone cyst of the pelvis with serial embolization. Orthopedics. 2012;35:e963–8.
26. Varshney MK, Rastogi S, Khan SA, Trikha V. Is sclerotherapy better than intralesional excision for treating aneurysmal bone cysts? Clin Orthop Relat Res. 2010;468:1649–59.
27. Falappa P, Fassari FM, Fanelli A, et al. Aneurysmal bone cysts: treatment with direct percutaneous Ethibloc injection—long-term results. Cardiovasc Intervent Radiol. 2002;25: 282–90.
28. de Gauzy JS, Abid A, Accadbled F, Knorr G, Darodes P, Cahuzac JP. Percutaneous Ethibloc injection in aneurysmal bone cysts. Skeletal Radiol. 2000;29:211–6.
29. Yildirim E, Ersözlü S, Kirbaş I, Ozgür AF, Akkaya T, Karadeli E. Treatment of pelvic aneurysmal bone cysts in two children: selective arterial embolization as an adjunct to curettage and bone grafting. Diagn Interv Radiol. 2007;13(1):49–52.
30. Topouchian V, Mazda K, Hamze B, Laredo JD, Penneçot GF. Aneurysmal bone cysts in children: complications of fibrosing agent injection. Radiology. 2004;232(2):522–6.
31. Adamsbaum C, Mascard E, Guinebretière JM, Kalifa G, Dubousset J. Intralesional Ethibloc injections in primary aneurysmal bone cysts: an efficient and safe treatment. Skeletal Radiol. 2003;32(10):559–66.

32. Clayer M. Injectable form of calcium sulphate as treatment of aneurysmal bone cysts. ANZ J Surg. 2008;78:366–70.
33. Bush CH, Adler Z, Drane WE, Tamurian R, Scarborough MT, Gibbs CP. Percutaneous radionuclide ablation of axial aneurysmal bone cysts. AJR Am J Roentgenol. 2010;194(1):W84–90.
34. Carpenter B, Motley T. Bone matrix therapy for aneurysmal bone cysts. J Am Podiatr Med Assoc. 2005;95(4):394–7.
35. Capanna R, Van Horn JR, Biagini R, Ruggieri P. Aneurysmal bone cyst of the sacrum. Skeletal Radiol. 1989;18(2):109–13.
36. Vester H, Wegener B, Weiler C, Baur-Melnyk A, Jansson V, Dürr HR. First report of a solid variant of aneurysmal bone cyst in the os sacrum. Skeletal Radiol. 2010;39(1):73–7.
37. Pogoda P, Linhart W, Priemel M, Rueger JM, Amling M. Aneurysmal bone cysts of the sacrum clinical report and review of the literature. Arch Orthop Trauma Surg. 2003; 123(5):247–51.
38. Green JA, Bellemore MC, Marsden FW. Embolization in the treatment of aneurysmal bone cysts. J Pediatr Orthop. 1997;17(4):440–3.
39. Brastianos P, Gokaslan Z, McCarthy EF. Aneurysmal bone cysts of the sacrum: a report of ten cases and review of the literature. Iowa Orthop J. 2009;29:74–8.
40. Dormans JP, Hanna BG, Johnston DR, Khurana JS. Surgical treatment and recurrence rate of aneurysmal bone cysts in children. Clin Orthop. 2004;421:205–11.
41. Ozaki T, Hillmann A, Lindner N, Winkelmann W. Cementation of primary aneurysmal bone cyst. Clin Orthop Relat Res. 1997;337:240–8.
42. Capanna R, Sudanese A, Baldini N, Campanacci M. Phenol as an adjuvant in the control of local recurrence of benign neoplasms of bone treated by curettage. Ital J Orthop Traumatol. 1985;11(3):381–8.
43. Cummings JE, Smith RA, Heck Jr RK. Argon beam coagulation as adjuvant treatment after curettage of aneurysmal bone cysts: a preliminary study. Clin Orthop Relat Res. 2010;468(1):231–7.
44. Rosenthal RK, Folkman J, Glowacki J. Demineralized bone implants for nonunion fractures, bone cysts, and fibrous lesions. Clin Orthop Relat Res. 1999;364:61–9.
45. Donati D, Frisoni T, Dozza B, DeGroot H, Albisinni U, Giannini S. Advance in the treatment of aneurysmal bone cyst of the sacrum. Skeletal Radiol. 2011;40(11):1461–6.
46. Lange T, Stehling C, Frohlich B, et al. Denosumab: a potential new and innovative treatment option for aneurysmal bone cysts. Eur Spine J. 2013;22:1417–22.
47. Pelle DW, Ringler JW, Peacock JD, Kampfschulte K, Scholten II DJ, Davis MM, Mitchell DS, Steensma MR. Targeting receptor-activator of nuclear kap-paB ligand in aneurysmal bone cysts: verification of target and therapeutic response. Transl Res. 2014;164:139–48
48. Skubitz KM, Peltola JC, Santos ER, Cheng EY. Response of aneurysmal bone cyst to denosumab. Spine (Phila Pa 1976). 2015;40(22):E1201–4.
49. Ghermandi R, Terzi S, Gasbarrini A, Boriani S. Denosumab: non-surgical treatment option for selective arterial embolization resistant aneurysmal bone cyst of the spine and sacrum. Case report. Eur Rev Med Pharmacol Sci. 2016;20(17):3692–5.
50. Marcove RC, Sheth DS, Takemoto S, Healey JH. The treatment of aneurysmal bone cyst. Clin Orthop. 1995;311:157–63.
51. Frassica FJ, Frassica DA, Wold LE, Beabout JW, Sim FH. Postradiation sarcoma of bone. Orthopedics. 1993;16:105–6.
52. Mavrogenis AF, Angelini A, Pala E, Calabro T, Bianchi G, Casadei R, Ruggieri P. Radiation-induced sarcomas. J Long-Term Eff Med Implants. 2011;21(3):233–40.
53. Mavrogenis AF, Stavropoulos NA, Angelini A, Papagelopoulos PJ, Ruggieri P. Post-radiation sarcomas. Acta Orthopaedica et Traumatologica Hellenica. 2012;63(4):161–5.
54. Capanna R, Campanacci DA, Manfrini M. Unicameral and aneurysmal bone cysts. Orthop Clin North Am. 1996;27:605–14.
55. Kyriakos M, Hardy D. Malignant transformation of aneurysmal bone cyst, with an analysis of the literature. Cancer. 1991;68:1770–80.

Schwannoma of the Sacrum

12

Andreas F. Mavrogenis, Georgios N. Panagopoulos, Andrea Angelini, and Pietro Ruggieri

12.1 Introduction

Nerve sheath tumors comprise only a small portion of the wide variety of lesions that occur in the sacrum [1–5]. Schwannomas (neurilemomas) are benign, slow-growing neurogenic tumors arising from Schwann cells of the peripheral nerve sheath. Sacral schwannomas are exceedingly rare, with merely around 50 cases reported in related literature [6]. Due to their largely indolent nature, the mobility of the sacral nerve roots, and the generous width of the sacral canal, sacral schwannomas frequently grow to a considerable size prior to detection; hence, giant sacral schwannomas are often described in related reports [7, 8]. Although benign, these tumors may occasionally pose a surgical challenge, as en bloc resection may be associated with disproportionally high surgical morbidity [9].

12.2 Epidemiology

Sacral schwannomas are decisively more rare than the common spinal schwannomas [6], accounting for less than 1–5% of all spinal schwannomas [6]. Schwannomas usually occur in individuals between 20 and 50 years of age with no gender predilection; they are associated with von Recklinghausen's disease (neurofibromatosis

A.F. Mavrogenis, M.D., Ph.D. • G.N. Panagopoulos, M.D.
First Department of Orthopaedics, National and Kapodistrian University of Athens, Athens, Greece
e-mail: afm@otenet.gr

A. Angelini, M.D., Ph.D. • P. Ruggieri, M.D., Ph.D. (✉)
Department of Orthopedics and Orthopedic Oncology, University of Padova, Padova, Italy
e-mail: andrea.angelini83@yahoo.it; pietro.ruggieri@unipd.it

P. Ruggieri et al. (eds.), *Tumors of the Sacrum*,
DOI 10.1007/978-3-319-51202-0_12

type II) in 18% of cases [10]. Schwannoma can involve the sacrum in one of three ways: (1) secondary erosion by an extraosseous tumor; (2) tumor arising from a nerve coursing through a canal and causing erosion of the bone, creating a dumbbell-shaped configuration; or (3) tumor arising centrally (intramedullary or intraosseous) [11]. The first two mechanisms are more common. Intraosseous schwannomas are exceptional, accounting for less than 0.2% of all primary bone tumors, with fewer than 200 cases described in literature, in all locations [12–21]. Intraosseous schwannomas have also been described in a setting of neurofibromatosis type III (schwannomatosis) [21]. Giant intraosseous sacral schwannomas were first reported by De Santo et al. in 1940 [17], and so far, approximately 50 cases have been reported [6, 18, 19].

12.3 Presentation and Diagnosis

Most patients with a sacral schwannoma remain asymptomatic for a long period of time. If present, symptoms are generally mild, and it is not until the tumor becomes very large that patients notice pain or swelling [9, 19]. In a report, a patient was harboring a sacral schwannoma for more than 25 years before the onset of symptoms [22]. The mean duration of symptoms prior to diagnosis ranges from 1 to 7 years [18, 20, 23, 24]. Pain is the most common presenting symptom. It may be either localized, low-back, or radicular pain extending in the distribution of one or more lumbosacral nerve roots. It may also be associated with sensory defects, such as paresthesias or dysesthesias. Urinary hesitancy and retention, weak stream and overflow, or unconscious incontinence may be present if bladder innervation is compromised. Patients may also present with recurrent bouts of cystitis [6]. Complaints of constipation or an unpleasant feeling of rectal fullness or pain (tenesmus) are alternative modes of presentation [6, 9, 23]. Potential physical signs previously described include lower extremity muscle weakness, atrophy, decreased deep tendon reflexes (particularly the Achilles tendon reflex), as well as diminished saddle and lower extremity sensation [9, 19].

Rectal examination is an important diagnostic maneuver in the setting of a suspected sacral tumor. The mass is often palpable, permitting a further restriction of differential diagnosis [24]. Neurogenic tumors are usually soft, firm, and off the midline, whereas chordomas are often solid and irregular tumors occurring in the midline of the axial skeleton [9]. A decisive aid in the definitive diagnosis of a sacral schwannoma is biopsy. However, its use has been somewhat controversial. Some authors sustain that biopsy is unreliable for the diagnosis of giant nerve sheath tumors because of the secondary degenerative changes frequently present and underline the potential risk of complications associated with the procedure, such as infection or bleeding [18, 25–27]. Others, however, believe that biopsy is essential for determining the treatment of choice or surgery type, as well as to exclude some tumors that would not benefit from a surgical procedure, such as lymphoma [28–30]. In the latter case, biopsy should be performed with oncological principles. The biopsy tract should be marked for possible resection, if pathology results yield the presence of a malignant tumor, such as a sacral chordoma.

12.4 Imaging

In radiographs, the lesions are lytic, with a narrow sclerotic margin usually present at the periphery. The bone contour may be expanded, but there is no periosteal new bone formation. The cortex may be thinned or partially eroded, but no true cortical destruction or extension into soft tissue is usually seen. Central calcification or ossification is absent [31]. However, radiography is almost always nonspecific, and the overlying bowel shadow may frequently obscure bony details. Therefore, CT and MR imaging provide a more complete and detailed assessment of the sacrum, also demonstrating the relationship of the tumor with the anatomical structures present within the pelvis. CT is superior in demonstrating bony detail, whereas MR imaging allows for a better contrast for the study of soft tissue and provides a better display in multiplanar views [8, 32]. On MR imaging, schwannomas are isointense to muscle on T1-weighted and hyperintense on T2-weighted images. After administration of contrast medium, central enhancement is typical [6]. In contrast, malignant peripheral nerve sheath tumors tend to have content with heterogeneous contrast enhancement [6]. Si et al. [8] performed a retrospective study on 49 patients with sacral tumors aiming to define CT and MR imaging features that can safely differentiate between sacral chordoma, sacral giant cell tumor, and giant sacral schwannoma. According to the authors, middle age, a midline and lower sacral location with irregular and fuzzy bone residues, fresh bleeding, and ascending extension in the sacral canal are characteristic features of sacral chordoma; in contrast, younger age, eccentric or upper sacral location, incomplete bony shell, polycystic areas, fluid-fluid levels, and involvement of the sacroiliac joints are features pointing toward a giant cell tumor; finally, pressure bone erosion instead of bone destruction, large and central cystic areas, and absence of adjacent muscle or sacroiliac joint involvement are more likely to represent a giant sacral schwannoma [8].

12.5 Pathology

Schwannomas are composed entirely of cells with the immunophenotype and ultrastructural features of Schwann cells. Macroscopically, intraosseous schwannomas are soft, tan-gray lesions with sparse, yellowish, patchy areas. Cystic and myxoid changes, as well as bleeding, are frequently seen. When the lesion is located in a neural canal or foramen, a capsule may be discernible [11]. The microscopic features of intraosseous schwannoma are similar to those of their more common soft tissue counterparts [14]. There are, however, numerous schwannoma variants. In their classic form, the tumors have two basic patterns: hypercellular or dense (Antoni A) and hypocellular or loose (Antoni B). In Antoni A areas, schwannoma cells are compactly arranged to form focally palisading structures (Verocay bodies).

In Antoni B areas, schwannoma cells are widely separated by a loose intervening collagenous matrix. Lesions may exhibit some nuclear atypia, with occasional mitoses. Long-standing schwannomas often show stromal and vascular degenerative changes including central tissue loss with cystic formation, necrosis without nuclear palisading, nuclear atypia, widespread hyalinization, and calcification [33]. Cellular schwannomas differ from the classic type in that the dense Antoni A pattern comprises 90% or more of the tumor area with a more uniform pattern, a lack of Verocay bodies, and a frequent lymphocytic infiltration [29]. A sacral melanocytic schwannoma has only been reported once [34]. Differential diagnosis should include neurofibroma and malignant nerve sheath tumors. Neurofibroma is another benign nerve sheath tumor that rarely involves the sacral region. It is composed of cells with a polymorphic cellular phenotype. These include Schwann and perineural cells as well as endoneurial fibroblasts [35]. Malignant nerve sheath tumors, such as malignant schwannoma or neurofibrosarcoma, very rarely occur in the sacrum, as well. Intrafascicular spread, local invasion, a fibrous pseudocapsule, gross areas of necrosis, numerous mitoses, and pleomorphism are hallmark features. Previous local radiotherapy may be a contributing factor to the development of malignant nerve sheath tumors [36, 37].

Immunohistochemically, tumor cells are positive for vimentin and S-100 protein. Differential diagnosis should include desmoplastic fibroma, well-differentiated fibrosarcoma, fibrous dysplasia, and nonossifying fibroma. Schwannoma should also be distinguished from a malignant spindle cell neoplasm [11]. Cytogenetic analysis of schwannomas has determined the occurrence of a complete or partial loss of chromosome 22, which bears the tumor suppressor gene *NF2*, as the most frequent abnormality [38].

12.6 Treatment

The mainstay of treatment for the patients with Schwannomas is surgical excision. Given the benign behavior of the tumors, excision can be accomplished by enucleation or curettage. However, sacral excision is usually difficult due to large size, robust blood supply, and frequent proximity to critical structures [9]. Furthermore, available studies suggest that intralesional curettage alone is probably unacceptable as it has a significantly high recurrence rate. In a series published by Abernathy et al. [18], 13 patients with sacral schwannoma were treated with intralesional excision; their local recurrence rate was reported to be as high as 54%, with four patients ultimately requiring reoperation. This data underscores the need for a more aggressive approach, more similar to that employed for malignant sacral tumors. Thus, most authors recommend en bloc resection as the most appropriate procedure for sacral schwannomas [17–19, 39].

An important aspect of the surgical treatment of sacral schwannomas is the choice of the surgical approach needed for efficient en bloc resection. This is often dictated by the exact anatomical distribution of the tumor, with emphasis on the amount of intrasacral and intrapelvic extension of the lesion. According to

Abernathy et al. [18], tumor extension can occur in three directions: (1) in a cephalad direction into the spinal canal, often intradurally; (2) track through the sacral foramina; or (3) erode through the walls of the sacrum. Based on the anatomic extension of the tumor, Klimo et al. [9] proposed a classification of sacral nerve sheath tumors in an attempt to aid the selection of the appropriate surgical approach. According to their work, a type I sacral nerve sheath tumor is one that is confined to the sacrum; a type II (most common) has eroded either the anterior or posterior sacral wall and spread to adjacent spaces; and a type III is confined to the presacral space. They proposed the use of a posterior approach for type I, an anterior approach for type III, and a combined anterior-posterior approach for type II tumors. In a similar fashion, based on an extensive series of 48 patients who underwent surgery for sacral neurogenic tumors, Wei et al. [40] proposed an extended version of the previously mentioned classification system. According to this revised scheme, tumors are classified into four types with respect to tumor growth patterns. Type I tumors are confined to the intrasacral canal and manifest as an enlarged and swollen sacral canal; type II tumors extend through the intrasacral foramina into the presacral space, typically forming a giant presacral mass; type III tumors grow toward both the presacral area and the posterior subcutaneous tissue, forming a mass both anterior and posterior to the sacrum; and type IV tumors are confined to the presacral space, with no tumor observed within the sacral canal. For type I, as well as type II and type III cases in which the tumor extends below S1, the authors employ a posterior approach. For type II and III cases, in which the tumor expanded higher than S1, a combined anterior-posterior approach is recommended. Finally, for type IV cases, the authors propose a single anterior approach [40].

Two operating teams can typically perform a combined, simultaneous abdominosacral resection, with the patient in the left lateral position; this allows full pelvic exposure and facilitates retraction of the sigmoid colon [41–43]. The "anterior" team would access the presacral space, displace the ureters laterally, expose the pelvic vasculature, and retract the rectum anteriorly. The "posterior" team would fully expose the sacrum, identify the sciatic nerve, and perform a lumbosacral laminectomy, to expose the sacral nerve roots. The sacrum would be then transected proximal to the schwannoma. An issue that should be addressed intraoperatively is the potential need for spino-pelvic reconstruction after tumor resection, if spinal stability is compromised. Adequate pelvic stability is usually maintained with transection at the S1–S2 interspace, or even at the L5–S1 interspace, if the lumbosacral facets are preserved [42, 44]. However, the amount of bony destruction should be individually assessed, and fusion should be performed when the continuity of the sacroiliac joint is disrupted.

Every effort should be made to preserve the involved sacral nerve roots. Unilateral preservation of the S2 and S3 can preserve urinary and rectal continence. Preservation of these roots bilaterally should ensure urinary and anorectal continence. Identification and preservation of the pudendal nerve (S2–S4) should ensure erectile function. Bilateral sacrifice of all sacral nerves except the S1 will result in loss of bowel, bladder, and sexual function [45–48]. In anterior surgery, care should be taken for a meticulous dissection and separation of the iliac arteries and veins and rectum from the tumor. Infection, profuse bleeding, and wound breakdown are further potentially catastrophic complications.

Adjuvant therapies such as embolization and cryosurgery have also been described for sacral Schwannomas. Embolization is a useful adjuvant treatment to reduce intraoperative blood loss during sacral surgery [49, 50]. Radiotherapy is generally avoided in the treatment of benign tumors, primarily because of the risk of radiation-induced sarcomas or of malignant degeneration of the nerve sheath tumor [9]. However, conventional external beam radiation therapy has been previously reported in a patient with an incompletely excised sacral schwannoma [51]. On the other hand, stereotactic radiosurgery has recently become an alternative therapy for spinal tumors and could also presumably become a cytoreductive adjuvant therapy for sacral nerve sheath tumors in the future.

Conflict-of-Interest Statement No benefits have been or will be received from a commercial party related directly or indirectly to the subject matter of this article.

References

1. Unni KK, Dahlin DC. Dahlin's bone tumors: general aspects and data on 11,087 cases. 5th ed. Philadelphia: Lippincott-Raven; 1996.
2. Mavrogenis AF, Patapis P, Kostopanagiotou G, Papagelopoulos PJ. Tumors of the sacrum. Orthopedics. 2009;32(5):342.
3. Randall RL. Giant cell tumor of the sacrum. Neurosurg Focus. 2003;15(2):E13.
4. Turcotte RE, Sim FH, Unni KK. Giant cell tumor of the sacrum. Clin Orthop Relat Res. 1993;291:215–21.
5. Turner ML, Mulhern CB, Dalinka MK. Lesions of the sacrum. Differential diagnosis and radiological evaluation. JAMA. 1981;245(3):275–7.
6. Cagli S, Isik HS, Yildirim U, Akinturk N, Zileli M. Giant sacral schwannomas. J Neuro-Oncol. 2012;110(1):105–10. doi:10.1007/s11060-012-0941-1.
7. Kagaya H, Abe E, Sato K, Shimada Y, Kimura A. Giant cauda equina schwannoma. A case report. Spine (Phila Pa 1976). 2000;25(2):268–72.
8. Si MJ, Wang CS, Ding XY, Yuan F, Du LJ, Lu Y, Zhang WB. Differentiation of primary chordoma, giant cell tumor and schwannoma of the sacrum by CT and MRI. Eur J Radiol. 2013;82(12):2309–15. doi:10.1016/j.ejrad.2013.08.034.
9. Klimo Jr P, Rao G, Schmidt RH, Schmidt MH. Nerve sheath tumors involving the sacrum. Case report and classification scheme. Neurosurg Focus. 2003;15(2):E12.
10. Ozturk C, Mirzanli C, Karatoprak O, Tezer M, Aydogan M, Hamzaoglu A. Giant sacral schwannoma: a case report and review of the literature. Acta Orthop Belg. 2009;75(5):705–10.
11. Dorfman HD, Czerniak B. Bone tumors. St. Louis: Mosby; 1998.
12. Agha FP, Lilienfeld RM. Roentgen features of osseous neurilemmoma. Radiology. 1972;102(2):325–6. doi:10.1148/102.2.325.
13. Benazzo F, Marullo M, Rossi SM, Viola E. Giant intraosseous schwannoma of the ileopubic ramus. Orthopedics. 2013;36(7):e982–5. doi:10.3928/01477447-20130624-34.
14. de la Monte SM, Dorfman HD, Chandra R, Malawer M. Intraosseous schwannoma: histologic features, ultrastructure, and review of the literature. Hum Pathol. 1984;15(6):551–8.
15. Sun Z, Sun L, Li T, Ma X, Zhang Z. Intraosseous trigeminal schwannoma of mandible with intracranial extension. J Laryngol Otol. 2011;125(4):418–22. doi:10.1017/S0022215110002707.

16. Verma A, Banerjee K, Verma A, Singh S, Rao J, Om P. Maxillary neurilemmoma-Rarest of the rare tumour: Report of 2 cases. Int J Surg Case Rep. 2013;4(11):1044–7. doi:10.1016/j.ijscr.2013.09.006.
17. DeSanto D, Burgess E. Primary and secondary neurilemmoma of bone. Surg Gynecol Obstet. 1940;71:454–61.
18. Abernathey CD, Onofrio BM, Scheithauer B, Pairolero PC, Shives TC. Surgical management of giant sacral schwannomas. J Neurosurg. 1986;65(3):286–95. doi:10.3171/jns.1986.65.3.0286.
19. Turk PS, Peters N, Libbey NP, Wanebo HJ. Diagnosis and management of giant intrasacral schwannoma. Cancer. 1992;70(11):2650–7.
20. Dominguez J, Lobato RD, Ramos A, Rivas JJ, Gomez PA, Castro S. Giant intrasacral schwannomas: report of six cases. Acta Neurochir. 1997;139(10):954–9. discussion 959–960
21. Kashima TG, Gibbons MR, Whitwell D, Gibbons CL, Bradley KM, Ostlere SJ, Athanasou NA. Intraosseous schwannoma in schwannomatosis. Skelet Radiol. 2013;42(12):1665–71. doi:10.1007/s00256-013-1712-6.
22. Lin PP, Horenstein MG, Healey JH. Sacral mass in a 56-year-old woman. Clin Orthop Relat Res. 1997;(344):333–7, 341–3.
23. Feldenzer JA, McGauley JL, McGillicuddy JE. Sacral and presacral tumors: problems in diagnosis and management. Neurosurgery. 1989;25(6):884–91.
24. Stewart RJ, Humphreys WG, Parks TG. The presentation and management of presacral tumours. Br J Surg. 1986;73(2):153–5.
25. Bastounis E, Asimacopoulos PJ, Pikoulis E, Leppaniemi AK, Aggouras D, Papakonstadinou K, Papalambros E. Benign retroperitoneal neural sheath tumors in patients without von Recklinghausen's disease. Scand J Urol Nephrol. 1997;31(2):129–36.
26. Guz BV, Wood Jr DP, Montie JE, Pontes JE. Retroperitoneal neural sheath tumors: cleveland clinic experience. J Urol. 1989;142(6):1434–7.
27. Luken 3rd MG, Michelsen WJ, Whelan MA, Andrews DL. The diagnosis of sacral lesions. Surg Neurol. 1981;15(5):377–83.
28. Ogose A, Hotta T, Morita T, Higuchi T, Umezu H, Imaizumi S, Hatano H, Kawashima H, Gu W, Endo N. Diagnosis of peripheral nerve sheath tumors around the pelvis. Jpn J Clin Oncol. 2004;34(7):405–13. doi:10.1093/jjco/hyh072.
29. Patocskai EJ, Tabatabaian M, Thomas MJ. Cellular schwannoma: a rare presacral tumour. Can J Surg. 2002;45(2):141–4.
30. Ogose A, Hotta T, Sato S, Takano R, Higuchi T. Presacral schwannoma with purely cystic form. Spine (Phila Pa 1976). 2001;26(16):1817–9.
31. Abdelwahab IF, Hermann G, Stollman A, Wolfe D, Lewis M, Zawin J. Case report 564: giant intraosseous schwannoma. Skelet Radiol. 1989;18(6):466–9.
32. Nyapathy V, Murthy UK, Chintamani J, Sridhar DY. A case report of a giant presacral cystic schwannoma with sigmoid megacolon. J Radiol Case Rep. 2009;3(12):31–7. doi:10.3941/jrcr.v3i12.225.
33. Maneschg C, Rogatsch H, Bartsch G, Stenzl A. Treatment of giant ancient pelvic schwannoma. Tech Urol. 2001;7(4):296–8.
34. Killeen RM, Davy CL, Bauserman SC. Melanocytic schwannoma. Cancer. 1988;62(1):174–83.
35. Topsakal C, Erol FS, Ozercan I, Murat A, Gurates B. Presacral solitary giant neurofibroma without neurofibromatosis type 1 presenting as pelvic mass—case report. Neurol Med Chir (Tokyo). 2001;41(12):620–5.
36. Isler MH, Fogaca MF, Mankin HJ. Radiation induced malignant schwannoma arising in a neurofibroma. Clin Orthop Relat Res. 1996;325:251–5.
37. Grnja V, Allen 3rd WE, Osborn DJ, Kier EL. Sacral neurofibrosarcoma: an angiographic evaluation. Case report. J Neurosurg. 1974;40(6):767–71. doi:10.3171/jns.1974.40.6.0767.
38. Kanamori M, Yasuda T, Hori T, Suzuki K. Giant invasive sacral schwannoma showing chromosomal numerical aberrations [−14, +18, +22]. Asian Spine J. 2013;7(3):227–31. doi:10.4184/asj.2013.7.3.227.

39. Muramatsu K, Ihara K, Kato Y, Yoshida Y, Taguchi T. Intrasacral schwannoma: clinical presentation, diagnosis and management. Br J Neurosurg. 2008;22(6):790–2. doi:10.1080/02688690802108798.
40. Wei G, Xiaodong T, Yi Y, Ji T. Strategy of surgical treatment of sacral neurogenic tumors. Spine (Phila Pa 1976). 2009;34(23):2587–92. doi:10.1097/BRS.0b013e3181bd4a2b.
41. Wanebo HJ, Whitehill R, Gaker D, Wang GJ, Morgan R, Constable W. Composite pelvic resection. An approach to advanced pelvic cancer. Arch Surg. 1987;122(12):1401–6.
42. Karakousis CP. Sacral resection with preservation of continence. Surg Gynecol Obstet. 1986;163(3):270–3.
43. Localio SA, Eng K, Ranson JH. Abdominosacral approach for retrorectal tumors. Ann Surg. 1980;191(5):555–60.
44. Huth JF, Dawson EG, Eilber FR. Abdominosacral resection for malignant tumors of the sacrum. Am J Surg. 1984;148(1):157–61.
45. Xu WP, Song XW, Yue SY, Cai YB, Wu J. Primary sacral tumors and their surgical treatment. A report of 87 cases. Chin Med J. 1990;103(11):879–84.
46. Wuisman P, Harle A, Matthiass HH, Roessner A, Erlemann R, Reiser M. Two-stage therapy in the treatment of sacral tumors. Arch Orthop Trauma Surg. 1989;108(4):255–60.
47. Smith PH, Ballantyne B. The neuroanatomical basis for denervation of the urinary bladder following major pelvic surgery. Br J Surg. 1968;55(12):929–33.
48. Payer M. Neurological manifestation of sacral tumors. Neurosurg Focus. 2003;15(2):E1. doi:10.3171/foc.2003.15.2.1.
49. Gottfried ON, Schmidt MH, Stevens EA. Embolization of sacral tumors. Neurosurg Focus. 2003;15(2):E4.
50. Kollender Y, Meller I, Bickels J, Flusser G, Issakov J, Merimsky O, Marouani N, Nirkin A, Weinbroum AA. Role of adjuvant cryosurgery in intralesional treatment of sacral tumors. Cancer. 2003;97(11):2830–8. doi:10.1002/cncr.11383.
51. Kotoura Y, Shikata J, Yamamuro T, Kasahara K, Iwasaki R, Nakashima Y, Yamabe H. Radiation therapy for giant intrasacral schwannoma. Spine (Phila Pa 1976). 1991;16(2):239–42.

Benign Cartilaginous Tumors of the Sacrum

13

Andrea Angelini and Pietro Ruggieri

13.1 Introduction

Primary benign bone tumors of the sacrum are extremely rare, and cartilaginous lesions have been reported only as case reports or small series. The histotypes affecting the sacrum and reported in literature were osteochondroma, chondroblastoma, chondromyxoid fibroma, and periosteal chondroma. Since clinical, imaging, and histologic characteristics vary immensely, as well as type of treatment, each of these lesions will be discussed in separate paragraphs.

13.2 Osteochondroma

Osteochondroma is caused by a misplaced fragment of the growth plate and the consequent abnormal overgrowth of cartilage in unusual site. The result is a progressive endochondral ossification into a bony subperiosteal protuberance, covered by cartilaginous cap, that projects from the bone surface [1]. The lesion has a thin outer cortex and an internal cancellous structure in continuity with the medulla of the bone from which it arises [2, 3], rich of fatty or hematopoietic marrow [4]. Osteochondroma may be solitary or multiple (associated with an autosomal disorder called hereditary multiple exostoses) [3, 5].

Osteochondroma rarely involves the spine (approximately 3% of cases) [3, 6–8], with solitary lesions involving 1.3–4.1% and HME involving 3–9% of the cases [2, 8–13]. Sacrum is involved less commonly than mobile spine, with an occurrence of about 0.5% of all spinal osteochondromas (Table 13.1) [2, 6–9, 13–19]. Swelling is

A. Angelini, M.D., Ph.D. • P. Ruggieri, M.D., Ph.D. (✉)
Department of Orthopaedics and Orthopedic Oncology, University of Padova, Padova, Italy
e-mail: andrea.angelini83@yahoo.it; pietro.ruggieri@unipd.it

P. Ruggieri et al. (eds.), *Tumors of the Sacrum*,
DOI 10.1007/978-3-319-51202-0_13

Table 13.1 Osteochondroma of the sacrum: review of the literature

Study	Year	Patients (*n*)	Age/ gender	Treatment	Approach and location	Outcome
Pugh et al. [14]	1946	1	–	–	–	–
Sung et al. [7]	1987	2	–	Surgery	PA, below S3	Good, no LR
Hanakita et al. [15]	1988	1	42/F	Surgery, hemilaminectomy L4-S1	PA, L5-S1 lamina	Good, no LR
Gille et al. [16]	2004	1	45/F	Surgery, lumbotomy	PA, S1	
Bess et al. [8]	2005	1	34/F	Surgery, MHE	PA, L5-S1 articular process	Good, no LR
Agrawal et al. [17]	2005	1	14/M	Surgery	PA, right ala sacrum	Good, no LR
Samartzis et al. [6]	2006	1	11/M	Surgery, en bloc excision with S1-S4 laminectomy	PA, S2 lamina	Good, no LR
Chin et al. [18]	2010	1	54/F	Surgery, en bloc excision	Abdominal-retroperitoneal approach, sacrum	Good, no LR
Kuraishi et a. [2]	2014	1	63/F	Surgery, hemilaminectomy right L5-S1	PA, S1 articular process	Good, no LR
Baruah et al. [19]	2015	1	21/M	Surgery, en bloc excision	PA, S3-S4 lamina	Good, no LR
Sciubba et al. [13]	2015	1	48/M	Surgery, en bloc excision	PA, S1	Good, no LR
		1	48/M	Surgery, en bloc excision	PA, S1	LR
		1	21/M	Surgery, en bloc excision	PA, S1	Good, no LR
		1	17/M	Surgery, en bloc excision	PA, S1	Good, no LR
		1	13/M	Surgery, en bloc excision	PA, L5-S3	Good, no LR

F Female, *M* Male, *MHE* multiple hereditary exostosis, *PA* posterior approach, *LR* Local recurrence

one of the main symptoms, slowly increasing during skeletal growth. Osteochondroma is usually painless considering that usually grows posteriorly into the soft tissue, out of the spinal canal, whereas rarely it grows anteriorly causing spinal cord or nerve root compression [8, 19–22]. Similar to other benign tumors, osteochondromas have predilection for young male patients younger than 20 years of age [9]. Due to the unusual site, half of the described cases were treated in adult age [2, 8, 13, 15, 16, 18].

X-rays and computed tomography (CT) scans show the pathognomonic features of bone components with pedunculated or sessile base. However, plain X-rays are usually insufficient because of overlapping of other osseous structures [6, 15, 17]. MRI is important to visualize the size of the cartilaginous cap and the eventual neural structures compression. Differential diagnosis from other neoplasms involving the sacrum is not difficult. Parosteal chondrosarcomas are suspected if increasing size is noticed after skeletal maturity [1, 3, 12]. Malignant transformations to chondrosarcoma range between 10 and 20% in hereditary multiple exostosis and 1–5% in solitary osteochondromas [3, 12, 16]. When the cartilaginous cap is greater than 1–3 cm, in presence of new onset of symptoms or when the tumor rapidly increases in size, malignant changes should be suspected [13].

The mainstay of treatment is observation because most lesions are asymptomatic. En bloc surgical excision of sacral osteochondroma with free margins or marginal margins usually constitutes adequate treatment for symptomatic tumors although it is important to consider the risk of injuring nearby pelvic organs and neurovascular structures [23]. Tumors of the sacrum can be removed through anterior, posterior, or combined approaches [24]. The choice of the appropriate approach is dictated by the location of the tumor and the anatomic peculiarity and hypervascularity of the sacrum. Complete excision of the cartilaginous cap and its overlying periosteum is recommended to reduce the risk of local recurrence [3, 6, 25, 26]. Some authors suggest a frozen section biopsy to confirm margin free of tumor [19].

The outcome and prognosis after surgery of sacral osteochondromas are excellent. The risk of recurrence after treatment of osteochondroma of the spine or the sacrum is not well known because of the rare occurrence. Based on literature review, Gille et al. estimated 4% risk of recurrence in spine, slightly higher than the estimated 2% recurrence in long bones [16]. A tumor recurrence may represent a suspicious of malignancy [3, 12].

13.3 Chondroblastoma

Chondroblastoma is a rare benign cartilage-producing tumor consisting of about 1% of all bone tumors [3]. Chondroblastoma is usually found in the epiphyseal or epimetaphyseal areas of long bones, in males (male:female ratio 2:1), and could be found in any ages, even if it occurs most frequently between 10 and 25 years old. The incidence of vertebral chondroblastoma is 1.4% of all chondroblastomas, and less than five cases of sacral involvement have been reported in literature (only one clearly described) [27]. The radiological findings of vertebral chondroblastomas are nonspecific and biopsy should be performed considering possible more frequent differential diagnosis: aneurysmal bone cyst, giant cell tumor, chondromyxoid fibroma, osteoid osteoma, osteoblastoma, chondrosarcoma, chordoma, and metastasis [3]. Chondroblastomas of the spine behave more aggressively than those of long bones with a higher rate of local recurrence (about one-third of patients) [27–30]. Some authors suggested that this may be related to the frequent extension to adjacent soft tissue and the spinal canal, which precludes complete tumor resection [31,

32]. Three cases of tumor-related death have been reported due to direct invasion to adjacent soft-tissue and neurological structures [27, 30, 33]. Therefore, complete excision and long-term follow-up are generally recommended as the treatment modality for vertebral or sacral chondroblastomas.

13.4 Chondromyxoid Fibroma

Chondromyxoid fibroma (CMF) is a rare benign cartilaginous tumor generally observed between 5 and 30 years of age. It accounts for about 0.5% of all primary bone tumors [3, 34]. CMF of the sacrum is exceedingly rare, with less than ten cases reported in the literature (Table 13.2) [35–43]. Many of them demonstrate expansile or erosive imaging pattern, with cortical destruction, sclerotic and lobulated borders, septation, and intralesional calcifications [34]. Because of these radiographic similarities with more aggressive sacral pathology, differentiating CMF from chondrosarcoma, chordoma, and giant cell tumor on the basis of imaging alone is not possible [40]. CT-guided biopsy with histologic evaluation is mandatory for diagnosis. Although follow-up and detailed documentation are rather lacking in the treatment of sacral CMF, surgery in terms of total en bloc resection or intralesional curettage represents the current accepted management options. Radiation therapy has been used for sacral CMF in only one patient who died of complications before 4 months of follow-up [37]. The risk of local recurrence for CMF ranges between 4 and 80% [41], but higher risk can be expected in younger age group with spine

Table 13.2 Chondromyxoid fibroma of the sacrum: review of the literature

Study	Year	Patients (*n*)	Age/gender	Treatment	Outcome
Markley et al. [35]	1982	1	–	–	–
Shulman et al. [36]	1985	1	15/M	Surgery, anterior-posterior resection	–
Zillmer et al. [37]	1989	1	58/F	Surgery and radiation therapy	Died of complications
Rodgers et al. [38]	1997	1	17/F	Surgery, curettage, and graft	Good, no LR
Wu et al. [39]	1998	1	59/F	Surgery, resection, and lumbopelvic fixation	–
Brat et al. [40]	1999	1	30/M	Surgery, partial sacrectomy	Good, no LR
Mehta et al. [41]	2006	1	26/F	Surgery, resection, and curettage	–
Ahuja et al. [42]	2011	1	59/F	Surgery, curettage, graft, and lumbopelvic fixation	Good, no LR
Minasian et al. [43]	2016	1	35/F	Surgery, partial sacrectomy	Good, no LR

lesions despite extensive curettage [36]. The longest reported follow-up for sacral CMF was a patient treated with curettage and bone grafting, who was found to be recurrencefree at 8-year follow-up [38]. Other authors reported no evidence of recurrence at about 1 year of follow-up after wide resection [40, 42].

13.5 Periosteal or Juxtacortical Chondroma

Periosteal chondroma in the spine is extremely rare and only two cases affecting the sacrum have been reported until now [44, 45]. Periosteal chondroma is a slow-growing benign cartilaginous tumor of bone surface with periosteal origin. Radiologically, it often demonstrates a periosteal shelf of bone and a superficial erosion of the cortex with endosteal sclerosis. Chondrosarcoma is the major differential diagnosis in cases of periosteal chondroma, followed by periosteal osteosarcoma (chondroblastic type), osteochondroma, osteoblastoma, and aneurysmal bone cyst [44, 46]. Akiyama et al. [45] reported a case with large periosteal chondroma that arose on the endopelvic surface of the sacrum, which was difficult to distinguish from chondroid chordoma. The treatment of choice for an asymptomatic tumor is observation as well as for osteochondromas, considering surgery only in presence of symptoms [17]. Singh et al. [44] performed an en bloc excision with good results in terms of pain relief and return to normal activities, without signs of local recurrence after 4 years of follow-up. Akiyama et al. [45] performed intralesional excision with curettage of the underlying cortical bone, and there has been no local recurrence at about 3 years of follow-up.

Conflict of Interest Statement No benefits have been or will be received from a commercial party related directly or indirectly to the subject matter of this article.

References

1. Solomon L, Warwick D, Osteochondroma Nayagam S. Apley's system of orthopaedics and fractures. 9th ed. London: Hodder Arnold; 2010. p. 199–200.
2. Kuraishi K, Hanakita J, Takahashi T, Watanab M, Honda F. Symptomatic osteochondroma of lumbosacral spine: report of 5 cases. Neurol Med Chir. 2014;54(5):408–12.
3. Unni K, editor. Dahlin's bone tumors: general aspects and data on 11,087 cases. Philadelphia: Lippincott-Raven; 1996.
4. Rodallec M, Feydy A, Larousserie F, Anract P, Campagna R, Babinet A, et al. Diagnostic imaging of solitary tumors of the spine: what to do and say. Radiographics. 2008;28:1019–41.
5. Wise C, Clines G, Massa H, et al. Identification and localization of the gene for EXTL, a third member of the multiple exostoses gene family. Genome Res. 1997;7:10–6.
6. Samartzis D, Marco RA. Osteochondroma of the sacrum: a case report and review of the literature. Spine. 2006;31(13):E425–9.
7. Sung H, Shu W, Wang H, et al. Surgical treatment of primary tumors of the sacrum. Clin Orthop Relat Res. 1987;215:91–8.
8. Bess RS, Robbin MR, Bohlman HH, Thompson GH. Spinal exostoses analysis of twelve cases and review of the literature. Spine. 2005;7:774–80.

9. Albrecht S, Crutchfeld JS, SeGall GK. On spinal osteochondromas. J Neurosurg. 1992;77:247–52.
10. Robbins SE, Laitt RD, Lewis T. Hereditary spinal osteochondromas in diaphyseal aclasia. Neuroradiology. 1996;38:59–61.
11. Royster RM, Kujawa P, Dryer RF. Multilevel osteochondroma of the lumbar spine presenting as spinal stenosis. Spine. 1991;16:992–3.
12. Schajowicz F. Tumors and tumorlike lesions of bone and joints. New York: Springer; 1994. p. 141–256.
13. Sciubba DM, Macki M, Bydon M, Germscheid NM, Wolinsky JP, Boriani S, Bettegowda C, Chou D, Luzzati A, Reynolds JJ, Szövérfi Z, Zadnik P, Rhines LD, Gokaslan ZL, Fisher CG, Varga PP. Long-term outcomes in primary spinal osteochondroma: a multicenter study of 27 patients. J Neurosurg Spine. 2015;22(6):582–8.
14. Pugh H, Crile GJ, Robnett A. Exostosis of sacrum: report of a case. US Nav Med Bull. 1946;46:269–72.
15. Hanakita J, Suzuki T. Solitary sacral osteochondroma compressing the cauda equina—case report. Neurol Med Chir. 1988;28:1010–3.
16. Gille O, Pointillart V, Vital JM. Course of spinal solitary osteochon-droma. Spine. 2004;30:E13–9.
17. Agrawal A, Dwivedi S, Joshi R, Gangane N. Osteochondroma of the sacrum with a correlative radiographic and histological evaluation. Paediatr Neurosurg. 2005;41:46–8.
18. Chin K, Kim J. A rare anterior sacral osteochondroma presenting as sciatica in an adult: a case report and review of the literature. Spine J. 2010;10(5):e1–4.
19. Baruah RK, Das H, Haque R. Solitary sacral osteochondroma without neurological symptoms: a case report and review of the literature. Eur Spine J. 2015;24(Suppl 4):S628–32.
20. Ohtori S, Yamagata M, Hanaoka E, Suzuki H, Takahashi K, Sameda H, Moriya H. Osteochondroma in the lumbar spinal canal causing sciatic pain: report of two cases. J Orthop Sci. 2003;8:112–5.
21. Fiumara E, Scarabino T, Guglielmi G, Bisceglia M, D'angelo V. Osteochondroma of L-5 vertebra a rare cause of sciatic pain. Case report. J Neurosurg. 1999;91(2 suppl):219–22.
22. Govender S, Parbhoo AH. Osteochondroma with compression of the spinal cord. A report of two cases. J Bone Joint Surg Br. 1999;81-B:667–9.
23. Bottner F, Rodl R, Kordish I, Winklemann W, Gosheger G, Lindner N. Surgical treatment of symptomatic osteochondroma: a three- to eight-year follow-up study. J Bone Joint Surg Br. 2003;85:1161–5.
24. Ruggieri P, Angelini A, Ussia G, Montalti M, Mercuri M. Surgical margins and local control in resection of sacral chordomas. Clin Orthop Relat Res. 2010;468(11):2939–47.
25. Boriani S, Weinstein JN, Biagini R. Primary bone tumors of the spine. Spine. 1997;22:1036–44.
26. Weinstein JN, McLain RF. Primary tumors of the spine. Spine. 1987;12:843–51.
27. Akai M, Tateishi A, Machinami R, Iwano K, Asao T. Chondroblastoma of the sacrum: a case report. Acta Orthop Scand. 1986;57:378–81.
28. Ilaslan H, Sundaram M, Unni KK. Vertebral chondroblastoma. Skelet Radiol. 2003;32:66–71.
29. Bloem JL, Mulder JD. Chondroblastoma: a clinical and radiological study of 104 cases. Skelet Radiol. 1985;14:1–9.
30. Hoe el JC, Brasse F, Schmi M, et al. About one case of vertebral chondroblastoma. Pediatr Radiol. 1987;17:392–6.
31. Kim J, Kumar R, Raymond AK, Ayala AG. Non-epiphyseal chondroblastoma arising in the iliac bone, and complicated by an aneurysmal bone cyst: a case report and review of the literature. Skelet Radiol. 2010;39(6):583–7.
32. Leung LY, Shu SJ, Chan MK, Chan CH. Chondroblastoma of the lumbar vertebra. Skelet Radiol. 2001;30:710–3.
33. Chung OM, Yip SF, Ngan KC, Ng WF. Chondroblastoma of the lumbar spine with cauda equina syndrome. Spinal Cord. 2003;41:359–64.

34. Wilson AJ, Kyriakos M, Ackerman LV. Chondromyxoid fibroma: radiographic appearance in 38 cases and in a review of the literature. Radiology. 1991;179:513–8.
35. Makley JT, Cohen AM, Baada E. Sacral tumours: hidden problems. Orthopedics. 1982;5:996–1003.
36. Shulman L, Bale P, de Silva M. Sacral chondromyxoid fibroma. Pediatr Radiol. 1985;15: 138–40.
37. Zillmer DA, Dorfman HD. Chondromyxoid fibroma of bone: thirtysix cases with clinicopathologic correlation. Hum Pathol. 1989;20:952–64.
38. Rodgers WB, Kennedy JG, Zimbler S. Chondromyxoid fibroma of the ala of the sacrum presenting as a cause of lumbar pain in an adolescent. Eur Spine J. 1997;6:351–3.
39. Wu CT, Inwards CY, O'Laughlin S, Rock MG, Beabout JW, Unni KK. Chondromyxoid fibroma of bone: a clinicopathologic review of 278 cases. Hum Pathol. 1998;29:438–46.
40. Brat HG, Renton P, Sandison A, Cannon S. Chondromyxoid fibroma of the sacrum. Eur Radiol. 1999;9:1800–3.
41. Mehta S, Szklaruk J, Faria SC, Raymond AK, Whitman GJ. Radiologicpathologic conferences of the University of Texas M.D. Anderson Cancer Center: chondromyxoid fibroma of the sacrum and left iliac bone. AJR Am J Roentgenol. 2006;186:467–9.
42. Ahuja SK, McCanna SP, Horn EM. Treatment strategy for chondromyxoid fibroma of the sacrum. J Clin Neurosci. 2011;18:1550–2.
43. Minasian T, Claus C, Hariri OR, Piao Z, Quadri SA, Yuhan R, Leong D, Tashjian V. Chondromyxoid fibroma of the sacrum: a case report and literature review. Surg Neurol Int. 2016;7(Suppl 13):S370–4.
44. Singh AP, Singh AP, Mahajan S. Periosteal chondroma of the sacrum. Can J Surg. 2008; 51(5):E105–6.
45. Akiyama T, Yamamoto A, Kashima T, Ishida T, Shinoda Y, Goto T, Nakamura K, Kawano H. Juxtacortical chondroma of the sacrum. J Orthop Sci. 2008;13(5):476–80.
46. Boriani S, Bacchini P, Bertoni F, et al. Periosteal chondroma. A review of twenty cases. J Bone Joint Surg Am. 1983;65:205–12.

Part III

Malignant Lesions

Metastases of the Sacrum

14

Andreas F. Mavrogenis, Georgios N. Panagopoulos,
Andrea Angelini, and Pietro Ruggieri

14.1 Introduction

The most common malignancy to occur in the sacrum is metastatic bone disease [1–3]. The most common primary cancers are breast, lung, prostate, renal, and thyroid cancer [4–7]. Other less common primary lesions include lymphoma, myeloma/plasmacytoma, melanoma, and tumors of unknown origin [8]. Spread is mainly by hematogenous dissemination, although direct extension in case of recurrent rectal tumors and drop metastases of intradural tumors has also been described [9, 10].

Bone metastases are the final common pathway of many malignancies and can result in skeletal events such as pathological fracture, spinal cord compression, bone pain, and hypercalcemia, which are frequently detrimental for the patients' outcome and quality of life. In the sacrum, metastatic disease frequently grows insidiously, causing ambiguous symptoms in the early stages and possibly resulting in a delayed diagnosis, when the tumor has already extended beyond bony margins and around sacral nerve roots [8, 11]. Pain is the most common presenting symptom, either local, mechanical, or radicular in nature, typically followed by progressive neurological deficits, eventually leading to bladder, bowel, and/or sexual dysfunction [12–14]. The treatment of sacral metastatic lesions is usually palliative, aiming primarily at pain control and preservation of neurological function. Commonly employed treatment modalities include radiotherapy and spinal stereotactic surgery, sacroplasty, embolization, ablation techniques, as well as targeted medical therapy.

A.F. Mavrogenis, M.D., Ph.D. • G.N. Panagopoulos, M.D.
First Department of Orthopaedics, National and Kapodistrian University of Athens, Athens, Greece
e-mail: afm@otenet.gr

A. Angelini, M.D., Ph.D. • P. Ruggieri, M.D., Ph.D. (✉)
Department of Orthopedics and Orthopedic Oncology, University of Padova, Padova, Italy
e-mail: andrea.angelini83@yahoo.it; pietro.ruggieri@unipd.it

P. Ruggieri et al. (eds.), *Tumors of the Sacrum*,
DOI 10.1007/978-3-319-51202-0_14

14.2 Epidemiology

As the incidence of cancer continues to increase, and patients with cancer live longer, the incidence of metastatic bone disease is steadily increasing [15, 16]. In the USA, nearly 1.4 million people are diagnosed with cancer every year. Of these, half of patients suffer a cancer that frequently metastasizes to bone. Over 400,000 Americans are estimated to develop skeletal metastases annually [17–20]. Spinal metastases develop in 5–10% of all cancer patients during the course of their illness, with sacral deposits representing the minority of spinal secondaries [3, 9]. However, if seen as a whole, metastatic deposits represent the most common malignant tumor of the sacrum [1, 6, 7]. The most common cancers to metastasize to the sacrum are breast, prostate, thyroid, lung, and renal cancer. In autopsy studies, the incidence of metastatic deposits in breast and prostate cancers is as high as 73% [21]. A quarter of patients with skeletally metastatic renal cell cancer will have proximal femoral metastases [20, 22–27].

14.3 Biology of the Metastatic Process

The ability of tumor cells to invade within their host organ and their ability to metastasize to distant sites are the main biological hallmarks of malignancy. The metastatic spread of tumor cells to the skeleton is a complex multistep process highly dependent on the properties and characteristics of tumor cells and bone microenvironment. To successfully metastasize, cancer cells must complete a number of important steps. Neoplastic cells must proliferate within the host organ and gain the ability to invade the surrounding tissue and matrix; they must invade blood vessels, whether induced by angiogenic properties of the tumor cells or normal vessels at the site; they should then enter the circulatory system and survive both intracellular and extracellular influences attempting to destroy them; they must adhere to and migrate across sinusoidal walls at distant sites; finally, they should form deposits capable of surviving in the new environment [28]. Many theories have been proposed over the years in an attempt to explain propensity for metastatic spread to bone. Batson first hypothesized, in 1940, that the vertebral system of veins acts like a conduit for cancer cell dissemination to the skeletal system [29]. In 1989, Paget proposed the "seed and soil" hypothesis to explain the metastatic tropism of tumor cells for specific organs [30]. More recently, the model of the pre-metastatic niche has been formulated. This model proposes that a primary tumor is capable to prepare a conductive microenvironment at a distant site before the disseminated tumor cells arrive at the site and establish metastases. The concept of pre-metastatic niche, hence, involves the action of the primary tumor on the destination site of metastasis through production of tumor-derived growth factors, such as TGF-β, vascular endothelial growth factor A (VEGF-A) and placental growth factor (PGF). In response to these factors, hematopoietic progenitor cells (HPCs), macrophages, and other tumor-associated immune cells gather at the metastatic site and prime the "soil" for the arrival of the tumor cells, helping adhesion and invasion [31–33].

14.4 Tissue of Origin Considerations

Among tumors with a unique propensity for skeletal metastases, cancer of the breast, prostate, thyroid, and kidney are worth mentioning separately because of their specific features.

Breast cancer is the most common cancer among women, with 1.3 million cases diagnosed each year worldwide; in this group, it also constitutes the leading cause of cancer death [34]. At the time of diagnosis, about 5% of all breast cancers are metastatic, with bone being the most common location of distant spread. In fact, in 35% of women with metastatic breast cancer, the only burden of metastatic disease is represented by bone metastases [22]. Importantly, women with bone-only metastatic breast cancer have a significantly better prognosis compared to women with visceral metastases [35, 36]. Furthermore, a significant portion of women with bone metastases from breast cancer (approximately 41%) have a solitary metastatic lesion, which is associated with increased survival compared to women with multiple bone deposits [37]. The most common type of metastatic bone disease from breast cancer is generally classified as osteolytic, estimated at 80–90%, causing bone destruction. However, osteoblastic or mixed lesions are not exceptional [38]. Bone metastases are disproportionately common among estrogen-receptor-positive breast tumors. It is important to note that women with estrogen-receptor-positive bone-only metastatic breast cancer can live many years with good quality of life, typically treated only with oral endocrine therapy. Thus, aggressive management of bony metastases and emphasis to the prevention of skeletal complications within this group of women are imperative [22]. After obtaining promising results in multiple clinical trials, zoledronic acid or denosumab is recommended in all patients with metastatic breast cancer and bone metastases, whether symptomatic or not [39].

Prostate cancer is the most common malignancy diagnosed in men and constitutes a model for epithelial malignancy that is likely to metastasize to bone [40]; 7.7% of men with prostate cancer have evidence of bone metastasis at diagnosis [41]. Studies have shown that nearly 90% of men who develop metastases from prostate cancer will have bone involvement [42]. Skeletal metastases from prostate carcinoma are typically osteoblastic, with sclerotic lesions most commonly seen in the pelvis and vertebral bodies. The most common diagnostic test used to screen for bone metastases in newly diagnosed prostate cancer patients is the technetium bone scan. Androgen deprivation therapy (ADT) is a well-accepted care standard in men diagnosed with prostate cancer and metastatic disease of bone. However, ADT demonstrates concomitant effects on bone density and general skeletal health that can compound the risk of skeletal events in men with metastatic bone disease [22]. Addition of primary site radiation to ADT has been shown to increase metastasis-free survival [43].

All variants of thyroid carcinoma can metastasize to bone, but the well-differentiated carcinomas (papillary, follicular, and Hürthle cell types) have a unique propensity to do so [44, 45]. Among the well-differentiated variants, follicular carcinoma is particularly prone to metastasize to bone. In thyroid cancer, after metastases to the neck lymph nodes, the skeleton and lungs are the most frequent sites of metastases, with skeletal lesions occurring even more than 20 years after treatment of the primary lesion [46]. Radiographically, metastatic thyroid carcinoma typically presents as a destructive, lytic bone lesion. Metastatic thyroid carcinoma has easily recognizable microscopic features and can be clinically associated with thyrotoxicosis [47]. Immunohistochemistry for thyroglobulin or TTF-1 in follicular and papillary carcinomas, and calcitonin in medullary carcinomas, can aid microscopic diagnosis. Management of these patients implicates a multidisciplinary approach, involving surgery, radiation, and medical therapy.

Renal cell carcinoma is another prototype of tumor that frequently presents as a skeletal (often solitary) metastasis, with a clinically occult primary tumor [48]. Nearly 30% of patients with renal cell carcinomas have metastatic disease at presentation [49]. Renal cell carcinomas are known to metastasize to unusual distant sites such as the skin, tongue, eye, heart muscle, acral skeleton, and breast [50, 51]. Although osteoblastic lesions have been described, the vast majority are lytic [52]. Nephrectomy or metastasectomy is often performed in patients with disseminated disease to reduce the tumor burden, with the hope that remaining foci may stabilize or regress. Resection of solitary skeletal metastasis significantly prolongs survival [53, 54]. Biological targeted therapy is also available against metastatic renal cell carcinoma (mRCC). As of 2014, there are seven FDA-approved drugs for use in mRCC utilizing four different mechanisms of action. Bevacizumab (Avastin) is an IgG_1 monoclonal antibody that binds VEGF. Axitinib (Inlyta) and Pazopanib (Votrient) are both kinase inhibitors effective against tyrosine kinases associated with VEGF receptors. Sunitinib (Sutent) and Sorafenib (Nexavar) are also kinase inhibitors active against intracellular kinase Raf-1, PDGF, and VEGF. Temsirolimus (Torisel) and Everolimus (Afinitor) are inhibitors of mTOR, a kinase involved in regulation of cell proliferation, survival, and transcription of HIF [55–58].

14.5 Presentation and Diagnosis

Sacral neoplasms generally grow insidiously, causing ambiguous symptoms in the early stages and frequently result in delayed diagnosis. Thus, presence of metastatic deposits in the sacrum often signifies advanced disease [11]. In a case series of 34 patients with sacral metastases [59], 61% of patients had distal organ involvement, whereas 41% demonstrated widespread spinal metastases. In a similar study of 19 patients [60], at the time of diagnosis, 68% of patients had extraspinal metastases and 53% involvement of multiple spinal levels.

Typically, the initial symptom at presentation of patients with sacral metastases is pain. This may be local pain due to periosteal stretching and local inflammation, mechanical pain as a result of instability, or radicular pain from nerve root irritation, compression, or neoplastic infiltration [11, 59]. Radicular pain may radiate unilaterally or bilaterally into the buttocks, posterior thigh or leg, external genitalia, and perineum. More commonly, sensory multiradicular deficit evolves in an insidious manner, slowly progressing to a motor deficit and eventually causing bladder, bowel, or sexual dysfunction [61].

Imaging of the sacrum with standard radiographs only is difficult. Typically, CT is done to define the osseous anatomy, whereas MR imaging gives more information on soft tissue extension, nerve root and visceral tumor involvement. A bone scan or PET CT can elucidate the presence of monostotic or polyostotic disease. A biopsy is usually necessary to confirm diagnosis and plan subsequent treatment. Failure to rule out other potential etiologies of osseous lesions creates the potential for misdiagnosis and mismanagement. The gold standard of biopsy is closed, imaging (preferable CT) guided; open biopsy may be indicated if results of the former are nondiagnostic or controversial. Whether closed or open, the soft tissue tract through which a biopsy is performed is considered contaminated with potentially malignant cells, and needs to be positioned in a manner that will facilitate its ultimate excision in continuity with the final tumor specimen. To that end, biopsy incisions should be minimized while providing access to diagnostic tissue and oriented longitudinally, in line with an extensile surgical approach. Generally, the surgeon who will perform the definitive tumor resection should perform or direct the biopsy procedure. Poorly planned incisional biopsies or incomplete debulking performed prior to referral to an orthopedic oncology unit have been shown to increase the risk of local recurrence and metastasis [62, 63].

14.6 Treatment

The treatment of sacral metastatic lesions is usually palliative, aiming primarily at pain control and preservation of neurological function. There is a paucity of studies dealing with the management of these lesions, since most papers refer to primary sacral tumors [9, 10, 59, 60, 64–77]. There is also no consensus or precise strategy algorithm as to which method is the most appropriate, making management highly individualized on a patient-to-patient basis, depending to an extent on institutional preferences (Table 14.1) [9, 10, 59, 60, 64–77]. Modalities commonly employed include radiation therapy and stereotactic surgery, surgery, sacroplasty, embolization, as well as various ablation techniques [9, 10, 59, 60, 64–77].

Radiation therapy is an integral part of treatment for patients with metastatic bone disease, both in the upfront and adjuvant setting. Radiation therapy is frequently chosen as a first-line initial therapy for radiosensitive sacral metastases, in patients without evidence of spinal instability or acute neurological deterioration, where pain reduction and neurological improvement are feasible [78, 79]. It must be taken into account that radiosensitivity varies among primary cancer types. In general, prostate and lymphoid tumors are radiosensitive, and breast cancer is 70% sensitive and 30% resistant, whereas gastrointestinal tumors, renal cell carcinomas, and melanomas are radioresistant [3]. Patients are unlikely to experience complete relief immediately, but should expect pain relief within 4–8 weeks following treatment. An emerging form of radiation therapy, which allows more precise radiation delivery and high-dose hypofractionation, is spinal stereotactic radiosurgery (SRS).

Table 14.1 Summary of the most important published studies involving patients with metastases of the sacrum

Study	Patients (number)	Age/Gender	Primary tumor	Metastasis level	Neoadjuvant treatments	Procedure	Survival
Ozdemir et al. [59]	65; 34 sacral metastases	21M/25F; mean age, 49 years (range, 12–83 years)	Breast (9), MM (7), prostate (4), lung (3), colon (3), leiomyosarcoma (2), lymphoma (2), ovary (1), RCC (1), thyroid (1), larynx (1)	N/A	N/A	Resection or curettage and PMMA	36 months (30–120)
Turgut et al. [64]	1	63M	Merkel cell cancer	L5–S1	None	L5 laminectomy and subtotal resection	2 months
Lee et al. [65]	1	51F	Meningioma	Left sacrum and ilium	None	2-stage excision	N/A
Kollender et al. [9]	14; 5 sacral metastases	7M/7F; mean age, 42 years (range, 14–74 years)	RCC (2), MC (2), colon (1)	Mid sacrum (2), left sacrum (2), entire sacrum (1)	All RT; embolization (2)	Decompression and cryosurgery	6–36 months
Nader et al. [60]	19	N/A	RCC (13), breast (2), melanoma (1), MM (1), colon (1), liposarcoma (1)	S1 (18), S2 (13), S3 (3), S4 (2), L/S (4), SIJ (4), other spine (10), extraspinal (13)	N/A	Laminectomy (18), vertebrectomy (13), instrumentation (12)	22 months (5–38)
Menegaz et al. [66]	1	45F	Chorioncarcinoma	L2–S1	None	CMT and RT	7 months
Uemura et al. [67]	1	76M	HCC	Left and right sacrum	Embolization and RT	Sacroplasty	72 days
Gerszten et al. [68]	393; 500 lesions; 103 sacral metastases	251M/142F; mean age, 56 years (range, 18–85 years)	RCC (93), breast (83), lung (80), colon (32), sarcoma (26), prostate (24), MM (18), unknown (14), SCC (12), thyroid (11), other (69)	Sacral (103)	RT (344)	Radiosurgery	21 months (3–53)
Akasu et al. [69]	44	35M/9F; mean age, 55 years (range, 32–73 years)	Recurrent rectal cancer	Pelvic (12), solitary pelvic (24), distant (8)	RT (13)	Sacral resection	2.3 years (1–16)
Fujibayashi et al. [70]	5	4M/1F; mean age, 47 years (range, 29–77 years)	Lung (2), renal (2), paraganglioma (1)	LS joint, sacrum	N/A	Instrumentation	28 months (3–72)

Table 14.1 (continued)

Study	Patients (number)	Age/Gender	Primary tumor	Metastasis level	Neoadjuvant treatments	Procedure	Survival
Kakutani et al. [71]	1	52M	Melanoma	Left S1–4 and ilium	None	CMT and RT	9 months
Zhang et al. [72]	2	1M/1F; age, 62 and 38 years	Lymphoma, lung	S1 and T12, L1–3; S1	CMT and RT	S1 percutaneous sacroplasty	N/A
Albareda et al. [73]	1	62F	Endometrial	S4	None	En bloc resection	26 months
Toro et al. [74]	1	65M	HCC	Right S1–5, left S1–2	None	Sacroplasty	N/A
Dozois et al. [75]	9	7M/2F; mean age, 63 years (range, 38–78 years)	Recurrent rectal	S2 (6), S1 (2), L/S (1)	RT (7), CMT (1)	High sacrectomy	30% at 5 years
Nebreda et al. [76]	1	48F	Small-cell lung cancer	Left S1–2 and SIJ	CMT and SRS	PMMA	40 days
Feiz-Erfan et al. [10]	25	21M/4F; mean age, 57 years (range, 25–71 years)	RCC (15), prostate (3), other (7)	Solitary sacrum (12), multiple sites (13)	RT (11), CMT (9), embolization (12), other (5)	En bloc resection and instrumentation	11 months (5.4–16.6)
Moussazadeh et al. [77]	25; 31 procedures	10M/15F, mean age, 65 years, (range, 32–84 years)	Sacral mets (15), w/previous RT for pelvic cancer (4), chordomas (3), osteoporotic (5), other (4)	N/A	RT (22)	Sacroplasty w/ PMMA	15 died at 4.3 months

RCC renal cell carcinoma, *MM* multiple myeloma, *SCC* squamous cell carcinoma, *MC* metastatic carcinoma, *HCC* hepatocellular carcinoma, *CMT* chemotherapy, *RT* radiation therapy, *SIJ* sacro-iliac joint, *PMMA* polymethylmethacrylate bone cement, *SRS* stereotactic radiation surgery, *N/A* not available

SRS allows administering a tumoricidal radiation dose even for radioresistant tumors, with minimal exposure of the surrounding normal tissues. Current commercial spinal SRS systems include the CyberKnife® (Accuray Incorporated, Sunnyvale, California) and Novalis® (BrainLAB, Heinstetten, Germany) [3]. Unlike conventional radiation therapy in which a full dose is delivered to both the vertebral body and the spinal cord or cauda equina, SRS can deliver a high-dose single fraction to the target tissue while sparing most of the adjacent neural elements, thus significantly reducing the possibility of radiation-induced myelopathy or injury to the nerve roots. Other major benefits of SRS include the relatively short treatment time, which can be in an outpatient setting and the minimal or complete absence of side effects.

The role of surgery in metastatic disease of the sacrum is not clearly defined. Indications for surgical intervention include progressive neurological dysfunction or persistent pain that is unresponsive to radiation therapy, the need for a diagnostic biopsy, and pathological sacro-pelvic instability [3, 59]. If nonsurgical measures fail and the patient is suffering from symptomatic sacral disease, surgery can be a reasonable therapeutic option [10]. Metastatic disease in the sacrum generally does not cause mechanical instability, as this segment is rigidly fixed to the pelvis by the bilateral sacroiliac joints and their accompanying ligaments. In cases of massive tumor destruction of the S1 body and/or L5–S1 junction, fixation from the low lumbar spine into the sacrum and pelvis may be required to restore spinopelvic continuity. If instability occurs in the sacrum, reconstruction often includes low lumbar pedicle-based instrumentation systems along with sacral pedicle instrumentation and iliac bolts, with or without additional sacroiliac screws. A posterior midline sacral laminectomy may be necessary in case of sacral nerve root compression. In any case, care must be taken in the decision-making process, as sacral resections are challenging operations with a high incidence of potential complications, especially in patients with an already limited life expectancy [80]. On the other hand, resective surgery in carefully selected patients with sacral metastases may result in a palliative benefit. Removal of secondary lesions of renal cell carcinoma tends to be associated with an increase in overall survival. A minimal disease burden (single-site metastasis) may signify that there is a greater chance for surgery to achieve definitive local control [10].

Sacroplasty is a therapeutic option more extensively described in the degenerative/osteoporotic literature, now gaining favor in cases of metastatic disease without instability or neurologic compromise [81–83]. The technique is similar to vertebroplasty, involving cement augmentation of a metastatic lesion under CT guidance. Potential complications include hemorrhage, infection, dural tears with cerebrospinal fluid leak, direct injury of nerve roots or the lumbosacral plexus, cement leakage or ectopic cement injection (into the sacroiliac joint), migration, and embolization. Clinical data on the procedure is promising, demonstrating immediate improvement in mobility and significant pain relief in most patients undergoing the procedure [67, 72, 74, 76].

Embolization of sacral tumors is another useful therapy, which may be primary (single or repeat treatment sessions), adjuvant to surgical treatment, or palliative. Preoperative selective arterial embolization of hypervascular metastatic lesions reduces intraoperative blood loss and improves the surgeon's ability to subsequently perform surgical resection. Studies have shown that embolization may cause tumor growth arrest, relieve pain, and reduce hospital stay [84–90]. The timing of preoperative embolization is also important. Typically, best results are achieved when surgery is performed within 24–48 h after embolization. Serial embolization can also be performed if there is persistent pain and/or evidence of progressive disease on imaging. It is typically performed in 4–6-week intervals until symptomatic improvement occurs or the tumor's vascularity disappears. Complication rate is generally low. Risks of the procedure include nerve palsy, subcutaneous or muscle necrosis, postembolization syndrome (fever, pain, malaise), ischemic pain (usually transitory), infection, and tumor bleeding [87–90].

Over the last few decades, percutaneous ablation has emerged as an effective, minimally invasive, local treatment alternative to conventional methods, aiming to provide either palliation of painful bone lesions or local control of oligometastatic disease. Various image-guided ablation technologies have been applied to the treatment of bone metastases with varied levels of published evidence. Thermal ablation methods include radiofrequency ablation (RFA), cryoablation, microwave ablation, laser ablation, and more recently MRI-guided extracorporeal-focused ultrasound (MRgFUS) [91]. RFA and other ablation techniques are safe and reproducible, with promising results (pain relief 75–95%) [92]. Potential complications include skin burns and injury to heat-sensitive structures, such as nerves and bowel [93].

Finally, modern targeted medical therapy aims to control pain and reduce skeletal events of metastatic cancers. Such agents are mainly represented by bisphosphonates and denosumab. Bisphosphonates inhibit normal and pathological osteoclast-mediated bone resorption by direct inhibition of osteoclast activity by cellular mechanisms that affect osteoclast attachment, differentiation, and survival. They also reduce osteoclast activity indirectly, through effects on osteoblasts. In 2002, intravenous zoledronic acid was approved to treat patients with multiple myeloma and bone metastases from any solid tumor including prostate cancer. Denosumab is a human monoclonal antibody for the treatment of osteoporosis, induced bone loss, bone metastases, rheumatoid arthritis, multiple myeloma, and giant cell tumor of bone. It is designed to target RANKL (RANK ligand), a protein that acts as the primary signal to promote bone loss. Denosumab has been approved by the US Food and Drug Administration (FDA) for the prevention of skeletal related events in patients with bone metastases from solid tumors. Potential drawbacks of both drug families notably include the risk for osteonecrosis of the jaw and for the development of atypical femoral fractures [93–95].

Conflict of Interest Statement No benefits have been or will be received from a commercial party related directly or indirectly to the subject matter of this article.

References

1. Mavrogenis AF, Patapis P, Kostopanagiotou G, Papagelopoulos PJ. Tumors of the sacrum. Orthopedics. 2009;32(5):342.
2. Unni KK, Inwards CY, Mayo Foundation for Medical Education and Research. Dahlin's bone tumors: general aspects and data on 10,165 cases. 6th ed. Philadelphia: Wollters Kluwer Health/Lippincott Williams & Wilkins; 2010.
3. Quraishi NA, Giannoulis KE, Edwards KL, Boszczyk BM. Management of metastatic sacral tumours. Eur Spine J. 2012;21(10):1984–93. doi:10.1007/s00586-012-2394-9.
4. Steinmetz MP, Mekhail A, Benzel EC. Management of metastatic tumors of the spine: strategies and operative indications. Neurosurg Focus. 2001;11(6):e2.
5. Raque Jr GH, Vitaz TW, Shields CB. Treatment of neoplastic diseases of the sacrum. J Surg Oncol. 2001;76(4):301–7.
6. Llauger J, Palmer J, Amores S, Bague S, Camins A. Primary tumors of the sacrum: diagnostic imaging. AJR Am J Roentgenol. 2000;174(2):417–24. doi:10.2214/ajr.174.2.1740417.

7. Diel J, Ortiz O, Losada RA, Price DB, Hayt MW, Katz DS. The sacrum: pathologic spectrum, multimodality imaging, and subspecialty approach. Radiographics. 2001;21(1):83–104. doi:10.1148/radiographics.21.1.g01ja0883.
8. Quraishi NA, Giannoulis KE, Manoharan SR, Edwards KL, Boszczyk BM. Surgical treatment of cauda equina compression as a result of metastatic tumours of the lumbo-sacral junction and sacrum. Eur Spine J. 2013;22(Suppl 1):S33–7. doi:10.1007/s00586-012-2615-2.
9. Kollender Y, Meller I, Bickels J, Flusser G, Issakov J, Merimsky O, Marouani N, Nirkin A, Weinbroum AA. Role of adjuvant cryosurgery in intralesional treatment of sacral tumors. Cancer. 2003;97(11):2830–8. doi:10.1002/cncr.11383.
10. Feiz-Erfan I, Fox BD, Nader R, Suki D, Chakrabarti I, Mendel E, Gokaslan ZL, Rao G, Rhines LD. Surgical treatment of sacral metastases: indications and results. J Neurosurg Spine. 2012;17(4):285–91. doi:10.3171/2012.7.SPINE09351.
11. Feldenzer JA, McGauley JL, McGillicuddy JE. Sacral and presacral tumors: problems in diagnosis and management. Neurosurgery. 1989;25(6):884–91.
12. Miralbell R, Louis DN, O'Keeffe D, Rosenberg AE, Suit HD. Metastatic ependymoma of the sacrum. Cancer. 1990;65(10):2353–5.
13. Payer M. Neurological manifestation of sacral tumors. Neurosurg Focus. 2003;15(2):E1. doi:10.3171/foc.2003.15.2.1.
14. Hall JH, Fleming JF. The "lumbar disc syndrome" produced by sacral metastases. Can J Surg. 1970;13(2):149–56.
15. Weber KL, Randall RL, Grossman S, Parvizi J. Management of lower-extremity bone metastasis. J Bone Joint Surg Am. 2006;88(Suppl 4):11–9. doi:10.2106/JBJS.F.00635.
16. Chang S, Long SR, Kutikova L, Bowman L, Finley D, Crown WH, Bennett CL. Estimating the cost of cancer: results on the basis of claims data analyses for cancer patients diagnosed with seven types of cancer during 1999 to 2000. J Clin Oncol. 2004;22(17):3524–30. doi:10.1200/JCO.2004.10.170.
17. Yu HH, Tsai YY, Hoffe SE. Overview of diagnosis and management of metastatic disease to bone. Cancer Control. 2012;19(2):84–91.
18. Jacofsky DJ, Haidukewych GJ. Management of pathologic fractures of the proximal femur: state of the art. J Orthop Trauma. 2004;18(7):459–69.
19. Aaron AD. The management of cancer metastatic to bone. JAMA. 1994;272(15):1206–9.
20. Heymann D, editor. Bone cancer: progression and therapeutic approaches. New York: Elsevier; 2010.
21. Weiss L, Gilbert HA. Bone metastasis. Metastasis, vol. vol 4. Boston: G. K. Hall Medical Publishers; 1981.
22. Randall RL. In: Metastatic bone disease: an integrated approach to patient care. New York, NY: Springer; 2016.
23. Jensen AO, Jacobsen JB, Norgaard M, Yong M, Fryzek JP, Sorensen HT. Incidence of bone metastases and skeletal-related events in breast cancer patients: a population-based cohort study in Denmark. BMC Cancer. 2011;11:29. doi:10.1186/1471-2407-11-29.
24. Norgaard M, Jensen AO, Jacobsen JB, Cetin K, Fryzek JP, Sorensen HT. Skeletal related events, bone metastasis and survival of prostate cancer: a population based cohort study in Denmark (1999–2007). J Urol. 2010;184(1):162–7. doi:10.1016/j.juro.2010.03.034.
25. Cetin K, Christiansen CF, Jacobsen JB, Norgaard M, Sorensen HT. Bone metastasis, skeletal-related events, and mortality in lung cancer patients: a Danish population-based cohort study. Lung Cancer. 2014;86(2):247–54. doi:10.1016/j.lungcan.2014.08.022.
26. Yong M, Jensen AO, Jacobsen JB, Norgaard M, Fryzek JP, Sorensen HT. Survival in breast cancer patients with bone metastases and skeletal-related events: a population-based cohort study in Denmark (1999–2007). Breast Cancer Res Treat. 2011;129(2):495–503. doi:10.1007/s10549-011-1475-5.
27. Oster G, Lamerato L, Glass AG, Richert-Boe KE, Lopez A, Chung K, Richhariya A, Dodge T, Wolff GG, Balakumaran A, Edelsberg J. Natural history of skeletal-related events in patients with breast, lung, or prostate cancer and metastases to bone: a 15-year study in two large US

health systems. Support Care Cancer. 2013;21(12):3279–86. doi:10.1007/s00520-013-1887-3.
28. Mundy GR. Metastasis to bone: causes, consequences and therapeutic opportunities. Nat Rev Cancer. 2002;2(8):584–93. doi:10.1038/nrc867.
29. Batson OV. The function of the vertebral veins and their role in the spread of metastases. Ann Surg. 1940;112(1):138–49.
30. Paget S. The distribution of secondary growths in cancer of the breast. 1889. Cancer Metastasis Rev. 1989;8(2):98–101.
31. Weilbaecher KN, Guise TA, McCauley LK. Cancer to bone: a fatal attraction. Nat Rev Cancer. 2011;11(6):411–25. doi:10.1038/nrc3055.
32. Psaila B, Lyden D. The metastatic niche: adapting the foreign soil. Nat Rev Cancer. 2009;9(4):285–93. doi:10.1038/nrc2621.
33. Oskarsson T, Batlle E, Massague J. Metastatic stem cells: sources, niches, and vital pathways. Cell Stem Cell. 2014;14(3):306–21. doi:10.1016/j.stem.2014.02.002.
34. Perou CM, Sorlie T, Eisen MB, van de Rijn M, Jeffrey SS, Rees CA, Pollack JR, Ross DT, Johnsen H, Akslen LA, Fluge O, Pergamenschikov A, Williams C, Zhu SX, Lonning PE, Borresen-Dale AL, Brown PO, Botstein D. Molecular portraits of human breast tumours. Nature. 2000;406(6797):747–52. doi:10.1038/35021093.
35. Wei S, Li Y, Siegal GP, Hameed O. Breast carcinomas with isolated bone metastases have different hormone receptor expression profiles than those with metastases to other sites or multiple organs. Ann Diagn Pathol. 2011;15(2):79–83. doi:10.1016/j.anndiagpath.2010.06.010.
36. Solomayer EF, Diel IJ, Meyberg GC, Gollan C, Bastert G. Metastatic breast cancer: clinical course, prognosis and therapy related to the first site of metastasis. Breast Cancer Res Treat. 2000;59(3):271–8.
37. Koizumi M, Yoshimoto M, Kasumi F, Ogata E. Comparison between solitary and multiple skeletal metastatic lesions of breast cancer patients. Ann Oncol. 2003;14(8):1234–40.
38. Akhtari M, Mansuri J, Newman KA, Guise TM, Seth P. Biology of breast cancer bone metastasis. Cancer Biol Ther. 2008;7(1):3–9.
39. Aapro M, Abrahamsson PA, Body JJ, Coleman RE, Colomer R, Costa L, Crino L, Dirix L, Gnant M, Gralow J, Hadji P, Hortobagyi GN, Jonat W, Lipton A, Monnier A, Paterson AH, Rizzoli R, Saad F, Thurlimann B. Guidance on the use of bisphosphonates in solid tumours: recommendations of an international expert panel. Ann Oncol. 2008;19(3):420–32. doi:10.1093/annonc/mdm442.
40. Bubendorf L, Schopfer A, Wagner U, Sauter G, Moch H, Willi N, Gasser TC, Mihatsch MJ. Metastatic patterns of prostate cancer: an autopsy study of 1,589 patients. Hum Pathol. 2000;31(5):578–83.
41. Sathiakumar N, Delzell E, Morrisey MA, Falkson C, Yong M, Chia V, Blackburn J, Arora T, Kilgore ML. Mortality following bone metastasis and skeletal-related events among men with prostate cancer: a population-based analysis of US Medicare beneficiaries, 1999–2006. Prostate Cancer Prostatic Dis. 2011;14(2):177–83. doi:10.1038/pcan.2011.7.
42. Wang W, Epstein JI. Small cell carcinoma of the prostate. A morphologic and immunohistochemical study of 95 cases. Am J Surg Pathol. 2008;32(1):65–71. doi:10.1097/PAS.0b013e318058a96b.
43. Mottet N, Peneau M, Mazeron JJ, Molinie V, Richaud P. Addition of radiotherapy to long-term androgen deprivation in locally advanced prostate cancer: an open randomised phase 3 trial. Eur Urol. 2012;62(2):213–9. doi:10.1016/j.eururo.2012.03.053.
44. Farooki A, Leung V, Tala H, Tuttle RM. Skeletal-related events due to bone metastases from differentiated thyroid cancer. J Clin Endocrinol Metab. 2012;97(7):2433–9. doi:10.1210/jc.2012-1169.
45. Hefer T, Joachims HZ, Hashmonai M, Ben-Arieh Y, Brown J. Highly aggressive behaviour of occult papillary thyroid carcinoma. J Laryngol Otol. 1995;109(11):1109–12.
46. Muresan MM, Olivier P, Leclere J, Sirveaux F, Brunaud L, Klein M, Zarnegar R, Weryha G. Bone metastases from differentiated thyroid carcinoma. Endocr Relat Cancer. 2008;15(1):37–49. doi:10.1677/ERC-07-0229.

47. Kasagi K, Takeuchi R, Miyamoto S, Misaki T, Inoue D, Shimazu A, Mori T, Konishi J. Metastatic thyroid cancer presenting as thyrotoxicosis: report of three cases. Clin Endocrinol. 1994;40(3):429–34.
48. Tongaonkar HB, Kulkarni JN, Kamat MR. Solitary metastases from renal cell carcinoma: a review. J Surg Oncol. 1992;49(1):45–8.
49. Szendroi A, Dinya E, Kardos M, Szasz AM, Nemeth Z, Ats K, Kiss J, Antal I, Romics I, Szendroi M. Prognostic factors and survival of renal clear cell carcinoma patients with bone metastases. Pathol Oncol Res. 2010;16(1):29–38. doi:10.1007/s12253-009-9184-7.
50. Jacobsen KD, Folleras G, Fossa SD. Metastases from renal cell carcinoma to the humerus or the shoulder girdle. Br J Urol. 1994;73(2):124–8.
51. Kobus RJ, Leinberry C, Kirkpatrick WH. Metastatic renal carcinoma in the hand: treatment with preoperative irradiation and ray resection. Orthop Rev. 1992;21(8):983–4, 990–5.
52. Sneag DB, Krajewski KM, Howard S, Jagannathan JP, Star KV, Ramaiya N. Sclerotic osseous metastases from renal cell carcinoma. Skelet Radiol. 2012;41(9):1169–75. doi:10.1007/s00256-012-1424-3.
53. Durr HR, Maier M, Pfahler M, Baur A, Refior HJ. Surgical treatment of osseous metastases in patients with renal cell carcinoma. Clin Orthop Relat Res. 1999;367:283–90.
54. Fottner A, Szalantzy M, Wirthmann L, Stahler M, Baur-Melnyk A, Jansson V, Durr HR. Bone metastases from renal cell carcinoma: patient survival after surgical treatment. BMC Musculoskelet Disord. 2010;11:145. doi:10.1186/1471-2474-11-145.
55. Banyra O, Tarchynets M, Shulyak A. Renal cell carcinoma: how to hit the targets? Cent European J Urol. 2014;66(4):394–404. doi:10.5173/ceju.2013.04.art2.
56. Curran Jr V. Managing the joint venture and its complications on the renal real estate process. Nephrol News Issues. 2008;22(1):28–29, 60.
57. Grunwald V, Soltau J, Ivanyi P, Rentschler J, Reuter C, Drevs J. Molecular targeted therapies for solid tumors: management of side effects. Onkologie. 2009;32(3):129–38. doi:10.1159/000194949.
58. Simpson D, Curran MP. Temsirolimus: in advanced renal cell carcinoma. Drugs. 2008;68(5):631–8.
59. Ozdemir MH, Gurkan I, Yildiz Y, Yilmaz C, Saglik Y. Surgical treatment of malignant tumours of the sacrum. Eur J Surg Oncol. 1999;25(1):44–9. doi:10.1053/ejso.1998.0598.
60. Nader R, Rhines LD, Mendel E. Metastatic sacral tumors. Neurosurg Clin N Am. 2004;15(4):453–7. doi:10.1016/j.nec.2004.04.009.
61. Sciubba DM, Gokaslan ZL. Diagnosis and management of metastatic spine disease. Surg Oncol. 2006;15(3):141–51. doi:10.1016/j.suronc.2006.11.002.
62. Babu NV, Titus VT, Chittaranjan S, Abraham G, Prem H, Korula RJ. Computed tomographically guided biopsy of the spine. Spine (Phila Pa 1976). 1994;19(21):2436–42.
63. Settle WJ, Ebraheim NA, Coombs R, Saunders RC, Jackson WT. CT-guided biopsy of metastatic sacral tumors. Orthopedics. 1990;13(7):753–8.
64. Turgut M, Gokpinar D, Barutca S, Erkus M. Lumbosacral metastatic extradural Merkel cell carcinoma causing nerve root compression–case report. Neurol Med Chir (Tokyo). 2002;42(2):78–80.
65. Lee YY, Wen-Wei Hsu R, Huang TJ, Hsueh S, Wang JY. Metastatic meningioma in the sacrum: a case report. Spine (Phila Pa 1976). 2002;27(4):E100–3.
66. Menegaz RA, Resende AD, da Silva CS, Barcelos AC, Murta EF. Metastasis of choriocarcinoma to lumbar and sacral column. Eur J Obstet Gynecol Reprod Biol. 2004;113(1):110–3. doi:10.1016/j.ejogrb.2003.09.029.
67. Uemura A, Matsusako M, Numaguchi Y, Oka M, Kobayashi N, Niinami C, Kawasaki T, Suzuki K. Percutaneous sacroplasty for hemorrhagic metastases from hepatocellular carcinoma. AJNR Am J Neuroradiol. 2005;26(3):493–5.
68. Gerszten PC, Burton SA, Ozhasoglu C, Welch WC. Radiosurgery for spinal metastases: clinical experience in 500 cases from a single institution. Spine (Phila Pa 1976). 2007;32(2):193–9. doi:10.1097/01.brs.0000251863.76595.a2.

69. Akasu T, Yamaguchi T, Fujimoto Y, Ishiguro S, Yamamoto S, Fujita S, Moriya Y. Abdominal sacral resection for posterior pelvic recurrence of rectal carcinoma: analyses of prognostic factors and recurrence patterns. Ann Surg Oncol. 2007;14(1):74–83. doi:10.1245/s10434-006-9082-0.
70. Fujibayashi S, Neo M, Nakamura T. Palliative dual iliac screw fixation for lumbosacral metastasis. Technical note. J Neurosurg Spine. 2007;7(1):99–102. doi:10.3171/SPI-07/07/099.
71. Kakutani K, Doita M, Nishida K, Miyamoto H, Kurosaka M. Radiculopathy due to malignant melanoma in the sacrum with unknown primary site. Eur Spine J. 2008;17(Suppl 2):S271–4. doi:10.1007/s00586-007-0561-1.
72. Zhang J, Wu CG, Gu YF, Li MH. Percutaneous sacroplasty for sacral metastatic tumors under fluoroscopic guidance only. Korean J Radiol. 2008;9(6):572–6. doi:10.3348/kjr.2008.9.6.572.
73. Albareda J, Herrera M, Lopez Salva A, Garcia Donas J, Gonzalez R. Sacral metastasis in a patient with endometrial cancer: case report and review of the literature. Gynecol Oncol. 2008;111(3):583–8. doi:10.1016/j.ygyno.2008.04.005.
74. Toro A, Pulvirenti E, Manfre L, Di Carlo I. Sacroplasty in a patient with bone metastases from hepatocellular carcinoma. A case report. Tumori. 2010;96(1):172–4.
75. Dozois EJ, Privitera A, Holubar SD, Aldrete JF, Sim FH, Rose PS, Walsh MF, Bower TC, Leibovich BC, Nelson H, Larson DW. High sacrectomy for locally recurrent rectal cancer: can long-term survival be achieved? J Surg Oncol. 2011;103(2):105–9. doi:10.1002/jso.21774.
76. Nebreda C, Vallejo R, Aliaga L, Benyamin R. Percutaneous sacroplasty and sacroiliac joint cementation under fluoroscopic guidance for lower back pain related to sacral metastatic tumors with sacroiliac joint invasion. Pain Pract. 2011;11(6):564–9. doi:10.1111/j.1533-2500.2010.00439.x.
77. Moussazadeh N, Laufer I, Yamada Y, Bilsky MH. Separation surgery for spinal metastases: effect of spinal radiosurgery on surgical treatment goals. Cancer Control. 2014;21(2):168–74.
78. Maranzano E, Trippa F, Chirico L, Basagni ML, Rossi R. Management of metastatic spinal cord compression. Tumori. 2003;89(5):469–75.
79. Loblaw DA, Laperriere NJ. Emergency treatment of malignant extradural spinal cord compression: an evidence-based guideline. J Clin Oncol. 1998;16(4):1613–24.
80. Randall RL, Bruckner J, Lloyd C, Pohlman TH, Conrad III EU. Sacral resection and reconstruction for tumors and tumor-like conditions. Orthopedics. 2005;28(3):307–13.
81. Masala S, Konda D, Massari F, Simonetti G. Sacroplasty and iliac osteoplasty under combined CT and fluoroscopic guidance. Spine (Phila Pa 1976). 2006;31(18):E667–9. doi:10.1097/01.brs.0000231962.04739.ac.
82. Hirsch JA, Barr JD, Zoarski GH. Sacroplasty: beyond the beginning. J Neurointerv Surg. 2013;5(5):395. doi:10.1136/neurintsurg-2012-010434.
83. Bayley E, Srinivas S, Boszczyk BM. Clinical outcomes of sacroplasty in sacral insufficiency fractures: a review of the literature. Eur Spine J. 2009;18(9):1266–71. doi:10.1007/s00586-009-1048-z.
84. Hess T, Kramann B, Schmidt E, Rupp S. Use of preoperative vascular embolisation in spinal metastasis resection. Arch Orthop Trauma Surg. 1997;116(5):279–82.
85. Prabhu VC, Bilsky MH, Jambhekar K, Panageas KS, Boland PJ, Lis E, Heier L, Nelson PK. Results of preoperative embolization for metastatic spinal neoplasms. J Neurosurg. 2003;98(2 Suppl):156–64.
86. Sundaresan N, Choi IS, Hughes JE, Sachdev VP, Berenstein A. Treatment of spinal metastases from kidney cancer by presurgical embolization and resection. J Neurosurg. 1990;73(4):548–54. doi:10.3171/jns.1990.73.4.0548.
87. Rossi G, Mavrogenis AF, Rimondi E, Braccaioli L, Calabro T, Ruggieri P. Selective embolization with N-butyl cyanoacrylate for metastatic bone disease. J Vasc Interv Radiol. 2011;22(4):462–70. doi:10.1016/j.jvir.2010.12.023.
88. Facchini G, Di Tullio P, Battaglia M, Bartalena T, Tetta C, Errani C, Mavrogenis AF, Rossi G. Palliative embolization for metastases of the spine. Eur J Orthop Surg Traumatol. 2016;26(3):247–52.
89. Rossi G, Mavrogenis AF, Casadei R, Bianchi G, Romagnoli C, Rimondi E, Ruggieri P. Embolisation of bone metastases from renal cancer. Radiol Med. 2013;118(2):291–302. doi:10.1007/s11547-012-0802-4.

90. Rossi G, Mavrogenis AF, Rimondi E, Ciccarese F, Tranfaglia C, Angelelli B, Fiorentini G, Bartalena T, Errani C, Ruggieri P, Mercuri M. Selective arterial embolisation for bone tumours: experience of 454 cases. Radiol Med. 2011;116(5):793–808. doi:10.1007/s11547-011-0670-0.
91. Kurup AN, Callstrom MR. Ablation of skeletal metastases: current status. J Vasc Interv Radiol. 2010;21(8 Suppl):S242–50. doi:10.1016/j.jvir.2010.05.001.
92. Goetz MP, Callstrom MR, Charboneau JW, Farrell MA, Maus TP, Welch TJ, Wong GY, Sloan JA, Novotny PJ, Petersen IA, Beres RA, Regge D, Capanna R, Saker MB, Gronemeyer DH, Gevargez A, Ahrar K, Choti MA, de Baere TJ, Rubin J. Percutaneous image-guided radiofrequency ablation of painful metastases involving bone: a multicenter study. J Clin Oncol. 2004;22(2):300–6. doi:10.1200/JCO.2004.03.097.
93. Mavrogenis AF, Angelini A, Vottis C, Pala E, Calabro T, Papagelopoulos PJ, Ruggieri P. Modern palliative treatments for metastatic bone disease: awareness of advantages, disadvantages, and guidance. Clin J Pain. 2016;32(4):337–50. doi:10.1097/AJP.0000000000000255.
94. Puhaindran ME, Farooki A, Steensma MR, Hameed M, Healey JH, Boland PJ. Atypical subtrochanteric femoral fractures in patients with skeletal malignant involvement treated with intravenous bisphosphonates. J Bone Joint Surg Am. 2011;93(13):1235–42. doi:10.2106/JBJS.J.01199.
95. Michaelson MD, Smith MR. Bisphosphonates for treatment and prevention of bone metastases. J Clin Oncol. 2005;23(32):8219–24. doi:10.1200/JCO.2005.02.9579.

Chordoma of the Sacrum

15

Andrea Angelini and Pietro Ruggieri

15.1 Introduction

Chordoma is a relatively rare, slow-growing, primary bone tumor with an overall incidence of approximately one per million population and accounts for 1–4% of all malignant bone lesions [1, 2]. Although rare, it represents the most frequent primary malignant bone tumor affecting the sacrum [3]. It has a slowly aggressive and locally invasive behavior, and it is considered a low-grade malignant neoplasm. In fact, it is poorly sensitive to conventional radiotherapy and chemotherapy. Surgical resection of sacral chordoma remains the standard for local disease control, even if it is associated with significant morbidity and repercussions for patient's quality of life due to the close relationship with relevant neurovascular structures [4]. An increasing number of novel (radio)surgical and pharmacological strategies are currently being investigated [5–7] and may have a role in addressing microscopic disease.

15.2 Embryology

The current line of thinking is that chordoma cells originate from remnants of the embryonic notochord [8–11]. For the purpose of clarifying the pathophysiology, one must first gain an understanding of the ontogenesis of the axial skeleton as it matures from the notochord to its ultimate configuration in the adult. During embryogenesis, in the third week of human development, gastrulation takes place with the formation of the three primary germ layers (ecto-, meso-, and endoderm). The stem cells for all major structural elements of the vertebral column are derived from the mesoderm [12]. One of the key events following this phenomenon is the

A. Angelini, M.D., Ph.D. • P. Ruggieri, M.D., Ph.D. (✉)
Department of Orthopaedics and Orthopedic Oncology, University of Padova, Padova, Italy
e-mail: andrea.angelini83@yahoo.it; pietro.ruggieri@unipd.it

P. Ruggieri et al. (eds.), *Tumors of the Sacrum*,
DOI 10.1007/978-3-319-51202-0_15

formation of the notochord in the Carnegie stages 7 through 9 (crown-rump [CR] length of 0.4–2.5 mm), an elongated rod of cells subadjacent to the neural tube with a caudo-cranial extension [13]. The notochord plays a critical role by producing and secreting important signaling factors (e.g., sonic hedgehog [14], bone morphogenetic protein [15, 16]) to the surrounding tissue in order to guide organogenesis and the formation of the axial skeleton [17]. Primary neurulation, the process of the flat neural plate folding into the cylindrical neural tube, occurs in response to soluble growth factors secreted by the notochord (Fig. 15.1). As a result of the cellular shape changes, the neural plate folds creating the U-shape neural groove. This neural groove sets the boundary between the right and left sides of the embryo. Then, the closure of the neural tube disconnects the neural crest from the epidermidis, and segmentation commences in the axial and paraxial mesenchyme with the formation of somites (Carnegie stage 11, CR 2.5–4.5 mm) [18–21]. In axial

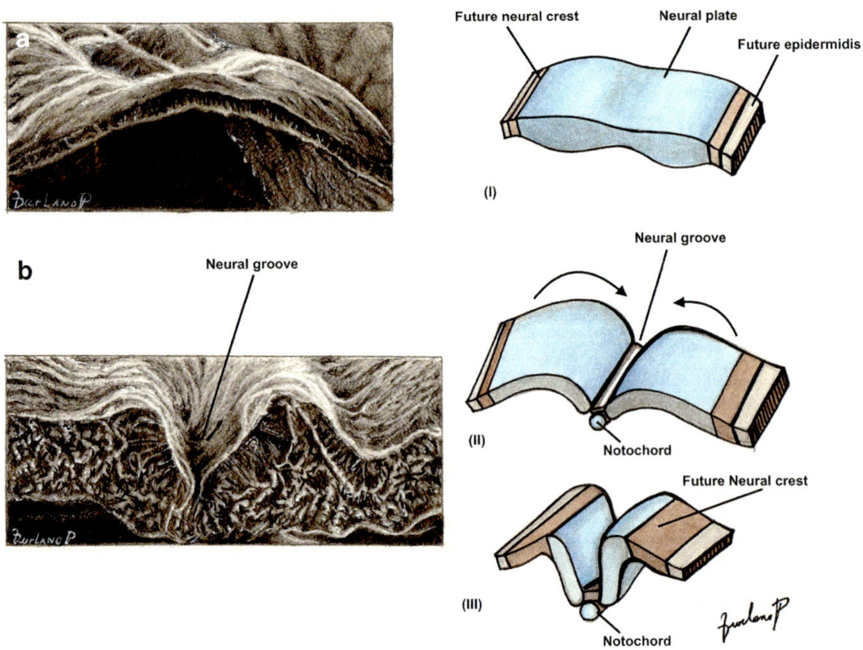

Fig. 15.1 Artistic drawings show embryogenesis of the vertebral column: primary neurulation. (**a**) Shaping. Schematic transverse sections showing neuroectodermal tissues differentiate from the ectoderm and thicken into the neural plate (*I*); (**b**) Folding and elevation. The neural plate bends dorsally creating the U-shaped neural groove. Notochord is shown at the ventral part of the neural groove (*II*). The two ends eventually joining at the neural plate borders, which are now referred to as the neural crest (*III*); (**c**) Convergence. Bending of the neural plate with convergence of the neural folds up to the complete closure of the neural tube (*IV*); (**d**) Closure. The closure of the neural tube disconnects the neural crest from the epidermidis (*V*). Neural crest cells differentiate to form most of the peripheral nervous system and notochord degenerates (*VI*)

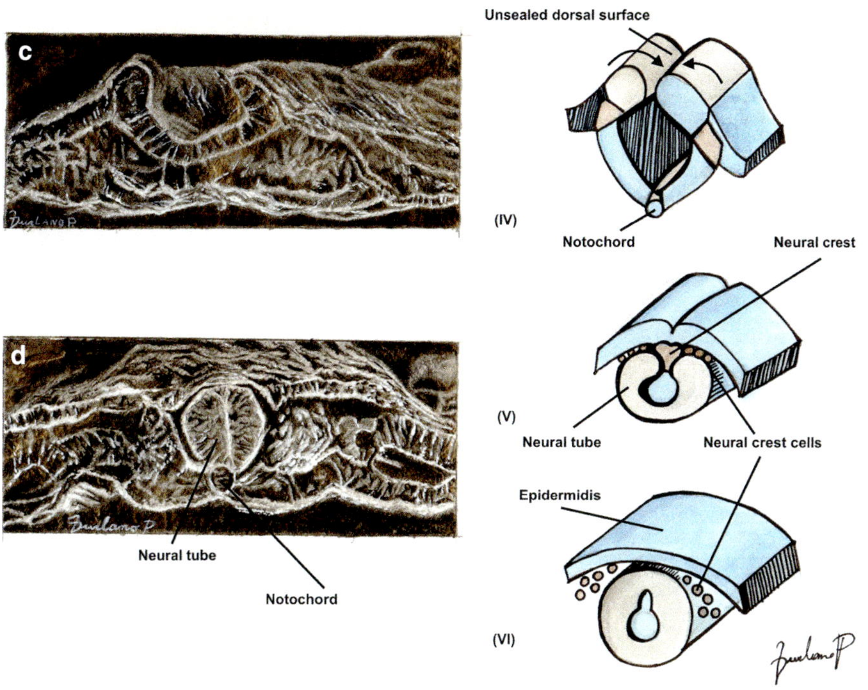

Fig. 15.1 (continued)

section, the mesoderm-derived tissue which bilaterally propagates alongside the notochord evolves by an epithelial-to-mesenchymal transition to form the ventral sclerotomes [22]. The mesenchymal cells are specified based on their location within the somite. they retain the ability to become any kind of somite-derived structure until relatively late in the process of somitogenesis [23] and gradually assume a concentric arrangement around the notochord, forming a perichordal sheath [18, 24, 25]. These mesenchymal cells of the perichordal sheath become cartilaginous (chondroblasts/chondrocytic cells) via a condensation process guided by secreted factors derived from the notochord originating primordial vertebral body [26, 27]. Concurrently with the vertebral body morphogenesis, the confined notochordal cells progressively degenerate and probably undergo apoptosis or differentiate into the chondrocyte-like cells [28]. Occasionally notochord cells remain in the nucleus pulpous of the mature intervertebral disk (Fig. 15.2) or can be witnessed in notochord-like tissue in the intravertebral region, in which case they are described as "benign notochordal cell tumors" (BNCT) [29]. The complete formation of the vertebral segments is expected to be at Carnegie stage 20–22 (CR 18–30 mm) (Fig. 15.3).

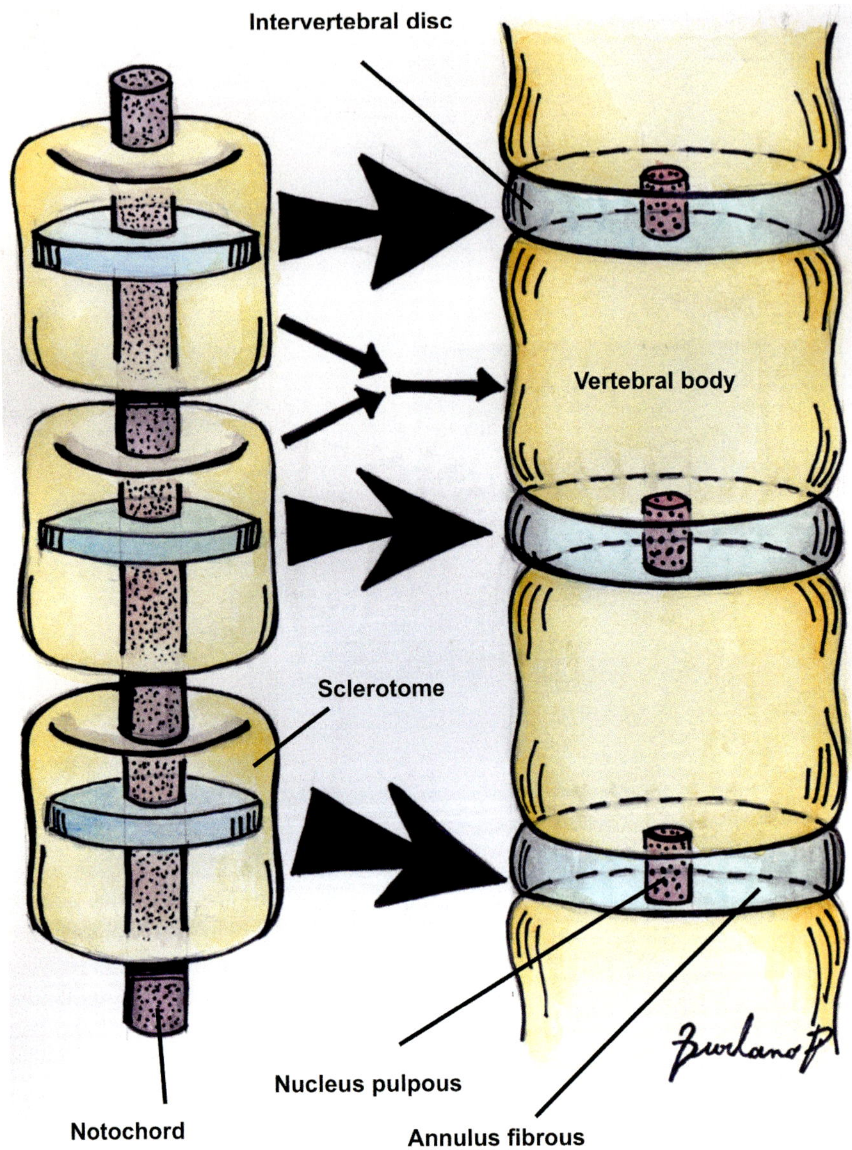

Fig. 15.2 Artistic drawing show notochord cells remain in the nucleus pulposus of the mature intervertebral disk. During resegmentation of the sclerotomes to form the vertebrae, each one splits into cranial and caudal segments, and cells remaining in the plane of division coalesce to form the annulus fibrous of the intervertebral disk

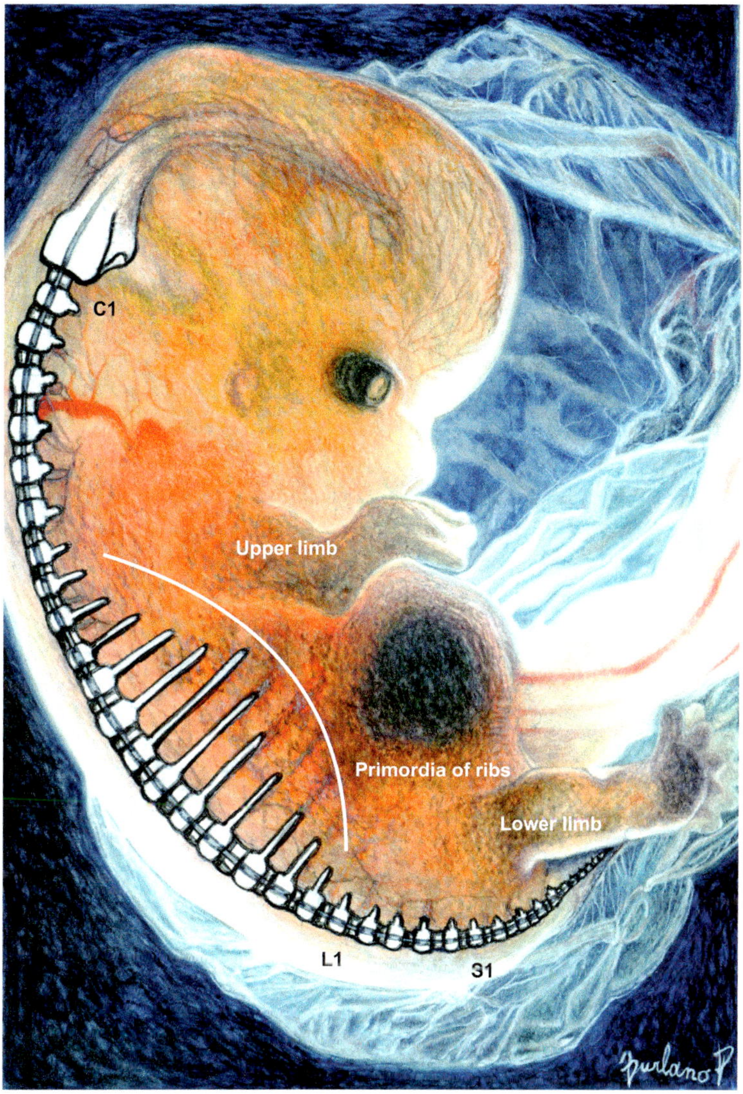

Fig. 15.3 Artistic drawing of a human embryo at Carnegie stage 20 show all of the vertebral segments have formed

15.3 Pathogenesis

The pathophysiology underlying this lethal disease is demonstrated to be complex. Starting from the histological characterization performed by Virchow in 1857 [30] up to the discovery of brachyury's involvement, numerous progresses have been performed in the pathogenesis of this tumor. Examination of human embryos and fetus showed that notochordal cell nests topographically correspond and distribute to the sites of occurrence of chordoma and histological appearance of tumor cells led to hypothesize the notochordal origin [31, 32]. Molecular research has so far yielded significant findings on the mechanisms underlying the initiation and further progression of chordoma cells. The most compelling evidence of the notochordal hypothesis derived from researches focused on a transcription factor named "brachyury." It is an important transcription factor in notochord development, but duplicated regions contained only the brachyury gene have been discovered in familial chordoma [33–36]. The remarkable overexpression revealed this transcription factor to be a crucial aspect of chordoma, although it is still unclear what role brachyury has in the pathogenesis [37]. Some other notochordal factors (Shh, Wnt, galectin-3, NCAM) seem to be relevant in notochord formation and in chordoma, as well as the other overexpression of cell cycle regulatory pathways and an activated receptor tyrosine kinase pathway [11]. The molecular biology process behind the initiation and progression of a chordoma needs to be revealed for a better understanding of the disease and to develop more effective therapies [38].

15.4 Epidemiology

Chordomas are classified on the basis of their location along the spine in sacrococcygeal, clival, cervical, thoracic, and lumbar (listed by the most frequent site) [1–3]. Recent studies reported an almost equal distribution in the clivus (32%), mobile spine (32.8%), and sacrum 29.2% [39]. Other epidemiological studies report that the sacrococcygeal area is the most common affect (40–50%) compared to clivus (35–40%) and vertebral bodies (20–40%) [40, 41]. Sacrococcygeal chordomas have very low incidence in patients below 40 years old and are more frequent in males (male to female ratio 2:1) [42–45].

15.5 Presentation and Diagnosis

Chordomas of the sacrum often present with non-specific symptoms which can delay diagnosis, such as localized deep pain or radiculopathies related to the spinal level at which they occur [46–49]. In advanced disease the tumors can present at the time of diagnosis as a slow-growing palpable mass associated with rectal or urinary dysfunction [46, 47, 50]. The average duration of symptoms is about 14 months (range, 4–24 months) [45]. Diagnosis is further complicated by the fact that lytic sacral lesions might be overlooked on plain radiographs of the pelvis, and CT or MRI studies are often not performed without a clinical suspicion of sacral tumor [45, 49]. Differential diagnosis for lumbosacral chordomas includes pilonidal sinus disease, deep abscesses, rectal sarcomas, and several retrorectal tumors (teratomas, extraperitoneal adenomucinosis, cystic lymphangiomas, neurogenic tumors, and cysts, developmental tailgut cysts, sacral myelomeningocele, rectal duplication) [51–53]. Most sacrococcygeal chordomas can protrude anteriorly into the pelvis, and rectal examination may be useful for clinical detection of sacral mass even if the tumor is limited by presacral fascia [54].

15.6 Imaging

Chordomas are midline lesions and often appear radiographically as destructive lytic bone lesions. Unlike other primary tumor (osteosarcomas and chondrosarcomas) of the spine, chordomas locally invade the intervertebral disk space as they spread to adjacent vertebral bodies [49]. Computed tomography (CT) and magnetic resonance imaging (MRI) are the gold standard for diagnosis. The tumors are often associated with soft tissue mass (Fig. 15.4). Calcification and bony expansion are

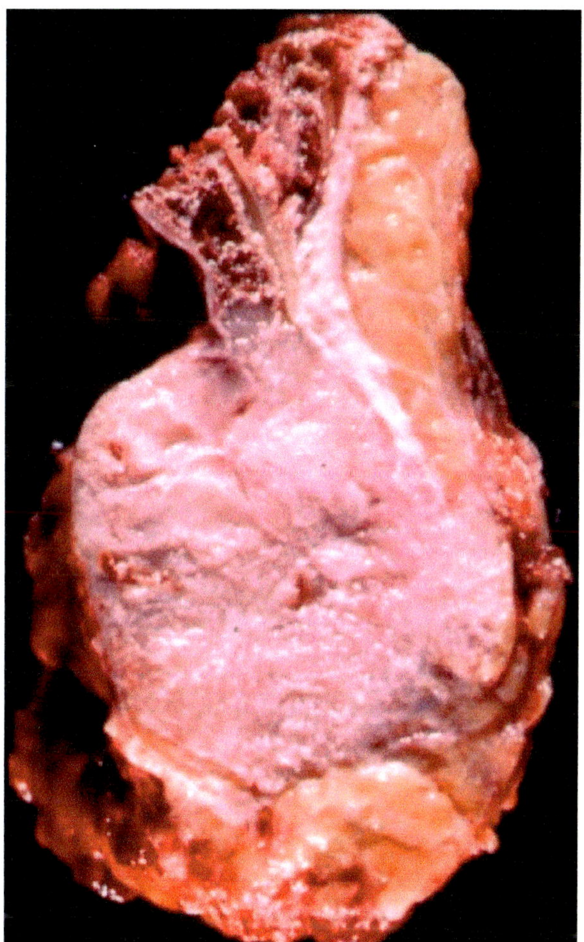

Fig. 15.4 Sagittal view of a specimen from a proximal sacral resection show the large involvement of soft tissue

present in 30–70% of the cases and appear isointense or hypointense on T1-weighted MRI images and hyperintense on T2-weighted MRI images and enhance with gadolinium [55]. On bone scan, chordomas show reduced or normal uptake of radioisotope when juxtaposed to other bone tumors [56]. Careful preoperative assessment of imaging within the multidisciplinary team is essential in planning surgical approach and discussing strategy of treatment.

15.7 Pathology

Chordomas were first described histologically by Virchow in 1857, when he identified the typical "physaliferous" tumor cell chordomas [30]. Physaliferous cells appear as large white cells with round nuclei and abundant vacuolated cytoplasm separated by fibrous septa into lobules [41, 42] and are typical of classic chordomas. Chordomas are classified as classical (or conventional), chondroid, or dedifferentiated [41]. Classic chordomas are pathologically identified by their typical cells and immunoreactivity for S-100, epithelial membrane antigen (MUC1), and cytokeratins [57, 58]. Brachyury staining is used to discriminate chordomas from other chondroid lesions [59]. Chondroid chordoma is a histological variant that account for 5–15% of all chordomas [41]. It shows histological features resembling chondrosarcoma, with hyaline cartilage associated with expression of chordoma markers [60, 61]. Dedifferentiated chordomas account for less than 10% of all chordomas and are characterized by sarcomatous areas with spindle cells such as fibrosarcoma, osteosarcoma, or rhabdomyosarcoma [62–66]. It is characterized by a fulminant clinical course resulting in metastases and/or death within 1 year of diagnosis in most of the cases [64–68].

15.8 Treatment

The most accredited treatment consists of surgical resection with wide margins, as no chemotherapy has been demonstrated to be effective against chordoma and conventional radiotherapy is only partially effective [5, 11, 69–74]. Complex pelvic anatomy coupled with the need of wide margins means that surgery is challenging to preserve essential neural function and avoid injury to visceral and vascular structures during resection. Frequently, margins are positive (marginal or contaminated) [11, 70, 71, 75, 76], and adjuvant treatment strategies must be considered.

15.8.1 Sacral Resection

In the 1970s, Stener and Gunterberg [77] first introduced the idea of wide en bloc surgical resection for the treatment of sacral tumors. Since then, en bloc resection has remained the mainstay of treatment of sacral chordoma worldwide, as reported by a large multicentric study based on the AOSpine Tumor Knowledge Forum Primary Spinal Tumor database [78]. En bloc sacrectomy is a highly demanding surgical procedure, consisting of a partial or total amputation of the sacrum. It is associated with significant soft tissue and skin defects, which may require reconstruction with myocutaneous flaps to reduce risk of wound infection and breakdown. However, it is attainable in more than 50% of sacral chordomas and offers the best long-term oncological outcomes when wide margins are obtained [69, 79].

The surgical approach is often planned according to tumor extension and level of resection. Usually all resections distal to S3 level could be approached posteriorly only [70, 80, 81], whereas proximal resections need a combined anterior-posterior approach [69–71, 78, 79, 82]. Advantages of the posterior approach are a single stage procedure and shorter operating time, whereas the combined approach enables the visceral organs to be dissected away from the tumor and protected during the osteotomy. Some exceptions have been reported in literature, using tools and innovative surgical techniques to perform proximal resections by a posterior approach only in selected cases [83, 84].

Unilateral or bilateral sacrifice of the nerve roots is necessary distal to resection, with corresponding functional damage [77, 82, 85–88]: motor and sensory deficits in the lower limbs are mainly related to the sacrifice of S1 and L5 nerve roots; sacrectomies that spare the S2 nerve root are associated with abnormal bladder and bowel function, even if better results can be expected if an S3 nerve root is also preserved; sexual dysfunction with relative saddle anesthesia is associated with bilateral S3 lesions, whereas unilateral sacrifice from S2 to S5 reduces but does not abolish urogenital and rectal functions. Numerous complications other than neurological deficits have been reported in literature, such as wound dehiscence, infection, iatrogenic visceral injury, hematoma, massive bleeding, liquoral fistula, flap necrosis, stress fractures, and other less frequently reported [70, 89]. Chen et al. [90] reported that albumin <3.0 g/dL, operating time (>6 h), and previous surgery were statistically significant risk factors for wound infection.

15.8.2 Radiotherapy

The use of radiotherapy (RT) as primary or adjuvant treatment for chordoma has been debated for several years and remains controversial. The majority of older publications that used conventional photon radiotherapy did not exceed 60 Gy, and investigators report poor local control in sacral chordomas [91, 92]. In fact, the problem of tolerance dose of the organs and tissues surrounding the sacrum results in the limitation of total RT dose that can safely be delivered to the tumor [93, 94]. Advances in radiation technology and treatment have led to more strategic targeting of neoplasms with higher doses of radiation. There is some consensus that the combination therapy of surgical resection and radiation therapy may be associated with higher rates of local control and overall survival [95].

- Intensity-modulated radiation therapy (IMRT) and stereotactic delivery techniques can custom modulate each photon beam to conform to the tumor volume by minimizing the dose to surrounding tissues [92]. Some authors report the experience in sacral chordomas, finding that local control was significantly higher in patients treated with radiation dose delivered higher than 60 Gy (range 60–78 Gy) [96, 97].
- Radiosurgery is a technique characterized by a very high dose of RT in a single fraction (or hypofractionated) thanks to the use of image-guided technology coupled with IMRT. The use of radiosurgery for chordoma has shown promising preliminary results for local control [98, 99].
- Proton beam and heavy-ion particle radiation therapy are characterized by delivering a high-specific radiation dose to the tumor target volume and small dose to uninvolved normal tissue (low risk of radiation toxicity to neural tissue) [94, 100, 101]. Hadrons (high-dose protons or charged particles, including carbon ions, helium, or neon) provide biological and physical advantages in terms of their high relative biological effectiveness and reduced oxygen-enhancement ratio in the tumor region [102]. In fact, studies exploiting the use of hadron therapy in chordomas of the sacrococcygeal region show local control at 5 years of 60–70% [99, 103–105]. Compared with protons and photons, carbon ions have a relative higher biological effectiveness with a larger mean energy per unit length of their trajectory [91, 106]. Therefore, carbon-ion radiotherapy has been considered for treatment of unresectable chordoma [107]. Promising local control rate and better preservation of bladder-bowel function with the use of carbon-ion radiotherapy has been reported compared with surgery [107–109], whereas good results have also been reported as adjuvant treatment [110]. Unfortunately, the availability of hadron-based therapy is limited because of the associated construction and operational expenses [111, 112], even if the cost is expected to decrease rapidly [113].

Although there is limited literature comparing the effectiveness of newer radiation therapy modalities coupled with surgery, preliminary promising results have been reported with hadron therapy than with photon-based radiation [114–116]. However, at this time, single-fraction photon RT and proton-beam and carbon-ion RT with wide en bloc excision both are the accepted treatment standard in the management of chordomas at many quaternary-care cancer centers, showing higher local control rates than conventional IMRT [116]. One of the critiques of RT is that it can cause pathological fracture of residual sacral bone [69, 70, 117].

15.8.3 Chemotherapy and Medical Treatment

No conventional chemotherapy has proven to be effective in terms of overall survival and local control in patients with sacral chordoma. The advent of molecular targeted therapies and the discovery of molecular profiling of chordomas have offered some encouraging alternatives to conventional chemotherapy for the management of advanced disease. Chordomas overexpress platelet-derived growth factor receptor (PDGFR)B, PDGFRA, and KIT receptors, suggesting a role for imatinib therapy [118–120], a tyrosine kinase inhibitor (TKI) with specificity for the kinase domain of PDGFR and KIT receptors. Another TKI, sunitinib, has shown clinical efficacy [121], even if reports are limited by small patient numbers and short follow-up. Additional molecular pathways such as mTOR and MAPK signaling pathways seem to be involved, meaning a possible role of other targeting therapies such as mTOR inhibitors (everolimus, temsirolimus) [122, 123].

In a small series of patients with chordoma, strong expression of epidermal growth factor receptor (EGFR) and c-MET was described [124]. EGFR is a tyrosine kinase receptor implicated in cell proliferation through the binding of several ligands. This led to the report of a patient's response to cetuximab and gefitinib [125]. Newer EGFR inhibitors, erlotinib and lapatinib, confirmed this efficacy [126, 127]. A recent analysis showed that activation of phosphorylated signal transducer and activator of transcription 3 (STAT3) is associated with poor prognosis [128]. The use of STAT3 inhibitors in chordoma cell lines in vitro showed strong inhibition of cell growth and proliferation [129]. Phase II studies are now ongoing, combining imatinib and everolimus or using lapatinib in HER2-positive advanced chordomas.

15.9 Oncologic Outcome

Several prognostic factors associated with poor survival have been reported: age [78, 130, 131], tumor size [46, 71, 72, 131–133], preoperative C-reactive protein >1.0 mg/dL [134], tumor site regarding the proximal extent of the tumor, local invasion into other tissues [131, 135], inadequate surgical margins [46, 69, 70–72, 75, 133, 136–138], content of extracellular matrix and high Ki-67 index [138], histological category such as dedifferentiated chordomas [41, 139], and local recurrence [46, 138, 140]. Patient survival seems to be less affected by distant metastasis than by local progression of the disease, underlining the role of local control to improve oncological outcomes.

Local recurrence (LR) after surgical treatment is common (43–85%) despite resection with adequate margins [71, 72]. Some authors suggested that infiltration of the musculature adjacent to the sacrum and/or involvement of the sacroiliac joints increases the tendency to local recurrence, even after apparently successful en bloc resection [135, 141, 142]. This hypothesis could also justify also the observation of similar recurrence rate between major resections of proximal part of the sacrum and small resections distal to S3 level [70, 71]. Therefore, in cases of infiltration of the sacroiliac joint, we should consider the tumor at an advanced stage with increased risk of satellite lesions which may promote disease recurrence. The factors associated with higher risk of local recurrence are: old age [82, 140], higher sacral localization [140], inadequate surgical margins [46, 69, 70, 78], and previous intralesional surgery [69–71, 78]. Adjuvant radiotherapy may improve oncological outcomes in patients with inadequate surgical margins or dedifferentiated disease, but optimal radiotherapeutic regimens with long-term survival have not been developed. In fact, despite combining en bloc resection with particle radiation therapy, frequent local recurrence remains a reality, and the 5- and 10-year overall survival rates are circa 65% and 35%, respectively [39, 143, 144].

Acknowledgements We would like to thank Pierpaolo Furlano for the production of research drawings which formed the basis of the final drawings in this chapter.

Conflict-of-Interest Statement No benefits have been or will be received from a commercial party related directly or indirectly to the subject matter of this article.

References

1. Healey JH, Lane JM. Chordoma: a critical review of diagnosis and treatment. Orthop Clin North Am. 1989;20:417–26.
2. Smoll NR, Gautschi OP, Radovanovic I, Schaller K, Weber DC. Incidence and relative survival of chordomas: the standardized mortality ratio and the impact of chordomas on a population. Cancer. 2013;119:2029–37.
3. Fabbri N, Ruggieri P. Chordoma. In: Picci P, et al., editors. Atlas of musculoskeletal tumors and tumor like lesions. Switzerland: Springer; 2014. p. 233–8.
4. Casali PG, Stacchiotti S, Sangalli C, Olmi P, Gronchi A. Chordoma. Curr Opin Oncol. 2007;19:367–70.
5. Garofalo F, di Summa PG, Christoforidis D, Pracht M, Laudato P, Cherix S, Bouchaab H, Raffoul W, Demartines N, Matter M. Multidisciplinary approach of lumbo-sacral chordoma: from oncological treatment to reconstructive surgery. J Surg Oncol. 2015; 112(5):544–54.
6. Amichetti M, Cianchetti M, Amelio D, Enrici RM, Minniti G. Proton therapy in chordoma of the base of the skull: a systematic review. Neurosurg Rev. 2009;32:403–16.
7. Staab A, Rutz HP, Ares C, et al. Spot-scanning-based proton therapy for extracranial chordoma. Int J Radiat Oncol Biol Phys. 2011;81:e489–96.
8. Luschka H. Die Altersveränderungen der Zwischenwirbelknorpel. Virchows Arch A Pathol Anat Histol. 1856;9:311–27.
9. Kyriakos M, Totty WG, Lenke LG. Giant vertebral notochordal rest: a lesion distinct from chordoma: discussion of an evolving concept. Am J Surg Pathol. 2003;27:396–406.
10. Walcott BP, Nahed BV, Mohyeldin A, Coumans JV, Kahle KT, Ferreira MJ. Chordoma: current concepts, management, and future directions. Lancet Oncol. 2012;13(2):e69–76.
11. Yakkioui Y, van Overbeeke JJ, Santegoeds R, van Engeland M, Temel Y. Chordoma: the entity. Biochim Biophys Acta. 2014;1846(2):655–69.
12. O'Rahilly R, Meyer DB. The timing and sequence of events in the development of the human vertebral column during the embryonic period proper. Anat Embryol. 1979;157(2):167–76.
13. Schoenwolf GC, Larsen WJ. Third week: becomming trilaminar and establishing body axis, Larsen's human embryology. Philadelphia: Elsevier/Churchill Livingstone; 2009.
14. Bumcrot DA, McMahon AP. Somite differentiation. Curr Biol. 1995;5:612–4.
15. Bami M, Mavrogenis AF, Angelini A, Milonaki M, Mitsiokapa E, Stamoulis D, Soucacos PN. Bone morphogenetic protein signaling in musculoskeletal cancer. J Cancer Res Clin Oncol. 2016;142(10):2061–72.
16. Liem Jr KF, Jessell TM, Briscoe J. Regulation of the neural patterning activity of sonic hedgehog by secreted BMP inhibitors expressed by notochord and somites. Development. 2000;127:4855–66.
17. Stemple DL. Structure and function of the notochord: an essential organ for chordate development. Development. 2005;132:2503–12.

18. Dietrich S, Schubert FR, Gruss P. Altered Pax gene expression in murine notochord mutants: the notochord is required to initiate and maintain ventral identity in the somite. Mech Dev. 1993;44:189–207.
19. Pourquie O, Coltey M, Teillet MA, Ordahl C, Le Douarin NM. Control of dorsoventral patterning of somitic derivatives by notochord and floor plate. Proc Natl Acad Sci U S A. 1993;90:5242–6.
20. Alvares LE, Lours C, El-Hanfy A, Dietrich S. Microsurgical manipulation of the notochord. Methods Mol Biol. 2008;461:289–303.
21. Claudio DS. Grafting of somites. Methods Mol Biol. 2008;461:277–87.
22. Resende TP, Ferreira M, Teillet MA, Tavares AT, Andrade RP, Palmeirim I. Sonic hedgehog in temporal control of somite formation. Proc Natl Acad Sci U S A. 2010;107(29): 12907–12.
23. Gilbert SF. Developmental biology. Sunderland: Sinauer Associates; 2010.
24. Moore KL, Persaud TVN, Torchia MG. The developing human: clinically oriented embryology. Philadelphia: Saunders/Elsevier; 2008.
25. Bogduk N. Embryology and development, Clinical anatomy of the lumbar spine and sacrum. Edinburgh: Elsevier/Churchill Livingstone; 2005. p. 149–63.
26. Oka Y, Sato Y, Tsuda H, Hanaoka K, Hirai Y, Takahashi Y. Epimorphin acts extracellularly to promote cell sorting and aggregation during the condensation of vertebral cartilage. Dev Biol. 2006;291(1):25–37.
27. Rodrigo I, Hill RE, Balling R, Münsterberg A, Imai K. Pax1 and Pax9 activate Bapx1 to induce chondrogenic differentiation in the sclerotome. Development. 2003;130(3):473–82.
28. Hunter CJ, Matyas JR, Duncan NA. The notochordal cell in the nucleus pulposus: a review in the context of tissue engineering. Tissue Eng. 2003;9(4):667–77.
29. Yamaguchi T, Suzuki S, Ishiiwa H, Ueda Y. Intraosseous benign notochordal cell tumours: overlooked precursors of classic chordomas? Histopathology. 2004;44(6):597–602.
30. Virchow R. Untersuchungen uber die Entwickelung des Schadelgrundes im gesunden und krankhaften Zustande, und uber den Einfluss derselben auf Schadelform, Gesichtsbildung und Gehirnbau. Berl: G. Rimer; 1857. p. 47.
31. Ribbert H. Uber die Eccondrosis physaliphora spheno-occipitalis. Zentralbl Allg Pathol Anat. 1894;5:457.
32. Salisbury JR. The pathology of the human notochord. J Pathol. 1993;171:253–5.
33. Vujovic S, Henderson S, Presneau N, et al. Brachyury, a crucial regulator of notochordal development, is a novel biomarker for chordomas. J Pathol. 2006;209:157–65.
34. Shen J, Li C-D, Yang H-L, et al. Classic chordoma coexisting with benign notochordal cell rest demonstrating different immunohistological expression patterns of brachyury and galectin-3. J Clin Neurosci. 2011;18:96–9.
35. Choi K-S, Cohn MJ, Harfe BD. Identification of nucleus pulposus precursor cells and notochordal remnants in the mouse: implications for disk degeneration and chordoma formation. Dev Dyn. 2008;237:3953–8.
36. Yang XR, Ng D, Alcorta DA, et al. T (brachyury) gene duplication confers major susceptibility to familial chordoma. Nat Genet. 2009;41:1176–8.
37. Nibu Y, José-Edwards DS, Di Gregorio A. From notochord formation to hereditary chordoma: the many roles of Brachyury. Biomed Res Int. 2013;2013:826435.
38. Gulluoglu S, Turksoy O, Kuskucu A, Ture U, Bayrak OF. The molecular aspects of chordoma. Neurosurg Rev. 2016;39(2):185–96.
39. McMaster ML, Goldstein AM, Bromley CM, Ishibe N, Parry DM. Chordoma: incidence and survival patterns in the United States, 1973–1995. Cancer Causes Control. 2001;12:1–11.
40. Jemal A, Siegel R, Ward E, et al. Cancer statistics, 2007. CA Cancer J Clin. 2007;57:43–66.
41. Chugh R, Tawbi H, Lucas DR, et al. Chordoma: the nonsarcoma primary bone tumor. Oncologist. 2007;12:1344–50.
42. Papagelopoulos PJ, Mavrogenis AF, Galanis EC, Savvidou OD, Boscainos PJ, Katonis PG, Sim FH. Chordoma of the spine: clinicopathological features, diagnosis, and treatment. Orthopedics. 2004;27(12):1256–63.

43. Anson KM, Byrne PO, Robertson ID, Gullan RW, Montgomery AC. Radical excision of sacrococcygeal tumours. Br J Surg. 1994;81:460–1.
44. Smith J, Ludwig RL, Marcove RC. Sacrococcygeal chordoma. A clinic radiological study of 60 patients. Skeletal Radiol. 1987;16:37–44.
45. Kayani B, Hanna SA, Sewell MD, Saifuddin A, Molloy S, Briggs TW. A review of the surgical management of sacral chordoma. Eur J Surg Oncol. 2014;40(11):1412–20.
46. Bergh P, Kindblom LG, Gunterberg B, Remotti F, Ryd W, Meis-Kindblom JM. Prognostic factors in chordoma of the sacrum and mobile spine: a study of 39 patients. Cancer. 2000;88:2122–34.
47. Kaiser TE, Pritchard DJ, Unni KK. Clinicopathologic study of sacrococcygeal chordoma. Cancer. 1984;53:2574–8.
48. Gray SW, Singhabhandhu B, Smith RA, Skandalakis JE. Sacrococcygeal chordoma: report of a case and review of the literature. Surgery. 1975;78:573–82.
49. Fourney DR, Gokaslan ZL. Current management of sacral chordoma. Neurosurg Focus. 2003;15:9.
50. Ozaki T, Hillmann A, Winkelmann W. Surgical treatment of sacrococcygeal chordoma. J Surg Oncol. 1997;64(4):274–9.
51. Dahan H, Arrive L, Wendum D, et al. Retrorectal developmental cysts in adults: Clinical and radiologic-histopathologic review, differential diagnosis, and treatment. Radiographics. 2001;21:575–84.
52. Williams LS, Rojiani AM, Quisling RG, et al. Retrorectal cyst-hamartomas and sacral dysplasia: MR appearance. AJNR Am J Neuroradiol. 1998;19:1043–5.
53. Lim KE, Hsu WC, Wang CR. Tailgut cyst with malignancy: MR imaging findings. AJR Am J Roentgenol. 1998;170:1488–90.
54. Bjornsson J, Wold LE, Ebersold MJ, Laws ER. Chordoma of the mobile spine. A clinicopathologic analysis of 40 patients. Cancer. 1993;71:735–40.
55. Llauger J, Palmer J, Amores S, et al. Primary tumors of the sacrum: diagnostic imaging. AJR Am J Roentgenol. 2000;174:417–24.
56. Rossleigh MA, Smith J, Yeh SD. Scintigraphic features of primary sacral tumors. J Nucl Med. 1986;27:627–30.
57. Crapanzano JP, Ali SZ, Ginsberg MS, Zakowski MF. Chordoma: a cytologic study with histologic and radiologic correlation. Cancer. 2001;93:40–51.
58. Mitchell A, Scheithauer BW, Unni KK, Forsyth PJ, Wold LE, McGivney DJ. Chordoma and chondroid neoplasms of the spheno-occiput. An immunohistochemical study of 41 cases with prognostic and nosologic implications. Cancer. 1993;72:2943–9.
59. Oakley GJ, Fuhrer K, Seethala RR. Brachyury, SOX-9, and podoplanin, new markers in the skull base chordoma vs chondrosarcoma differential: a tissue microarray-based comparative analysis. Mod Pathol. 2008;21:1461–9.
60. Paidakakos NA, Rovlias A, Rokas E, Theodoropoulos S, Katafygiotis P. Primary clear cell chondrosarcoma of the spine: a case report of a rare entity and a review of the literature. Case Rep Oncol Med. 2012;2012:693137.
61. Jeffrey PB, Biava CG, Davis RL. Chondroid chordoma. A hyalinized chordoma without cartilaginous differentiation. Am J Clin Pathol. 1995;103(3):271–9.
62. Saito A, Hasegawa T, Shimoda T, Toda G, Hirohashi S, Tajima G, et al. Dedifferentiated chordoma: a case report. Jpn J Clin Oncol. 1998;28:766–71.
63. Kim SC, Cho W, Chang UK, Youn SM. Two cases of dedifferentiated chordoma in the sacrum. Korean J Spine. 2015;12(3):230–4.
64. Meis JM, Raymond AK, Evans HL, Charles RE, Giraldo AA. "De-differentiated" chordoma: a clinicopathologic and immunohistochemical study of three cases. Am J Surg Pathol. 1987;11:516–25.
65. Bisceglia M, D'Angelo VA, Guglielmi G, Dor DB, Pasguinelli. De-differentiated chordoma of the thoracic spine with rhabdomyosarcomatous differentiations: report of a case and review of the literature. Ann Diagn Pathol 2007;11:262–273.

66. Kishikawa H, Tanaka K. Chordoma: report of an autopsy case with fibrosarcoma. Acta Pathol Jpn. 1974;24:299–308.
67. Morimitsu Y, Aoki T, Yokoyama K, Hashimoto H. Sarcomatoid chordoma: chordoma with a massive spindle cell component. Skeletal Radiol. 2000;29:721–5.
68. Fukuda T, Aihara T, Ban S, Nakajima T, Machinami R. Sacrococcygeal chordoma with malignant spindle cell component: a report of two autopsy cases with a review of the literature. Acta Pathol Jpn. 1992;42:448–53.
69. Fuchs B, Dickey ID, Yaszemski MJ, Inwards CY, Sim FH. Operative management of sacral chordoma. J Bone Joint Surg Am. 2005;87:2211–6.
70. Ruggieri P, Angelini A, Ussia G, Montalti M, Mercuri M. Surgical margins and local control in resection of sacral chordomas. Clin Orthop Relat Res. 2010;468:2939–47.
71. Angelini A, Pala E, Calabrò T, Maraldi M, Ruggieri P. Prognostic factors in surgical resection of sacral chordoma. J Surg Oncol. 2015;112(4):344–51.
72. Jawad MU, Scully SP. Surgery significantly improves survival in patients with chordoma. Spine. 2010;35:117–23.
73. Romeo S, Hogendoorn PC. Brachyury and chordoma: the chondroid-chordoid dilemma resolved? J Pathol. 2006;209:143–6.
74. Park JB, Lee CK, Koh JS, Lee JK, Park EY, Riew KD. Overexpressions of nerve growth factor and its tropomyosin-related kinase A receptor on chordoma cells. Spine. 2007;32(18):1969–73.
75. Hulen CA, Temple T, Fox WP, Sama AA, Green BA, Eismont FJ. Oncologic and functional outcome following sacrectomy for sacral chordoma. J Bone Joint Surg Am. 2006;88-A:1532–9.
76. Randall RL, Bruckner J, Lloyd C, Pohlman TH, Conrad EU. Sacral resection and reconstruction for tumors and tumor-like conditions. Orthopaedics. 2005;28:307–13.
77. Stener B, Gunterberg B. High amputation of the sacrum for extirpation of tumors. Principles and technique. Spine. 1978;3:351–66.
78. Varga PP, Szövérfi Z, Fisher CG, Boriani S, Gokaslan ZL, Dekutoski MB, Chou D, Quraishi NA, Reynolds JJ, Luzzati A, Williams R, Fehlings MG, Germscheid NM, Lazary A, Rhines LD. Surgical treatment of sacral chordoma: prognostic variables for local recurrence and overall survival. Eur Spine J. 2015;24(5):1092–101.
79. Hsieh PC, Xu R, Sciubba DM, et al. Long-term clinical outcomes following en bloc resections for sacral chordomas and chondrosarcomas: a series of twenty consecutive patients. Spine. 2009;34:2233–9
80. Atalar H, Selek H, Yildiz Y, et al. Management of sacrococcygeal chordomas. Int Orthop. 2006;30:514–8.
81. Devin C, Chong PY, Holt GE, et al. Level-adjusted perioperative risk of sacral amputations. J Surg Oncol. 2006;94:203–11.
82. Samson IR, Springfield DS, Suit HD, Mankin HJ. Operative treatment of sacrococcygeal chordoma. A review of twenty-one cases. J Bone Joint Surg Am. 1993;75:1476–84.
83. Angelini A, Ruggieri P. A new surgical technique (modified Osaka technique) of sacral resection by posterior-only approach: description and preliminary results. Spine. 2013;38(3):E185–92.
84. Osaka S, Yoshida Y, Ryu J. Longitudinal osteotomy of lateral sacrum for malignant iliac tumor using modified threadwire saw. J Surg Oncol. 2007;95(3):258–60.
85. Gunterberg B, Kewenter J, Petersen I, Stener B. Anorectal function after major resections of the sacrum with bilateral or unilateral sacrifice of sacral nerves. Br J Surg. 1976;63(7):546–54.
86. Gunterberg B, Norlén L, Stener B, Sundin T. Neurourologic evaluation after resection of the sacrum. Invest Urol. 1975;13(3):183–8.
87. Gunterberg B, Petersen I. Sexual function after major resection of the sacrum with bilateral or unilateral sacrifice of sacral nerves. Fertil Steril. 1976;27:1146–53.

88. Zoccali C, Skoch J, Patel AS, Walter CM, Maykowski P, Baaj AA. Residual neurological function after sacral root resection during en-bloc sacrectomy: a systematic review. Eur Spine J. 2016;25. [Epub ahead of print].
89. Angelini A, Drago G, Trovarelli G, Calabrò T, Ruggieri P. Infection after surgical resection for pelvic bone tumors: an analysis of 270 patients from one institution. Clin Orthop Relat Res. 2014;472(1):349–59.
90. Chen KW, Yang HL, Lu J, et al. Risk factors for postoperative wound infections of sacral chordoma after surgical excision. J Spinal Disord Tech. 2011;24:230–4.
91. Pennicooke B, Laufer I, Sahgal A, Varga PP, Gokaslan ZL, Bilsky MH, Yamada YJ. Safety and local control of radiation therapy for chordoma of the spine and sacrum: a systematic review. Spine. 2016;41(Suppl 20):S186–92.
92. Rich TA, Schiller A, Suit HD, Mankin HJ. Clinical and pathologic review of 48 cases of chordoma. Cancer. 1985;56:182–7.
93. Catton C, O'Sullivan B, Bell R, et al. Chordoma: long-term follow-up after radical photon irradiation. Radiother Oncol. 1996;41:67–72.
94. Cummings BJ, Hodson DI, Bush RS. Chordoma: the results of megavoltage radiation therapy. Int J Radiat Oncol Biol Phys. 1983;9:633–42.
95. Rotondo RL, Folkert W, Liebsch NJ, et al. High-dose proton-based radiation therapy in the management of spine chordomas: outcomes and clinicopathological prognostic factors. J Neurosurg Spine. 2015;23:788–97.
96. Zabel-du Bois A, Nikoghosyan A, Schwahofer A, et al. Intensity modulated radiotherapy in the management of sacral chordoma in primary versus recurrent disease. Radiother Oncol. 2010;97:408–12.
97. Hug EB, Fitzek MM, Liebsch NJ, et al. Locally challenging osteo- and chondrogenic tumors of the axial skeleton: results of combined proton and photon radiation therapy using three-dimensional treatment planning. Int J Radiat Oncol Biol Phys. 1995;31:467–76.
98. Yamada Y, Laufer I, Cox BW, et al. Preliminary results of high-dose single-fraction radiotherapy for the management of chordomas of the spine and sacrum. Neurosurgery. 2013;73:673–80.
99. Brown JM, Koong AC. High-dose single-fraction radiotherapy: exploiting a new biology? Int J Radiat Oncol Biol Phys. 2008;71:324–5.
100. Suit HD, Goitein M, Munzenrider J, et al. Definitive radiation therapy for chordoma and chondrosarcoma of base of skull and cervical spine. J Neurosurg. 1982;56:377–85.
101. Austin-Seymour M, Munzenrider JE, Goitein M, et al. Progress in low-LET heavy particle therapy: intracranial and paracranial tumors and uveal melanomas. Radiat Res Suppl. 1985;8:219–26.
102. Tobias CA, Blakely EA, Alpen EL, et al. Molecular and cellular radiobiology of heavy ions. Int J Radiat Oncol Biol Phys. 1982;8:2109–20.
103. DeLaney TF, Liebsch NJ, Pedlow FX, et al. Long-term results of phase II study of high dose photon/proton radiotherapy in the management of spine chordomas, chondrosarcomas, and other sarcomas. J Surg Oncol. 2014;110:115–22.
104. McDonald MW, Linton OR, Shah MV. Proton therapy for reirradiation of progressive or recurrent chordoma. Int J Radiat Oncol Biol Phys. 2013;87:1107–14.
105. Indelicato DJ, Rotondo RL, Begosh-Mayne D, et al. A prospective outcomes study of proton therapy for chordomas and chondrosarcomas of the spine. Int J Radiat Oncol Biol Phys. 2016;95:297–303.
106. Scholz M, Kraft G. Track structure and the calculation of biological effects of heavy charged particles. Adv Space Res. 1996;18:5–14.
107. Imai R, Kamada T, Tsuji H, et al. Carbon ion radiotherapy for unresectable sacral chordomas. Clin Cancer Res. 2004;10:5741–6.
108. Nishida Y, Kamada T, Imai R, et al. Clinical outcome of sacral chordoma with carbon ion radiotherapy compared with surgery. Int J Radiat Oncol Biol Phys. 2011;79:110–6.
109. Imai R, Kamada T, Sugahara S, et al. Carbon ion radiotherapy for sacral chordoma. Br J Radiol. 2011;84(Spec. No. 1):S48–54.

110. Uhl M, Welzel T, Jensen A, Ellerbrock M, Haberer T, Jäkel O, Herfarth K, Debus J. Carbon ion beam treatment in patients with primary and recurrent sacrococcygeal chordoma. Strahlenther Onkol. 2015;191(7):597–603.
111. Lundkvist J, Ekman M, Ericsson SR, Jönsson B, Glimelius B. Proton therapy of cancer: potential clinical advantages and cost-effectiveness. Acta Oncol. 2005;44:850–61.
112. Durante M, Loeffler JS. Charged particles in radiation oncology. Nat Rev Clin Oncol. 2010;7:37–43.
113. Mohan R, Bortfeld T. Proton therapy: clinical gains through current and future treatment programs. Front Radiat Ther Oncol. 2011;43:440–64.
114. Goitein M, Cox JD. Should randomized clinical trials be required for proton radiotherapy? J Clin Oncol. 2008;26:175–6.
115. Park L, Delaney TF, Liebsch NJ, et al. Sacral chordomas: impact of high-dose proton/photon-beam radiation therapy combined with or without surgery for primary versus recurrent tumor. Int J Radiat Oncol Biol Phys. 2006;65:1514–21.
116. Suit H, Kooy H, Trofimov A, et al. Should positive phase III clinical trial data be required before proton beam therapy is more widely adopted? No. Radiother Oncol. 2008;86:148–53.
117. Patt JC. CORR Insights(®): sacral insufficiency fractures are common after high-dose radiation for sacral chordomas treated with or without surgery. Clin Orthop Relat Res. 2016;474(3):773–5.
118. Negri T, Casieri P, Miselli F, et al. Evidence for PDGFRA, PDGFRB and KIT deregulation in an NSCLC patient. Br J Cancer. 2007;96:180–1.
119. Casali PG, Messina A, Stacchiotti S, et al. Imatinib mesylate in chordoma. Cancer. 2004;101:2086–97.
120. Stacchiotti S, Marrari A, Tamborini E, et al. Response to imatinib plus sirolimus in advanced chordoma. Ann Oncol. 2009;20:1886–94.
121. George S, Merriam P, Maki RG, et al. Multicenter phase II trial of sunitinib in the treatment of nongastrointestinal stromal tumor sarcomas. J Clin Oncol. 2009;27:3154–60.
122. Tamborini E, Virdis E, Negri T, et al. Analysis of receptor tyrosine kinases (RTKs) and downstream pathways in chordomas. Neuro-Oncology. 2010;12:776–89.
123. Stacchiotti S, Longhi A, Ferraresi V, et al. Phase II study of imatinib in advanced chordoma. J Clin Oncol. 2012;30:914–20.
124. Weinberger PM, Yu Z, Kowalski D, et al. Differential expression of epidermal growth factor receptor, c-Met, and HER2/neu in chordoma compared with 17 other malignancies. Arch Otolaryngol Head Neck Surg. 2005;131:707–11.
125. Hof H, Welzel T, Debus J. Effectiveness of cetuximab/gefitinib in the therapy of a sacral chordoma. Onkologie. 2006;29:572–4.
126. Singhal N, Kotasek D, Parnis FX. Response to erlotinib in a patient with treatment refractory chordoma. Anticancer Drugs. 2009;20:953–5.
127. Stacchiotti S, Tamborini E, Lo Vullo S, et al. Phase II study on lapatinib in advanced EGFR-positive chordoma. Ann Oncol. 2013;24:1931–6.
128. Yang C, Schwab JH, Schoenfeld AJ, et al. A novel target for treatment of chordoma: signal transducers and activators of transcription 3. Mol Cancer Ther. 2009;8:2597–605.
129. Yang C, Hornicek FJ, Wood KB, et al. Blockage of Stat3 with CDDO-Me inhibits tumor cell growth in chordoma. Spine. 2010;35:1668–75.
130. Thieblemont C, Biron P, Rocher F, Bouhour D, Bobin JY, Gérard JP, et al. Prognostic factors in chordoma: role of postoperative radiotherapy. Eur J Cancer. 1995;31A:2255–9.
131. McGirt MJ, Gokaslan ZL, Chaichana KL. Preoperative grading scale to predict survival in patients undergoing resection of malignant primary osseous spinal neoplasms. Spine J. 2011;11(3):190–6. doi:10.1016/j.spinee.2011.01.013.
132. Ozger A, Eralp L, Sungur M, Atalar AC. Surgical management of sacral chordoma. Acta Orthop Belg. 2010;76:243–53.
133. Lee J, Bhatia N, Hoang B, Ziogas A, Zell J. Analysis of prognostic factors for patients with chordoma with use of the California Cancer Registry. J Bone Joint Surg Am. 2012;94:356–63.

134. Hobusch GM, Bodner F, Walzer S, Marculescu R, Funovics PT, Sulzbacher I, Windhager R, Panotopoulos J. C-reactive protein as a prognostic factor in patients with chordoma of lumbar spine and sacrum—a single center pilot study. World J Surg Oncol. 2016;14:111.
135. Hanna SA, Aston WJ, Briggs TW, Cannon SR, Saifuddin A. Sacral chordoma: can local recurrence after sacrectomy be predicted? Clin Orthop Relat Res. 2008;466(9):2217–23.
136. Boriani S, Bandiera S, Biagini R, Bacchini P, Boriani L, Cappuccio M, Chevalley F, Gasbarrini A, Picci P, Weinstein JN. Chordoma of the mobile spine: fifty years of experience. Spine. 2006;31(4):493–503.
137. Stacchiotti S, Casali PG, Lo Vullo S, Mariani L, Palassini E, Mercuri M, et al. Chordoma of the mobile spine and sacrum: a retrospective analysis of a series of patients surgically treated at two referral centers. Ann Surg Oncol. 2010;17:211–9.
138. von Witzleben A, Goerttler LT, Lennerz J, Weissinger S, Kornmann M, Mayer-Steinacker R, von Baer A, Schultheiss M, Möller P, Barth TF. In chordoma, metastasis, recurrences, Ki-67 index, and a matrix-poor phenotype are associated with patients' shorter overall survival. Eur Spine J. 2016;25:4016–24.
139. Ridenour 3rd RV, Ahrens WA, Folpe AL, Miller DV. Clinical and histopathologic features of chordomas in children and young adults. Pediatr Dev Pathol. 2010;13(1):9–17.
140. Cheng EY, Ozerdemoglu RA, Transfeldt EE, Thompson Jr RC. Lumbosacral chordoma. Prognostic factors and treatment. Spine. 1999;24:1639–45.
141. Chen KW, Yang HL, Lu J, Liu JY, Chen XQ. Prognostic factors of sacral chordoma after surgical therapy: a study of 36 patients. Spinal Cord. 2009;48:166–71.
142. Ishii K, Chiba K, Watanabe M, Yabe H, Fujimura Y, Toyama Y. Local recurrence after S2-3 sacrectomy in sacral chordoma. Report of four cases. J Neurosurg. 2002;97(1 Suppl):98–101.
143. Dorfman HD, Czerniak B. Bone cancers. Cancer. 1995;75:203–10.
144. Mukherjee D, Chaichana KL, Parker SL, Gokaslan ZL, McGirt MJ. Association of surgical resection and survival in patients with malignant primary osseous spinal neoplasms from the surveillance, epidemiology, and end results (SEER) database. Eur Spine J. 2012;22:1375.

Osteosarcoma of the Sacrum 16

Andrea Angelini, Douglas G. Letson, and Pietro Ruggieri

16.1 Introduction

Osteosarcoma and Ewing's sarcoma are the most common primary malignant bone tumors in childhood and adolescence, most occurring during the first two decades [1, 2]. Osteosarcoma rarely involves the spine (1–3% of all osteosarcomas), and the sacrum is one of the most common spinal locations [2–9]. Osteosarcoma is the third most frequent primary malignant tumor of the sacrum after chordoma and Ewing's sarcoma. Secondary osteosarcoma may occur in patients that received pelvic radiation treatment or as sarcomatous degeneration in patients with polyostotic Paget's disease [10–15].

There have been several articles on the treatment of patients with osteosarcoma of the spine [4–7, 16–32]; however, those publications included case reports or selected patients from small series, making the optimal evidence-based therapeutic approach very difficult. Wuisman et al. [23] reported a case of sacral osteosarcoma and performed a review of all reported cases since 1984–2001: they were able to find only 11 patients [7, 18, 25–32]. In the last 15 years, still some data appear in the literature, indicating that the combination of chemotherapy with adequate surgical procedures (hemi/total sacrectomies) may increase survival in this poor prognostic tumor site [4, 20–22, 24].

A. Angelini, M.D., Ph.D. • P. Ruggieri, M.D., Ph.D. (✉)
Department of Orthopaedics and Orthopedic Oncology, University of Padova, Padova, Italy
e-mail: andrea.angelini83@yahoo.it; pietro.ruggieri@unipd.it

D.G. Letson, M.D.
Department of Surgery, University of South Florida, H. Lee Moffitt Cancer Center, Tampa, FL, USA
e-mail: Douglas.Letson@moffitt.org

P. Ruggieri et al. (eds.), *Tumors of the Sacrum*,
DOI 10.1007/978-3-319-51202-0_16

16.2 Epidemiology, Presentation, and Diagnosis

Patients with primary spinal osteosarcoma are older than those with osteosarcoma of the extremity (mean age of about 38 years old) [5, 6, 8, 33]. Exposure to radiation is a proven exogenous risk factor for secondary osteosarcoma of the bone. Incidence of sarcomas postirradiation therapy comprises about 0.1% of all cancer cases, and the sarcomas usually appear 10–20 years posttreatment (thus radiation-induced sarcoma is typical of adult age) [10–15]. It has been demonstrated that osteosarcoma could be related to pelvic radiation therapy [10, 13–14].

As well as for other sacral tumors, early diagnosis is difficult and pain and swelling are the most frequent symptoms of sacral osteosarcoma. Neurological symptoms are associated with large tumors. A detailed history with a complete physical exam should be performed prior to any evaluation. Ozaki et al. reported in 2002 their experience in 15 osteosarcomas of the sacrum and 7 of the mobile spine [4]: the duration of symptoms between onset and diagnosis ranged from 2 to 18 months, and the most common was represented by pain (almost all) followed by neurological disorder (half of the cases). The median tumor size in sacral tumors was 8.0 cm. Other reports were results in terms of diagnostic delay and tumor size [8, 34]. The laboratory findings may show an increase in alkaline phosphatase (AP) and lactic dehydrogenase in the serum (about 30% of cases) [35–38]. In some cases mild anemia and high erythrocyte sedimentation rate may also be present at diagnosis [35, 36].

16.3 Imaging

Most spinal osteosarcomas are pathologically osteoblastic, resulting in typical mineralized lesions on radiographs and CT, even if rarely osteolytic lesions also occurred [4, 29, 37, 39]. Computed tomography (CT), magnetic resonance imaging (MRI), angiography, and dynamic bone scintigraphy are used to evaluate the extension of tumors and the involvement of surrounding structures such as vessels, nerves, and soft tissues [40, 41]. CT of the lung is part of the basal staging. MRI is also useful in the assessment of patients with intraosseous tumor spread, particularly in the sacrum or sacroiliac joint, or in the identification of neural compression [8].

Nuclear medicine imaging techniques (bone scans and PET/CT) are being used increasingly to aid in the initial staging/metastatic evaluation and response to therapy. Isotope scans with technetium [41] or thallium [42] are a standard part of the staging because they show the intense hotspot of the tumor and are very sensitive in detecting any skip or distant bony metastases [43]. 18-Fluorodeoxy-glucose positron emission tomography (18FDG-PET) combined with a whole-body CT is being increasingly used in staging and also in treatment monitoring [44–46]. On 18FDG-PET/CT, there is increased uptake within the tumor, which decreases following effective neoadjuvant therapy [44–46]. Whole-body MRI and PET/CT are currently being evaluated for the detection of metastatic disease [47].

Biopsy is a key diagnostic method for sacral osteosarcomas and should be carefully planned according to the definitive surgery, in order to avoid improper treatments or negative effects on survival [48–50]. Conventional high-grade osteosarcoma is the most frequent variant at histopathologic evaluation. Multicentric osteosarcoma is a rare type of the disease characterized by a synchronous or metachronous appearance of multiple skeletal lesions. Some cases with sacral involvement have been reported [51, 52] with extremely poor prognosis. On the other hand, low-grade osteosarcoma of the sacrum (well-differentiated intraosseous osteosarcoma) has been described in only one report in literature [53].

16.4 Treatment

In recent years, multidisciplinary approach and aggressive adjuvant/neoadjuvant chemotherapy have increased the oncologic outcome of patients with osteosarcoma [5, 6, 35, 37, 54–60], even if spinal involvement has been linked with a very poor prognostic outlook with median survival times of only 10–23 months. Much like with Ewing's sarcoma, a combination of chemotherapy with surgery (when possible) is also the standard therapy in tumors involving the axial skeleton. Some authors suggested that patients with osteosarcoma of the spine should be treated with a combination of chemotherapy and at least marginal surgery [4]. Postoperative radiotherapy can also be applied in the treatment program and may be of benefit in selected patients.

16.4.1 Chemotherapy

Currently, chemotherapy is undoubtedly the method that is likely to cure the greatest proportion of patients with osteosarcoma. However the association with surgery is essential for the local control and the management program of all patients. In fact, in the presence of effective chemotherapy, osteosarcoma is rarely cured without surgical resection [5, 17, 61]. Doxorubicin, cisplatin, high-dose methotrexate, ifosfamide, and etoposide have antitumor activity in osteosarcoma and are frequently used with different protocols as the basis of treatment [54, 57–59, 62]. The selection of postoperative adjuvant chemotherapy based on the degree of the tumor necrosis induced by preoperative therapy improves the patient survival rate [59, 62]. New drugs such as bisphosphonates, interferon, interleukin, and monoclonal antibodies have been trialed in preclinical and clinical studies, showing encouraging results [59]. Specific aspects on protocol of treatment are analyzed in the dedicated chapter.

16.4.2 Sacrectomy

Recent progression of surgical techniques may enable total sacrectomy to improve the survival of patients [63–68]. Patients whose tumors can be completely resected with adequate margins should be approached with curative intent. Simon et al. [29] reported a patient disease-free almost 5 years after surgical excision alone. However, the surgical intervention is quite challenging given the magnitude of treatment, the significant compromise of neurological status, and the high risk of complications [69–72]. To date, the question whether this type of surgery is really beneficial to the affected patients is still debated. Ozaki et al. [4] show that complete tumor resection may improve their prognosis. In the author's experience, most patients have unresectable or partially resectable tumors, or metastases at presentation, and thus are not good candidates for a surgical treatment (or adequate margins cannot be achieved). Obviously sacral resection in low-grade tumors should be considered the mainstay of treatment and has been successfully reported [53].

There is no absolute contraindication for surgical resection because the decision is dictated by local practice and the surgical expertise of the tumor center. Relative contraindications for resection are large extraosseous extension, major neurovascular involvement, high mortality/morbidity risk with extensive surgery, and unavailability of experienced multidisciplinary team.

16.5 Radiation Therapy

In general, radiotherapy has a limited role in the management of osteosarcoma because of the relative radioresistance and the need for a large dose of radiation to achieve clinical response, but there are anatomical locations in which the possibility of complete surgical resection is unfeasible [73–75]. However, the effect of chemotherapy alone is usually temporary, and there is a need of intensive treatment for local control. In these cases, radiation therapy may be an option to try to extend the progression-free interval. Another possible scenario is the use of adjunctive irradiation in patients who underwent intralesional or inadequate surgery, in which the overall survival was better compared with patients that not received further local treatments [4, 6].

Radiotherapy may provide significant palliation in patients with unresectable sacral osteosarcomas (or patients that refused surgery), even if some cases successfully treated with combination of chemotherapy and radiation have been reported in literature [6, 59, 76, 77].

Considering that high-dose conventional radiation cannot usually be given in the sacrum and new radiation therapy techniques (e.g., proton beam and heavy ion carbon therapy) are available, the role of radiation therapy in osteosarcoma may need to be reinvestigated with modern techniques that may extend indications [78]. Targeted internal radiotherapy with Sm-153-EDTMP could be an additional treatment option for some patients with inoperable tumors [79, 80].

16.6 Oncologic Outcome

Although multimodal treatment, osteosarcoma of the sacrum has a significantly worse outcome than it affects other sites [5, 6, 35, 58, 59]. In the recent ESMO guidelines, primary metastases, axial or proximal extremity tumor site, large tumor size, elevated serum AP or LDH, and older age are considered adverse prognostic or predictive factors [58].

The median survival for patients with osteosarcoma of the spine has been reported in the range of 6–10 months [5–7, 16]. Shives et al. [6] reported that only 7 of 26 patients treated for their spinal osteosarcomas up to 1980 survived for 1 year. In a large retrospective series of spinal osteosarcomas (15 with tumors of the sacrum and 7 with tumors at other sites), 86% of the patients survived 1 year, but only 3 were alive at 6 years of follow-up [4]. Li et al. [20] reported a series including two cases of osteosarcoma of the sacrum treated with hemisacrectomy and adjuvant chemotherapy: one was alive with disease with local recurrence after resection with marginal margins at 49 months of follow-up, whereas the other was alive with no evidence of disease at 24 months (wide margin). Guo et al. [21] reported a series on en bloc sacrectomies including two patients affected by osteosarcoma: one was alive with disease with local recurrence at 11 months of follow-up and the other alive with no evidence of disease at 20 months. Arkader et al. [22] reported two cases of sacral osteosarcoma in pediatric age, disease-free at 8 years of follow-up after sacrectomy and chemotherapy. Sundaresan et al. [7] suggested that the combination of surgery, chemotherapy, and radiation may increase survival, showing three patients who survived longer than 36 months without evidence of disease.

Conflict-of-Interest Statement No benefits have been or will be received from a commercial party related directly or indirectly to the subject matter of this article.

References

1. Longhi A, Errani C, De Paolis M, Mercuri M, Bacci G. Primary bone osteosarcoma in the pediatric age: state of the art. Cancer Treat Rev. 2006;32:423–36.
2. Unni KK. Dahlin's bone tumors general aspects and data on 11,087 cases. 5th ed. Philadelphia: Lippincott-Raven; 1996.
3. Weinstein JN, McLain RF. Primary tumors of the spine. Spine. 1987,12:843–51.
4. Ozaki T, Flege S, Liljenqvist U, Hillmann A, Delling G, Salzer-Kuntschik M, Jürgens H, Kotz R, Winkelmann W, Bielack SS. Osteosarcoma of the spine: experience of the Cooperative Osteosarcoma Study Group. Cancer. 2002;94(4):1069–77.
5. Barwick KW, Huvos AG, Smith J. Primary osteogenic sarcoma of the vertebral column: a clinicopathologic correlation of ten patients. Cancer. 1980;46:595–604.
6. Shives TC, Dahlin DC, Sim FH, Pritchard DJ, Earle JD. Osteosarcoma of the spine. J Bone Joint Surg Am. 1986;68:660–8.
7. Sundaresan N, Rosen G, Huvos AG, Krol G. Combined treatment of osteosarcoma of the spine. Neurosurgery. 1988;23:714–9.
8. Green R, Saifuddin A, Cannon S. Pictorial review: imaging of primary osteosarcoma of the spine. Clin Radiol. 1996;51:325–9.
9. Kurugoglu S, Adaletli I, Mihmanli I, Kanberoglu K. Lumbosacral osseous tumors in children. Eur J Radiol. 2008;65(2):257–69.
10. Weatherby RP, Dahlin DC, Ivins JC. Postradiation sarcoma of bone: review of 78 Mayo Clinic cases. Mayo Clin Proc. 1981;56(5):294–306.
11. Iyer R, Jhingran A. Radiation injury: imaging findings in the chest, abdomen and pelvis after therapeutic radiation. Cancer Imaging. 2006;6:S131–9.

12. Longhi A, Barbieri E, FAbbri N. Radiation-induced osteosarcoma arising 20 years after the treatment of Ewing's sarcoma. Tumorigenesis. 2003;89:569–72.
13. Kwon JW, Huh SJ, Yoon YC, et al. Pelvic bone complications after radiation therapy of uterine cervical cancer: evaluation with MRI. AJR Am J Roentgenol. 2008;191(4):987–94.
14. Noh JM, Huh SJ. Two cases of post-radiation osteosarcoma of the sacrum after pelvic irradiation for uterine cervical cancer. Eur J Gynaecol Oncol. 2007;28(6):497–500.
15. Torreggiani WC, Al-Ismail K, Munk PL, Lee MJ. Musculoskeletal case 18. Radiation-induced osteosarcoma of the sacrum. Can J Surg. 2001;44(5):334–5; 346.
16. Mnaymneh W, Brown M, Tejada F, Morrison G. Primary osteogenic sarcoma of the second cervical vertebra. Case report. J Bone Joint Surg Am. 1979;61:460–2.
17. Ogihara Y, Sekiguchi K, Tsuruta T. Osteogenic sarcoma of the fourth thoracic vertebra. Long-term survival by chemotherapy only. Cancer. 1984;53:2615–8.
18. Spiegel DA, Richardson WJ, Scully SP, Harrelson JM. Long- term survival following total sacrectomy with reconstruction for the treatment of primary osteosarcoma of the sacrum. A case report. J Bone Joint Surg Am. 1999;81:848–55.
19. Kawahara N, Tomita K, Fujita T, Maruo S, Otsuka S, Kinoshita G. Osteosarcoma of the thoracolumbar spine: total en bloc spondylectomy. A case report. J Bone Joint Surg Am. 1997;79:453–8.
20. Li D, Guo W, Tang X, Yang R, Tang S, Qu H, Yang Y, Sun X, Du Z. Preservation of the contralateral sacral nerves during hemisacrectomy for sacral malignancies. Eur Spine J. 2014;23(9):1933–9.
21. Guo W, Tang X, Zang J, Ji T. One-stage total en bloc sacrectomy: a novel technique and report of 9 cases. Spine. 2013;38(10):E626–31.
22. Arkader A, Yang CH, Tolo VT. High long-term local control with sacrectomy for primary high-grade bone sarcoma in children. Clin Orthop Relat Res. 2012;470(5):1491–7.
23. Wuisman P, Lieshout O, van Dijk M, van Diest P. Reconstruction after total en bloc sacrectomy for osteosarcoma using a custom-made prosthesis: a technical note. Spine. 2001;26(4):431–9.
24. Zileli M, Hoscoskun C, Brastianos P, Sabah D. Surgical treatment of primary sacral tumors: complications associated with sacrectomy. Neurosurg Focus. 2003;15:E9.
25. Huth JF, Dawson EG, Eilber FR. Abdominosacral resection for malignant tumors of the sacrum. Am J Surg. 1984;148:157–61.
26. Kawai A, Huvos AG, Meyers PA, et al. Osteosarcoma of the pelvis. Clin Orthop. 1998;348:196–207.
27. Krajbich JI, Gillespie R. Complete en bloc resection of the sacrum for osteogenic sarcoma. In: Brown KLB, editor. Complications of limb salvage. Montreal: ISOLS; 1991. p. 395–6.
28. Ritschl P, Missaghi SM, Wurnig C, et al. Operative procedures in tumors of the sacrum: results of 26 cases. Chir Organi Mov. 1990;75(Suppl):111–3.
29. Simon RG, Irwin RB. An unusual presentation of telangiectatic osteosarcoma. Am J Orthop. 1996;25:375–9.
30. Simpson AHRW, Porter A, Davis A, et al. Cephalad sacral resection with a combined extended ilioinguinal and posterior approach. J Bone Joint Surg Am. 1995;77:405–11.
31. Stener B, Guntherberg B. High amputation of the sacrum for extirpation of tumors. Spine. 1978;3:351–66.
32. Tolo VT, Atkinson JB, Sato JK. Resection of sacral Ewing's sarcoma and osteosarcoma in children. In: Brown KLB, editor. Complications of limb salvage. Montreal: ISOLS; 1991. p. 365–70.
33. Murphey MD, Andrews CL, Flemming DJ, Temple HT, Smith WS, Smirniotopoulos JG. From the archives of the AFIP. Primary tumors of the spine: radiologic pathologic correlation. Radiographics. 1996;16:1131–58.
34. Pollock BH, Krischer JP, Vietti TJ. Interval between symptom onset and diagnosis of pediatric solid tumors. J Pediatr. 1991;119:725–32.
35. Link MP, Goorin AM, Horowitz M, et al. Adjuvant chemotherapy of high- grade osteosarcoma of the extremity: updated results of the Multi-Institutional Osteosarcoma Study. Clin Orthop Relat Res. 1991;270:8–14.

36. Hannisdal E, Solheim OP, Theodorsen L, Host H. Alterations of blood analyses at relapse of osteosarcoma and Ewing's sarcoma. Acta Oncol. 1990;29:585–7.
37. Ferrari S, Bacci G, Picci P, et al. Long-term follow-up and post relapse survival in patients with non-metastatic osteosarcoma of the extremity treated with neoadjuvant chemotherapy. Ann Oncol. 1997;8:765.
38. Thorpe WP, Reilly JJ, Rosenborg SA. Prognostic significance of alkaline phosphatase measurements in patients with osteogenic sarcoma receiving chemotherapy. Cancer. 1979;43:2178–81.
39. deSantos LA, Edeiken B. Purely lytic osteosarcoma. Skeletal Radiol. 1982;9:1–7.
40. Thornton E, Krajewski KM, O'Regan KN, Giardino AA, Jagannathan JP, Ramaiya N. Imaging features of primary and secondary malignant tumours of the sacrum. Br J Radiol. 2012;85(1011):279–86.
41. Aisen AM, Martel W, Braunstein EM, McMillin KI, Phillips WA, Kling TF. MRI and CT evaluation of primary bone and soft-tissue tumors. AJR Am J Roentgenol. 1986;146:749–56.
42. Wittig JC, Bickels J, Priebat D, Jelinek J, Kellar-Graney K, Shmookler B, et al. Osteosarcoma: a multidisciplinary approach to diagnosis and treatment. Am Fam Physician. 2002;65:1123–32.
43. McKillop JH, Etcubanas E, Goris ML. The indications for and limitations of bone scintigraphy in osteogenic sarcoma: a review of 55 patients. Cancer. 1981;46:2603–6.
44. McCarville MB, Christie R, Daw NC, Spunt SL, Kaste SC. PET/CT in the evaluation of childhood sarcomas. AJR Am J Roentgenol. 2005;184:1293–304.
45. Volker T, Denecke T, Steffen I, Misch D, Schonberger S, et al. Positron emission tomography for staging of pediatric sarcoma patients: results of a prospective multicenter trial. J Clin Oncol. 2007;25:5435–41.
46. Schulte M, Brecht-Krauss D, Werner M, Hartwig E, Sarkar MR, Keppler P, et al. Evaluation of neoadjuvant therapy response of osteogenic sarcoma using FDG PET. J Nucl Med. 1999;40:1637–43.
47. Hogendoorn PC, Athanasou N, Bielack S, De Alava E, Dei Tos AP, Ferrari S, et al. Bone sarcomas: ESMO Clinical Practice Guidelines for diagnosis, treatment and follow-up. Ann Oncol. 2010;21(Suppl. 5):v204–13.
48. Mankin HJ, Mankin CJ, Simon MA. The hazards of the biopsy, revisited: members of the Musculoskeletal Tumor Society. J Bone Joint Surg. 1996;78:656–63.
49. Mavrogenis AF, Angelini A, Vottis C, Palmerini E, Rimondi E, Rossi G, Papagelopoulos PJ, Ruggieri P. State-of-the-art approach for bone sarcomas. Eur J Orthop Surg Traumatol. 2015;25(1):5–15.
50. Mavrogenis AF, Angelini A, Errani C, Rimondi E. How should musculoskeletal biopsies be performed? Orthopedics. 2014;37(9):585–8.
51. Mahoney JP, Spanier SS, Morris JL. Multifocal osteosarcoma: a case report with review of the literature. Cancer. 1979;44:1897–907.
52. Yamamoto T, Fujita I, Kurosaka M, Mizuno K. Sacral radiculopathy secondary to multicentric osteosarcoma. Spine. 2001;26(15):1729–32.
53. Liuhong W, Minming Z. Well-differentiated intraosseous osteosarcoma in the sacrum: a case report. Iran J Radiol. 2013;10(3):175–8.
54. Ferrari S, Smeland S, Mercuri M, et al. Neoadjuvant chemotherapy with high-dose Ifosfamide, high-dose methotrexate, cisplatin, and doxorubicin for patients with localized osteosarcoma of the extremity: a joint study by the Italian and Scandinavian Sarcoma Groups. J Clin Oncol. 2005;23:8845–52.
55. Winkler K, Beron G, Delling G, Heise U, Kabisch H, Purfurst C, et al. Neoadjuvant chemotherapy of osteosarcoma: results of a randomized cooperative trial (COSS-82) with salvage chemotherapy based on histological tumor response. J Clin Oncol. 1988;6:329–37.
56. Winkler K, Bielack S, Delling G, Saltzer-Kuntschik M, Kotz R, Greenshaw C, et al. Effect of intraarterial versus intravenous cisplatin in addition to systemic doxorubicin, high-dose methotrexate, and ifosfamide on histologic tumor response in osteosarcoma (study COSS-86). Cancer. 1990;66:1703–10.

57. Bacci G, Mercuri M, Briccoli A, Ferrari S, Bertoni F, Donati D, et al. Osteogenic sarcoma of the extremity with detectable lung metastases at presentation. Results of treatment of 23 patients with chemotherapy followed by simultaneous resection of primary and metastatic lesions. Cancer. 1997;79:245–54.
58. ESMO/European Sarcoma Network Working Group. Bone sarcomas: ESMO Clinical Practice Guidelines for diagnosis, treatment and follow-up. Ann Oncol. 2014;25(Suppl 3):iii113–23.
59. Ta HT, Dass CR, Choong PF, Dunstan DE. Osteosarcoma treatment: state of the art. Cancer Metastasis Rev. 2009;28(1–2):247–63.
60. Gherlinzoni F, Picci P, Bacci G, et al. Limb sparing versus amputation in osteosarcoma. Correlation between local control, surgical margins and tumor necrosis: Istituto Rizzoli experience. Ann Oncol. 1992;3(Suppl 2):S23–7.
61. Jaff N, Carrasco H, Raymond K, Ayala A, Eftekhari F. Cancure in patients with osteosarcoma be achieved exclusively with chemotherapy and abrogation of surgery. Cancer. 2003;95:2202–10.
62. Carrle D, Bielack SS. Current strategies of chemotherapy in osteosarcoma. Int Orthop. 2006;30:445–51.
63. Angelini A, Ruggieri P. A new surgical technique (modified Osaka technique) of sacral resection by posterior-only approach: description and preliminary results. Spine. 2013;38(3):E185–92.
64. Ruggieri P, Angelini A, Ussia G, Montalti M, Mercuri M. Surgical margins and local control in resection of sacral chordomas. Clin Orthop Relat Res. 2010;468(11):2939–47.
65. Tomita K, Kawahara N, Hata M, Mizuno K. Indication and operative method of sacral amputation. In: Kaneda K, editor. Orthopaedic surgery now, no. 22. Surgical techniques for disorders of the thoracolumbar, lumbar and lumbosacral spine. Tokyo: Medical View, Inc.; 1996. p. 188–97.
66. Wuisman P, Lieshout O, Sugihara S, van Dijk M. Total sacrectomy and reconstruction: oncologic and functional outcome. Clin Orthop Relat Res. 2000;381:192–203.
67. Tomita K, Tsuchiya H. Total sacrectomy and reconstruction for huge sacral tumors. Spine. 1990;15:1223–7.
68. Shikata J, Yamamuro T, Kotoura Y, Mikawa Y, Iida H, Maetani S. Total sacrectomy and reconstruction for primary tumors. Report of two cases. J Bone Joint Surg Am. 1988;70:122–5.
69. Ruggieri P, Angelini A, Pala E, Mercuri M. Infections in surgery of primary tumors of the sacrum. Spine. 2012;37(5):420–8.
70. Capanna R, Briccoli A, Casadei R, et al. Sacral resections: experiences of the I.O.R. bone tumor center. Chirurgia Delgi Organi di Movimento. 1990;75(Suppl):114–6.
71. Samson IR, Springfield DS, Suit HD, et al. Operative treatment of sacrococcygeal chordoma: a review of twenty-one cases. J Bone Joint Surg Am. 1993;75:1476–84.
72. Sung HW, Shu WP, Wang HM, et al. Surgical treatment of primary tumors of the sacrum. Clin Orthop. 1987;215:91–8.
73. Delaney TF, Park L, Goldberg SI, et al. Radiotherapy for local control of osteosarcoma. Int J Radiat Oncol Biol Phys. 2005;61:492–8.
74. Mialou V, Philip T, Kalifa C, et al. Metastatic osteosarcoma at diagnosis: prognostic factors and long-term outcome—the French pediatric experience. Cancer. 2005;104(5):1100–9.
75. Loeb DM, Garrett-Mayer E, Hobbs RF, et al. Dose finding study of 153Sm-EDTMP in patients with poor-prognosis osteosarcoma. Cancer. 2009;115(11):2514–22.
76. Aledavood SA, Amirabadi A, Memar B. Non surgical treatment of sacral osteosarcoma. Iran J Cancer Prev. 2012;5(1):46–9.
77. Mahajan A, Woo SY, Kornguth DG, et al. Multimodality treatment of osteosarcoma: radiation in a high-risk cohort. Pediatr Blood Cancer. 2008;50(5):976–82.
78. Blattmann C, Oertel S, Schulz-Ertner D, et al. Non-randomized therapy trial to determine the safety and efficacy of heavy ion radiotherapy in patients with non-resectable osteosarcoma. BMC Cancer. 2010;10:96.
79. Franzius C, Bielack S, Sciuk J, Vollet B, Jurgens H, Schober O. High-activity samarium-153-EDTMP therapy in unresectable osteosarcoma. Nuklearmedizin. 1999;38:337–40.
80. Bruland OS, Skretting A, Solheim OP, Aas M. Targeted radiotherapy of osteosarcoma using 153 Sm-EDTMP. A new promising approach. Acta Oncol. 1996;35:381–4.

Ewing's Sarcoma of the Sacrum

17

Andrea Angelini, Douglas G. Letson, and Pietro Ruggieri

17.1 Introduction

Ewing's Sarcoma (ES) is a small round cells malignant tumor that accounts for 6–8% of all primary bone tumors. Together with osteosarcoma, they are the most common primary malignant bone tumors in children, most occurring during the first two decades [1, 2]. Primary ES of the spine and sacrum presents unique anatomic limitations specific to the neurological structures, vertebral column, and pelvic involvement, that challenge our ability to offer good local control. The use of multidrug chemotherapy, together with radiation therapy (RT) and surgery for local control, has significantly improved the prognosis of ES, even if it is still considered worse in the spine compared to other site [3–5]. Owing to the rarity of sacral tumors, the observations on long-term function and survival after treatment for high-grade sarcomas are limited to case reports or small series [6–10], surgical techniques [6, 11–14], or cooperative studies reporting cohorts that include but are not limited to sacrum [11, 15–22].

17.2 Epidemiology, Presentation, and Diagnosis

Primary Ewing sarcoma rarely affects the spine, and accounts for approximately 3.5–5% of the entire skeleton, falling down to 1% if the sacrum is excluded [3, 7, 20, 23–27]. Early diagnosis of sacral tumors is usually difficult because

A. Angelini, M.D., Ph.D. • P. Ruggieri, M.D., Ph.D. (✉)
Department of Orthopaedics and Orthopedic Oncology, University of Padova,
Via N. Giustiniani, 3, Padova 35128, Italy
e-mail: andrea.angelini83@yahoo.it; pietro.ruggieri@unipd.it

D.G. Letson, M.D.
Department of Surgery, University of South Florida, H. Lee Moffitt Cancer Center,
Tampa, FL 33602, USA
e-mail: Douglas.Letson@moffitt.org

P. Ruggieri et al. (eds.), *Tumors of the Sacrum*,
DOI 10.1007/978-3-319-51202-0_17

patients with a sacral tumor usually do not see a doctor until the symptoms become severe. Night or rest pain, swelling, and low-grade fewer are the most common presenting symptoms in early stages, followed by radiculopathy and major neurological compromise, such as bowel and bladder dysfunction. When delayed diagnosis occurs, tumor may reach a large size due to the lack of anatomic barriers or tumor growth into the pelvic region [2, 12]. Serum HDL and erythrocyte sedimentation rate are frequently increased, sometimes associated to leukocytosis and anemia.

17.3 Imaging

ES is a predominantly lytic lesion and may be seen on plain radiographs, better on lateral sacral view than anterior-posterior view. CT scans and MRI play a predominant role in evaluating the features, soft tissue and intramedullary/epidural extent of the lesion, and in developing a preoperative surgical plan [28]. ES may present with either a hot or cold bone scan [29]. CT-guided needle biopsy followed by immediate initiation of chemotherapy and corticosteroids for patients with stable neurologic deficits should be preferred to surgical decompression in conjunction with biopsy [17]. PET and dynamic MRI seem not to be predictive for tumor response to primary chemotherapy [30, 31].

17.4 Pathology

The histopathological diagnosis of Ewing's sarcoma family tumors is based on the current criteria defined by the World Health Organization (WHO). Histologically, ES comprises small round blue cells originating from bone and soft tissues; the expression of neural markers distinguishes conventional ES from malignant primitive neuroectodermal tumors (PNET). The majority of cases share a cytogenetic translocation *t*(11;22) (q24;q12) with occasional variations and a characteristic immunohistochemical staining profile.

17.5 Treatment

The current treatment for ES includes multiagent neoadjuvant and adjuvant chemotherapy, with local control performed by surgical resection (when technically achievable) in combination with radiation therapy [5, 15, 32, 33]. Although Ewing sarcoma is highly sensitive to radiation therapy, at today surgery should be considered as treatment for local control. However, it is unclear whether and to what extent sacrectomy with wide margins provides local disease control, as well as the improvement of efficacy supported by new technologies in the field of radiation therapy [14, 17, 18, 34, 35].

17.5.1 Sacrectomy

Some authors consider that wide resection of the primary malignant sacral tumor is the only way to reduce local recurrence and cure the patient [12, 14, 26, 36], but this correlation is not clearly confirmed. As conclusion of a systematic review of the literature, en bloc resection of ES of the spine is weakly recommended as it provides improved local control, but not improved overall survival [15]. On the other hand, surgery with inadequate margins (both piecemeal excision and en bloc resection with intralesional margins) is associated with high recurrence rate and worse prognosis [16].

Clinical outcomes following sacral surgery parallel the level of neurologic sacrifice. Total or partial sacrectomy is a demanding procedure and may result in nerve root sacrifice, potentially causing major neurologic deficits and functional compromise, with high risk of complications (ranging from 32 to 67%, mainly infection) and a technical challenge in the reconstruction [6, 14, 21, 34, 37–40]. Patients who are able to retain one S3 nerve root and bilateral S2 nerve roots almost always regain functional bowel, bladder, and sexual capacity, while patients with higher levels of neurologic sacrifice have lesser capacity for these functions. Arkader et al. observed that despite the neurologic deficits and the associated psychological impact, survivor patients with sacrectomy are active participants in society [34].

17.5.2 Chemotherapy

Chemotherapy is critical in the treatment of ES [2, 5, 15], therefore sacrectomy without effective chemotherapy most likely would be insufficient to achieve disease-free status. Multiagent neoadjuvant chemotherapy is considered the standard in patients with ES, increasing the likelihood of local control and facilitating eventual surgical approaches [1, 2, 5, 15]. When ES is surgically treated, one of the most important prognostic predictive factors is the pathological evaluation of chemotherapy-induced tumor necrosis [5, 41]. Specific aspects on protocol of treatment are analyzed in the dedicated chapter.

17.5.3 Radiation Therapy

If en bloc resection is not feasible due to the lack of the criteria to perform wide resection or to unaccepted functional loss, the combination of radiation therapy (RT) and chemotherapy seems to be the best option rather than intralesional surgery [17, 18]. Previous experience has suggested that debulking procedures followed by RT do not improve outcomes in patients with Ewing tumor compared with RT alone [42], and intralesional dissection might result in tumor seeding [43]. With the advantages of new technologies, RT provides reasonable local control for ES of the spine with acceptable long-term toxicity in survivors, justifying its evaluation in alternative to surgical treatment [17–18].

17.6 Oncologic Outcome

The overall survival of primary high-grade malignant sacral tumors depends on the tumor type, presence of metastasis, response to chemotherapy, local control, and/or quality of surgical margins [11–15, 20–22, 34, 41]. The local recurrence rate is relatively high after surgery due to the location, the complex anatomy, and the difficulty in achieving safe margins. Bacci et al. [41] reported a series of spinal ES that includes 17 patients with sacral involvement. Authors reported their results with local recurrence rate of 29% and 5-year event-free survival rate of 0%, concluding that tumors primarily located in the sacrum have a much poorer outcome compared to those located in other bones. Guo et al. [14] reported a series on en bloc sacrectomies with only one patient affected by ES, that died of disease at 13 months of follow-up. Li et al. [13] reported a series including three cases of ES of the sacrum treated with hemisacrectomy, with two patients alive with no evidence of disease at 43 and 69 months of follow-up. Bradway and Pritchard underlined the importance of surgical resection considering that 6 out of 15 patients with sacral involvement remained alive compared to none of four patients with lumbar lesions [44]. Arkader et al. [34] reported a disease-free survival rate of 75% in children with osteosarcoma and ES of the sacrum, suggesting that sacrectomy has the potential to be curative. However, other authors reported good local control in nine cases with sacral involvement treated with radiotherapy only for local control (except one treated with surgery and radiation therapy), with 5-year EFS of 44% [17].

Conflict of Interest Statement No benefits have been or will be received from a commercial party related directly or indirectly to the subject matter of this article.

References

1. Iwamoto Y. Diagnosis and treatment of Ewing's sarcoma. Jpn J Clin Oncol. 2007;37:79–89.
2. Lahl M, Fisher VL, Laschinger K. Ewing's sarcoma family of tumors: an overview from diagnosis to survivorship. Clin J Oncol Nurs. 2008;12:89–97.
3. Rosen G, Caparros B, Nirenberg A, Marcove RC, Huvos AG, Kosloff C, Lane J, Murphy ML. Ewing's sarcoma: ten-year experience with adjuvant chemotherapy. Cancer. 1981;47:2204–13.
4. Nesbit Jr ME, Gehan EA, Burgert Jr EO, Vietti TJ, Cangir A, Tefft M, Evans R, Thomas P, Askin FB, Kissane JM, et al. Multimodal therapy for the management of primary, nonmetastatic Ewing's sarcoma of bone: a long-term follow-up of the First Intergroup study. J Clin Oncol. 1990;8:1664–74.
5. Gaspar N, Hawkins DS, Dirksen U, et al. Ewing sarcoma: current management and future approaches through collaboration. J Clin Oncol. 2015;33:3036–46.
6. Ohata N, Ozaki T, Kunisada T, Morimoto Y, Tanaka M, Inoue H. Extended total sacrectomy and reconstruction for sacral tumor. Spine (Phila Pa 1976). 2004;29:E123–6.
7. Hashimoto M, Akabane Y, Tate E. Ewing's sarcoma of the sacrum. Radiat Med. 1999;17:451–3.
8. Kakogawa J, Nako T, Kawamura K, Nakamura S, Mochiduki A, Kanayama N, Tanaka M. Successful pregnancy after sacrectomy combined with chemotherapy and radiation for

Ewing sarcoma: case report and literature review. J Pediatr Adolesc Gynecol. 2015;28(3):e79–81.
9. Kier A, Timchur MD, McCarthy PW. A case report of an uncommon cause of cauda equina symptoms. J Manip Physiol Ther. 2007;30(6):459–65.
10. Baker ND, Dorfman DM. Ewing's sarcoma of the sacrum. Skeletal Radiol. 1996;25(3):302–4.
11. Fourney DR, Rhines LD, Hentschel SJ, Skibber JM, Wolinsky JP, Weber KL, Suki D, Gallia GL, Garonzik I, Gokaslan ZL. En bloc resection of primary sacral tumors: classification of surgical approaches and outcome. J Neurosurg Spine. 2005;3:111–22.
12. Wuisman P, Lieshout O, Sugihara S, van Dijk M. Total sacrectomy and reconstruction: oncologic and functional outcome. Clin Orthop Relat Res. 2000;381:192–203.
13. Li D, Guo W, Tang X, Yang R, Tang S, Qu H, Yang Y, Sun X, Du Z. Preservation of the contralateral sacral nerves during hemisacrectomy for sacral malignancies. Eur Spine J. 2014;23(9):1933–9.
14. Guo W, Tang X, Zang J, Ji T. One-stage total en bloc sacrectomy: a novel technique and report of 9 cases. Spine (Phila Pa 1976). 2013;38(10):E626–31.
15. Sciubba DM, Okuno SH, Dekutoski MB, Gokaslan ZL. Ewing and osteogenic sarcoma: evidence for multidisciplinary management. Spine. 2009;34:58–68.
16. Boriani S, Amendola L, Corghi A, Cappuccio M, Bandiera S, Ferrari S, Picci R, Difiore M, Gasbarrini A. Ewing's sarcoma of the mobile spine. Eur Rev Med Pharmacol Sci. 2011;15(7):831–9.
17. Indelicato DJ, Keole SR, Shahlaee AH, Morris CG, Gibbs Jr CP, Scarborough MT, Pincus DW, Marcus Jr RB. Spinal and paraspinal Ewing tumors. Int J Radiat Oncol Biol Phys. 2010;76(5):1463–71.
18. Hesla AC, Tsagozis P, Jebsen N, Zaikova O, Bauer H, Brosjö O. Improved prognosis for patients with Ewing sarcoma in the sacrum compared with the innominate bones: the scandinavian sarcoma group experience. J Bone Joint Surg Am. 2016;98(3):199–210.
19. Dickey ID, Hugate Jr RR, Fuchs B, Yaszemski MJ, Sim FH. Reconstruction after total sacrectomy: early experience with a new surgical technique. Clin Orthop Relat Res. 2005;438:42–50.
20. Randall RL, Bruckner J, Lloyd C, Pohlman TH, Conrad 3rd EU. Sacral resection and reconstruction for tumors and tumor-like conditions. Orthopedics. 2005;28:307–13.
21. Sar C, Eralp L. Surgical treatment of primary tumors of the sacrum. Arch Orthop Trauma Surg. 2002;122:148–55.
22. Zileli M, Hoscoskun C, Brastianos P, Sabah D. Surgical treatment of primary sacral tumors: complications associated with sacrectomy. Neurosurg Focus. 2003;15:E9.
23. Whitehouse GH, Griffiths GJ. Roentgenologic aspects of spinal involvement by primary and metastatic Ewing's tumor. J Can Assoc Radiol. 1976;27:290–7.
24. Wilkins RM, Pritchard DJ, Burgert Jr EO, Unni KK. Ewing's sarcoma of bone. Experience with 140 patients. Cancer. 1986;58:2551–5.
25. Grubb MR, Currier BL, Pritchard DJ, Ebersold MJ. Primary Ewing's sarcoma of the spine. Spine (Phila Pa 1976). 1994;19:309–13.
26. Kozlowski K, Barylak A, Campbell J, Hoeffel JD, Beluffi G, Masel J, Panuel M, Pelizza A, Taccone A, Arico M. Primary sacral bone tumours in children (report of 16 cases with a short literature review). Australas Radiol. 1990;34:142–9.
27. Lam CH, Naqib MG. Nonteratomatous tumors in the pediatric sacral region. Spine (Phila Pa 1976). 2002;27:E284–7.
28. Huang WY, Tan WL, Geng DY, Zhang J, Wu G, Zhang BY, Li YX, Yin B. Imaging findings of the spinal peripheral Ewing's sarcoma family of tumours. Clin Radiol. 2014;69(2):179–85.
29. Bushnell D, Shirazi P, Khedkar N, Blank J. Ewing's sarcoma seen as a "cold" lesion on bone scans. Clin Nucl Med. 1983;8(4):173–4.
30. Raciborska A, Bilska K, Drabko K, et al. Response to chemotherapy estimates by FDG PET is an important prognostic factor in patients with Ewing sarcoma. Clin Transl Oncol. 2016;18(2):189–95.

31. Gaston LL, Di Bella C, Slavin J, Hicks RJ, Choong PF. 18F-FDG PET response to neoadjuvant chemotherapy for Ewing sarcoma and osteosarcoma are different. Skeletal Radiol. 2011;40:1007–15.
32. Sewell MD, Tan KA, Quraishi NA, Preda C, Varga PP, Williams R. Systematic review of en bloc resection in the management of ewing's sarcoma of the mobilespine with respect to local control and disease-free survival. Medicine (Baltimore). 2015;94(27):e1019.
33. Dominkus M, Darwish E, Funovics P. Reconstruction of the pelvis after resection of malignant bone tumours in children and adolescents. Recent Results Cancer Res. 2009;179:85–111.
34. Arkader A, Yang CH, Tolo VT. High long-term local control with sacrectomy for primary high-grade bone sarcoma in children. Clin Orthop Relat Res. 2012;470(5):1491–7.
35. Rock J, Kole M, Yin FF, Ryu S, Guttierez J, Rosen-Blum M. Radiosurgical treatment for Ewing's sarcoma of the lumbar spine: case report. Spine. 2002;27:471–5.
36. Kelley SP, Ashford RU, Rao AS, Dickson RA. Primary bone tumours of the spine: a 42-year survey from the Leeds Regional Bone Tumour Registry. Eur Spine J. 2007;16:405–9.
37. Davidge KM, Eskicioglu C, Lipa J, Ferguson P, Swallow CJ, Wright FC. Qualitative assessment of patient experiences following sacrectomy. J Surg Oncol. 2010;101:447–50.
38. Sciubba DM, Nelson C, Gok B, McGirt MJ, McLoughlin GS, Noggle JC, Wolinsky JP, Witham TF, Bydon A, Gokaslan ZL. Evaluation of factors associated with postoperative infection following sacral tumor resection. J Neurosurg Spine. 2008;9:593–9.
39. Angelini A, Pala E, Calabrò T, Maraldi M, Ruggieri P. Prognostic factors in surgical resection of sacral chordoma. J Surg Oncol. 2015;112(4):344–51.
40. Ruggieri P, Angelini A, Pala E, Mercuri M. Infections in surgery of primary tumors of the sacrum. Spine (Phila Pa 1976). 2012;37(5):420–8.
41. Bacci G, Boriani S, Balladelli A, Barbieri E, Longhi A, Alberghini M, Scotlandi K, Forni C, Pollastri P, Vanel D, Mercuri M. Treatment of nonmetastatic Ewing's sarcoma family tumors of the spine and sacrum: the experience from a single institution. Eur Spine J. 2009;18(8):1091–5.
42. Schuck A, Ahrens S, Paulussen M, et al. Local therapy in localized Ewing tumors: results of 1058 patients treated in the CESS 81, CESS 86, and EICESS 92 trials. Int J Radiat Oncol Biol Phys. 2003;55:168–77.
43. Samartzis D, Marco RA, Benjamin R, et al. Multilevel en bloc spondylectomy and chest wall excision via a simultaneous anterior and posterior approach for Ewing sarcoma. Spine. 2005;30:831–7.
44. Bradway JK, Pritchard DJ. Ewing's tumor of the spine. In: Sudersan N, Schmidek HH, Schiller AL, Rosenthal DI, editors. Tumors of the spine, diagnosis and clinical management. Philadelphia: WB Sauders; 1990. p. 235–9.

Lymphoma and Myeloma of the Sacrum

18

Andreas F. Mavrogenis, Georgios N. Panagopoulos,
Andrea Angelini, Pier Luigi Zinzani, and Pietro Ruggieri

18.1 Introduction

Neoplasms of the sacrum are relatively uncommon, representing 1–2% of all musculoskeletal tumors [1]. They can be classified as primary or metastatic, the former being either benign or malignant. The most common malignancy of the sacrum is metastatic disease, whereas the most common primary sacral tumor is chordoma; more rare sacral malignancies include hematologic neoplasms, Ewing's sarcoma, chondrosarcoma, and osteosarcoma [2].

Hematologic malignancies, more frequently multiple myeloma and lymphoma, occur relatively frequently in the sacrum, accounting for 18% of all primary malignant sacral tumors [3]. Traditional treatment for hematologic neoplasms affecting bone consists of chemotherapy and/or radiation therapy [4]. As medical treatment of these conditions improves and patients' survival extends, skeletal lesions caused by hematologic malignancies are more likely to necessitate some form of orthopaedic surgery or interventional procedure, with either curative or palliative intent.

A.F. Mavrogenis, M.D., Ph.D. • G.N. Panagopoulos, M.D.
First Department of Orthopaedics, National and Kapodistrian University of Athens, Athens, Greece
e-mail: afm@otenet.gr

A. Angelini, M.D., Ph.D. • P. Ruggieri, M.D., Ph.D. (✉)
Department of Orthopedics and Orthopedic Oncology, University of Padova, Padova, Italy
e-mail: andrea.angelini83@yahoo.it; pietro.ruggieri@unipd.it

P.L. Zinzani, M.D., Ph.D.
Institute of Hematology "L. E A. Seràgnoli", University of Bologna, Bologna, Italy

P. Ruggieri et al. (eds.), *Tumors of the Sacrum*,
DOI 10.1007/978-3-319-51202-0_18

18.2 Lymphoma

Primary lymphoma of bone is rare, accounting for 3–7% of bone tumors and less than 2% of adult lymphomas [5, 6]. Although there is no universal definition, by convention, an interval of 4–6 months between skeletal manifestation of the lesion and the development of extraskeletal disease is required for the tumor to be considered a primary tumor in bone [5]. Because of the infrequency of primary bone lymphoma and the disagreement as to its clinical definition, there have been few published series documenting patients' outcomes, clinical characteristics, and biological aspects [5–17].

The great majority of bone lymphomas are diffuse large B-cell Non-Hodgkin lymphomas. In three published large series of primary bone lymphoma, this histotype was represented in at least 70, 79, and 83% of cases [7–9]. More than 50% of primary lymphomas of bone occur in patients older than 60 years, with a slight male predominance [8]. The vertebrae, femur, and pelvis are the most frequently involved bones, accounting for approximately 29%, 12%, and 13% of lesions, respectively. Lesion multifocality is seen in approximately 15% of cases [8].

The incidence of primary sacral lymphoma is unknown, due to its rarity, with only a few case reports dedicated to the subject [2, 10]. Similarly to other sacral lesions, persistent low back pain from a sacral insufficiency fracture, and referred pain to a leg or buttock from nerve root irritation, are the usual presenting symptoms [2]. Neurological signs are rarely seen prior to diagnosis or tend to manifest late in the course of disease. If the lesion has expanded into the presacral space, rectal exam may reveal the presence of a palpable soft tissue mass.

Radiographic features are usually non-specific and tend to overlap with those of other tumors. As a rule of thumb, lymphoma of bone will present as a lytic destructive lesion with a permeative or moth-eaten pattern [5]. CT and MR imaging are helpful in evaluating the extent of bone involvement and cortical erosion, as well as the soft tissue extension of the tumor. Bone scan or PET/CT are useful to document additional foci of bone or extraskeletal involvement [11].

The Ann Arbor staging system developed for Hodgkin's disease has also been used in staging non-Hodgkin lymphomas [12]. This staging system focuses on the number of tumor sites (nodal and extranodal), location, and presence/absence of systemic symptoms [12]. Percutaneous biopsy of sacral lesions is a reasonable first-line diagnostic tool. Fine-needle aspiration biopsy sampling performed using CT, fluoroscopic, or ultrasound guidance has been reported to be successful [13]; although the use of fine-needle biopsy in musculoskeletal tumors is not recommended. Because there is a 7% rate of false-negative findings, a negative biopsy result should prompt a repeated biopsy procedure, preferably using a core or trephine tool, or an open biopsy [2].

Immunohistochemistry is usually essential for diagnosis. Lymphoma must be distinguished from other hematopoietic neoplasms, such as plasma cell myeloma, Langerhans cell histiocytosis, and mastocytosis. The differential diagnosis should also include round-cell tumors, such as Ewing's sarcoma, rhabdomyosarcoma, and metastatic small cell carcinoma. Most untreated diffuse large B-cell lymphomas are

CD20-positive. If this is negative, PAX5 or CD79 will usually be positive. Once the diagnosis is confirmed, further prognostic tests, such as Ki-67, CD10, BCL6, and MUM1, are usually requested to subclassify the disease and guide treatment [14]. Radiation therapy and chemotherapy are the standard treatments for primary lymphoma of bone. A general algorithm for stage I/II, nonbulky disease involves 3–4 cycles of rituximab plus cyclophosphamide, vincristine, doxorubicin, and prednisone (CHOP), followed by involved field radiation therapy (IFRT) [15–17].

18.3 Multiple Myeloma

Multiple myeloma is a monoclonal, neoplastic proliferation of plasma cells that involves the bone marrow and occasionally extraskeletal sites, whose prominent feature is the widespread presence of lytic bone lesions [14]. It is one of the most frequently occurring hemapoietic malignancies (10%), accounting for approximately 1% of all malignant neoplasms in White and 2% in Black patients [14]. It is also the most frequent neoplasm to present with skeletal lesions, with the skull, vertebral bodies, pelvis, and proximal parts of long bones being the most commonly involved sites [18, 19]. Peak incidence is between ages 65 and 74 years, with a median age at diagnosis ranging from 66 to 69 years [20, 21].

It is currently accepted that myeloma is always preceded by (or evolves from) a premalignant condition clinically recognized as monoclonal gammopathy of undetermined significance (MGUS) [22]. MGUS is usually asymptomatic and present in 3–4% of the general population older than 50 years. It is associated with a risk of progression to multiple myeloma of approximately 1% per year [23]. Smoldering multiple myeloma (SMM) is an intermediate stage between MGUS and multiple myeloma and is associated with a higher risk of progression of approximately 10% per year [24].

The most common presenting symptoms of multiple myeloma are fatigue and bone pain [25]. Anemia is detected in 75% of patients, whereas osteolytic skeletal lesions are present in 80% of cases [21]. Other findings may include hypercalcemia, renal failure, proteinuria, and a history of recurrent infections [14]. The cardinal diagnostic feature of multiple myeloma is the detection of monoclonal (M) protein on serum or urine protein electrophoresis (82% of patients) [25]. Serum immunofixation, serum-free light chain (FLC) assay, or 24 h urine studies can further increase sensitivity of detection [26]. The M protein type is IgG in approximately 50%, IgA in 20%, immunoglobulin light chain only in 20%, IgD in 2%, and IgM in 0.5% [25]. About 2–3% of multiple myeloma has no detectable M protein and is referred to as nonsecretory multiple myeloma [27].

The baseline diagnostic work-up required for the diagnosis of multiple myeloma includes a complete blood cell count, measurement of serum calcium and creatinine levels, serum and urinary protein electrophoresis with immunofixation, serum FLC assay, and bone marrow examination [21]. Plain radiography of the entire skeleton (skeletal survey) to detect osteolytic bone lesions usually completes the diagnostic work-up [28]. From a biopsy standpoint, diagnosis of multiple myeloma requires the presence of clonal bone marrow plasma cells of ≥10%, or biopsy-proven bony or extramedullary plasmacytoma [29]. Skeletal lesions typically represent multifocal, sharply demarcated, lytic, often called punched-out lesions. CT and MR imaging are useful adjuncts in the spine, or when skeletal survey is initially negative.

Although multiple myeloma is still considered by many to be a single disease, it is in reality a collection of several cytogenetically distinct plasma cell neoplasms. These distinct forms of myeloma are designated as solitary plasmacytoma of bone, extramedullary plasmacytoma, nonsecretory myeloma, plasma cell leukemia, and osteosclerotic myeloma (POEMS) [14]. Amyloidosis associated with multiple myeloma can also cause bone lesions (amyloidomas) [30]. Although median survival in patients with multiple myeloma is approximately 5–7 years, there is major variation in survival depending on host factors, tumor burden (stage), biology (cytogenetic abnormalities), and response to therapy [31]. Based on these premises, risk stratification is carried out, which will subsequently lead to treatment. Molecular classification is important, as high-risk cytogenetic features are likely to modify therapy accordingly.

Until 2000, the mainstay of therapy for multiple myeloma was the use of alkylators and corticosteroids, and in selected patients, high-dose chemotherapy with autologous stem cell transplant (ASCT) [21]. Subsequently, alternative agents, such as thalidomide, bortezomib, and lenalidomide, have emerged as effective agents that have significantly improved clinical outcome [32–35]. More recently, carfilzomib, pomalidomide, panobinostat, daratumumab, ixazomib, and elotuzumab have been approved for the treatment of multiple myeloma in the United States, substantially expanding the number of treatment regimens available for patients in all stages of the disease [21]. In patients diagnosed with multiple myeloma, development of end-organ damage (myeloma-defining events) is the hallmark indication for treatment initiation [20]. Evidence of end-organ damage is traditionally represented by the acronym CRAB (hyper**C**alcemia, **R**enal insufficiency, **A**nemia, lytic **B**one lesions) [18, 36, 37]. Multiple myeloma without end-organ damage is referred to as smoldering multiple myeloma (SMM) and should be monitored closely, as these patients have a risk of progression of approximately 10% per year for the first 5 years, 3% per year for the next 5 years, and 1% per year thereafter [24].

The most important phases of therapy are initial therapy, ASCT (if eligible), consolidation/maintenance therapy, and treatment of relapse [21]. Transplant-eligible patients typically receive approximately four cycles of initial therapy followed by stem cell collection and ASCT. Delayed ASCT, with stem cell collection after four cycles of initial therapy and cryopreservation for future use, is also possible. Pre-transplant conditioning (total body irradiation and/or melphalan) is necessary prior to ASCT [38]. ASCT has been shown to increase median survival in MM by approximately 12 months [39]. The upper limit for ASCT is 65 years in most countries (75 years in the US) [20, 21]. Transplant-ineligible patients are usually treated for 12–18 months. After initial therapy, with or without ASCT, consolidation/maintenance therapy should be considered. Treatment at relapse or progression is more complicated and may include re-induction and repeat ASCT, or treatment with novel drugs [20].

Supportive care is also paramount in patients with multiple myeloma. Hypercalcemia is usually treated with hydration, steroids, and bisphosphonates (pamidronate or zoledronic acid). Pamidronate at 60–90 mg intravenously over 2–4 h, or zoledronic acid at 4 mg intravenously over 15 min, will normalize the calcium levels within 24–72 h in most patients [40, 41]. In refractory patients, salmon calcitonin may be used. A small percentage of patients with multiple myeloma may develop hyperviscosity syndrome (especially in the IgA subtype). This should be promptly treated with plasmapheresis [42]. Prevention of recurrent infections is another important issue. Patients with MM should receive pneumococcal and influenza vaccinations. Intravenously administered gammaglobulin every 3–4 weeks is indicated if patients have recurrent serious infections associated with severe hypogammaglobulinemia [21]. Prophylaxis against herpes zoster reactivation and *Pneumocystis jiroveci* should also be considered [43].

Maybe the most important element in the supportive care of patients with multiple myeloma is the use of bisphosphonates to prevent and/or reduce the number of skeletal events and, ultimately, the associated pain and morbidity. Zoledronic acid or pamidronate once monthly at least for the first 1–2 years is recommended for almost all patients with multiple myeloma who have evidence of myeloma-associated bone disease [44–48]. All patients should receive a dental examination before initiation of bisphosphonates, and invasive dental procedures should be done with caution because of the risk of osteonecrosis of the jaw [49]. Local radiation therapy is also used in patients with pain refractory to analgesics and systemic therapy, as well as in case of spinal cord compression with extramedullary tumor extension. Vertebroplasty and kyphoplasty are frequently used for vertebral pathological fractures [50]. Prophylactic nailing is also commonly performed for pathological or impending fractures of long bones. Sacroplasty is also evolving as an acceptable and efficient treatment of MM-induced sacral insufficiency fractures. Even though published series are limited, results intended primarily as pain relief seem to be promising [51–53].

Treatment is different in the case of localized disease, such as solitary plasmacytoma or extraosseous plasmacytoma. These cases can be treated either with curatively intended radiation therapy to the involved field with cumulative doses of ≥45 Gy [54, 55], or resected surgically [4, 20]. Although cure is the primary goal of treatment in solitary plasmacytoma, a progression to multiple myeloma may occur in 30–60% of cases within the next 3–5 years, thereby requiring regular follow-up [56].

Conflict of Interest Statement No benefits have been or will be received from a commercial party related directed or indirectly to the subject matter of this article.

References

1. Capanna R, Briccoli A, Campanacci L. Benign and malignant tumors of the sacrum. In: Frymoyer J, Ducker T, Hadler N, editors. The adult spine: principles and practice. Philadelphia: Lippincott-Raven; 1997. p. 2367–405.

2. Liu JK, Kan P, Schmidt MH. Diffuse large B-cell lymphoma presenting as a sacral tumor. Report of two cases. Neurosurg Focus. 2003;15(2):E10.
3. Mavrogenis AF, Patapis P, Kostopanagiotou G, Papagelopoulos PJ. Tumors of the sacrum. Orthopedics. 2009;32(5):342.
4. Mavrogenis AF, Angelini A, Pala E, Zinzani P, Ruggieri P. The role of surgery for haematologic neoplasms of bone. Acta Orthop Belg. 2012;78(3):382–92.
5. Dorfman HD, Czerniak B. Bone tumors. St. Louis: Mosby; 1998.
6. Kitsoulis P, Vlychou M, Papoudou-Bai A, Karatzias G, Charchanti A, Agnantis NJ, Bai M. Primary lymphomas of bone. Anticancer Res. 2006;26(1A):325–37.
7. Alencar A, Pitcher D, Byrne G, Lossos IS. Primary bone lymphoma—the University of Miami experience. Leuk Lymphoma. 2010;51(1):39–49. doi:10.3109/10428190903308007.
8. Jawad MU, Schneiderbauer MM, Min ES, Cheung MC, Koniaris LG, Scully SP. Primary lymphoma of bone in adult patients. Cancer. 2010;116(4):871–9. doi:10.1002/cncr.24828.
9. Ramadan KM, Shenkier T, Sehn LH, Gascoyne RD, Connors JM. A clinicopathological retrospective study of 131 patients with primary bone lymphoma: a population-based study of successively treated cohorts from the British Columbia Cancer Agency. Ann Oncol. 2007;18(1):129–35. doi:10.1093/annonc/mdl329.
10. Nayil K, Makhdoomi R, Ramzan A, Malik R, Alam S, Wani A, Chhiber S. Primary sacral lymphoma: a case report and review of the literature. Turk Neurosurg. 2011;21(4):659–62. doi:10.5137/1019-5149.JTN.3001-10.1.
11. Mikhaeel NG. Primary bone lymphoma. Clin Oncol (R Coll Radiol). 2012;24(5):366–70. doi:10.1016/j.clon.2012.02.006.
12. Carbone PP, Kaplan HS, Musshoff K, Smithers DW, Tubiana M. Report of the committee on Hodgkin's disease staging classification. Cancer Res. 1971;31(11):1860–1.
13. Gupta S, Takhtani D, Gulati M, Khandelwal N, Gupta D, Rajwanshi A, Gupta S, Suri S. Sonographically guided fine-needle aspiration biopsy of lytic lesions of the spine: technique and indications. J Clin Ultrasound. 1999;27(3):123–9.
14. Ewton A. Hematopoietic tumors. In: Czerniak B, editor. Dorfman and Czerniak's bone tumors. 2nd ed. Philadelphia: Elsevier/Saunders; 2016. p. 817–902.
15. Coiffier B. Treatment paradigms in aggressive non-Hodgkin's lymphoma in elderly patients. Clin Lymphoma. 2002;3(Suppl 1):S12–8.
16. Coiffier B, Lepage E, Briere J, Herbrecht R, Tilly H, Bouabdallah R, Morel P, Van Den Neste E, Salles G, Gaulard P, Reyes F, Lederlin P, Gisselbrecht C. CHOP chemotherapy plus rituximab compared with CHOP alone in elderly patients with diffuse large-B-cell lymphoma. N Engl J Med. 2002;346(4):235–42. doi:10.1056/NEJMoa011795.
17. Jaffe ES. The 2008 WHO classification of lymphomas: implications for clinical practice and translational research. Hematology Am Soc Hematol Educ Program. 2009:523–531. doi: 10.1182/asheducation-2009.1.523.
18. Kyle RA, Rajkumar SV. Multiple myeloma. Blood. 2008;111(6):2962–72. doi:10.1182/blood-2007-10-078022.
19. Swerdlow SH, International Agency for Research on Cancer, World Health Organization. WHO classification of tumours of haematopoietic and lymphoid tissues. World Health Organization classification of tumours. 4th ed. Lyon: International Agency for Research on Cancer; 2008.
20. Rollig C, Knop S, Bornhauser M. Multiple myeloma. Lancet. 2015;385(9983):2197–208. doi:10.1016/S0140-6736(14)60493-1.
21. Rajkumar SV, Kumar S. Multiple myeloma: diagnosis and treatment. Mayo Clin Proc. 2016;91(1):101–19. doi:10.1016/j.mayocp.2015.11.007.
22. Kyle RA, Therneau TM, Rajkumar SV, Offord JR, Larson DR, Plevak MF, Melton 3rd LJ. A long-term study of prognosis in monoclonal gammopathy of undetermined significance. N Engl J Med. 2002;346(8):564–9. doi:10.1056/NEJMoa01133202.
23. Landgren O, Kyle RA, Pfeiffer RM, Katzmann JA, Caporaso NE, Hayes RB, Dispenzieri A, Kumar S, Clark RJ, Baris D, Hoover R, Rajkumar SV. Monoclonal gammopathy of undeter-

mined significance (MGUS) consistently precedes multiple myeloma: a prospective study. Blood. 2009;113(22):5412–7. doi:10.1182/blood-2008-12-194241.
24. Kyle RA, Remstein ED, Therneau TM, Dispenzieri A, Kurtin PJ, Hodnefield JM, Larson DR, Plevak MF, Jelinek DF, Fonseca R, Melton 3rd LJ, Rajkumar SV. Clinical course and prognosis of smoldering (asymptomatic) multiple myeloma. N Engl J Med. 2007;356(25):2582–90. doi:10.1056/NEJMoa070389.
25. Kyle RA, Gertz MA, Witzig TE, Lust JA, Lacy MQ, Dispenzieri A, Fonseca R, Rajkumar SV, Offord JR, Larson DR, Plevak ME, Therneau TM, Greipp PR. Review of 1027 patients with newly diagnosed multiple myeloma. Mayo Clin Proc. 2003;78(1):21–33. doi:10.4065/78.1.21.
26. Katzmann JA, Dispenzieri A, Kyle RA, Snyder MR, Plevak MF, Larson DR, Abraham RS, Lust JA, Melton 3rd LJ, Rajkumar SV. Elimination of the need for urine studies in the screening algorithm for monoclonal gammopathies by using serum immunofixation and free light chain assays. Mayo Clin Proc. 2006;81(12):1575–8. doi:10.4065/81.12.1575.
27. Chawla SS, Kumar SK, Dispenzieri A, Greenberg AJ, Larson DR, Kyle RA, Lacy MQ, Gertz MA, Rajkumar SV. Clinical course and prognosis of non-secretory multiple myeloma. Eur J Haematol. 2015;95(1):57–64. doi:10.1111/ejh.12478.
28. Regelink JC, Minnema MC, Terpos E, Kamphuis MH, Raijmakers PG, Pieters-van den Bos IC, Heggelman BG, Nievelstein RJ, Otten RH, van Lammeren-Venema D, Zijlstra JM, Arens AI, de Rooy JW, Hoekstra OS, Raymakers R, Sonneveld P, Ostelo RW, Zweegman S. Comparison of modern and conventional imaging techniques in establishing multiple myeloma-related bone disease: a systematic review. Br J Haematol. 2013;162(1):50–61. doi:10.1111/bjh.12346.
29. Rajkumar SV, Dimopoulos MA, Palumbo A, Blade J, Merlini G, Mateos MV, Kumar S, Hillengass J, Kastritis E, Richardson P, Landgren O, Paiva B, Dispenzieri A, Weiss B, LeLeu X, Zweegman S, Lonial S, Rosinol L, Zamagni E, Jagannath S, Sezer O, Kristinsson SY, Caers J, Usmani SZ, Lahuerta JJ, Johnsen HE, Beksac M, Cavo M, Goldschmidt H, Terpos E, Kyle RA, Anderson KC, Durie BG, Miguel JF. International Myeloma Working Group updated criteria for the diagnosis of multiple myeloma. Lancet Oncol. 2014;15(12):e538–48. doi:10.1016/S1470-2045(14)70442-5.
30. Klenke FM, Wirtz C, Banz Y, Keel MJ, Klass ND, Novak U, Benneker LM. Multiple myeloma-associated amyloidoma of the sacrum: case report and review of the literature. Global Spine J. 2014;4(2):109–14. doi:10.1055/s-0033-1360724.
31. Russell SJ, Rajkumar SV. Multiple myeloma and the road to personalised medicine. Lancet Oncol. 2011;12(7):617–9. doi:10.1016/S1470-2045(11)70143-7.
32. Singhal S, Mehta J, Desikan R, Ayers D, Roberson P, Eddlemon P, Munshi N, Anaissie E, Wilson C, Dhodapkar M, Zeddis J, Barlogie B. Antitumor activity of thalidomide in refractory multiple myeloma. N Engl J Med. 1999;341(21):1565–71. doi:10.1056/NEJM199911183412102.
33. Richardson PG, Schlossman RL, Weller E, Hideshima T, Mitsiades C, Davies F, LeBlanc R, Catley LP, Doss D, Kelly K, McKenney M, Mechlowicz J, Freeman A, Deocampo R, Rich R, Ryoo JJ, Chauhan D, Balinski K, Zeldis J, Anderson KC. Immunomodulatory drug CC-5013 overcomes drug resistance and is well tolerated in patients with relapsed multiple myeloma. Blood. 2002;100(9):3063–7. doi:10.1182/blood-2002-03-0996.
34. Richardson PG, Barlogie B, Berenson J, Singhal S, Jagannath S, Irwin D, Rajkumar SV, Srkalovic G, Alsina M, Alexanian R, Siegel D, Orlowski RZ, Kuter D, Limentani SA, Lee S, Hideshima T, Esseltine DL, Kauffman M, Adams J, Schenkein DP, Anderson KC. A phase 2 study of bortezomib in relapsed, refractory myeloma. N Engl J Med. 2003;348(26):2609–17. doi:10.1056/NEJMoa030288.
35. Kumar SK, Rajkumar SV, Dispenzieri A, Lacy MQ, Hayman SR, Buadi FK, Zeldenrust SR, Dingli D, Russell SJ, Lust JA, Greipp PR, Kyle RA, Gertz MA. Improved survival in multiple myeloma and the impact of novel therapies. Blood. 2008;111(5):2516–20. doi:10.1182/blood-2007-10-116129.
36. Kyle RA, Rajkumar SV. Criteria for diagnosis, staging, risk stratification and response assessment of multiple myeloma. Leukemia. 2009;23(1):3–9. doi:10.1038/leu.2008.291.

37. Dimopoulos M, Kyle R, Fermand JP, Rajkumar SV, San Miguel J, Chanan-Khan A, Ludwig H, Joshua D, Mehta J, Gertz M, Avet-Loiseau H, Beksac M, Anderson KC, Moreau P, Singhal S, Goldschmidt H, Boccadoro M, Kumar S, Giralt S, Munshi NC, Jagannath S, International Myeloma Workshop Consensus P. Consensus recommendations for standard investigative workup: report of the International Myeloma Workshop Consensus Panel 3. Blood. 2011;117(18):4701–5. doi:10.1182/blood-2010-10-299529.
38. Moreau P, Facon T, Attal M, Hulin C, Michallet M, Maloisel F, Sotto JJ, Guilhot F, Marit G, Doyen C, Jaubert J, Fuzibet JG, Francois S, Benboubker L, Monconduit M, Voillat L, Macro M, Berthou C, Dorvaux V, Pignon B, Rio B, Matthes T, Casassus P, Caillot D, Najman N, Grosbois B, Bataille R, Harousseau JL, Intergroupe Francophone du M. Comparison of 200 mg/m(2) melphalan and 8 Gy total body irradiation plus 140 mg/m(2) melphalan as conditioning regimens for peripheral blood stem cell transplantation in patients with newly diagnosed multiple myeloma: final analysis of the Intergroupe Francophone du Myelome 9502 randomized trial. Blood. 2002;99(3):731–5.
39. Blade J. Autologous transplantation in multiple myeloma. Haematologica. 2006;91(9):1157.
40. Gucalp R, Theriault R, Gill I, Madajewicz S, Chapman R, Navari R, Ahmann F, Zelenakas K, Heffernan M, Knight RD. Treatment of cancer-associated hypercalcemia. Double-blind comparison of rapid and slow intravenous infusion regimens of pamidronate disodium and saline alone. Arch Intern Med. 1994;154(17):1935–44.
41. Major PP, Coleman RE. Zoledronic acid in the treatment of hypercalcemia of malignancy: results of the international clinical development program. Semin Oncol. 2001;28(2 Suppl 6):17–24.
42. Gertz MA, Kyle RA. Hyperviscosity syndrome. J Intensive Care Med. 1995;10(3):128–41.
43. Oken MM, Pomeroy C, Weisdorf D, Bennett JM. Prophylactic antibiotics for the prevention of early infection in multiple myeloma. Am J Med. 1996;100(6):624–8.
44. Berenson J. Pamidronate in the treatment of osteolytic bone lesions in multiple myeloma patients–the American experience. Br J Clin Pract Suppl. 1996;87:5–7. Discussion 13–4
45. Berenson JR. Bone disease in myeloma. Curr Treat Options Oncol. 2001;2(3):271–83.
46. Berenson JR, Hillner BE, Kyle RA, Anderson K, Lipton A, Yee GC, Biermann JS, American Society of Clinical Oncology Bisphosphonates Expert P. American Society of Clinical Oncology clinical practice guidelines: the role of bisphosphonates in multiple myeloma. J Clin Oncol. 2002;20(17):3719–36.
47. Rosen LS, Gordon D, Kaminski M, Howell A, Belch A, Mackey J, Apffelstaedt J, Hussein M, Coleman RE, Reitsma DJ, Seaman JJ, Chen BL, Ambros Y. Zoledronic acid versus pamidronate in the treatment of skeletal metastases in patients with breast cancer or osteolytic lesions of multiple myeloma: a phase III, double-blind, comparative trial. Cancer J. 2001;7(5):377–87.
48. Morgan GJ, Davies FE, Gregory WM, Cocks K, Bell SE, Szubert AJ, Navarro-Coy N, Drayson MT, Owen RG, Feyler S, Ashcroft AJ, Ross F, Byrne J, Roddie H, Rudin C, Cook G, Jackson GH, Child JA, National Cancer Research Institute Haematological Oncology Clinical Study G. First-line treatment with zoledronic acid as compared with clodronic acid in multiple myeloma (MRC Myeloma IX): a randomised controlled trial. Lancet. 2010;376(9757):1989–99. doi:10.1016/S0140-6736(10)62051-X.
49. Dickinson M, Prince HM, Kirsa S, Zannettino A, Gibbs SD, Mileshkin L, O'Grady J, Seymour JF, Szer J, Horvath N, Joshua DE. Osteonecrosis of the jaw complicating bisphosphonate treatment for bone disease in multiple myeloma: an overview with recommendations for prevention and treatment. Intern Med J. 2009;39(5):304–16. doi:10.1111/j.1445-5994.2008.01824.x.
50. Fourney DR, Schomer DF, Nader R, Chlan-Fourney J, Suki D, Ahrar K, Rhines LD, Gokaslan ZL. Percutaneous vertebroplasty and kyphoplasty for painful vertebral body fractures in cancer patients. J Neurosurg. 2003;98(1 Suppl):21–30.
51. Butler CL, Given II CA, Michel SJ, Tibbs PA. Percutaneous sacroplasty for the treatment of sacral insufficiency fractures. AJR Am J Roentgenol. 2005;184(6):1956–9. doi:10.2214/ajr.184.6.01841956.

52. Wee B, Shimal A, Stirling AJ, James SL. CT-guided sacroplasty in advanced sacral destruction secondary to tumour infiltration. Clin Radiol. 2008;63(8):906–12. doi:10.1016/j.crad.2008.02.010.
53. Basile A, Tsetis D, Cavalli M, Fiumara P, Di Raimondo F, Coppolino F, Coppolino C, Mundo E, Desiderio C, Granata A, Patti MT. Sacroplasty for local or massive localization of multiple myeloma. Cardiovasc Intervent Radiol. 2010;33(6):1270–7. doi:10.1007/s00270-009-9761-x.
54. Dimopoulos MA, Moulopoulos A, Delasalle K, Alexanian R. Solitary plasmacytoma of bone and asymptomatic multiple myeloma. Hematol Oncol Clin North Am. 1992;6(2):359–69.
55. Hu K, Yahalom J. Radiotherapy in the management of plasma cell tumors. Oncology (Williston Park). 2000;14(1):101–8, 111. Discussion 111–2, 115
56. Reed V, Shah J, Medeiros LJ, Ha CS, Mazloom A, Weber DM, Arzu IY, Orlowski RZ, Thomas SK, Shihadeh F, Alexanian R, Dabaja BS. Solitary plasmacytomas: outcome and prognostic factors after definitive radiation therapy. Cancer. 2011;117(19):4468–74. doi:10.1002/cncr.26031.

Chondrosarcoma of the Sacrum

19

Andrea Angelini, Andreas F. Mavrogenis, and Pietro Ruggieri

19.1 Introduction

Primary malignant tumors of the sacrum are rare [1–3]. The most frequent are chordomas followed by hematologic neoplasms, osteosarcomas, Ewing's sarcomas, and in very rare cases, chondrosarcomas [3]. Chondrosarcomas (CS) can be classified as a primary malignant bone tumor (>90%) when they arise de novo or as a secondary malignant transformation of an underlying enchondroma or osteochondroma (<10%). They are further classified as central (intramedullary) or peripheral (on bony surface). Studies for patients with CSs of the sacrum are limited (Table 19.1) [4–10]. Most of the studies reported on patients with CSs in various skeletal sites, and tumor location is not always clearly described [11–13]. Therefore, the outcome of the patients with CS in this location is unclear.

A. Angelini, M.D., Ph.D. • P. Ruggieri, M.D., Ph.D. (✉)
Department of Orthopaedics and Orthopedic Oncology, University of Padova, Padova, Italy
e-mail: andrea.angelini83@yahoo.it; pietro.ruggieri@unipd.it

A.F. Mavrogenis, M.D., Ph.D.
First Department of Orthopaedics, National and Kapodistrian University of Athens, Athens, Greece
e-mail: afm@otenet.gr

P. Ruggieri et al. (eds.), *Tumors of the Sacrum*,
DOI 10.1007/978-3-319-51202-0_19

Table 19.1 Summary of the most relevant studies involving patients with chondrosarcoma of the sacrum

Study	Patients	Age-gender	Primary tumor	Sacral level	Adjuvant treatments	Procedure/margins	Survival
Bergh et al. [4] (2001)	11	N/A	CS (high proportion of grade 2 and grade 3 CS)	N/A	N/A	None (4 cases)	DWD (8 cases)
						Resection (2)	NED (2 cases)
						Ext Hemipelvectomy (4)	NEDLR (1 case)
						Sacrectomy (1)[a]	
Fourney et al. [5] (2005)	1	39M	CS	L5–S1	None	Resection/W	DWD 33 months
	1	37M	CS	Hemisacrum	None	Ext Hemipelvectomy/M	AWD 78 months
	1	59M	CS	Hemisacrum + SIJ	None	Resection/M	AWD 65 months
Hsieh et al. [6] (2009)	1	46F	CS	N/A	None	Resection/M	NED 32 months
Chan et al. [7] (2014)	1	62M	Well-differentiated CS	S1–S5	Rxt	Debulking/IL	NED 1.5 years
Possover et al. [8] (2014)	1	33F	Grade I CS	L5–S3 + SIJ	None	Resection/W[b]	NED 17 months
Li et al. [9] (2014)	1	46F	CS	N/A	None	Hemisacrectomy/W	AWD 25 months
	1	35F	CS	N/A	None	Hemisacrectomy/W	NED 29 months
	1	51M	CS	N/A	None	Hemisacrectomy/M	DWD 21 months
	1	38F	CS	N/A	None	Hemisacrectomy/M	NED 23 months
	1	42M	CS	N/A	None	Hemisacrectomy/W	NED 69 months
Zang et al. [10] (2015)	1	43F	CS	S1–S3	None	Debulking/IL	NED 29 months

CS chondrosarcoma, *Cht* chemotherapy, *Rxt* radiation therapy, *SIJ* sacroiliac joint, *NED* no evidence of disease, *DWD* died with disease, *AWD* alive with disease, *N/A* not available

[a]Surgical margins were wide in five cases and intralesional in two

[b]Resection has been performed under laparoscopic control

19.2 Epidemiology, Presentation, and Diagnosis

CS predominantly arises in elderly patients (range, 30–70 years) with a peak incidence in the sixth decade [14]. CSs can occur in all bones, but rarely involve the spine: the prevalence is reported between 6.5 and 12% in the mobile spine and approximately 2–5% within the sacrum [3, 4, 15–17]. Considering only the spine, roughly 19–20% of CSs arise in the cervical spine, 30–48% in the thoracic spine, 20–33% in the lumbar spine, and 16–20% in the sacrum [4, 15, 18].

Primary CS is usually eccentric and involves the proximal part of the sacrum, destroying the sacroiliac joint [4, 5]. Secondary CS can develop from benign lesions most frequently in diffuse disease such as enchondromatosis, Maffuci syndrome, or Ollier's disease [19].

Clinical occurrence of CS varies widely. Tumor remains clinically silent for a long time before the patients finally experience pain in the area of the lesion, or pain can be present for weeks to years. Swelling and sacral mass at presentation, as well as neurological symptoms, are associated with large tumors. Radicular symptoms are seen in roughly 24% of patients [18]. In huge tumors, skin ulceration and hemoserous discharge may be observed [7].

19.3 Imaging

An adequate staging of sacral CS includes complete imaging assessment and histologic evaluation. CS presents radiographically as a mixed lytic with typical dense areas of calcifications in the extraosseous soft tissue component of the tumor [20, 21]. CT scan and MRI show the same appearance of CS of the extremities. Additional imaging studies include a CT scan of the chest, abdomen, and pelvis. Bone scan could be useful in distinguishing central to peripheral CS [21] as well as for early diagnosis of silent lesions in the rest of the spinal column. The appropriate imaging studies allow for a better understanding of the extent of the lesion as well as a differential diagnosis, but biopsy is a key diagnostic method for sacral CS and should be carefully planned according to the definitive surgery.

19.4 Pathology

Histologically, CSs show abundant blue-gray cartilage matrix production and irregularly shaped cartilage lobules varying in size and shape. These lobules may be separated by fibrous bands or permeate bony trabeculae. Mitotic figures, hypercellularity, mild to moderate nuclear atypia, double-nucleated cells, and myxoid changes in the stroma can be observed [15, 16, 19, 20, 22]. CSs are pathologically classified as conventional (80–85%), clear cell (1–2%), myxoid (8–10%), mesenchymal (3–10%), and dedifferentiated (5–10%) subtype [19, 22]. Moreover, they are grade on a scale of 1 (low grade) to 3 (high grade) based on nuclear size, nuclear staining, and cellularity [22, 23].

19.5 Treatment

Sacral CSs are rare and thus difficult to manage. In general, surgery is the most accredited treatment modality, as no chemotherapy has been demonstrated to be effective against CS as well as conventional radiotherapy [5, 6, 15, 16, 18]. Resection with wide margins is the procedure of choice in sacral CS, since this is the most effective way of reducing recurrence rate [6].

19.5.1 Surgical Treatment

Surgical treatment consisting of either curettage (debulking procedures) or en bloc resection has been described for both primary and recurrent tumors [5, 6, 10]. Sacral tumors are often large and achieving adequate surgical margins during resection is challenging, because of difficulties in accessing the lesion, risks for damages of neighboring organs, and risks for massive blood loss due to an extensive vascularity. Moreover, CS usually involves the sacroiliac joint [9, 24]. Therefore, the surgical expertise required to remove these tumors is usually found only at centralized tumor treatment centers [4]. Nevertheless, in some cases, intralesional curettage, or debulking procedures, are more appropriate [7, 10], as well as been reported for CS of the mobile spine [25].

Results following curettage are contradictory, probably due to the different behavior of tumor in relation to histologic grade. In the mobile spine, two groups reported their large experience showing local recurrence or progression of disease in all cases treated with curettage, with poor oncologic outcome [15, 25]. York et al. found a recurrence rate of 69% and 20% in patients treated with intralesional or wide margins, respectively [18]. Good results with intralesional excision combined with radiotherapy have been reported in cases of low-grade well-differentiated chondrosarcoma [7]. Other case reports reported no evidence of disease or recurrence in patients treated intralesionally for sacral CS [10].

The role of en bloc resection in the treatment of sacral CSs has been well-established, even if the surgical planning should be customized on the patient [4–6]. Patients whose tumors can be completely resected with adequate margins should be approached with curative intent. Fourney et al. reported on three patients with sacral CS in their series on en bloc resections of sacral tumors. All patients had local recurrence with poor oncologic outcome after resection, but a previous inadequate treatment was performed in all cases [5]. This report underlines the important role of negative margins and the need of a specialized tumor center. Possover et al. [8] reported a case of ilio-sacral CS treated with laparoscopic-assisted posterior resection, concluding that primary anterior laparoscopic approach appears to be a good way for preparation sacral resection.

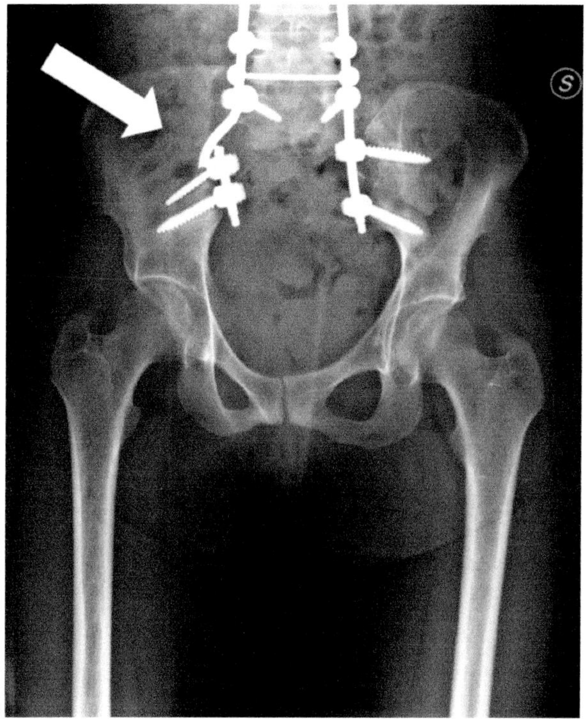

Fig. 19.1 Patient with chondrosarcoma of the sacrum treated with total sacrectomy and reconstruction. Plain radiograph show the breakage of the implant at 8 months of follow-up (*white arrow*) that has been surgically revised

In the Author's experience, eight patients with sacral CS have been treated since 1975–2012. Surgery has been considered for six out of eight cases and consists of sacral resection (four cases), intralesional curettage (one case), and excision with laminectomy (one case), whereas one patient with mesenchymal CS received both radiotherapy and chemotherapy and one patient with grade I CS refused treatments. Two patients had local recurrence and died of disease at 2.5 and 7 years of follow-up. Moreover, although en bloc sacral resections can improve the clinical outcome, the procedures do not come without complications [26–28]. In our experience, 67% of the cases surgically treated reported a complication (three deep infections and one revision for breakage of the spino-pelvic reconstruction (Fig. 19.1).

19.5.2 Radiotherapy and Chemotherapy

Chondrogenic tumors are considered relatively radioresistant. Radiation therapy can be considered after resection with inadequate margins as local adjuvant, when resection is not feasible or would cause unacceptable morbidity, and as palliative procedure for pain relief [13, 29]. The use of low adjuvant dose of radiotherapy (in the dose range of <70 Gy) combined with surgery could be useful to improve local control without a compromise of nerve function [30, 31]. CSs are heterogeneous group of tumors with different histology, biological behavior, and chemosensitivity. Conventional chemotherapy has been undertaken in patients with high-grade lesions with scarce benefit and several attempts are ongoing to explore alternative target therapies in CS [32, 33].

19.6 Oncologic Outcome

The survival of patients with pelvic, sacral, and spinal CSs is substantially lower to those with tumors of the appendicular skeleton (ranging from 25 to 54%) and appears to be related to the histological grade of the tumor, age at diagnosis, previous inadequate treatment, surgical margins, and high recurrence rate [11–13, 23, 34–38]. Previous study on pelvic CS reported that histological grade is the single most important predictor of the overall survival of the patients: the higher the histological grade, the lower the survival to death, local recurrence, and metastasis [4, 13]. The other major prognostic factor is the surgical margin: an inadequate margin or incomplete surgical resection is associated with local recurrence, and worse overall survival [4, 15, 18, 39], whereas patients who undergo successful en bloc excision have recurrence rates as low as 20%.

Conflict of Interest Statement No benefits have been or will be received from a commercial party related directed or indirectly to the subject matter of this article.

References

1. Dreghorn CR, Newman RJ, Hardy GJ, et al. Primary tumors of the axial skeleton. Experience of the Leeds Regional Bone Tumor Registry. Spine. 1990;15:137–40.
2. Weinstein JN, McLain RF. Primary tumors of the spine. Spine. 1987;12:843–51.
3. Mavrogenis AF, Patapis P, Kostopanagiotou G, Papagelopoulos PJ. Tumors of the sacrum. Orthopedics. 2009;32(5):342.
4. Bergh P, Gunterberg B, Meis-Kindblom JM, Kindblom LG. Prognostic factors and outcome of pelvic, sacral, and spinal chondrosarcomas: a center-based study of 69 cases. Cancer. 2001;91(7):1201–12.
5. Fourney DR, Rhines LD, Hentschel SJ, Skibber JM, Wolinsky JP, Weber KL, Suki D, Gallia GL, Garonzik I, Gokaslan ZL. En bloc resection of primary sacral tumors: classification of surgical approaches and outcome. J Neurosurg Spine. 2005;3(2):111–22.
6. Hsieh PC, Xu R, Sciubba DM, McGirt MJ, Nelson C, Witham TF, Wolinksy JP, Gokaslan ZL. Long-term clinical outcomes following en bloc resections for sacral chordomas and chondrosarcomas: a series of twenty consecutive patients. Spine (Phila Pa 1976). 2009;34(20):2233–9.
7. Chan H, Wang C, Azuhairy A, Hau A, Zulkiflee O. Giant sacral chondrosarcoma in an elderly male: a case report. Malays Orthop J. 2014;8(1):79–81.
8. Possover M, Uehlinger K, Ulrich EG. Laparoscopic assisted resection of a ilio-sacral chondrosarcoma: a single case report. Int J Surg Case Rep. 2014;5(7):381–4.

9. Li D, Guo W, Tang X, Yang R, Tang S, Qu H, Yang Y, Sun X, Du Z. Preservation of the contralateral sacral nerves during hemisacrectomy for sacral malignancies. Eur Spine J. 2014;23(9):1933–9.
10. Zang J, Guo W, Yang R, Tang X, Li D. Is total en bloc sacrectomy using a posterior-only approach feasible and safe for patients with malignant sacral tumors? J Neurosurg Spine. 2015;22(6):563–70.
11. Angelini A, Guerra G, Mavrogenis AF, Pala E, Picci P, Ruggieri P. Clinical outcome of central conventional chondrosarcoma. J Surg Oncol. 2012;106(8):929–37.
12. Giuffrida AY, Burgueno JE, Koniaris LG, et al. Chondrosarcoma in the United States (1973–2003): an analysis of 2,890 cases from the SEER database. J Bone Joint Surg Am. 2009;91:1063–72.
13. Mavrogenis AF, Angelini A, Drago G, Merlino B, Ruggieri P. Survival analysis of patients with chondrosarcomas of the pelvis. J Surg Oncol. 2013;108(1):19–27.
14. Rodallec MH, Feydy A, Larousserie F, Anract P, Campagna R, Babinet A, Zins M, Drapé JL. Diagnostic imaging of solitary tumors of the spine: what to do and say. Radiographics. 2008;28:1019–41.
15. Shives TC, McLeod RA, Unni KK, Schray MF. Chondrosarcoma of the spine. J Bone Joint Surg Am. 1989;71(8):1158–65.
16. Gitelis S, Bertoni F, Picci P, Campanacci M. Chondrosarcoma of bone. The experience at the Istituto Ortopedico Rizzoli. J Bone Joint Surg Am. 1981;63(8):1248–57.
17. Camins MB, Duncan AW, Smith J, Marcove RC. Chondrosarcoma of the spine. Spine (Phila Pa 1976). 1978;3(3):202–9.
18. York JE, Berk RH, Fuller GN, Rao JS, Abi-Said D, Wildrick DM, Gokaslan ZL. Chondrosarcoma of the spine: 1954–1997. J Neurosurg. 1999;90(1 Suppl):73–8.
19. Unni KK. Chondrosarcoma. In: Dahlin's bone tumors: general aspects and data on 11,087 cases. 5th ed. Philadelphia: Lippincott-Raven; 1996. p. 71–108.
20. Marco RA, Gitelis S, Brebach GT, Healey JH. Cartilage tumors: evaluation and treatment. J Am Acad Orthop Surg. 2000;8(5):292–304.
21. Llauger J, Palmer J, Amores S, Bague S, Camins A. Primary tumors of the sacrum: diagnostic imaging. AJR Am J Roentgenol. 2000;174(2):417–24.
22. Bertoni F, Bacchini P, Hogendoorn PCW. Chondrosarcoma. In: CDM F, Unni KK, Mertens F, editors. World Health Organization classification of tumours of soft tissue and bone. Pathology and genetics of tumours of soft tissue and bone. Lyon: IARC Press; 2002. p. 247–58.
23. Rosenthal DI, Schiller AL, Mankin HJ, et al. Chondrosarcoma: correlation of radiological and histological grade. Radiology. 1984;150:21–6.
24. Mankin HJ, Hornicek FJ, Temple HT, et al. Malignant tumors of the pelvis: an outcome study. Clin Orthop Relat Res. 2004;425:212–7.
25. Boriani S, De Iure F, Bandiera S, Campanacci L, Biagini R, Di Fiore M, Bandello L, Picci P, Bacchini P. Chondrosarcoma of the mobile spine: report on 22 cases. Spine (Phila Pa 1976). 2000;25(7):804–12.
26. Ruggieri P, Angelini A, Pala E, Mercuri M. Infections in surgery of primary tumors of the sacrum. Spine (Phila Pa 1976). 2012;37:420–8.
27. Chen KW, Yang HL, Lu J, Wang GL, Ji YM, Bao ZH, et al. Risk factors for postoperative wound infections of sacral chordoma after surgical excision. J Spinal Disord Tech. 2011;24:230–4.
28. Angelini A, Drago G, Trovarelli G, Calabrò T, Ruggieri P. Infection after surgical resection for pelvic bone tumors: an analysis of 270 patients from one institution. Clin Orthop Relat Res. 2014;472(1):349–59.
29. Rhomberg W, Eiter H, Böhler F, Dertinger S. Combined radiotherapy and razoxane in the treatment of chondrosarcomas and chordomas. Anticancer Res. 2006;26(3B):2407–11.
30. Holliday EB, Mitra HS, Somerson JS, Rhines LD, Mahajan A, Brown PD, Grosshans DR. Postoperative proton therapy for chordomas and chondrosarcomas of the spine: adjuvant versus salvage radiation therapy. Spine (Phila Pa 1976). 2015;40(8):544–9.

31. DeLaney TF, Liebsch NJ, Pedlow FX, Adams J, Weyman EA, Yeap BY, Depauw N, Nielsen GP, Harmon DC, Yoon SS, Chen YL, Schwab JH, Hornicek FJ. Long-term results of Phase II study of high dose photon/proton radiotherapy in the management of spine chordomas, chondrosarcomas, and other sarcomas. J Surg Oncol. 2014;110(2):115–22.
32. van Maldegem AM, Gelderblom H, Palmerini E, et al. Outcome of advanced, unresectable conventional central chondrosarcoma. Cancer. 2014;120:3159–64.
33. Grignani G, Palmerini E, Stacchiotti S, et al. A phase 2 trial of imatinib mesylate in patients with recurrent nonresectable chondrosarcomas expressing platelet-derived growth factor receptor-α or -β: an Italian Sarcoma Group study. Cancer. 2011;117:826–31.
34. Evans HL, Ayala AG, Romsdahl MM. Prognostic factors in chondrosarcoma of bone: a clinicopathologic analysis with emphasis on histologic grading. Cancer. 1977;40:818–31.
35. Marcove RC, Miké V, Hutter RV, et al. Chondrosarcoma of the pelvis and upper end of the femur. An analysis of factors influencing survival time in one hundred and thirteen cases. J Bone Joint Surg Am. 1972;54:561–72.
36. Lee FY, Mankin HJ, Fondren G, et al. Chondrosarcoma of bone: an assessment of outcome. J Bone Joint Surg Am. 1999;81:326–38.
37. Ozaki T, Hillmann A, Lindner N, Blasius S, Winkelmann W. Chondrosarcoma of the pelvis. Clin Orthop. 1997:226–39.
38. Sheth DS, Yasko AW, Johnson ME, Ayala AG, Murray JA, Romsdahl MM. Chondrosarcoma of the pelvis. Prognostic factors for 67 patients treated with definitive surgery. Cancer. 1996;78:745–50.
39. Schoenfeld AJ, Hornicek FJ, Pedlow FX, Kobayashi W, Raskin KA, Springfield D, DeLaney TF, Nielsen GP, Mankin HJ, Schwab JH. Chondrosarcoma of the mobile spine: a review of 21 cases treated at a single center. Spine (Phila Pa 1976). 2012;37(2):119–26.

Part IV

Treatments

Anatomy and Surgical Approaches to the Sacrum

20

Sean Accardo and Ricardo Gonzalez

20.1 Introduction

The treatment of tumors of and around the sacrum is complex, even in the most experienced hands. As such, a thorough understanding of the anatomy of the sacrum and its relations to the vast array of surrounding structures is of utmost importance. With this understanding, and the histology and location of the tumor being treated, the needed surgical approach can be chosen: from limited anterior sacroiliac exposure for benign tumors to combined anterior and posterior approaches for total sacrectomy in the treatment of large sacral chordomas.

In this chapter, we set out to describe the bony anatomy of the sacrum and how it relates to the pelvis, and its contents, as a whole. The relevant neurovascular structures within and adjacent to the sacrum will also be detailed. Additionally, surgical approaches to the sacrum will be described. Both anterior and posterior approaches, as well as combined approaches, will be detailed. Finally, consideration will be paid for how these approaches affect soft tissue reconstruction.

S. Accardo, M.D. • R. Gonzalez, M.D. (✉)
Sarcoma Department, H. Lee Moffitt Cancer Center,
12902 Magnolia Drive, Tampa, FL 33602, USA
e-mail: Saccardo@gmail.com; Ricardo.Gonzalez@moffitt.org

P. Ruggieri et al. (eds.), *Tumors of the Sacrum*,
DOI 10.1007/978-3-319-51202-0_20

20.2 Anatomy of the Sacrum

20.2.1 Bony Anatomy

The sacrum is a large bone of the axial skeleton, formed from the fusion of the S1 through S5 sacral vertebrae. It is triangular in shape and articulates with four other bones: the L5 vertebra, the left and right innominate bones, and the coccyx. Centrally there is the sacral canal, through which the continued lumbosacral dural sac sits, transmitting the sacral nerve roots. Of note, the dural sac most often ends at the S2 sacral body, with the remainder of the sacral nerve roots exiting caudally. The lateral projections of the sacrum, whose articular cartilage-covered lateral surface forms the sacral surface of the sacroiliac joint, are referred to as the sacral alae. Anteriorly, within the pelvis, the sacrum is curved in shape in both the axial and sagittal planes and tilted such that the super portion of the sacrum faces slightly anterior; this allowed for expanded volume within the pelvis. There are four pairs of anterior sacral foramina, out of which exit the sacral nerve roots. These lie directly lateral to the transverse sacral ridges, which demarcate the fusion lines between the fused sacral vertebrae.

Dorsally, the sacrum is narrower when compared to the anterior surface and also convex is shape. In the midline is the median sacral crest, which is delineated by up to four tubercles that represent the fused sacral vertebrae's spinous processes. Lateral to the median sacral crest is a relatively flat surface formed from the fused transverse processes that are the origin of the multifidus muscle. Lateral to this surface are the four pairs of posterior sacral foramina, out of which exits the posterior sacral nerves. The most lateral portion of the posterior sacrum is overhung, but not the posterior ilium and posterior inferior iliac spine. Most caudally, the sacral hiatus is present, near the articulation with the coccyx, and represents the most caudal extent of the sacral canal.

The lateral surfaces of the sacrum are somewhat triangular in shape, with the cranial portion being broader than the caudal portion. The majority of the lateral sacrum is comprised of the sacral portion of the sacroiliac joint, is convoluted in geography, and is covered in articular cartilage. The thin, inferior-most edge of the lateral sacrum is called the inferior lateral angle, off of which a bony projection comes. Inferior to this is where the fifth sacral nerve exits. The inferolateral-most portion of the sacrum is the attachment point for the sacrospinous and sacrotuberous ligaments, along with some origin fibers of the gluteus maximus and coccygeus.

20.2.2 Ligamentous Anatomy

There are three general areas of ligamentous attachment to the sacrum: cranially at the lumbosacral articulation, laterally at the sacroiliac joints, and inferiorly with the sacrospinous and sacrotuberous attachments.

The lumbosacral articulation lies at the L5–S1 intervertebral disk. The usual ligamentous attachments of the lumbar spine exist between the L5 vertebra and the S1 portion of the sacrum.

There are three ligaments, per side, that constitute the sacroiliac ligament complex: the anterior sacroiliac ligament, the interosseous sacroiliac ligament, and the posterior sacroiliac ligaments. Anteriorly, the anterior sacroiliac ligament is a thin structure that traverses the entirety of the sacroiliac joint capsule. It is not separable from the joint capsule itself. The interosseous ligament lies just anterior to the posterior ligament complex and is formed by near horizontal fibers that directly connect the ilium to the sacrum. The posterior sacroiliac ligament complex is the most substantial of the ligaments attaching the sacrum to the ilium. This complex is composed of a short posterior sacroiliac ligament, which lies just posterior to the interosseous ligament and has horizontal fibers, and the long posterior sacroiliac ligament, which runs vertically cranially from the posterior superior iliac spine to caudally at the lateral portion of the S3 and S4 segments.

The sacrospinous and sacrotuberous ligaments originate from the inferior lateral portion of the sacrum, with the sacrotuberous ligament sharing some origin fibers with the posterior sacroiliac ligaments. The ischial attachments of the sacrospinous and sacrotuberous ligaments are the ischial spine and the ischial tuberosity, respectively.

20.3 Surgical Approaches to the Sacrum

20.3.1 Anterior Approach to the Sacroiliac Joint

The anterior approach to the sacroiliac joint is a reliable, reproducible, and safe approach that can provide direct access to the entire anterior joint and lateral sacral ala. This can be a useful approach for resection, curettage, and adjuvant treatment of lateral sacral tumors that are being treated using marginal or intralesional treatment principles.

20.3.1.1 Description of Approach

The patient is positioned supine on the operating table, with the option of placing a bump under the ipsilateral buttock. An incision is made along the margin of the iliac crest starting several centimeters proximal and posterior to the anterior superior iliac spine and extending 2–3 cm distal to the anterior superior iliac spine. Once through subcutaneous fat, incise the fascia and periosteum overlying the outer table of the iliac crest, and carry this subperiosteal dissection over the brim of the iliac crest. This, in effect, is dissecting the attachment of the abdominal wall musculature to allow for suitable closure. At this point, the iliacus, whose origin is the inner table of the ilium, is encountered and can be freed from the inner table bluntly. This is often best done using a Cobb elevator and a laparotomy sponge. This dissection is carried all the way to the sacroiliac joint. Several perforating blood vessels will be encountered, which will need to be cauterized or controlled with firm placement of bone wax. This dissection can be carried all the way to the lateral border of the sacral foramina; dissection should not be carried medial to this point, unless necessary, as there is considerable risk of damage to the anterior sacral nerve roots. Cranially, caution should be exercised, as the L5 nerve root can be encountered as it crosses the brim of the sacral ala. Hohmann retractors can be placed directly into the sacrum medially, as long as care is taken not to inadvertently place the point of the retractor into the sacral foramen. Closure is fairly simple, requiring only reapproximation of the abdominal musculature fascia, subcutaneous tissue, and fat.

20.3.1.2 Dangers

Dangers in this approach are, as described above, the perforating nutrient vessels, sacral nerve roots, as well as the lateral femoral cutaneous nerve.

The perforating nutrient vessels can generally not be avoided, but are easily controlled with the use of bone wax or electrocautery.

The sacral nerve root can be avoided by not extending the dissection medially to the lateral border of the sacral foramina. However, they can still be at risk due to medial retractor placement into the sacral foramen.

The lateral femoral cutaneous nerve can be encountered if superficial dissection is carried out distally. Damage to this nerve can generally be avoided by carrying out dissection deep to the iliacus muscle and by not extending the dissection distal to the anterior superior iliac spine.

20.3.2 Anterior Midline Approach to the Sacrum

The anterior approach to the sacrum is the utilitarian approach for sacrectomy. The approach is utilized for higher resections of the sacrum, generally S2 and higher [1, 2].

20.3.2.1 Description of Approach

For the transperitoneal approach, the patient is positioned supine for this approach, on a radiolucent table. A standard midline incision is made. Dissection is carried through the rectus abdominis muscle, in line with the incision. The peritoneum is entered, and the bowel is mobilized cranially. The rectum is either freed and retracted or transected. The pelvic vasculature is identified and mobilized, as needed. The median sacral artery and vein are ligated about the level of planned osteotomy. The internal iliac artery, or its branches, can also be ligated as needed. The lateral gutters between the sacrum and pelvis are developed [2]. At this point, with the sacrum visualized, the resection can proceed at the level dictated by the planned resection. Closure occurs in the usual fashion needed for a standard laparotomy.

20.3.2.2 Dangers

Multiple dangers exist with the anterior approach: enteral injuries, iliac artery and vein injuries (including main and secondary branches), and injuries in the sacral venous plexus, sacral nerve root and its plexus, the obturator neurovascular bundle, the urinary bladder and ureters, and in males the spermatic cord and base of the phallus and in females the uterus. This all necessitates a thorough knowledge of the anatomy of the pelvis and its contents, along with a multidisciplinary approach to the planned procedure including general surgical oncology, orthopedic oncology, vascular surgery, urology, and gynecologic oncology.

20.3.3 Posterior Approach to the Sacroiliac Joint

The posterior approach to the sacroiliac joint, like the anterior sacroiliac approach, can provide good access to the sacroiliac joint for treatment of benign tumors of the lateral sacrum and posterior ilium.

20.3.3.1 Description of Approach

The patient is positioned prone on the operating room table. Either a curved or longitudinal incision over the posterior ilium, centered on the posterior iliac spine, can be utilized. The gluteal fascia is incised, and the gluteus muscle is elevated from the posterior ilium and sacrum. Care needs to be taken to attempt preservation of the inferior gluteal artery and nerve as they exit the greater sciatic notch. Once the gluteus maximus is elevated and retracted laterally and inferiorly, the greater sciatic notch, with the exiting piriformis muscle, will be exposed. The gluteus medius can be elevated as needed, allowing for palpation through the greater sciatic notch of the anterior sacroiliac joint. From here, the posterior sacroiliac ligament can be transected as needed, and the posterior ilium is fully exposed along with the posterolateral sacrum. Much of this portion of the sacrum is obstructed from view due to the overhanging posterior ilium. Closure of this approach involves repair of the posterior sacroiliac ligament, gluteus maximus muscle and fascia, and standard subcutaneous closure.

20.3.3.2 Dangers

Dangers in this approach mainly involve the inferior and superior gluteal neurovascular bundles, as lateral dissection can injure these important structures. If dissection needs to be carried out far laterally, these vessels should be identified and protected.

20.3.4 Posterior Midline Approach to the Sacrum

The posterior midline approach can be utilized when performing sacral amputations below the level of S2 [3]. The approach cannot be utilized alone when performing sacrectomy above that level, as mobilization of structures anterior to the sacroiliac joints cannot be exposed safely.

20.3.4.1 Description of Approach

For this approach, the patient is positioned prone. A midline incision is made directly over the sacrum, from the L5 spinous process to the coccyx. An ellipse of the skin can also be incorporated into the incision, as dictated by the tumor. Subcutaneous dissection is carried down to the fascia. By starting midline and dissecting subperiosteally along the sacrum, the dorsal neural foramina are identified. The dorsal nerve roots are often sacrificed. Dissection is carried out from cranial to caudal and midline to lateral. Once the entire sacrum is exposed, which requires elevation of the gluteus from the sacrum, the greater sciatic notches are identified.

The common attachment of the sacrospinous and sacrotuberous ligaments is identified and transected. At this point, an osteotomy can be performed as determined in the preoperative plan, either using lateral fluoroscopy or computer navigation. If a total sacrectomy is planned, the sacroiliac ligaments can be resected in total by incising them from their iliac attachment. A burr tip can be used to enter the sacral canal at the proximal-most extent of the resection in order to identify and protect most cranial sacral nerve roots. From here, the osteotomy can be completed, and the caudal aspect of the sacrum can be "rolled out," and anterior dissection can be performed to free the sacrum.

Alternately, after subcutaneous dissection to fascia, the gluteus musculature can be incised from its origin on the sacrum [4]. Care is taken to not damage the sciatic or pudendal nerves, which are in close proximity to the gluteal transection. The sciatic nerve is then identified exiting the greater sciatic notch. Transecting the sacrotuberous ligament from the ischial tuberosity, thereby exposing the ischiorectal fossa, can identify the pudendal nerve. From here the pudendal nerve lies on the lateral wall, where it can be identified and protected. The sacrospinous ligament can then be safely divided by retracting and protecting the now exposed pudendal nerve. Blunt dissection can then be carried out to develop the presacral space, and the anococcygeal raphe can be divided, allowing for complete access to the presacral space from posterior.

Closure of this approach is dependent on the amount of resection and need for soft tissue coverage, whether the rectum was excised [3]. Drains should be utilized in all cases to prevent hematoma formation, as a significant space is created with sacral resection.

20.3.4.2 Dangers

Dangers in this approach include injuries to the gluteal vessels, as in the posterior approach to the SI joint, and injury to the sciatic nerves. Additionally, if not carefully dissected, significant injury to the rectum and anus can occur [5]. This approach also necessitates a multidisciplinary team due to the multiple organ structures needing mobilization and manipulation during the approach.

20.3.5 Combined Approaches to the Sacrum

A combined approach can be utilized for treatment of malignant tumors of the sacrum, generally those requiring total sacrectomy, rectal involvement, or neurovascular involvement. [3]. When sacral resection above the S3 level is required, a combined approach is often necessary [6].

20.3.5.1 Description of Approach

The position of the patient can be in the lateral position, allowing for both anterior and posterior midline approaches to be performed without patient repositioning [4]. Often preferred, the alternate procedure is to perform each approach independently, repositioning after completion of one half of the resection [1]. Whether to start anteriorly or posteriorly is at the discretion of the surgeon; however, the anterior approach is often performed first to allow for harvest and passage of a rectus abdominis flap [3]. Starting with the anterior approach first also allows for ease of resection of the anterior sacroiliac ligaments that facilitates and expedites posterior resection.

Another option when performing the combined approach is to stage the resection, separating the two approaches by 1–2 days. This allows for a single position for each exposure as well as patient resuscitation between stages.

20.3.5.2 Dangers

The dangers of the combined approach include all those listed individually for the anterior and posterior approaches, including damage to the gluteal vessels, the sciatic nerves, and enteral injury from the posterior approach and enteral injuries, iliac artery and vein injuries, sacral venous plexus, sacral nerve root and its plexus, the obturator neurovascular bundle, urinary system injuries, in males the spermatic cord and base of the phallus and in females the uterus and adnexa from the anterior approach. Additionally, in these cases, especially when done as a single stage, the dangers of prolonged surgical case time are present including large blood loss, postoperative ileus, nerve damage, and increased surgical time [6, 7]. By staging the procedures, and allowing for patient resuscitation between stages, many of these prolonged case dangers can be avoided or mitigated.

20.3.6 Approach Considerations for Soft Tissue Reconstruction

Most frequently, a large inferior and posterior defect will be present when resecting large portions of the sacrum. Given the limited posterior coverage options, most often a transverse rectus abdominis (TRAM) flap is utilized. This flap can be harvested after the anterior approach and resection is performed, as harvest of this flap before intrapelvic work is performed puts the pedicle of the flap at risk of injury [1]. The standard midline laparotomy performed for most anterior approaches allowed for easy harvest of this flap, which can then be manually passed into the pelvis and left safely, after which the posterior approach and resection can proceed, allowing for combined resection and soft tissue reconstruction without the need for patient repositioning. The chapter on soft tissue reconstruction further details specifics on this topic.

20.4 Summary

Given the anatomical complexity and morbidity associated with resection of sacral tumors, a detailed understanding of the anatomy and surgical approaches is required when treating tumors of the sacrum. The anterior and posterior approaches to the sacroiliac joint allow for limited exposure of the lateral aspect of the sacrum along with the medial portion of the ilium; however, the advantage of these approaches is their relative simplicity and often avoids damage to surrounding structures. In certain instances, an isolated anterior or isolated posterior approach can be utilized to approach the sacrum. The anterior approach is fraught with danger to the abdominal and retroperitoneal viscera, the iliac vasculature, and the genitourinary system. However, the approach provides excellent exposure of the anterior sacral structures, allowing for anterior sacroiliac ligament release and anterior osteotomy for high-level sacral osteotomies. The posterior approach allows for exposure and resection, with relative ease, of the lower sacral levels; however, soft tissue compromise is often an issue, and the sciatic nerves, gluteal vasculature, and rectum and anus are often at risk. In spite of these risks, a combined anterior-posterior approach is often warranted. This is most effectively executed by performing the anterior approach, TRAM harvest as needed, followed by patient repositioning and posterior approach, completed resection, and soft tissue reconstruction. These prolonged, more complicated, procedures often necessitate collaboration between multiple surgeons, be it an orthopedic oncologist, general surgeon oncologist, vascular surgeon, urologist, or plastic surgeon. A well-experienced and well-informed team will most certainly add to the ease with which these complicated cases can be performed, while at the same time decreasing complications and untoward surgical events.

References

1. Sim F, et al. Master techniques in orthopaedic surgery: orthopaedic oncology and complex reconstructions. Philadelphia: Lippincott Williams and Wilkins; 2011.
2. Soloman MJ, Tan K, Bromilow RG, Al-mozany N, Lee PJ. Sacrectomy via the abdominal approach during pelvic exenteration. Dis Colon Rectum. 2014;57:272–7.
3. Takahashi HE, et al. Operative treatment of pelvis tumors. 1st ed. New York: Springer; 2003.
4. Malawer M, et al. Musculoskeletal cancer surgery: treatment of sarcoma and allied diseases. New York: Kluwer Academic; 2001.
5. Asavamongkolkul A, Waikakul S. Wide resection of sacral chordoma via a posterior approach. Int Orthop. 2012;36:607–12.
6. Fuchs B, Dickey ID, Yaszemski MJ, Inwards CY, Sim FH. Operative management of sacral chordoma. J Bone Joint Surg Am. 2005;87-A:2211–6.
7. Dubory A, Missenard G, Lambert B, Court C. "En bloc" resection of sacral chordomas by combined anterior and posterior surgical approach: a monocentric retrospective review about 29 cases. Eur Spine J. 2014;23:1940–8.

21 Tumors of the Sacrum: Diagnosis, Management, and Surgical Techniques

Eric T. Newman, Francis J. Hornicek, and Joseph H. Schwab

21.1 Introduction

Latin for "sacred bone" and so named for its recurrent role in ancient Greek and Egyptian mythology [1], the *os sacrum* remains the subject of much discourse and scholarship in modern-day musculoskeletal oncology. While certain sacral tumors, including hematologic malignancies, giant cell tumors, and the majority of metastatic lesions, may be managed medically, chordomas, chondrosarcomas, and other primary malignancies typically warrant resection. The surgical treatment of these tumors demands careful attention to the complex interplay of anatomic, biomechanical, and oncologic factors. However, with meticulous preoperative planning and input from a specialized multidisciplinary team, good functional and oncologic results can be obtained.

21.2 Anatomy

The surgical management of sacral tumors requires a detailed understanding of the bony, ligamentous, vascular, and nervous anatomy of the pelvis [2].

Bony anatomy: A single bone formed by the fusion of five vertebrae, the sacrum articulates laterally with the ileum via paired L-shaped facets. Inferior articulation (or fusion) with the coccyx involves the two horn-like coccygeal *cornua* and their sacral counterparts. Four pairs of anterior and four pairs of posterior foramina carry the anterior and posterior rami, respectively, of the S1–4 nerve roots, as they emerge from the sacral canal. The termination of the sacral canal, which itself is the caudal continuation of the vertebral canal, is the sacral hiatus.

E.T. Newman, M.D. • F.J. Hornicek, M.D., Ph.D. (✉) • J.H. Schwab, M.D., M.S.
Section of Orthopaedic Oncology, Department of Orthopaedic Surgery, Massachusetts General Hospital, 55 Fruit Street, Boston, MA 02114, USA
e-mail: Fhornicek@mgh.harvard.edu; Jhschwab@mgh.harvard.edu

P. Ruggieri et al. (eds.), *Tumors of the Sacrum*,
DOI 10.1007/978-3-319-51202-0_21

Ligamentous and articular anatomy: The articulation between L5 and S1 involves the two zygapophyseal joints and the intervertebral disk. The L5/S1 disk is wedge-shaped, thicker anteriorly than posteriorly, contributing to the lordosis at this level. Stout iliolumbar and lumbosacral ligaments, extending from the transverse processes of L5 to the ilium and sacrum, reinforce the lumbosacral junction. The synovial sacroiliac joints, prone to fibrosis and fusion with aging, are likewise stabilized by thick anterior and posterior ligaments. Finally, the sacrospinous and sacrotuberous ligaments serve to stabilize the bony pelvis, reinforce the lateral pelvic walls, and define the greater and lesser sciatic foramina.

Muscular anatomy: Relevant muscular anatomy about the sacrum includes the paired piriformis and coccygeus muscles, as well as the anococcygeal ligament. The piriformis originates on the anterior surface of the sacrum and exits the pelvis through the greater sciatic foramen, en route to its tendinous insertion on the greater trochanter. The piriformis serves as an important landmark within the greater sciatic foramen; contents of the suprapiriform foramen include the superior gluteal nerve and vessels, while structures exiting inferiorly include the inferior gluteal vessels, sciatic nerve, pudendal nerve, internal pudendal vessels, posterior femoral cutaneous nerve, and nerves to the obturator internus and quadratus femoris.

Contents of the lesser sciatic foramen, separated from its superior counterpart by the sacrospinous ligament, include the tendon of the obturator internus as it exits the pelvis and the pudendal nerve and internal pudendal vessels as they reenter the pelvis. The coccygeus, which originates on the inner surface of the sacrospinous ligament, inserts on the lateral borders of the sacrum and coccyx. The anococcygeal ligament is formed at the midline raphe of the left and right levator ani musculature, which constitutes the pelvic floor and helps to maintain anal and vaginal closure. Posteriorly, the anococcygeal ligament inserts on the coccyx.

Peritoneal anatomy: The sacrum is a retroperitoneal structure. It should be noted that the rectum is retroperitoneal as well; the upper two-thirds of this structure is draped anteriorly by peritoneum, while the lower one-third is completely uncovered by peritoneum.

Vascular anatomy: The internal iliac vascular system is relevant to surgery of the sacrum and pelvis. The paired internal iliac (hypogastric) arteries typically branch from the common iliac arteries at the level of L5/S1, anteromedial to the SI joint. At the superior border of the greater sciatic foramen, the internal iliac artery divides into anterior and posterior trunks, which each subsequently give rise to multiple named vessels. The posterior trunk supplies the posterior pelvic wall and gluteal region; branches include the iliolumbar artery, which ascends superiorly out of the posterior pelvis and gives off a spinal branch that passes through the L5/S1 intervertebral foramen; the lateral sacral artery, which gives multiple branches that pass into each anterior sacral foramina; and the superior gluteal artery, which exits the pelvis through the suprapiriform greater sciatic foramen and supplies the abductor musculature.

Relevant branches of the anterior trunk of the internal iliac include the internal pudendal artery, which runs through Alcock's canal with the pudendal nerve and supplies the external genitalia; the obturator artery, which exits the pelvis through the obturator foramen into the adductor compartment of the thigh; the inferior gluteal artery, which exits the pelvis through the infrapiriform greater sciatic foramen and supplies the gluteus maximus and piriformis; and multiple branches to the pelvic viscera. The median sacral artery, an unpaired, midline vessel, branches off the abdominal aorta just proximal to its bifurcation and travels down the anterior surface of the sacrum and coccyx.

Nervous anatomy: The sacral and coccygeal plexuses, formed by the anterior rami of S1-Co with contributions from L4 to L5, carry primarily somatosensory fibers, with sympathetic and parasympathetic components as well. As noted above, four paired anterior and four paired posterior foramina transmit the anterior and posterior rami of the S1–4 nerve roots. Each anterior ramus, except at the S4 level, in turn divides into ventral and dorsal divisions.

The sacral plexus gives rise to multiple somatic nerves, including the sciatic (L4–S2), superior and inferior gluteal, and pudendal nerves, as well as smaller motor branches to the quadratus femoris, gemelli, obturator internus, levator ani, and coccygeus muscles, and two sensory nerves (the posterior femoral cutaneous and perforating cutaneous). The pudendal nerve is of particular importance to surgery of the sacrum and pelvis. Arising from the ventral divisions of the anterior rami of S2–S4, the pudendal nerve exits the pelvis through the infrapiriform greater sciatic foramen, passes dorsal to the sacrospinous ligament, and reenters the pelvis through the lesser sciatic foramen. As it does so, it courses along the lateral wall of the ischioanal fossa within Alcock's canal (pudendal canal), inferior to the pelvic floor and accompanied by the internal pudendal vessels. The pudendal nerve innervates the levator ani as well as the skeletal muscle of the external anal and urethral sphincters and provides sensory innervation to much of the perineum and penis or clitoris. Compression or injury to the pudendal nerve or its sacral nerve roots can result in bowel, bladder, and sexual dysfunction.

In addition to its somatic nervous functions, the sacral plexus provides parasympathetic visceral innervation through its contributions to the inferior hypogastric plexus of the pelvis. Functions of parasympathetic pelvic innervation include vasodilation of the erectile tissue of the penis or clitoris, stimulation of bladder contraction during micturition, and modulation of activity of the descending colon and rectum. This parasympathetic outflow is carried by the pelvic splanchnic nerves, which originate primarily from the S2–S4 roots. The pelvic splanchnic nerves join fibers from the superior hypogastric plexus, which descends along the posterior abdominal wall and carries both sympathetic and parasympathetic fibers, to form the inferior hypogastric plexus.

Sympathetic functions of the inferior hypogastric plexus include innervation of smooth muscle within the pelvic vasculature, internal anal and urethral sphincters, and reproductive tract (i.e., critical for the processes of ejaculation). It should be noted that sympathetic fibers within the inferior hypogastric plexus are supplied by the roots of T10–L2, but *not* by sacral nerve roots. Finally, the somatic coccygeal plexus, with contributions from S4, S5, and Co, gives rise to the anococcygeal nerve, which contributes to motor and sensory innervation of the perineum.

21.3 Applied Surgical Anatomy: Biomechanical and Neurologic Considerations

The anatomic features of the pelvis inform the biomechanical and functional considerations relevant to planning for sacral resections. Partial transverse sacrectomies have been classified with respect to nerve root anatomy, wherein preservation of S3, S2, and S1 corresponds to low, middle, and high sacrectomies, respectively [3]. Level of resection is of critical importance not only with respect to margin status but also with respect to preservation of mechanical stability of the pelvis and maintenance of bowel, bladder, and sexual function.

21.3.1 Biomechanical Considerations

Spinopelvic fixation is typically performed after total sacrectomy; in the absence of reconstruction, as elaborated by one author, the resultant "flail axial skeleton precludes the ability to ambulate" [4]. On the other hand, low partial sacrectomy does not warrant reconstruction. However, the indications for reconstruction after high or middle partial sacrectomy are less clear. Early biomechanical work performed by Gutenberg [5] found that resection through (or just cephalad to) the S1 foramina weakened the pelvic ring by 50%, while resection between the S1 and S2 foramina resulted in only 30% weakening. A more recent cadaveric study, which purported to model physiologic loading more accurately, found that pelvises with sacral resections just caudal to the S1 foramina could withstand forces associated with postoperative mobilization, while those with resections just cephalad to the S1 foramina could not [6]. These authors highlighted the importance of (at least partial) preservation of the sacroiliac joint and noted that bone cuts just cephalad vs. just caudal to the S1 foramina are associated with preservation of 75% vs. 84%, respectively, of the sacroiliac joint—perhaps signifying a biomechanically significant "cutoff" point within that range. Clinical outcome data have largely confirmed these findings. One review found that three of nine sacrectomies involving the S1 body failed via fracture, ultimately requiring reconstruction [7]; another series from our institution, in which high-dose adjuvant radiation was utilized, reported a 76% rate of postoperative sacral insufficiency following high sacrectomy, as compared with 0% after low sacrectomy [8]. Not all authors advocate for reconstruction after total or high sacrectomy: Ruggieri et al. [9] have suggested that muscle and scar tissue may form a "biologic sling" between the unreconstructed pelvis and lower lumbar spine, which may migrate inferiorly toward the ilia. However, it is our preference to perform spinopelvic reconstruction for any sacrectomy cephalad to the S3 foramina when adjuvant radiotherapy (and the attendant risk of fracture) is utilized.

21.3.2 Neurologic Considerations

The S3 nerve roots have traditionally been thought to play a critical role in supplying normal bowel, bladder, and, to a lesser extent, sexual function. Sacrectomy with nerve root sacrifice cephalad to S3 may result in loss of normal bowel and bladder function in many, if not all, patients [3, 5, 7, 10, 11]. Specifically, S2 may allow for weak internal and external anal sphincter activity, but not for discrimination between different rectal contents or sensation of rectal distention, nor for maintenance of the micturition reflex. A review of 53 sacrectomies performed at the Mayo Clinic found that preservation of bilateral S3 nerve roots ensured maintenance of normal bowel and bladder function in 100% and 69% of patients, respectively; unilateral S3 preservation ensured maintenance of function in approximately two-thirds of patients. All patients with sacrifice of bilateral S2 roots had abnormal bowel and bladder function, and a minority of patients enjoyed normal bowel and bladder function with bilateral S3 sacrifice [7]. However, a more recent case series [10] found slightly improved outcomes with S3-sacrificing sacrectomies: normal bowel and bladder function in 63% and 71%, respectively. Preservation of the S2 nerve roots—and perhaps even S1 nerve roots alone—might be sufficient for maintenance of sexual function [5, 12–14]. Unilateral S1–5 resection, with preservation of contralateral nerve roots, has minimal impact on bowel, bladder, or sexual function [3, 5, 7].

Investigations of patient-reported outcomes at our center, utilizing PROMIS and other subjective patient response questionnaires, have confirmed the negative impact of more proximal resections, while demonstrating that postoperative bowel and bladder deficits exist along a spectrum. Phukan et al. [15], in a review of survey data from 33 patients, reported a stepwise decrease in voiding, continence, and defecation scores in patients with S4, S3, S2, and S1 partial sacrectomies, respectively. A similar downtrend in defecation scores among patients with S4, S3, and S2 partial sacrectomies was observed in a study of questionnaire data in 74 sacrectomy patients at our institution and two others [14]. Taken together, these results argue against a binary model of sacral nerve root contribution to bowel and bladder function: preservation of the S3 nerve roots, while ideal, may be neither sufficient nor necessary in all cases for maintenance of normal voiding and defecation.

Evaluation of PROMIS questionnaire data also demonstrated that high partial and total sacrectomies were consistently associated with chronic pain and significantly lower physical and mental health scores in patients with resections cephalad to S3 [14, 15]. As with bowel, bladder, and sexual function, therefore, chronic pain must be addressed in preoperative patient discussions as a known risk of high sacrectomy. Notably, however, quality of life and functional scores following *low* sacrectomy were in fact equivalent or superior to normative (general population) PROMIS data [15].

It should also be noted that the level of bony resection does not necessarily correlate with the extent of sacral root sacrifice: intraoperative margin considerations might require sacrifice of more cephalad nerve roots, or conversely, tumor location might allow for the sparing of nerve roots contralateral or caudal to the bone cut. Neurologic dysfunction might also result from disruption (caused by tumor or surgery) of the pudendal nerves or the inferior hypogastric plexus, even if the sacral nerve roots are preserved intraoperatively. Indeed, it has been demonstrated that the greatest predictor of postoperative bowel and bladder outcome is preoperative function [10]. Finally, sacral nerve root status is only one of a number of factors that may contribute to postoperative function. High partial sacrectomies may necessitate lumbo-pelvic fixation, which can be associated with sciatic nerve dysfunction or pain-generating hardware failure.

21.4 Clinical Management of Sacral Tumors

Sacral tumors may present with pain, perineal sensory changes, and sexual, bowel, and bladder dysfunction, the latter of which may be the result of either nervous or direct visceral compression. Additionally, sacral tumors may be quite large before symptoms arise. As for evaluation of any bone tumor, initial work-up should consist of history, physical examination, and imaging studies, including plain radiographs, computed tomography (CT) and magnetic resonance imaging (MRI) of the sacrum and pelvis, and CT of the chest and bone scan for staging. Complete imaging of the mobile spine should be performed as well; additional lesions may be present in 17% of patients with sacral chordomas [16].

Tissue is necessary for histologic analysis and should preferably be obtained through image-guided needle biopsy. Open incisional biopsy of chordomas, especially when performed outside of the ultimate treating center, is associated with a higher risk of local recurrence, metastasis, and tumor-related death [3, 17, 18]. Analysis of sacral mass biopsy tissue should include immunohistochemical staining for cytokeratins, EMA, vimentin, and brachyury, which stain strongly in chordoma tissue, as well as for Ki-67, which is associated with a poor prognosis when present with a high degree of proliferative activity in chordoma tissue [17]. Genetic analysis is also emerging as a component of the clinical work-up, as knowledge increases regarding the link between chordoma and brachyury, a notochordal "master regulator" transcription factor [19]. Genetic duplication of the brachyury locus is typical in familial chordomas, and a specific single-nucleotide variant in the gene has been identified in 86–94% of chordoma patients and associated with a sixfold increase in risk of chordoma development [19–21].

Tumor characteristics dictate surgical management, including extent of resection and use of adjuvants. Chordomas are the most common primary sacral malignancy; sacral chondrosarcomas, osteosarcomas, and Ewing sarcomas are seen as well. Benign primary tumors include giant cell tumors, aneurysmal bone cysts, and osteoid osteomas/osteoblastomas. Metastatic disease, multiple myeloma, and lymphomas are commonly encountered as well. Teratomas are the most common sacral tumors in children [22].

21.4.1 Management of Chordomas

Deriving from notochordal tissue, chordomas represent 1–4% of all primary malignant bone tumors, with an incidence of 0.08 per 100,000 [23, 24]. While chordomas have traditionally been thought to occur more commonly in the sacrum (50%) than in the skull base (35%) or the mobile spine (15%) [24], more recent data from the population-based SEER registry suggest that these tumors may occur with equal frequency in the skull base, mobile spine, and sacrum [23]. Reported overall 5-year survival in patients treated with sacral chordomas has ranged from 68% to 97% in the literature [9, 17, 23, 25–27], with median survival between 6 and 7 years in three large series [20, 23, 28].

Intralesional resection (or resection with inadequate margins) is associated with a higher rate of local recurrence—up to 83%—and, in some series, decreased survival [9, 11, 17, 20, 24–26, 28, 29]. Fuchs et al. [25], for instance, reported on 52 primary sacral chordomas treated surgically at the Mayo Clinic and noted that all 21 patients who underwent resection with wide margins were alive at 8-year follow-up, while two-thirds of patients with inadequate margins experienced local recurrence and two-thirds of those with local recurrence died within the study period. Bergh et al. [17] reported that local recurrence was associated with a 23-fold increased risk of metastases and a 21-fold increased risk of tumor-related death in a cohort of 39 chordoma patients, while Young et al. [30], reviewing 219 chordoma patients, reported a more modest 2.5-fold increased metastatic risk in cases of local recurrence, with an overall metastatic rate of 18%. Wide, *en bloc* resection is therefore recommended in the management of chordomas.

It has been suggested that tumor invasion into the piriformis or gluteus maximus musculature, or involvement of the sacroiliac joints, is an independent predictor of local recurrence, regardless of margin status at time of resection [29]. Indeed, local recurrences may tend to occur most frequently in the posterior musculature, and wider margins may be required posteriorly as compared with anteriorly, where the presacral fascia may pose a barrier to tumor spread [27, 29].

High-dose (70.2 Gy) proton/photon-beam radiotherapy is now standard in the management of chordomas and other spinal malignancies at our institution. For sacral tumors, preoperative radiation of either 19.8 or 50.4 Gy is administered, with the remainder administered postoperatively; in cases of positive surgical margins, localized boosts are utilized as well. A phase II clinical trial performed at our institution, evaluating 50 patients undergoing surgical resection of spinal chordomas and sarcomas (predominantly sacral), demonstrated that high-dose radiotherapy in addition to surgical resection was associated with a 74% rate of local control at 8-year follow-up [31, 32]. Notably, local control for primary tumors (94% at 5 years and 85% at 8 years) was far superior to that for locally recurrent tumors (~50% re-recurrence rate).

Chordomas, in particular, appear to benefit from high-dose radiation. A retrospective review of 127 spinal chordomas (including recurrent tumors) treated at our institution demonstrated 5-year overall survival and local control of 81% and 62%, respectively [26]. This study found further improvement in local control when surgical resection of primary chordoma was accompanied by neoadjuvant and adjuvant radiation, as opposed to adjuvant radiation alone: 85 vs. 56% at 5 years. Most strikingly, among the 28 patients with primary tumors in this series who underwent *en bloc* resection and received both neoadjuvant and adjuvant radiation, *no* cases of recurrence were observed.

Even in cases of margin-positive primary resection, good results may be salvaged: the use of adjuvant high-dose radiation achieved local control at 8.8 years in 10 of 11 patients with primary sacral chordomas resected with positive surgical margins (but in 0 of 5 patients with recurrent disease) treated at our institution [33]. Taken together, these results highlight not only the excellent outcomes achieved with wide resection plus neo- and adjuvant radiation, but also the critical importance of initiation of aggressive treatment at first presentation.

Additionally, in patients for whom surgical resection is not feasible due to risk of intraoperative nervous injury (i.e., high sacral tumors) or medical comorbidities, definitive management with high-dose radiation is reasonable. In a review of 24 spinal chordomas, of which 19 were located in the sacrum, treated at our institution with proton or photon radiotherapy alone, local control rates were 90.4% and 79.8% at 3 and 5 years, respectively. All surviving patients maintained ambulatory status [34]. A follow-up study noted ongoing tumor volumetric reduction up to 5 years after definitive radiation treatment [35]. Definitive carbon ion radiotherapy, which is characterized by a higher biological effectiveness than proton therapy and may be particularly effective against hypoxic tumors [36], may also be utilized. Five-year local control rates of 77–88% in patients with proximal, unresectable sacral chordomas have been published by a group in Japan [37, 38], while a group in Germany has reported 53% local control and 100% survival among a mixed cohort of primary and recurrent tumors treated with carbon ion radiotherapy [39].

However, high-dose radiation to the sacrum can be associated with significant adverse effects. Specifically, delivery of greater than 77 Gy, which is the standard dose at our institution in cases of definitive treatment with radiation alone, has been associated with higher rates of neuropathy and erectile dysfunction as compared with patients receiving ~70 Gy or less [26, 31, 32, 33, 38]. Sacral insufficiency fractures have been noted to occur in roughly half of all patients with sacral chordomas treated with definitive high-dose radiation [34, 35], and in over three-quarters of patients undergoing high sacrectomy with radiation [8]. For this reason, we avoid radiation doses greater than ~70 Gy in patients undergoing surgical resection.

Though the role of medical therapy in the clinical management of chordomas is currently limited, potential molecular targets for future drug development include the mechanistic target of rapamycin (mTOR) signaling pathway [40], as well as vascular endothelial growth factor (VEGF)-mediated angiogenesis and other receptor tyrosine kinase pathways [36].

21.4.2 Management of Other Sacral Malignancies

Chondrosarcoma of the sacrum represents approximately 20% of spinal chondrosarcomas and 5% of all chondrosarcomas [41], and is the second most commonly resected primary sacral tumor after chordoma [3, 32, 42]. As is the case with other sacral malignancies, *en bloc* resection with negative margins is likely associated with decreased rates of local recurrence and improved disease-free survival [41, 43, 44]. Chondrosarcomas, like chordomas, are treated with high-dose neo- and adjuvant radiation and wide surgical resection at our institution [32]. Spinal osteosarcoma is rare, but has been reported to occur in the sacrum in 31–68% of cases [45, 46]. At our institution, treatment includes *en bloc* resection, high-dose radiotherapy, and neo- and adjuvant chemotherapy [46], though outcome is poor and prognosis is worse for osteosarcoma of the sacrum as compared with that of the mobile spine [45].

Locally recurrent rectal cancer may be treated with aggressive re-resection, to include partial sacrectomy in cases of cortical invasion or tumor adherence to the bone. Overall mean survival of 22–40 months has been reported following re-resection with sacrectomy, with improved outcomes in cases of negative margins [47–49].

21.4.3 Management of Giant Cell Tumors

Traditionally, giant cell tumors (GCTs) of the sacrum have been treated with intralesional curettage, but high rates of recurrence—in up to one-third to one-half of cases—have been reported [50–52]. The authors of a review of a pooled cohort of 166 patients with sacral GCTs, therefore, recommended wide surgical resection for lower sacral lesions and for recurrent proximal sacral lesions [50]. Notably, this study reported a 23% disease-related mortality, of which approximately one-third was related to treatment complications, at 8-year follow-up. Radiation may be utilized in cases of large or challenging sacral GCTs, but is associated with high recurrence rates when used alone or as an adjuvant following curettage [50]. Radiation-related malignant transformation is also a concern [50, 52, 53]. Arterial embolization may represent a more successful nonoperative modality, and good results with respect to symptomatic improvement and low rates of recurrence have been reported with the use of serial arterial embolizations (typically performed every 4–6 weeks) as monotherapy for sacral GCTs [54–56]. Additionally, embolization may be performed concurrently with local intraarterial injection of cisplatin [56] or may be employed as a preoperative adjunct to limit surgical bleeding [51].

The development of denosumab has significantly increased the role of medical management in GCT treatment. A monoclonal antibody against receptor activator of nuclear factor-kappa B (RANK), denosumab inhibits the activation of osteoclast-like multinucleated cells, which express RANK ligand, thereby decoupling the osteoclastic pathway. Prolonged treatment results in marked depletion of giant cells and decreased cellularity overall on histologic analysis [57]. Phase II trials have demonstrated objective tumor response in 72–88% of patients, with significant improvements in pain reports as well [58, 59]. Among the subgroup of patients with tumors deemed operable but with high risk of morbidity, Chawla et al. [58] found that nearly three-quarters were able to avoid surgery altogether after denosumab treatment and that 62% of those who did ultimately undergo resection were managed with a smaller procedure than initially planned. At our institution, a 3–6 month course of denosumab "pretreatment" is typically pursued prior to surgical resection.

21.5 Total and Partial Sacrectomy: Surgical Techniques

Meticulous planning is necessary for successful surgical management of sacral tumors. Preoperative considerations include options for preservation of fertility, general and plastic surgery consultations, and vascular embolization, while intraoperative considerations include choice of approach (combined anterior and posterior vs. posterior only), use of computer-assisted navigation, and options for spinopelvic fixation, when needed.

21.5.1 Preoperative Preparation

We routinely refer reproductive-aged female patients for gynecologic evaluation prior to initiation of oncologic treatment. If desired, laparoscopic oophoropexy may be performed prior to radiotherapy, relocating the ovaries within the abdominal cavity such that they are outside of the planned radiation field, thereby preserving future fertility options. Preoperative consideration should also be given, in consultation with a general surgeon, to colostomy creation prior to or at the time of sacral resection. This decision is highly dependent on patient preference. Among a cohort of total and partial sacrectomy patients studied at our institution, no differences in quality of life metrics were observed between patients with and without colostomy creation [14].

Preoperative consultation with a plastic surgeon should also be pursued. Wound complications are frequent after sacral resections, especially in the setting of radiotherapy or poor patient nutritional status. Options for soft tissue wound closure include mobilization of a pedicled omental flap; transpelvic vertical rectus abdominis myocutaneous (VRAM) flap, fed by the inferior epigastric vessels; and local tissue advancement techniques. A reconstructive algorithm put forth by Miles et al. [60] recommended that bilateral gluteus advancement flaps, associated with the lowest complication rate among reconstructive options, should be the first choice for post-sacrectomy closure *if* the gluteal vessels are intact; transpelvic VRAM reconstruction should be performed in the setting of preoperative radiation, though it is contraindicated for patients with a prior laparotomy; and free flap coverage may be performed if other options are unavailable. In their review of outcomes following surgical management of sacral chordomas, Schwab et al. found a significant decrease in wound complications in patients in whom rectus flap coverage was performed, as compared to patients without flap coverage [11]. Reconstruction of the pelvic floor can also prove problematic; sacroperineal hernia is a rare complication but a risk in cases of large pelvic floor defects. Good results have been reported with reconstruction utilizing acellular dermal collage grafts [61] or mesh [62].

Intraoperative blood loss may be minimized by bilateral internal iliac ligation, which is the standard practice at our institution. However, preoperative embolization and intraoperative aortic balloon pump occlusion are options as well. Embolization of the internal iliac, median sacral, and other tumor-feeding arteries, typically within 24 hours of surgery, may be performed with Gelfoam (Pfizer Inc.), thereby potentially minimizing longer-term devascularization of healthy tissues [63]. Additionally, the use of an occlusive aortic balloon pump has been reported as a technique to reduce intraoperative blood loss in sacral tumor resections [64, 65]. In their review of 215 sacral resections, Tang et al. [64] found that balloon occlusion, utilized in 120 patients, was associated with significantly lower blood loss (2.2 vs. 3.9 liters).

21.5.2 Staged Anterior and Posterior Approaches for Total and Partial Sacrectomy

21.5.2.1 Anterior Approach

Following induction of general anesthesia, administration of antibiotics for coverage of both bowel and skin flora, and establishment of central venous access, the patient is positioned supine on a flexible Jackson table, broken in the middle to improve intraoperative sacral exposure. With the assistance of a general surgeon, a low midline incision is made from the pubis to the umbilicus and the peritoneal cavity is entered. A table-mounted retractor system is utilized. The rectosigmoid colon and left ureter are mobilized away from the tumor, pelvic side wall, and sacrum; this process is repeated on the right side. Great care must be taken not to inadvertently enter the tumor in the course of mobilizing the overlying tissues. For chordomas in particular, violation of the tumor pseudocapsule confers a poor chance for curative resection. Subsequently, following identification and mobilization of the common, internal, and external iliac vessels, the trunks of the left and right internal iliac arteries and veins are ligated just distal to their respective bifurcations; large branches, such as the gluteal and iliolumbar vessels, may be identified and individually ligated as well. Exposure of the anterior sacrum will typically also require ligation of the median sacral artery. The L5 nerve root, which is closely associated with the anterior surface of the sacral ala, is identified and protected. The L5 root may be traced distally to facilitate further exploration of the lumbosacral plexus and identification of the sciatic nerve within the greater sciatic foramen.

En bloc partial sacrectomy: If a partial sacrectomy is to be performed, a high-speed burr is used to create a transverse osteotomy through the anterior sacral cortex, cephalad to the tumor. An intraoperative radiograph is made to assess the level of the osteotomy. The osteotomy is started in the midline, advanced laterally toward the left and right SI joints (or toward the greater sciatic foramina, in cases of more distal resections), and continued posteriorly until the posterior sacral cortex is reached. As the osteotomy is extended laterally from the midline, exiting nerve roots cephalad to the level of the cut are protected and gently retracted laterally; the more proximal L5 nerve root will need to be retracted as well. Additionally, osteotomies at the S1–S2 level may place the superior gluteal vessels at particular risk [66]. A Cobb elevator can be used to deepen the osteotomy and score the posterior cortex. Throughout the creation of the osteotomy, hemostasis is maintained with silk ligatures, monopolar and bipolar electrocautery, thrombin hemostatic matrix, epinephrine-soaked sponges, and bone wax. Prior to closure, a Gore-Tex patch may be placed ventral to the sacrum but dorsal to the rectum and left in place until the second stage, at which point it will serve as a landmark for the safe anterior plane of dissection.

En bloc total sacrectomy: Following anterior approach and exposure, a spinal needle is placed into the L5/S1 disk space (for tumors that do not extend cephalad to S1), and correct level is confirmed on a lateral radiograph. As noted above, the L5 nerve roots and internal iliac vessels (in particular, the artery on the right) should be identified and protected in the course of dissection anterior to the L5–S1 junction and sacral ala. Discectomy is performed at this level with curettes, Kerrison rongeurs, and endplate elevators, extending dorsally to the posterior annulus. Using a high-speed burr, longitudinal osteotomies are created through the anterior cortices of the posterior ilia bilaterally. The resultant troughs are packed with bone wax for hemostasis; osteotomies will be completed posteriorly during the second stage procedure. The location of the iliac osteotomies with respect to the sacroiliac joints is dictated by tumor size and margin considerations. For small, midline sacral tumors, vertical osteotomies may even be created within the sacral ala, thereby preserving the sacroiliac joints.

Coverage with a pedicled rectus abdominis flap is standard practice at our institution. Following completion of the anterior osteotomy, the VRAM flap is harvested by the plastic surgeon. Typically, the flap, once raised, is dunked into the pelvis and secured with a PROLENE (Johnson & Johnson) suture to assist in subsequent orientation. Blake drains are placed within the anterior pelvis. The patient is taken to the intensive care unit for further resuscitation between stages. A vena cava filter is typically placed on the first postoperative day to obviate the need for chemical DVT prophylaxis. Additionally, we obtain a pelvic CT scan between stages for assessment of the anterior osteotomy position. The posterior procedure is performed 3–5 days later.

21.5.2.2 Posterior Approach

The patient is placed prone, in a position of neutral lumbar lordosis, and a midline incision is made. Alternatively, an upside-down "smile" incision may be utilized. For large tumors with dorsal extension into the superficial soft tissues, a skin paddle may be removed with the specimen. Biopsy tracts should also be ellipsed out with the incision. The spinous processes are exposed. Dissection proceeds laterally, elevating the paraspinal musculature proximally and, more distally and laterally, elevating or transecting the gluteus maximus to expose the ilium. The sacral ala is exposed, as are the adjacent transverse process and lamina of L5. After removal of the spinous processes with a Leksell rongeur, laminectomy just cephalad to the level of the planned sacral osteotomy is performed with a diamond-tipped burr and Leksell and Kerrison rongeurs. The dorsal aspect of the dura is dissected free of adhesions to the overlying lamina. The laminectomy may be widened laterally with a small osteotome. The bilateral nerve roots at L5 and any additional caudal levels to be preserved are exposed laterally and mobilized with a Kerrison rongeur and Stevens tenotomy scissors. The thecal sac is then circumferentially exposed at the level of the planned resection, just caudal to the axilla of the exiting nerve roots, and a right-angled clamp is passed ventral to the dura. The thecal sac is ligated with a 2–0 silk suture and clips and then sharply transected. Later in the procedure, after removal of the mass, the transected end of the thecal sac should be covered with dural sealant as well.

Dissection is carried laterally and caudally, elevating the gluteus maximus musculature; a ratcheted self-retaining retractor system is helpful in maintaining exposure. Extent of lateral exposure will be dictated, in part, by the soft tissue extension of the tumor. Dissection proceeds caudally along the lateral borders of the sacrum, exposing and identifying the piriformis and sacrotuberous and sacrospinous ligaments. Sizeable traversing vessels are typically encountered about these structures and will need to be ligated; the use of a bipolar hemostatic sealer can be of benefit here. The piriformis and ligaments are subsequently divided, allowing access into the pelvic cavity through the greater sciatic foramen. Now, using blunt dissection, a plane may be developed ventral to the tumor and dorsal to the rectum. The sciatic nerve should be identified and protected throughout. Dissection should be continued caudally until the tip of the coccyx is palpable.

En bloc partial sacrectomy: An intraoperative radiograph is made to assess the correct level for completion of the sacral osteotomy. A high-speed burr and Cobb elevator are used to complete the osteotomy in the midline. As the osteotomy is continued laterally, nerve roots cephalad to the level of resection should be identified, dissected free from overlying bone with a high-speed burr, and protected. The osteotomy is eventually completed laterally into the left and right sciatic foramina. The mass is now lifted caudally, carefully elevating it off of the adjacent rectum; a Gore-Tex patch, if placed ventral to the sacrum during the first stage, will serve to identify the safe plane between the sacrum and rectum. Nerve roots passing through the tumor are sacrificed. Vessels extending into the specimen are clamped and ligated. Remaining soft tissue attachments to the pelvic floor are transected, the specimen is passed off, and hemostasis of the resection bed is obtained.

En bloc total sacrectomy: Posterior exposure is performed. The thecal sac is ligated just cephalad to the L5/S1 disk space after laminectomy is performed at this level. The posterior L5/S1 discectomy is completed. The bilateral iliac osteotomies, initiated during the anterior approach, are completed posteriorly using a high-speed burr and Cobb elevator. The sacrum and mass are dissected free and lifted out of the wound, as described above.

Spinopelvic reconstruction: As discussed above, the extent of sacral resection impacts the degree of biomechanical instability imparted and therefore the need for spinopelvic fixation. Total sacrectomy warrants spinopelvic reconstruction. Multiple techniques for reconstruction of the bony defect after sacrectomy have been reported. Dickey et al. [4] described a triangular construct in which two segments of fibular autograft are oriented in an inverted "V," such that the apex is "docked" into the inferior endplate of L5 and each limb is buttressed against the inner table of the ilium along the iliopectineal line. The authors note that oval "receptacles" in the ilium need to be fashioned, utilizing a high-speed burr, during the anterior approach. This construct allows for the fibular graft to be oriented along the force transmission lines between the acetabulum and lumbar spine. As discussed below, vascularized fibular grafts can be used in a similar fashion.

Instrumentation is then performed: first, a wide osteotome is used to remove the dorsal cortex of the posterior superior iliac spines, which may be morselized for later use as bone graft. Two iliac screws are placed on each side; orienting the pedicle probe toward the ipsilateral greater trochanter assists with proper placement. Standard pedicle screws are placed bilaterally at L4 and L5. A total of four lumbo-pelvic rods are used: on each side, rods are fixed to the heads of the L4, L5, and proximal iliac screws. Rod-to-rod connectors are used to incorporate two additional parallel rods, one on each side. A horizontal transiliac rod is fixed to the two distal iliac screws. In cadaveric biomechanical testing, this dual-rod, double iliac screw construct has been shown to be stiffer than constructs involving single rods, single iliac screws, or Galveston rods (in which the distal end of the spinopelvic rod itself is driven between the inner and outer tables of the pelvis) [67]. Cross-link connectors may be used proximally between the parallel lumbo-pelvic rods, and distally between the lumbo-pelvic and transiliac rods, to provide additional stability. Burr decortication of the lumbar posterior elements is performed, and morselized autograft and allograft bone is laid down to promote fusion. We routinely make use of calcium phosphate scaffold graft as well.

Additionally, our practice is to perform limited spinopelvic reconstruction for middle partial sacrectomies cephalad to the S3 foramina, especially in cases of adjuvant radiation, which we feel significantly retards the fusion process. In these cases, L5-ilium instrumentation is performed with bilateral iliac screws, longitudinal rods, and horizontal transiliac rod. Complete exposure and thorough decortication of the remnant sacroiliac joints will increase the probability of successful fusion.

Vascularized autograft reconstruction: Though not routinely performed at our institution, the use of vascularized fibular autografts in reconstruction after total sacrectomy has been described. Choudry et al. [68] reported on the use of bilateral vascularized fibular grafts, fashioned into an inverted V at the spinopelvic junction as described above, with vascular anastomoses to the internal iliac vessels (presumably prohibiting intraoperative iliac ligation). In that study, bony fusion was observed on CT scan by 6 months. Anastomosis of free fibular grafts into the deep inferior epigastric pedicle of the mobilized VRAM flap has also been described [69]. This "vertical rectus abdominis musculocutaneous flow-through flap" technique has the advantage of permitting ligation of the internal iliac vessels during the anterior approach. These authors reported fusion on imaging within 3 months of surgery. It should be noted that the added complexity of these procedures, which in some cases required the use of a saphenous vein graft to increase fibular pedicle length, necessitated a three-stage procedure for some patients.

Computer-assisted navigation: Intraoperative CT-guided navigation is now routinely used at our institution. Following anterior sacral exposure during the first stage procedure, the anterior iliac crest is exposed through a small longitudinal incision. The navigation system tracker is affixed to two Steinmann pins driven through the iliac crest, between the inner and outer tables. Intraoperative CT scan is performed. Navigation subsequently aids in identification of the correct osteotomy level and assessment of anterior-posterior depth during creation of the osteotomy. During the posterior procedure, the tracker is affixed to one of the lumbar spinous processes, and CT scan is performed after laminectomy and nerve root exposure. Navigation is then used to confirm that the posterior osteotomy is performed at the same level as the anterior osteotomy.

21.5.2.3 Rebar Technique for Reconstruction After Curettage of Proximal Sacral Tumors

In select circumstances, benign tumors (i.e., GCTs) within the proximal sacrum treated with curettage of the S1 body may be amenable to reconstruction with an anterior "rebar" technique and limited posterior spinopelvic stabilization. We prefer, in these cases, to perform the posterior intralesional resection and spinopelvic instrumentation as a first stage. Laminectomies of the proximal sacrum and L5 are performed, the filum terminale and sacral nerve roots are dissected and protected, and a Gore-Tex patch is placed ventral to the nervous structures; residual, inaccessible anterior tumor is left for completion of resection in the second stage. As compared with that for a total sacrectomy, less extensive instrumentation is required: single, bilateral L5-ileum spinal rods, with a single horizontal transiliac rod, are sufficient. The second stage involves a standard transperitoneal approach and resection of the remnant anterior tumor and S1 body. A high-speed burr, curettes, and Kerrison rongeurs are used to excise the tumor in a piecemeal fashion. If the posterior approach was performed previously, the Gore-Tex patch, placed ventral to the sacral nerve roots, will be encountered and will signify the dorsal extent of safe dissection.

Anterior reconstruction commences with the placement of one or two large fragment screws into both the inferior endplate of L5 and the exposed superior endplate of S2. The screws may be placed in a retrograde or antegrade fashion to maximize cortical purchase, such that either the heads or the tips are exposed within the defect. Antibiotic-laden bone cement is then introduced into the defect and molded around the exposed screws. A Gore-Tex patch or segment of Esmarch tourniquet may be utilized as a temporary dorsal "backstop," preventing damage to the underlying nerve roots as the wet cement cures.

21.5.3 Posterior-Only Approach for Total Sacrectomy

While staged anterior-posterior approaches are the preferred option for total sacrectomy at our institution, other authors have advocated for posterior-only approaches. Good oncologic outcomes with low rates of bowel or vascular injury have been reported with posterior-only total sacrectomy [18, 70]. The use of radioopaque gauze, packed anteriorly to the sacrum, from above the iliac crests and through the greater sciatic foramina, has been described as a method of tamponading anterior bleeding and displacing the iliac vasculature and pelvic viscera away from the osteotomy sites [70]. Disadvantages of a posterior-only approach include blind dissection of the rectum off of the anterior surface of the sacrum and inability to ligate the internal iliac vasculature as a method of decreasing blood loss. Additionally, a posterior-only approach precludes the ability to harvest a rectus abdominis flap, though proponents have argued that preservation of the gluteal vessels (and internal iliac system as a whole) decreases soft tissue ischemia and allows for successful closure with gluteus maximus myocutaneous flaps [18]. Potential contraindications to posterior-only total sacrectomy include direct tumor invasion of the rectum or iliac vessels, or tumor extension cephalad to the L5/S1 disk space [18].

Our preference for malignant tumors, in which curative resection is the goal, is for staged anterior and posterior approaches for both total and partial sacrectomies. For benign tumors such as GCTs, for which intralesional margins are acceptable, a posterior approach may permit excellent nerve root visualization. However, in addition to the aforementioned benefits of decreased blood loss (after internal iliac ligation) and safer dissection about the rectum and pelvic vasculature, we feel that negative margins can be more reliably obtained from a combined approach. Tumor visualization is best when approached anteriorly, and "scoring" the anterior cortical osteotomy during the first stage prevents subsequent "lifting up" and splintering of the anterior cortex, which can occur in posterior-only osteotomies and which can result in less precise margins.

21.6 Complications

Complications following sacrectomies are common, including surgical site infection, hardware failure, vascular or visceral injury, and CSF leak and pseudomeningocele formation. Additionally, postoperative bowel, bladder, and sexual dysfunction are typically expected, as discussed above, following sacrifice of the upper sacral nerve roots. The rates of major complications are likely increased in total and high partial sacrectomies: 85% vs. 29% for resections above vs. below S2, respectively, in one series [71]. In a review of 46 patients undergoing partial or total sacrectomy, Sciubba et al. [72] reported postoperative infection in 39% of patients. Identified risk factors included prior lumbosacral surgery and number of surgeons scrubbed into the case, regardless of length of operation. While staphlococcus aureus was the most frequently cultured organism, the relatively high rate of gram-negative infections led the authors to posit that proximity to the rectum, especially in the context of bowel (or bladder) dysfunction, might increase the risk of surgical site infection after sacrectomy. Interestingly, another study of postoperative complications described two *delayed* rectal perforations, both within 2–3 weeks of sacrectomy, thought to result from bowel ischemia in the setting of internal iliac ligation [62]. This series, reporting on complications in 34 patients with primary sacral tumors, identified five infections, three cases of postoperative foot drop (likely resulting from L5 nerve root injury), one case of cutaneous CSF fistula formation, and three perioperative deaths, highlighting the significant risks associated with these surgeries. Hardware failure occurred after total sacrectomy in 16% of patients included in a systematic review [42], though our experience suggests that the use of adjuvant high-dose radiation significantly increases the risk of postoperative fracture (up to 57%) [8], as well as nonunion and hardware failure. Radiation likely increases the risk of infection as well. A large series from our institution identified wound infection or dehiscence in 20 of 118 patients (17%) undergoing resection of spinal chordomas, all of whom received radiation as well [26]. Specifically, wound complications were observed in 13 of 60 patients (22%) treated with neo- *and* adjuvant radiation, as compared with 7 of 58 patients (12%) treated with adjuvant radiation alone.

Conflict-of-Interest Statement No benefits have been or will be received from a commercial party related directly or indirectly to the subject matter of this article.

References

1. Sugar O. How the sacrum got its name. JAMA. 1987;257(15):2061–3.
2. Drake RL, Vogl W, Mitchell AW, Tibbitts R, Richardson P, Horn A. Gray's anatomy for students. Philadelphia: Churchill Livingstone; 2010.
3. Fourney DR, Rhines LD, Hentschel SJ, Skibber JM, Wolinsky JP, Weber KL, Suki D, Gallia GL, Garonzik I, Gokaslan ZL. En bloc resection of primary sacral tumors: classification of surgical approaches and outcome. J Neurosurg Spine. 2005;3(2):111–22.
4. Dickey ID, Hugate Jr RR, Fuchs B, Yaszemski MJ, Sim FH. Reconstruction after total sacrectomy: early experience with a new surgical technique. Clin Orthop Relat Res. 2005;438:42–50.
5. Gunterberg B. Effects of major resection of the sacrum clinical studies on urogenital and anorectal function and a biomechanical study on pelvic strength. Acta Orthop Scand. 1976;47(sup162):1–38.
6. Hugate Jr RR, Dickey ID, Phimolsarnti R, Yaszemski MJ, Sim FH. Mechanical effects of partial sacrectomy: when is reconstruction necessary? Clin Orthop Relat Res. 2006;450:82–8.
7. Todd Jr LT, Yaszemski MJ, Currier BL, Fuchs B, Kim CW, Sim FH. Bowel and bladder function after major sacral resection. Clin Orthop Relat Res. 2002;397:36–9.
8. Osler P, Bredella MA, Hess KA, Janssen SJ, Park CJ, Chen YL, DeLaney TF, Hornicek FJ, Schwab JH. Sacral insufficiency fractures are common after high-dose radiation for sacral chordomas treated with or without surgery. Clin Orthop Relat Res. 2016;474(3):766–72.
9. Ruggieri P, Angelini A, Ussia G, Montalti M, Mercuri M. Surgical margins and local control in resection of sacral chordomas. Clin Orthop Relat Res. 2010;468(11):2939–47.
10. Moran D, Zadnik PL, Taylor T, Groves ML, Yurter A, Wolinsky JP, Witham TF, Bydon A, Gokaslan ZL, Sciubba DM. Maintenance of bowel, bladder, and motor functions after sacrectomy. Spine J. 2015;15(2):222–9.
11. Schwab JH, Healey JH, Rose P, Casas-Ganem J, Boland PJ. The surgical management of sacral chordomas. Spine. 2009;34(24):2700–4.
12. Gunterberg B, Petersén I. Sexual function after major resections of the sacrum with bilateral or unilateral sacrifice of sacral nerves. Fertil Steril. 1976;27(10):1146–53.
13. Gunterberg B, Kewenter J, Petersen I, Stener B. Anorectal function after major resections of the sacrum with bilateral or unilateral sacrifice of sacral nerves. Br J Surg. 1976;63(7):546–54.
14. van Wulfften Palthe OD, Houdek MT, Rose PS, Yaszemski MJ, Sim FH, Boland PJ, Healey JH, Hornicek FJ, Schwab JH. How does the level of nerve root resection in en bloc sacrectomy influence patient-reported outcomes? Clin Orthop Relat Res. 2017;475(3):607–16.
15. Phukan R, Herzog T, Boland PJ, Healey J, Rose P, Sim FH, Yazsemski M, Hess K, Osler P, DeLaney TF, Chen YL. How does the level of sacral resection for primary malignant bone tumors affect physical and mental health, pain, mobility, incontinence, and sexual function? Clin Orthop Relat Res. 2016;474(3):687–96.
16. Sebro R, DeLaney TF, Hornicek F, Schwab J, Choy E, Nielsen GP, Rosenthal DI. Frequency and risk factors for additional lesions in the axial spine in subjects with chordoma: indications for screening. Spine. 2016;42(1):E37–40.
17. Bergh P, Kindblom LG, Gunterberg B, Remotti F, Ryd W, Meis-Kindblom JM. Prognostic factors in chordoma of the sacrum and mobile spine. Cancer. 2000;88(9):2122–34.
18. Clarke MJ, Dasenbrock H, Bydon A, Sciubba DM, McGirt MJ, Hsieh PC, Yassari R, Gokaslan ZL, Wolinsky JP. Posterior-only approach for en bloc sacrectomy: clinical outcomes in 36 consecutive patients. Neurosurgery. 2012;71(2):357–64.

19. Nelson AC, Pillay N, Henderson S, Presneau N, Tirabosco R, Halai D, Berisha F, Flicek P, Stemple DL, Stern CD, Wardle FC. An integrated functional genomics approach identifies the regulatory network directed by brachyury (T) in chordoma. J Pathol. 2012;228(3): 274–85.
20. Bettegowda C, Yip S, Lo SFL, Fisher CG, Boriani S, Rhines LD, Wang JY, Lazary A, Gambarotti M, Wang WL, Luzzati A. Spinal column chordoma: prognostic significance of clinical variables and T (brachyury) gene SNP rs2305089 for local recurrence and overall survival. Neuro Oncol. 2017;19(3):405–13.
21. Pillay N, Plagnol V, Tarpey PS, Lobo SB, Presneau N, Szuhai K, Halai D, Berisha F, Cannon SR, Mead S, Kasperaviciute D. A common single-nucleotide variant in T is strongly associated with chordoma. Nat Genet. 2012;44(11):1185–7.
22. Deutsch H, Mummaneni PV, Haid RW, Rodts GE, Ondra SL. Benign sacral tumors. Neurosurg Focus. 2003;15(2):1–3.
23. McMaster ML, Goldstein AM, Bromley CM, Ishibe N, Parry DM. Chordoma: incidence and survival patterns in the United States, 1973–1995. Cancer Causes Control. 2001;12(1):1–11.
24. Sundaresan N. Chordomas. Clin Orthop Relat Res. 1986;204:135–42.
25. Fuchs B, Dickey ID, Yaszemski MJ, Inwards CY, Sim FH. Operative management of sacral chordoma. J Bone Joint Surg Am. 2005;87(10):2211–6.
26. Rotondo RL, Folkert W, Liebsch NJ, Chen YLE, Pedlow FX, Schwab JH, Rosenberg AE, Nielsen GP, Szymonifka J, Ferreira AE, Hornicek FJ. High-dose proton-based radiation therapy in the management of spine chordomas: outcomes and clinicopathological prognostic factors. J Neurosurg Spine. 2015;23(6):788–97.
27. Yonemoto T, Tatezaki SI, Takenouchi T, Ishii T, Satoh T, Moriya H. The surgical management of sacrococcygeal chordoma. Cancer. 1999;85(4):878–83.
28. Varga PP, Szövérfi Z, Fisher CG, Boriani S, Gokaslan ZL, Dekutoski MB, Chou D, Quraishi NA, Reynolds JJ, Luzzati A, Williams R. Surgical treatment of sacral chordoma: prognostic variables for local recurrence and overall survival. Eur Spine J. 2015;24(5):1092–101.
29. Hanna SA, Aston WJS, Briggs TWR, Cannon SR, Saifuddin A. Sacral chordoma: can local recurrence after sacrectomy be predicted? Clin Orthop Relat Res. 2008;466(9):2217–23.
30. Young VA, Curtis KM, Temple HT, Eismont FJ, DeLaney TF, Hornicek FJ. Characteristics and patterns of metastatic disease from chordoma. Sarcoma. 2015;2015:7.
31. DeLaney TF, Liebsch NJ, Pedlow FX, Adams J, Dean S, Yeap BY, McManus P, Rosenberg AE, Nielsen GP, Harmon DC, Spiro IJ. Phase II study of high-dose photon/proton radiotherapy in the management of spine sarcomas. Int J Radiat Oncol Biol Phys. 2009;74(3):732–9.
32. DeLaney TF, Liebsch NJ, Pedlow FX, Adams J, Weyman EA, Yeap BY, Depauw N, Nielsen GP, Harmon DC, Yoon SS, Chen YL. Long-term results of Phase II study of high dose photon/proton radiotherapy in the management of spine chordomas, chondrosarcomas, and other sarcomas. J Surg Oncol. 2014;110(2):115–22.
33. Park L, DeLaney TF, Liebsch NJ, Hornicek FJ, Goldberg S, Mankin H, Rosenberg AE, Rosenthal DI, Suit HD. Sacral chordomas: impact of high-dose proton/photon-beam radiation therapy combined with or without surgery for primary versus recurrent tumor. Int J Radiat Oncol Biol Phys. 2006;65(5):1514–21.
34. Chen YL, Liebsch N, Kobayashi W, Goldberg S, Kirsch D, Calkins G, Childs S, Schwab J, Hornicek F, DeLaney T. Definitive high-dose photon/proton radiotherapy for unresected mobile spine and sacral chordomas. Spine. 2013;38(15):E930–6.
35. Kabolizadeh P, Chen YL, Liebsch N, Hornicek F, Schwab J, Choy E, Rosenthal D, Niemierko A, DeLaney TF. Updated outcome and analysis of tumor response in mobile spine and sacral chordoma treated with definitive high dose photon/proton radiotherapy. Int J Radiat Oncol Biol Phys. 2016;97(2):254–62.
36. Diaz RJ, Cusimano MD. The biological basis for modern treatment of chordoma. J Neuro-Oncol. 2011;104(2):411–22.
37. Imai R, Kamada T, Sugahara S, Tsuji H, Tsujii H. Carbon ion radiotherapy for sacral chordoma. Br J Radiol. 2011;84:S48–53.

38. Imai R, Kamada T, Araki N, Working Group for Bone and Soft Tissue Sarcomas. Carbon ion radiation therapy for unresectable sacral chordoma: an analysis of 188 cases. Int J Radiat Oncol Biol Phys. 2016;95(1):322–7.
39. Uhl M, Welzel T, Jensen A, Ellerbrock M, Haberer T, Jäkel O, Herfarth K, Debus J. Carbon ion beam treatment in patients with primary and recurrent sacrococcygeal chordoma. Strahlenther Onkol. 2015;191(7):597–603.
40. Schwab J, Antonescu C, Boland P, Healey J, Rosenberg A, Nielsen P, Iafrate J, Delaney T, Yoon S, Choy E, Harmon D. Combination of PI3K/mTOR inhibition demonstrates efficacy in human chordoma. Anticancer Res. 2009;29(6):1867–71.
41. Stuckey RM, Marco RA. Chondrosarcoma of the mobile spine and sacrum. Sarcoma. 2011;2011:4.
42. Bederman SS, Shah KN, Hassan JM, Hoang BH, Kiester PD, Bhatia NN. Surgical techniques for spinopelvic reconstruction following total sacrectomy: a systematic review. Eur Spine J. 2014;23(2):305–19.
43. Bergh P, Gunterberg B, Meis-Kindblom JM, Kindblom LG. Prognostic factors and outcome of pelvic, sacral, and spinal chondrosarcomas. Cancer. 2001;91(7):1201–12.
44. Hsieh PC, Xu R, Sciubba DM, McGirt MJ, Nelson C, Witham TF, Wolinksy JP, Gokaslan ZL. Long-term clinical outcomes following en bloc resections for sacral chordomas and chondrosarcomas: a series of twenty consecutive patients. Spine. 2009;34(20):2233–9.
45. Ozaki T, Flege S, Liljenqvist U, Hillmann A, Delling G, Salzer-Kuntschik M, Jürgens H, Kotz R, Winkelmann W, Bielack SS. Osteosarcoma of the spine. Cancer. 2002;94(4):1069–77.
46. Schoenfeld AJ, Hornicek FJ, Pedlow FX, Kobayashi W, Garcia RT, DeLaney TF, Springfield D, Mankin HJ, Schwab JH. Osteosarcoma of the spine: experience in 26 patients treated at the Massachusetts General Hospital. Spine J. 2010;10(8):708–14.
47. Dozois EJ, Privitera A, Holubar SD, Aldrete JF, Sim FH, Rose PS, Walsh MF, Bower TC, Leibovich BC, Nelson H, Larson DW. High sacrectomy for locally recurrent rectal cancer: can long-term survival be achieved? J Surg Oncol. 2011;103(2):105–9.
48. Wells BJ, Stotland P, Ko MA, Al-Sukhni W, Wunder J, Ferguson P, Lipa J, Last L, Smith AJ, Swallow CJ. Results of an aggressive approach to resection of locally recurrent rectal cancer. Ann Surg Oncol. 2007;14(2):390–5.
49. Zacherl J, Schiessel R, Windhager R, Herbst F, Karner-Hanusch J, Kotz R, Jakesz R, Teleky B. Abdominosacral resection of recurrent rectal cancer in the sacrum. Dis Colon Rectum. 1999;42(8):1035–9.
50. Leggon RE, Zlotecki R, Reith J, Scarborough MT. Giant cell tumor of the pelvis and sacrum: 17 cases and analysis of the literature. Clin Orthop Relat Res. 2004;423:196–207.
51. Raskin KA, Schwab JH, Mankin HJ, Springfield DS, Hornicek FJ. Giant cell tumor of bone. J Am Acad Orthop Surg. 2013;21(2):118–26.
52. Turcotte RE, Sim FH, Unni KK. Giant cell tumor of the sacrum. Clin Orthop Relat Res. 1993;291:215–21.
53. Goldenberg RR, Campbell CJ, Bonfiglio M. Giant-cell tumor of bone. J Bone Joint Surg Am. 1970;52(4):619–64.
54. Gottfried ON, Schmidt MH, Stevens EA. Embolization of sacral tumors. Neurosurg Focus. 2003;15(2):1–4.
55. Hosalkar HS, Jones KJ, King JJ, Lackman RD. Serial arterial embolization for large sacral giant-cell tumors: mid-to long-term results. Spine. 2007;32(10):1107–15.
56. Lin PP, Guzel VB, Moura MF, Wallace S, Benjamin RS, Weber KL, Morello FA, Gokaslan ZL, Yasko AW. Long-term follow-up of patients with giant cell tumor of the sacrum treated with selective arterial embolization. Cancer. 2002;95(6):1317–25.
57. Wojcik J, Rosenberg AE, Bredella MA, Choy E, Hornicek FJ, Nielsen GP, Deshpande V. Denosumab-treated giant cell tumor of bone exhibits morphologic overlap with malignant giant cell tumor of bone. Am J Surg Pathol. 2016;40(1):72–80.
58. Chawla S, Henshaw R, Seeger L, Choy E, Blay JY, Ferrari S, Kroep J, Grimer R, Reichardt P, Rutkowski P, Schuetze S. Safety and efficacy of denosumab for adults and skeletally mature

adolescents with giant cell tumour of bone: interim analysis of an open-label, parallel-group, phase 2 study. Lancet Oncol. 2013;14(9):901–8.
59. Ueda T, Morioka H, Nishida Y, Kakunaga S, Tsuchiya H, Matsumoto Y, Asami Y, Inoue T, Yoneda T. Objective tumor response to denosumab in patients with giant cell tumor of bone: a multicenter phase II trial. Ann Oncol. 2015;26(10):2149–54.
60. Miles WK, Chang DW, Kroll SS, Miller MJ, Langstein HN, Reece GP, Evans GR, Robb GL. Reconstruction of large sacral defects following total sacrectomy. Plast Reconstr Surg. 2000;105(7):2387–94.
61. Abhinav K, Shaaban M, Raymond T, Oke T, Gullan R, Montgomery ACV. Primary reconstruction of pelvic floor defects following sacrectomy using Permacol™ graft. Eur J Surg Oncol. 2009;35(4):439–43.
62. Zileli M, Hoscoskun C, Brastianos P, Sabah D. Surgical treatment of primary sacral tumors: complications associated with sacrectomy. Neurosurg Focus. 2003;15(5):1–8.
63. Yang HL, Chen KW, Wang GL, Lu J, Ji YM, Liu JY, Wu GZ, Gu Y, Sun ZY. Pre-operative transarterial embolization for treatment of primary sacral tumors. J Clin Neurosci. 2010;17(10):1280–5.
64. Tang X, Guo W, Yang R, Tang S, Dong S. Use of aortic balloon occlusion to decrease blood loss during sacral tumor resection. J Bone Joint Surg Am. 2010;92(8):1747–53.
65. Yang L, Chong-qi T, Hai-bo S, Lan Z, Tian-fu Y, Hong D, Fu-xing P. Applying the abdominal aortic-balloon occluding combine with blood pressure sensor of dorsal artery of foot to control bleeding during the pelvic and sacrum tumors surgery. J Surg Oncol. 2008;97(7):626–8.
66. Zoccali C, Skoch J, Patel A, Walter CM, Maykowski P, Baaj AA. The surgical neurovascular anatomy relating to partial and complete sacral and sacroiliac resections: a cadaveric, anatomic study. Eur Spine J. 2015;24(5):1109–13.
67. Mindea SA, Chinthakunta S, Moldavsky M, Gudipally M, Khalil S. Biomechanical comparison of spinopelvic reconstruction techniques in the setting of total sacrectomy. Spine. 2012;37(26):E1622–7.
68. Choudry UH, Moran SL, Karacor Z. Functional reconstruction of the pelvic ring with simultaneous bilateral free fibular flaps following total sacral resection. Ann Plast Surg. 2006;57(6):673–6.
69. Garvey PB, Clemens MW, Rhines LD, Sacks JM. Vertical rectus abdominis musculocutaneous flow-through flap to a free fibula flap for total sacrectomy reconstruction. Microsurgery. 2013;33(1):32–8.
70. Asavamongkolkul A, Waikakul S. Wide resection of sacral chordoma via a posterior approach. Int Orthop. 2012;36(3):607–12.
71. Devin C, Chong PY, Holt GE, Feurer I, Gonzalez A, Merchant N, Schwartz HS. Level-adjusted perioperative risk of sacral amputations. J Surg Oncol. 2006;94(3):203–11.
72. Sciubba DM, Nelson C, Gok B, McGirt MJ, McLoughlin GS, Noggle JC, Wolinsky JP, Witham TF, Bydon A, Gokaslan ZL. Evaluation of factors associated with postoperative infection following sacral tumor resection: clinical article. J Neurosurg Spine. 2008;9(6):593–9.

Computer Navigation in the Sacrum

22

David M. Joyce

22.1 Introduction

Computer navigation has been introduced as an intraoperative guidance option as an alternative for fluoroscopy because this two-dimensional (2D) imaging has limitation in orthopedic oncology surgery because of the difficulty in identifying the full geometric extent of the lesion as well as intraosseous involvement [1]. Computed tomography (CT)-based computer navigation aims to help the surgeon by increasing the spatial accuracy when performing surgery in and around the pelvis by augmenting a surgeon's visibility. The demanding three-dimensional (3D) configuration of the sacrum and pelvic anatomy, tumor size, structural alterations due to tumor, neoadjuvant therapy, rarity (leading to a lack of experience on part of the surgeon), and the morbidity associated with sacral and pelvic resection has in the past resulted with positive surgical margins in the majority of cases, with local recurrence approaching rates of 70–80% [2–9]. This has made limb salvage, improved function, and decreased morbidity hard to attain without sacrificing surgical margins until the advent and use of computer navigation for surgical resection. Computer navigation has increased the precision, accuracy and ability to preserve sacral and pelvic structures with the intention of not compromising oncologic outcomes in terms of margins and recurrence. It has improved the visualization of the surgical field through a virtual 3D reconstruction of the surgical field allowing for precise osteotomy resection levels [4]. Only computer navigation that is based on advanced imaging can be used for tumor resections in the sacrum and pelvis. Several studies looking at computer navigation have reported advantages to using this modality in pelvic and sacral tumors [2, 10, 11]. Knowing where a resection tool ends when a

D.M. Joyce, M.D.
Sarcoma Department, H. Lee Moffitt Cancer Center, Tampa, FL, USA
e-mail: David.Joyce@moffitt.org

P. Ruggieri et al. (eds.), *Tumors of the Sacrum*,
DOI 10.1007/978-3-319-51202-0_22

surgeon is unable to protect the tumor on the other side is of great benefit. Unfortunately, all too often in tumor resection we do not have direct line of sight and the benefit of navigation is that a virtual line of sight is obtained. This chapter intends to explain computer navigation in sacral oncology surgery with respect to its developmental history and clinical use.

22.2 History and Progression of Computer Navigation

Computer-assisted surgery specifically computer navigation is relatively new to the musculoskeletal oncology world. Computer-assisted surgery has been used for over 20 years for cranial biopsies and tumor resections in neurosurgery [12]. Computer navigation has also been used in spine, trauma, knee, and hip surgery and was originally developed for those surgical environments [13]. There are three types of computer navigation: imageless navigation, fluoroscopic navigation, and advanced imaging navigation consisting of computed tomography (CT) and magnetic resonance imaging (MRI). Computer navigation CT based was introduced for pedicle screw fixation in 1993 and has been used in total hip and total knee reconstructive surgery for component placement [14, 15]. In spine surgery, navigation has led to a benefit of decreased rate of misplaced pedicle screws to 5% with navigation compared to 16–40% misplaced screws with conventional techniques [10, 16, 17]. Another advantage is orthopedic hardware that can be placed accurately within 1 mm of the desired location [10, 18]. Langlotz et al. performed the first CT-based computer-assisted osteotomy in 1995 [19]. It wasn't until 2004 that the use of computer-navigated chisels was reportedly used to perform an osteotomy for a sacral tumor [20]. Computer navigation offers benefits to musculoskeletal oncology and sacrum surgery that the community is only beginning to realize [2, 10, 20–28].

Sacral and pelvic bone tumors are usually large at presentation and often invade and compromise important anatomical structures such as nerves and vessels specifically the femoral and sciatic nerves and sacral nerve roots, iliac vessels, and pelvic viscera along with invading into the sacral bone and foramina [3, 4, 29]. Obtaining negative margins in sacral and pelvic surgery is difficult and studies that have looked at sarcoma resection in the pelvis have reported higher positive margin rates and thus higher local recurrence rates compared to the treatment of sarcomas in the extremities [20, 30] suggesting it is harder to obtain adequate surgical margins in areas difficult to identify structures. The purpose of computer navigation in the musculoskeletal oncology setting is to first plan and then assist in executing a local wide excision with preservation of vital structures. As with all tumor surgery, removing all the tumor is first priority, but with computer navigation one can remove less normal tissue which aids in reconstruction without increasing the risk of inadvertent tumor violation [23]. Computer navigation used in the sacrum can help identify where the surgeon is and if the anatomy is distorted, which occurs often, by better understanding the relationship between malignant tumor and surrounding structures [23, 31, 32] thus allowing the surgeon to minimize the morbidity in the surgical field. This relatively new technology can aid a surgeon in saving nerves and thus preserving function and improving margins. This intraoperative system produces and allows for real-time visual feedback that can be seen on a monitor above the surgical field. It is this real-time feedback that augments and enhances the surgeon's direct interpretation of the visual and tactile perception of the surgical field. Unfortunately, little data exists on computer navigation and sacral surgery due to the rarity of both sacral tumors and the limited use of navigation in musculoskeletal oncology in the oncology community. This chapter is intended to present computer navigation and its use in sacral surgery; however, most of the data presented comes from computer navigation with respect to the pelvic (sacral included) surgery both oncologic and non-oncologic.

22.3 Computer Navigation Systems Overview

Several different computer navigation systems that exist in the commercial world consist of imageless navigation, fluoroscopic navigation, and advanced imaging navigation. It is most important to understand that most navigation was developed for spine, trauma, or hip and knee surgery for accuracy of hardware placement. Computer navigation has been used for pedicle screw application, component positioning in total hip and knee arthroplasty, and ACL reconstruction [15, 33–35]. Computer navigation has also been used for pelvic osteotomies, SI screw, and acetabular fracture screw placement [18, 36–38]. Most of the computer navigation for sacral and pelvic oncology surgery is commercially adapted software not developed for oncology. The commercially available computer navigation used for oncology is CT based but can be augmented with an MRI for the benefit of identifying marrow edema. While MRI and CT are excellent for identifying osseous tumor, infiltration margins are often difficult to identify intraoperatively in the pelvis [29]. Patients can undergo MRI and CT imaging and have these images fused if the surgeon elects and then uploads to the navigation system [39, 40]. CT is great for bone resection planning but MRI is essential to determine marrow infiltration and true bony involvement [11, 41]. Planning for resection can be done on the computer navigation system prior to surgery. This resection plan is then used after the patient is registered in the operating room.

22.4 Computer Navigation Requirements

In order to understand navigation and its benefits in the sacrum and pelvis with respect to oncology, one must understand the basics. Some form of 3D imaging (CT, MRI, PET CT) is required of the sacrum and preferably of the entire pelvis for proper registration prior to surgery. Some elect to also obtain an MRI for the possibility of CT-MRI fusion. At a minimum, a CT scan of the affected bone must be obtained that has 0.5–2 mm cuts, continuous with no overlap [20, 28, 31, 39, 40, 42]. If obtaining an MRI, similar slice thickness and scanning limits should be obtained.

If using fiducial markers, later discussed, the slice thickness should be less than the fiducial width size; otherwise, the possibility exists of missing the fiducial marker on scanning. After the preoperative CT scan, there are three required components to computer navigation in the setting of the sacrum or pelvis. These include a computer platform loaded with some form of computer navigation software; several exist commercially but none are specific for oncology [25, 26]. Second a tracking system is used, which can either consist of optical trackers (consisting of three OCD cameras) or electromagnetic trackers using a coil to detect changes in position [43]. At our institution, we use optical trackers and cameras (Figs. 22.1, 22.2, and 22.3). The last important component is referencing system and methods by which one references the patient's anatomy in all navigation systems. These include 2D and 3D fluoroscopic, imageless, kinematic, bone morphing or "pair matching," and ultrasound referencing [13] with the use of a pointer. For surgery of the pelvis and sacrum, our institution uses 3D fluoroscopy in the form of the Arcadis Orbic 3D system (Siemens) (Fig. 22.4) in order to properly register our patients with their preoperative CT scan, bone surface matching and paired-point matching can be later used for registration refinement. Other places use 2D fluoroscopy, fiducial markers, and some places described the use of the O-arm or intraoperative CT scan if fiducial markers are not used prior to a preoperative CT scan. It is important for one to understand the limitation of the navigation system one is using as well as having knowledge of accuracy

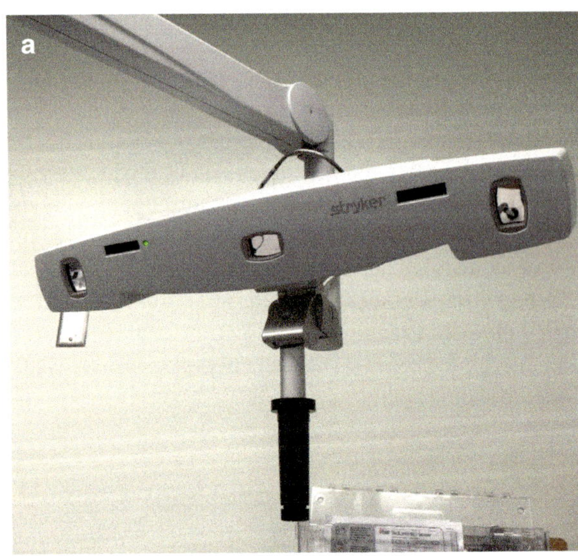

Fig. 22.1 (**a**) Optical Tracking System. (**b**) Optical Tracking System placed over the head of the bed for optimal "line of sight"

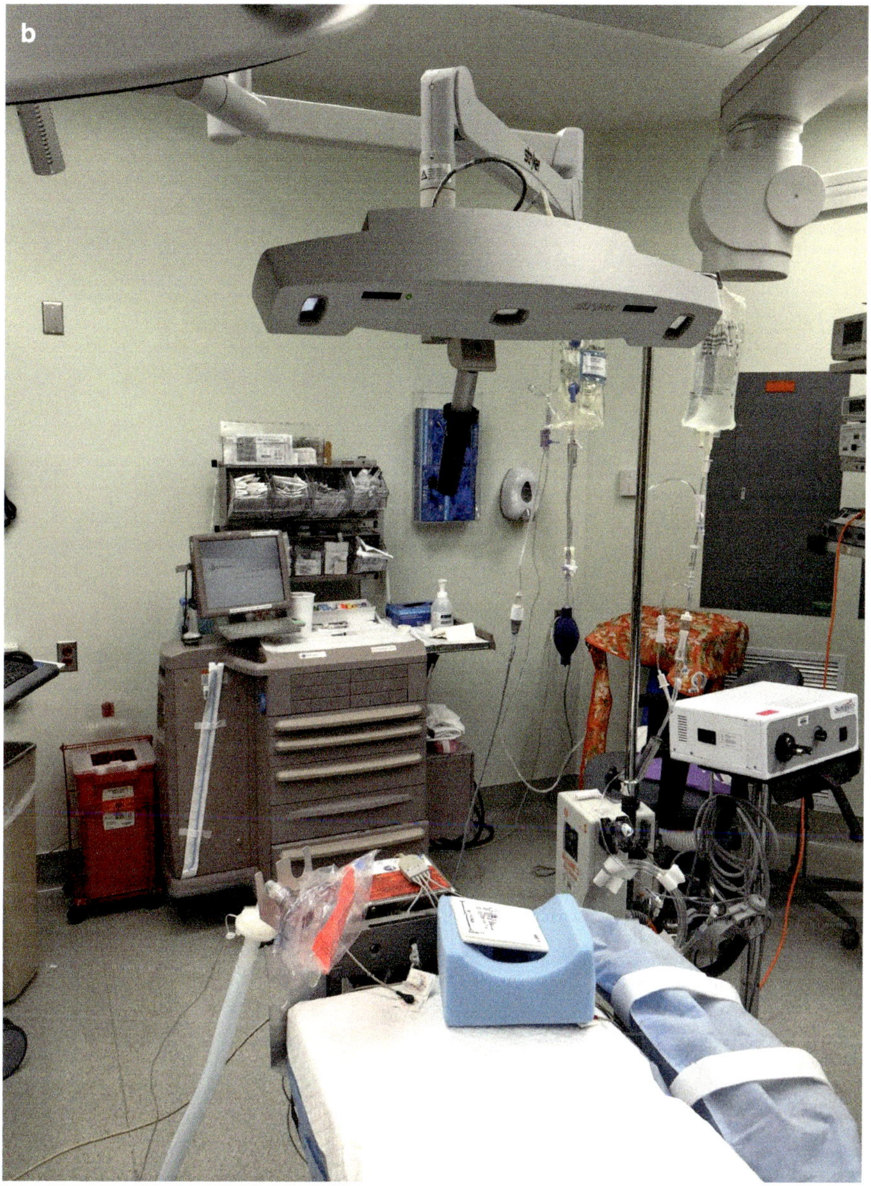

Fig. 22.1 (continued)

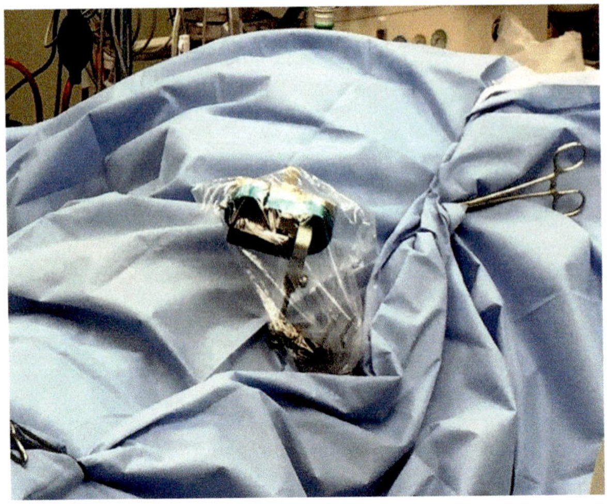

Fig. 22.2 Tracker attached to the pelvis with three pins with the patient in the prone position; the tracker is oriented to see the camera. It is important to appreciate line of sight and avoid drapes, tubing, and electrocautery wiring blocking the view of the camera

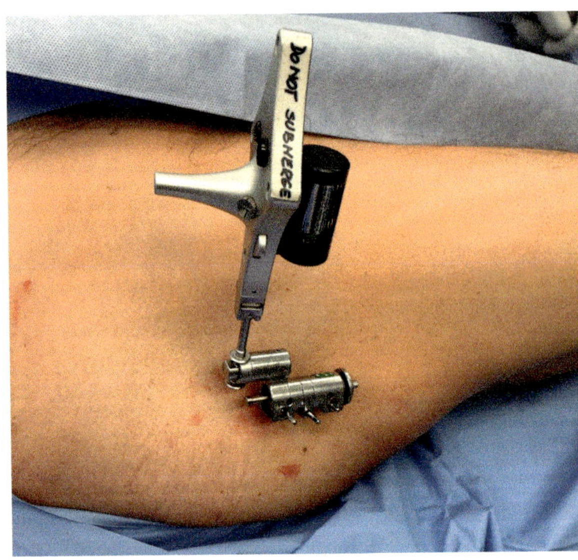

Fig. 22.3 Alternate tracker sometimes used if unable to register with the standard patient tracker

of the system and knowing what affects accuracy [13, 44–47]. There is no specific navigation software for oncologic surgery; most navigation systems used today are from commercially available systems that are then adapted for their use [25, 26], so it is important to understand each system limitations as they are different.

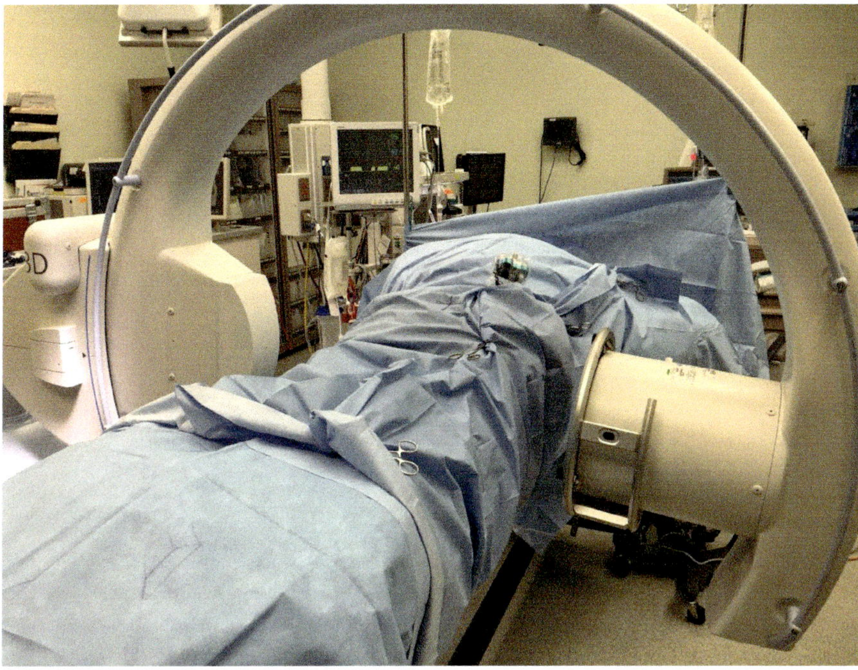

Fig. 22.4 Arcadis Orbic 3D fluoroscopic system

22.5 Computer Navigation Process

Preoperative Process: The use of computer navigation starts with obtaining 3D imaging of the tumor in question. Navigation of the pelvis and sacrum cannot be performed with imageless referencing, and thus all this navigation is based on CT, MRI, and CT-MRI fusion imaging. This is because "imageless navigation" uses the pelvic plane and bony landmarks for reference and soft tissue on the pelvis renders this method fairly inaccurate [48–50]. In order to use computer navigation, the entire bone must be imaged. While theoretically one could just image the sacrum, it is very hard to identify specific bony landmarks on the sacrum intraoperatively, and thus the entire pelvis is often imaged. Bone tumor resection requires several important steps in order to make the osteotomy almost effortless. Fluoro-CT matching and 3D fluoroscopy may allow for more accurate resections because soft tissue on the sacrum and pelvis can distort the ability to use surface matching and paired-point matching [24, 42]. Newer navigation systems exist with the use of cone-beam computed tomography or O-arm that allows 3D image quality with submillimeter spatial resolution with less radiation dose that can be used repeatedly in the operating room [27, 51]. The most important study to obtain is a preoperative CT with or without fiducial markers.

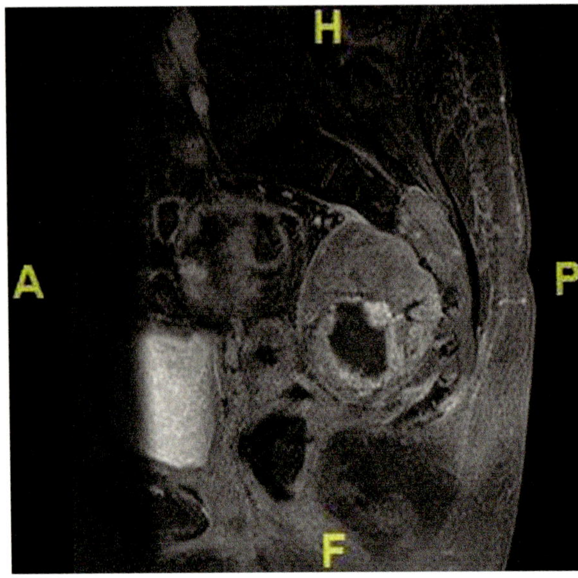

Fig. 22.5 Contrast MRI of the sacrum showing bone infiltration not easily appreciated on an X-ray

The purpose of navigation is to identify the bony margins for resection, and thus a CT scan is used because it is the best modality for cortical bone. MRI and CT have a high sensitivity and specificity for bony tumor infiltration but margins are difficult to identify intraoperatively and intralesional resection is very much possible in the sacrum [29]. Currently, surgeons not using navigation rely on two-dimensional imaging consisting of a CT and MRI obtained preoperatively and then analyze and reconstruct the images into a 3D model within their mind during the intraoperative resection leading to significant inaccuracies in tumor resection [31, 39, 40]. While CT is often better at visualizing cortical bone status, MRI (Fig. 22.5) is the best method for defining marrow involvement for bone tumors and soft tissue sarcomas when planning for resection margins [52]. A surgeon can measure on MRI the marrow infiltration and then recreate this measurement on the CT used in computer navigation as long as a similar slice thickness is used. In general, when we perform surgery in the pelvis and on the sacrum using computer navigation, we typically only use the CT imaging although some will use a CT-MRI fusion [1, 2, 11, 52]. We can see some of the soft tissue on CT although not as well as on an MRI. While we have not taken advantage of CT-MRI fusion, this modality is probably the best way to look at soft tissue when using computer navigation. CT-MRI fusion allows for determining the extent of tumor resection planes based on the bony involvement seen on the navigated software [25, 26]. CT-MRI fusion use has been described and was felt to be beneficial to the surgical procedure [24]. Most fiducial markers in the past were K-wires or titanium screws not allowing for the MRI to be used in preoperative imaging for navigation. Some studies have described using resorbable 1.5 mm pins placed beyond the tumor resection so that CT-MRI fusion and MRI images alone can be used for patient registration [52]. While MRI alone can be used as an intraoperative guide, its use in registration for navigation requires the use of paired-point registration but obtaining a registration error of <1 mm is hard without using fiducial markers

[2] and metal markers cannot be used due to artifact associated with MRI. An important point several authors make is that when using fiducial markers the slice cut must be less than the slice thickness of either the preoperative MRI or CT scan; otherwise, the possibility exists that one may miss the fiducial marker on the scan [52]. The image fusion process is not without its own contribution to registration errors because merging is still done visually by the surgeon leading to potential error even with the best processes producing errors of 6 mm or more [52, 53].

Next comes planning on part of the surgeon through the aid of MRI for soft tissue component and bony peritumoral edema and as well a CT for bone component to determine the resection level. A specific CT consisting of a protocol for navigational software must be obtained in order to be imported into the navigation or computer-assisted software. At a minimum, a CT scan of the entire affected bone must be obtained that has 0.5–2 mm cuts, continuous, and with no overlap [20, 28, 31, 39, 40, 42]. Virtual planning comes at the time when a CT scan is imported into the navigational software and the surgeon elects planes to determine the starting point and vector of the intended plane for future osteotomy or resection plane (Fig. 22.6). This all occurs prior to the patient coming to surgery and is determined by the interpretation of the preoperative imaging at a minimum consisting of a CT, but can include an MRI.

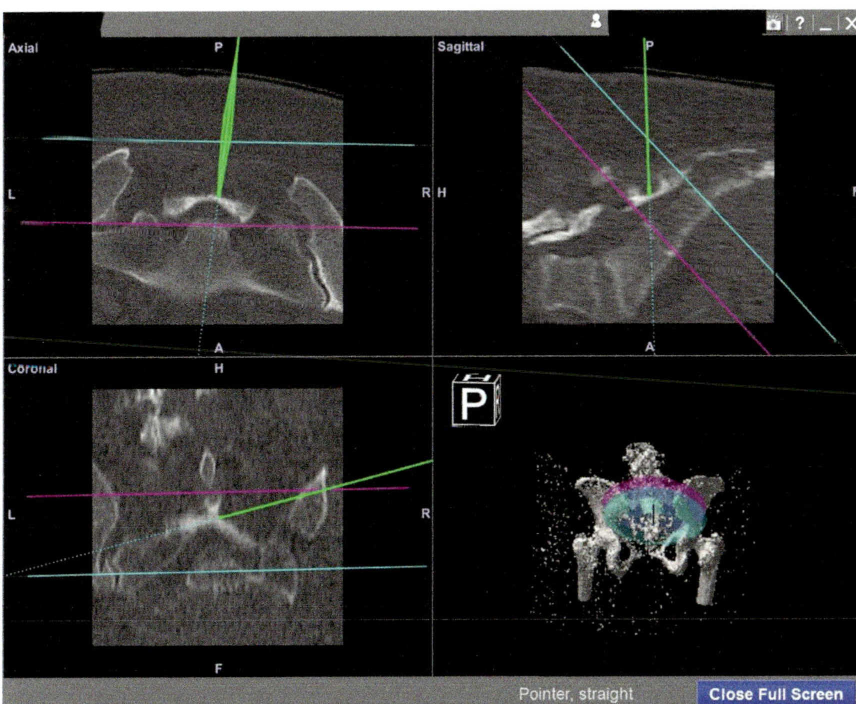

Fig. 22.6 Navigation screen showing tip of navigated instrument in *green*; the other planes represent the sacral joints in several different planes. This figure shows the navigated pointer and its use to identify the beginning of the resection level. The other planes were created during preoperative planning in order to avoid resection above or below these levels

Intraoperative Process: The intraoperative process consists of tracker placement, registration, and then resection. Intraoperative registration can occur at one of two time points, both of which are after the patient has been put under general anesthesia. Either at the beginning prior to major surgical incision or at the time prior to resection after all is exposed. This is determined by the technology available or the surgeon's preference on whether they think registration through "paired matching" based on surface landmarks will be accurate enough or whether a reconstruction by fluoroscopic "spin" with a C-arm would be more accurate.

When performing surgery with computer navigation, it is important to understand tracker placement. Optical trackers can have issues with line of sight (Figs. 22.1 and 22.2), and it is important to think about surgeon's and patient's positioning and use of navigated tools [54]. Currently, at our institution, we have used an optical tracker with infrared sensors but we were forced to be cognizant about tracker placement as well as tracker and tool direction. Often the longest pins are used and placed into a stable part of the pelvis away from the surgical site, usually on the contralateral side of the pelvis [55]. The tracker can be placed into the non-resected sacral or pelvic bone or can be placed into the resected bone if one chooses. However, if one needs to reconstruct or re-resect based on frozen margins, placing the pins in the resected section will not work. Although two pins can be used for tracker fixation, it is best to use three pins to better stabilize the tracker [56]. If the tracker pins become loose, it can affect the registration accuracy and the registration process will have to be performed again [20]. Also one must understand that the further the tracker is placed away from the resection plane or the bony sacrum or pelvis the more room there is for induced additional error in the system [45, 57]. The tracker should be placed far enough away from the surgical site so minimal disturbance happens to the system during surgery, i.e., leaning on the tracker with a retractor. We have placed pins and both removed and left the tracker attached during surgery prior to resection but after registration. After registration and prior to resection, we either place the tracker back on and or touch point on the pelvis or sacrum to confirm on the imaging that where we place the pointer is where we are on the computer navigation screen. Anecdotally, no difference in accuracy between the two methods has been seen although this hasn't been formally tested. Decreased accuracy will develop when the tracker or pins have been leaned on or when the pins become loose. When this happens, rescue points or respinning can be used to re-establish accuracy of the tracker. Rescue points are chosen on the computer navigation system prior to surgery. A minimum of four rescue points are chosen that are accessible, identifiable, and reproducible and are often prominent bone landmarks, i.e. ASIS, AIIS, PSIS, and pubic tubercle and pubic symphysis and one can use fiducial markers that are bioabsorbable.

One of the main logistical and timing issues in sacral surgery is often the need to flip the patient if using anterior and posterior approaches. This becomes a major issue with computer navigation as the most accurate way to match the CT with the patient in surgery is through a "spin" (Fig. 22.4). The benefit to navigation is that sometimes allows surgery to be performed through one approach. We often perform only one 3D fluoroscopic spin at the beginning of surgery with only tracker site incision opened up and the patient partially draped. The patient was covered with sterile sheets and the tracker with a sterile clear bag (Fig. 22.2). After the spin is completed with the Arcadis C-arm, we finish draping the patient which includes Ioband and thus only the pin sites were exposed to infection risk. This theoretically minimizes our risk of infection at the actual surgical site. This is probably less of a concern in sacral surgery unless one is performing lumbar-pelvis fixation. Each time the patient is flipped and repositioned the tracker must be replaced and new spin can be performed but it most likely places the patient at a theoretically increased infection risk although placing the patient on fresh surgical incision probably is a bigger risk. In this situation or having to flip back and forth more than once, screws can be placed in either planned resected bone or in other areas of the pelvis that can then be marked on the computer navigation software that can be used as well-defined rescue points, at least four of these have to be chosen. The benefit to fiducial markers is that another spin need not be performed but rather the fiducial markers can be marked as rescue points in order to alleviate the need for another spin.

Registration: All CT-based navigation systems require a registration process prior to navigated surgical resection [58]. Registration is the most significant and error prone step in navigation [59]. Originally, there were two registration algorithms developed for CT-based navigation paired-point matching and surface matching [58, 60] and now there is noninvasive registration of 3D data sets with the use of a navigated 2D fluoroscopy via contour matching first described in the spine [60]. This occurs after a tracker has been placed in a position that will be stable throughout surgery [20, 22]. This can be done in several different ways and is mostly based on the type of computer navigation software present at each institution with most systems being commercially available. Since 2008, we have used a commercially available system (OrthoMap, 3D, Styrker Orthopaedics, Mahwah, NJ) at our institution. This software package allows the surgeon to input data from both a CT and MRI obtained preoperatively several days before surgery. In the surgical suite, we take advantage of the Arcadis C-arm (Siemens), a 360 degree fluoroscopic image intensifier that allows the clinician to use a C-arm to perform a spin to obtain multiple multi-planar fluoroscopic images focused on the pubic symphysis (Fig. 22.4). This 3D fluoroscope turns around a surgical bed in a 190° arc acquiring up to 100 images of the iso-center with a dimension of 12.5 cm^3. With these axial cuts, 2D and 3D reformations can be transferred into the navigation system (Fig. 22.7) [61]. In order to use 3D fluoroscopy for registration, a radiolucent bed is required to allow the spin to occur. The limitation of this process is the small fluoroscope field (12.5 cm) and the need to spin around a radiolucent bed requiring that the surgeon use a centered anatomic structure of the patient in order to match the registration, i.e., the pubis. The C-arm obtains several hundred images that form a pseudo 3D CT image that is then matched with the pubic symphysis (Fig. 22.7) on the preoperative CT loaded into the navigation software to create a virtual model to guide the surgeon. This process can take up to 20–30 min to perform and requires sterilely covering the draped sterile field. The other intraoperative data we collect are surgeon-defined landmarks to confirm accuracy of the "spin" as well as defining optimal resection levels and implant positioning if needed. Image-to-image registration using 3D fluoroscopy [42] offers the benefit of not requiring fiducial markers along with a pre-resection surgery and can have improved registration accuracy over paired-point matching using bony landmarks. Although target registration error is the smallest when using the ilium (centered 3 cm above the acetabulum), one often has to use the pubis symphysis due the inability of a C-arm to be centered over ilium at the supra-acetabular location and complete an unimpeded revolution around the bed depending on the type of 2D fluoroscopic arm [42].

Other methods exist and include "paired-point matching and requires a minimum of 4 points or paired points" that are chosen on the CT image and then

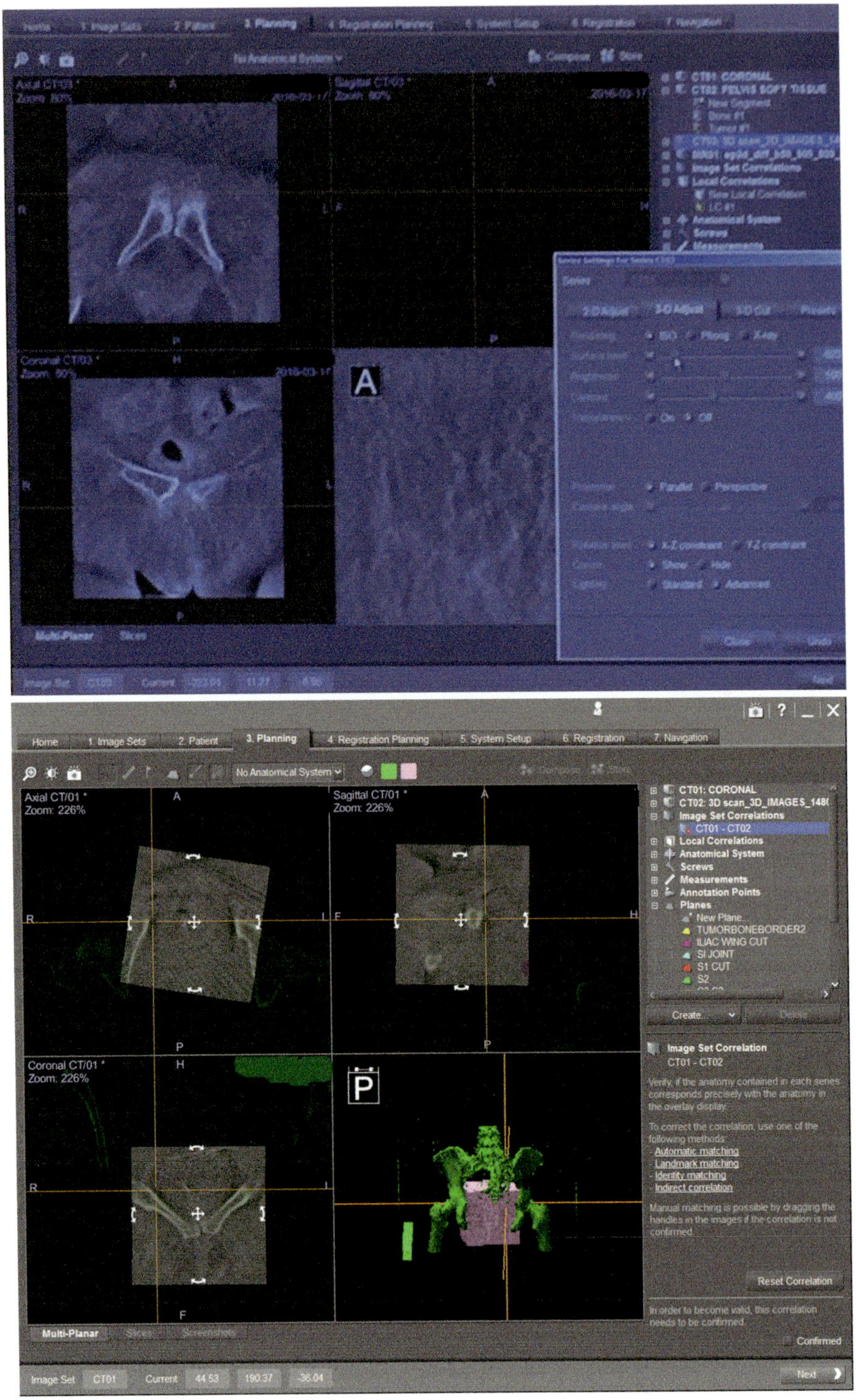

Fig. 22.7 This is a screenshot showing the navigational computer screen after uploading the imaging obtained from the Arcadis fluoroscopy machine. This imaging created by the navigational computer is used to merge the pubic symphysis seen on the preoperative CT scan and intraoperative "spin"

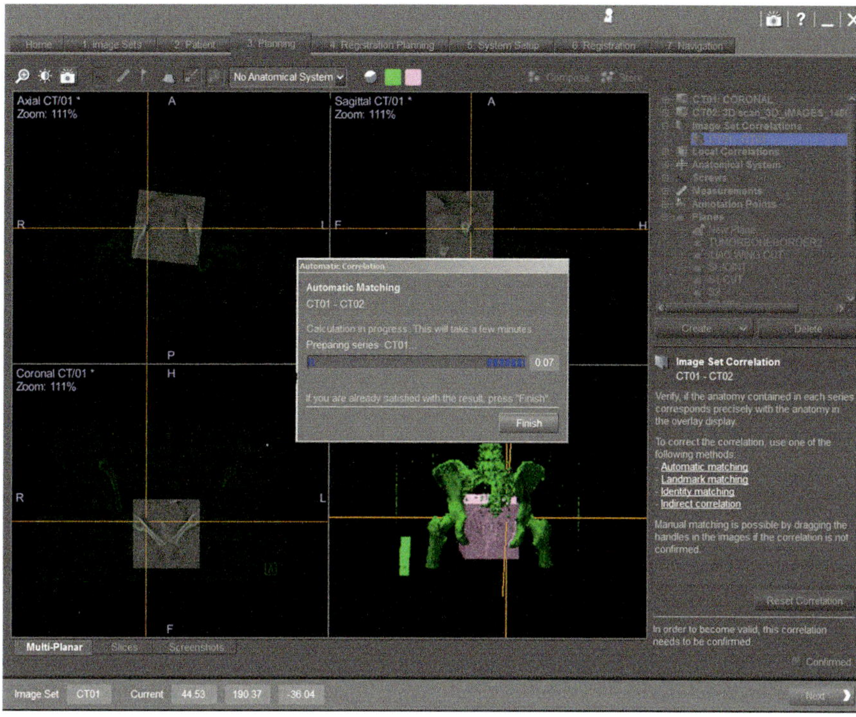

Fig. 22.7 (continued)

identified in the patient [22, 25, 26, 28]. This requires the surgeon to accurately identify both on the CT image and on the patient the corresponding points. Oftentimes, the pubic symphysis, ASIS, AIIS, pubic tubercle, and PSIS are used for the patient to image matching [55]. Many will confirm the registration process by palpating pubis and ilium [31, 55]. However, there are specific bony landmarks often that cannot be identified or palpated due to patient positioning.

Accuracy of the registration process can be improved by surface matching [23]. Surface matching was developed to avoid a second surgery and improve efficiency [58, 62]. The surgeon used the navigational probe to select in continuous succession a minimum of 50 points on the patient's exposed bone surface of the pelvis or sacrum [22, 28]. Cartilage, ligament, and soft tissue cannot be used for surface mapping due to the fact that they will not show up very well on a CT scan. CT images can be used for surface registration due to the nature of the bony cortex [25, 26]. MRI, on the other hand, can't be used for surface registration because the navigation system has a difficult time recognizing the cortical surface on the MRI [1, 52].

The registration error can be calculated by the navigation software and gives an indication of the mismatch between the true anatomy of the patient and the virtual image created by the preoperative CT scan. The goal is to obtain a registration error of <1 mm but some will accept below 2 mm [11, 22, 25, 26, 28, 63, 64]. Not too frequently a registration error of greater than 2 mm will be obtained. When this occurs, it often happens due to soft tissue being in the way of a bony landmark or that the paired points were not correctly matched from the preselected area on the preoperative CT scan. Having an obese patient can make it hard to identify the correct points. The surgeon will then have to repick points after confirming in the navigation system he has picked his correct landmarks on the CT scan. After this, the process is repeated again to correctly obtain point on the pelvis. Rarely does one have to abandon navigation. Because the "paired point" process can lead to user error, our institution chooses to use a "spin" method (discussed above) performed by recreating a bony landmark such as the pubic symphysis through the use of a C-arm taking several hundred images of the pubic symphysis that allow a virtual 3D image to be created that can be matched with the CT imaging. Tracker insertion and registration can take between 15 and 47 min but can often decrease from an average of 30–20 min after the surgeon has performed more navigated surgeries [28]. Time is then saved during surgery by not having to bring in C-arm or X-ray for multiple orthogonal images.

Fiducial markers are another way of enabling accuracy of registration; an implant such as a titanium implant, either a Kirschner wire [1] or screw, is placed into the patient's pelvis under anesthesia prior to obtaining a CT scan of the pelvis for navigation. These serve as fiducials for patient registration at the time of surgical resection [20]. Due to the possibility of needing to flip the patient, which can cause issue with registration and thus accuracy, surgeons in the past have placed fiducial markers consisting of K-wires (Titanium 1.8 mm) [20] into the pelvis prior to obtaining CT imaging for navigation. The points are chosen based on ease of access during surgery such as the iliac crests and posterior iliac spines [2, 20]. No more than four fiducial markers are needed for an accuracy of 1.5 mm [65]. Fiducials allow for better paired- point registration than would be obtained with identifying bony landmarks. This can then be augmented with surface fit registration. Planned registration landmarks should not be prominent osseous features that may be included in the resection [52].

To improve accuracy with paired-point matching, small pins or fiducial markers can be attached to the anatomical surface of interest but an additional surgery to place these markers must occur prior to the preoperative CT [42, 58]. Fiducial markers can make things easier or if the patient is needed to be flipped from supine to prone, not all the time can the surgery be performed only through a posterior approach [54, 66]. While not routinely done, there are reported series of performing a surgery prior to resection to place fiducial markers on or within the pelvis prior to obtaining a CT scan for navigational planning. It is important to understand that a surgery needs to be performed prior to obtaining the preoperative CT scan loaded into navigation. These offer the ability to identify a finer paired-matched point when performing registration. However, this places the patient as risk for infection although it is really mostly percutaneous. It also puts the patient through another anesthesia.

Performing the resection: After reconfirming ones observed accuracy from the registration process, bone cuts can be made several ways with navigation. Instrumentation exists that allows a tracker to be placed onto a designated tool, and custom tracker connectors can allow about any type of tool to be navigated as long as it can be calibrated. Several different tools can be used for navigation and can be navigated and include diathermy device [22, 28], osteotomes [21], chisels [10, 19, 20], drills [25, 26, 67], burrs [2, 11], screw driver [21], and oscillating saws (Fig. 22.8) [22, 24, 31, 68]. Two of the most common tools used include a navigated saw and navigated osteotome. The navigational saw involves placing a tracker on a conventional battery-driven saw that has a specific blade that is much narrower than a saw blade used to perform a knee

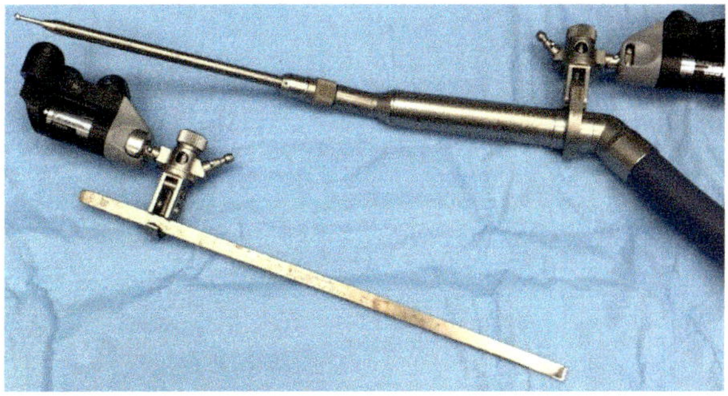

Fig. 22.8 Comparison of a navigated osteotome or chisel to a navigated burr. Make note the burr is not straight; the burr tip is referenced to the instrument tracker relative to space

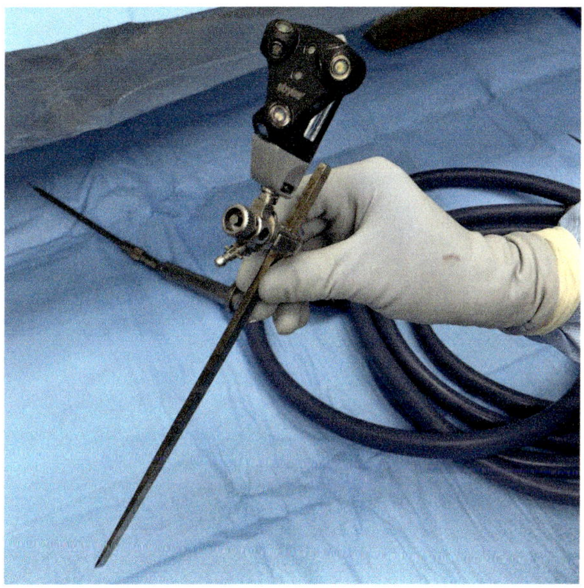

Fig. 22.9 Navigated osteotome 1/4 in. (1/4 to 1 in. can be navigated)

arthroplasty. The drawback of this saw blade is there is some significant flexibility in the system. Instability due to vibrations and flexibility produced by the oscillating saw can potentially induce error in the planned resection [51]. The operator can try to push the saw blade and cause flexion that can cause an inaccurate reading of the saw blade in space to the effect of several millimeters [39, 40, 68]. The saw also has to be started away from the cortex. The key is to let the saw blade do the work. The other limitation of the saw is the excursion of the blade and often cannot be used if the blade cannot oscillate or if oscillation will injure tissue or disrupt tumor [22]. There are significant improvements for angle of cut and location of the cut plane (2.8 mm) when using a navigated saw compared to the freehand process (5.7 mm) [69]. The other navigational tool at hand is the osteotome that allows the user to have non-flexible tool that gives reliable depth and trajectory feedback via the computer navigational screen to the surgeon (Fig. 22.9). The drawback of the osteotome is that using it can cause unwanted fractures in bone. Both the saw and the osteotome are ideal for uniplanar cuts but when a multi-planar three-dimensional cut is needed another method is used. The surgeon

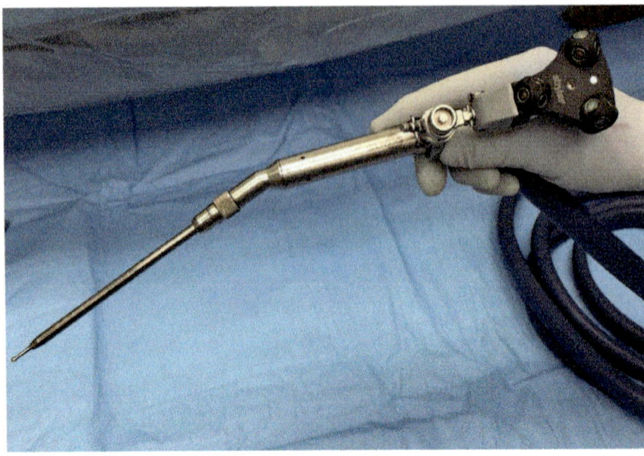

Fig. 22.10 Navigated burr used for resection in multiple planes; generally, the smallest size burr is used to avoid compromising margins

can use the navigation pointer/gun to mark "wayward" points along the bone for the planned resection performed with either a drill, burr, or osteotome. These points after being identified with the navigated pointer [1] can be marked with cautery or a sterile marker which has been described [4, 25, 26, 39, 40]. At this point, a drill or a burr can be used to create several holes along the planned cut. A burr has benefit over a drill in that it can be used to thin cortex on the far side before dropping into tumor or a critical structure that may exist on the opposite side (Fig. 22.10). The cut can then be completed with either an osteotome or burr at the discretion of the surgeon. Once the integrity of what bone in question is compromised, i.e., resected then the accuracy of the navigation is no longer valid. This occurs once the pelvis is disrupted in one area; there is too much flexibility in the system to assure that the second osteotomy is in the intended place [28]. Disruption of the ring can potentially disturb the accuracy of the spatial relationship and the registration of the patient [2]. One thing to be aware of is that the display of the instrument on the monitor and real localization may differ with respect to what is seen in the operative field [38].

22.6 Benefits of Navigation

Computer navigation is a real-time intraoperative virtual imaging system that allows the surgeon to identify location and planned resection in musculoskeletal oncology (Fig. 22.11). The system can allow the user to make uniplanar resections with confidence as it allows one to know the exit point of the cutting device (Fig. 22.12). Previously, these cuts would have been made visually or with the aid of two-dimensional radiograph or fluoroscopy. Those two modalities often do not allow the surgeon to know how far or deep one has a cut. In the past and still today with sacral surgery, a surgeon may attempt to place screws in the sacrum on the opposite side to be able to identify on a plain radiograph or fluoroscopic image in order to make a relatively safe blind cut. The issue with this cut is that x-ray and fluoroscopic image doesn't allow the surgeon to identify soft tissue component of the tumor on the other side. With the use of computer navigation the surgeon can now save nerves and blood

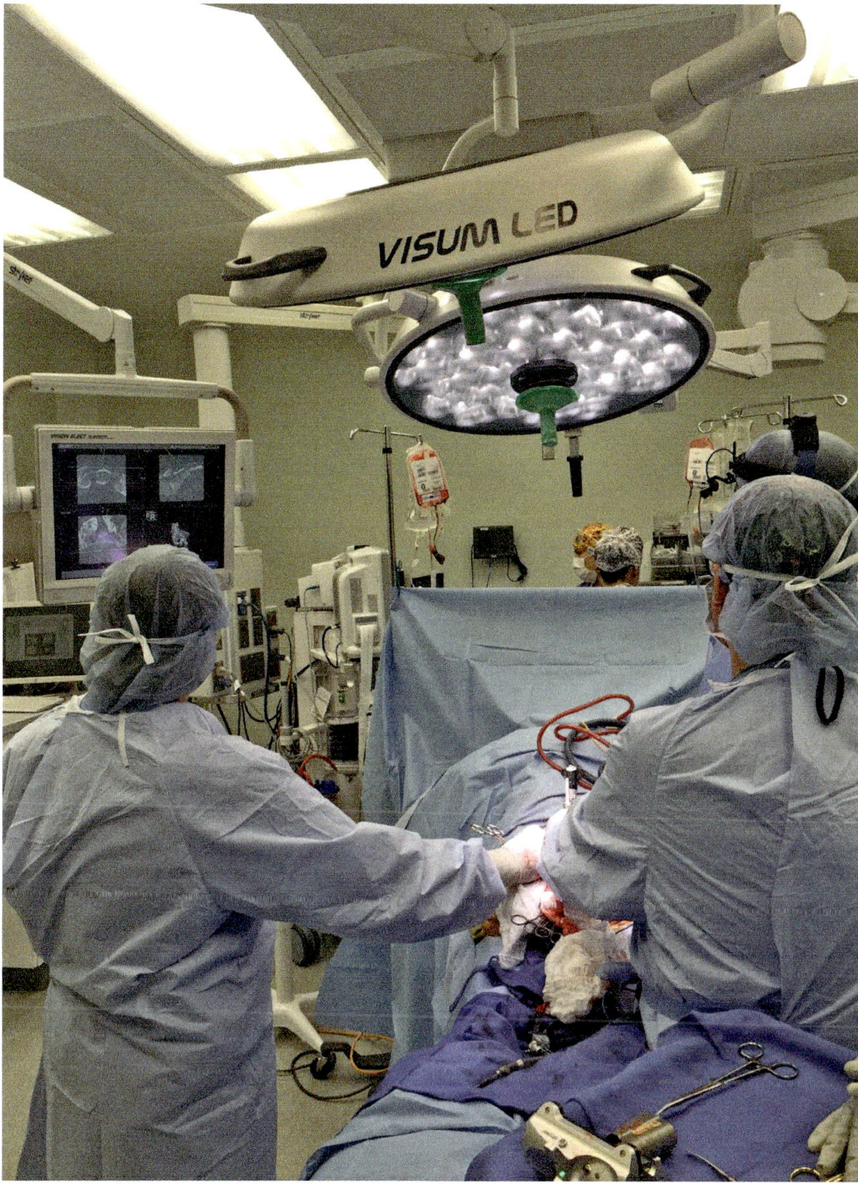

Fig. 22.11 Two surgeons watching the computer navigation screen while using a navigated burr on and in the sacrum for a chordoma resection

vessels and create multi-planar resections that allow for preservation of bone and thus improved the ability to implant attachment if needed. Musculoskeletal tumors are not one dimensional, they don't follow a single plane border, instead they are often lobulated three-dimensional masses thus making the resection harder. The other benefit of navigation is the ability to navigate multiple tools. A surgeon can now know the depth

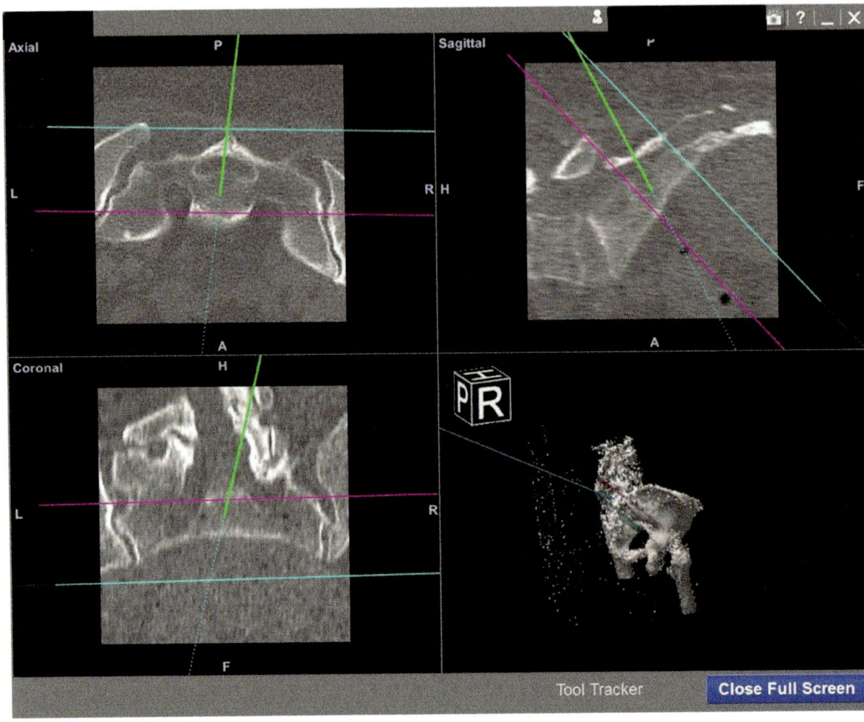

Fig. 22.12 The *green* tip represents the tip of the navigated burr and shows how deep it has gone

and direction of their tool in three-dimensional space. Computer navigation doesn't only have to be used for resection and reconstruction, stealth navigation with the O-arm and single K-wire for sacral and pelvic lesions that represent benign tumors and hematologic tumors were used for tumor ablation and kyphoplasty in benign and malignant non-primary bone tumors [27]. Another theoretical benefit of navigation compared is decreased fluoroscopic exposure times to the surgeon [61, 70].

Accuracy Benefits: Computer navigation surgery allows the surgeon several benefits with regard to surgery and margin status. In surgeries without navigation, surgeons often have to plan 2 cm margins in order to be assured that there is no tumor violation [66]. It is difficult to achieve negative margins in sacral surgery [66] and tumors involved with the sacrum have a higher prevalence of positive margins [71] leading to higher recurrence rates and poorer outcomes. Clinical studies have shown that navigated tools have assisted in attaining negative margins in pelvic and sacral tumors [2, 10, 24–26, 31, 72]. Freehand-navigated saw improves cutting accuracy [51, 73]. Computer-navigated surgery can increase precision of the osteotomies for tumor resection [1, 2, 10, 20, 25, 26]. Given the accuracy of navigated tools, bone loss related to the saw blade thickness can be accounted for and then adjusted for on computer navigation planning by shifting the planned resection planes by 1.5 mm [31]. In fact, most resection planes can be adjusted preoperatively based on known resection width tools such as the osteotome (0.6 mm) and oscillating saw blade (1.25 mm) which produced a loss of bone width of 2 mm due to oscillation [51].

The use of computer navigation allows for accurate identification of the local anatomy in a distorted environment and can define the extent of the tumor and resection margins [28, 39, 40]. Oftentimes, it is hard to identify the location and the extent of tumor infiltration intraoperatively [39, 40]. A surgeon without computer navigation can't see the infiltration of the tumor within the bone marrow intraoperatively and instead the surgeon must identify on MRI and CT the tumor infiltration related to bony landmarks and translate that into landmarks on the patient's pelvis or sacrum during surgery; this relationship between what is seen on preoperative imaging and what is identified in the patient can lead to errors that translate into positive margins in the non-computer-assisted surgery. Computer navigation allows a surgeon to identify the extent of the tumor infiltration on the virtual imaging that is shown on the computer navigation monitor and know that their resection will not go through tumor. The main benefit of improved accuracy through this modality is the ability to get closer to the tumor without compromising margins. The goal of navigation is to reduce the rate of intralesional resection, i.e., positive margins. One can study looking at navigation in the pelvis and sacrum reduced the intralesional rate to 8.7% ($n = 2$) with clear bone margins in all cases ($n = 31$) with a 13% local recurrence rate compared to the traditional method where intralesional rate and local recurrence rate were found to be 29% and 27%, respectively [22]. Only now are oncologic surgeons beginning to see the benefit of getting closer to the tumor without compromising the margins. Surgeons using computer navigation believe that it allows more complex resections and reconstructions than are possible with conventional surgery including preservation of sacral nerve root controlling bladder and bowel (42% of time), resect unresectable tumors (13%), and avoidance of hindquarter amputation (10%) [22].

In studies, there is a 52% probability of achieving a 1 cm margin in a triplane-simulated tumor model of the pelvis when performed by an experienced surgeon without computer navigation [30]. One experimental study showed that the cut planes with respect to the planned planes in the pelvis were significantly improved by using a navigated saw, averaging 2.8 mm compared to 11.2 mm for the freehand saw ($p < 0.001$) and there were no intralesional tumor resections compared to 22% ($N = 5$) intralesional procedures in the freehand group ($N = 23$) [68]. What was also found within this experimental study is that the maximum difference achieved between the cut and the desired safe margin of 10 mm was 6.5 mm for the navigated cut compared to the 13 mm cut [68]. In another experimental study in the setting of using intraoperative CT, the navigated sawbones cuts were 1.4 ± 1 mm entry cut and 1.9 ± 1.2 mm exit cut from the planned resection compared to non-navigated 2.8 ± 4.9 mm entry cut and 3.5 ± 4.6 mm exit cut in a pelvic bone model showing a significant ($p \leq 0.01$) difference in the two methods and the navigated cadaver study produced similar values for the navigated entry cut location of 1.5 ± 0.9 mm and navigated exit cut location of 2.1 ± 1.5 mm form the planned cuts using [51]. This showed that navigation used in pelvic tumor resection allowed an osteotomy within 5 mm of the planned resection [51]. The overall benefit to navigated surgery is the reproducibility of the surgical resection. In a study of 28 patients with 61 osteotomies, the quantitative difference between the planned osteotomies and performed osteotomies was 2.52 ± 2.32 mm for all patients and 2.82 ± 2.01 for the sacrum and pelvis [39, 40]. While not often used in the setting of sacral tumor allograft, reconstructions can benefit from the use of computer navigation. Inaccuracy with respect to measured dimensions exists in the selection of massive bone allograft of the pelvis using template comparison method [74]. Due to the reproducibility of the precision, some surgeons use navigation to resect the tumor and then use the navigation software to create an allograft piece of pelvis or sacrum to fill the defect created from the resection in order to reconstruct the pelvis. Navigation has been shown that it can also be used to cut a custom fitting allograft if reconstruction is to be performed [31]. One of the original purposes of navigation that is not often used in sacral resection is reconstruction of the appropriate hip center, leg length, and hip joint version. It allows a way to properly orient reconstruction components when no bony landmarks exist.

22.7 Limitations of Navigation

Limitations of Accuracy: Navigation is not a perfect system and the surgeon should understand what affects its accuracy in surgery [13]. Accuracy can be limited in several ways: the imaging system itself can limit accuracy, operator error of the tools, and registration of the tools and registration of the patient can limit accuracy. Inaccurate osteotomies or lack of precision for a cut can be manually caused by the surgeon due to saw blade bending when cutting bone [69]. Be aware that the instrument location seen on the display may not match the real localization on the patient [38]. Some studies have reported that the true accuracy in most studies only represent the accuracy of the intra-operative registration process as recorded by the navigation machine [24] and have even suggested that pathology margins are the best way to measure accuracy. Given that most inaccuracies occur due to the registration process which is operator dependent, a surgeon should understand the affect that they impart into the system. Getting good information out of computer navigation is dependent on putting good data into the system. Patients with significant BMI [28] can limit exposure and make it difficult to accurately identify bony landmarks for paired-point matching. Depending on age, a thick cartilage cap can lead to an inaccurate registration [28]. In fact, any soft tissue that impedes one's ability to get to cortical bone, such as tendon insertion, ligaments, articular cartilage, and soft tissue component of tumor can affect the accuracy of the resection due to compromised registration. Picking or creating a mobile segment of bone can lead to inaccurate resection [28], so it is important to appreciate what is mobile or what will be mobile. Once a single bone cut is created a certain amount of uncertainty is introduced into the system for the subsequent cut [2]. Disruption of the ring by ligament sectioning can potentially disturb the accuracy of the spatial relationship and the registration of the patient [2]. The use of navigation can only improve accuracy of bony resection and avoid inadvertent perforation of tumor with osteotome. Navigation is not the perfect system. Narrow soft tissue margins cannot be improved with navigation [22]. It does have several drawbacks including time for surgery [1, 21] due to the registration process [49]. The use of navigation is costly due to surgery time and system itself. It does have a learning curve associated with it but that time lessens as more experience is gained [22]. Although additional operating time is needed for navigation setup, defining the resection plane on preoperatively obtained images can reduce the overall surgical time as no resection margin has to be defined while in surgery [25, 26]. The cumulative accuracy of the entire navigation system can be a limiting factor [18, 20, 37, 58]. Infrared cameras in some studies were felt to be the main contributing factor of inaccuracy [75]. Image fusion involved in CT-MRI fusion is also a type of registration, although the registration is image to image instead of image to patient, process that leads registration error [52, 53]. This is often due to the fact that merging is performed on a visual basis.

22.8 Summary

Sacrum and pelvis three-dimensional anatomy is difficult to understand and master conceptually when trying to resect tumors [51, 76]. Pelvic area surgery is demanding due to anatomy and is difficult to get tumor-free margin leading to higher local recurrence [20, 23, 72, 77]. The purpose of navigation is to provide the surgeon an accurate three-dimensional virtual model of the tumor and pelvic structures including the sacrum that will correlate with the patient's anatomy at the time of surgery. With this 3D model, the surgeon can plan and map on the navigational software the surgical resection cuts that can be either uniplanar or multi-planar. If needed, although not usually with the sacrum, a custom prosthesis can be made based on the presurgical modeling if standard implants cannot be used. Most importantly, one can choose with the aid of computer navigation the number and vector of the surgical resection as well as a defined margin with respect to the tumor. Navigation serves as a planning tool. Surgery in the sacrum can be hard in normal anatomy and even harder when a tumor distorts the normal anatomy. Computer navigation is relatively new in the musculoskeletal world and has probably been used for tumor resection for less than 10 years. Computer navigation offers a lot of benefits; however, the system is not foolproof. Where computer navigation excels, there is the ability to "see beyond walls." Working on the sacrum is hard for several reasons; this includes the fact that there are nerves the surgeon would like to spare; it can be hard to identify what level of the sacrum one is at either on intraoperative fluoroscopy or by bony landmarks; and lastly, it is hard to know what lies on the other side of the sacral cut and which direction one is heading. With computer navigation one can literally see where one is heading to in real time and how close ones cut is coming to tumor on the other side. Navigation can only improve bone resection accuracy; it cannot improve the narrow margins associated with soft tissue components due the nature of soft tissue moving because of the inability to navigate soft tissue sarcoma [23, 78].

The future of computer-assisted surgery will include computer navigation but also will begin to include the benefit of robotic-assistive devices and patient-specific instrumentation [72]. Computer navigation is a passive system which only provides information or feedback while the future robotic-assisted surgeries will be performed with a more active system that physically guides and limits the surgeon from straying outside of predetermined resection planes [79]. Currently, systems exist to help with total knee and total hip arthroplasty that provide reproducibility and precision. The benefit to robotic-assisted surgery involves still maintaining control of saws and osteotomes while minimizing the effect of tool vibration and fatigue on part of the surgeons hand [80].

References

1. Cho HS, et al. Joint-preserving limb salvage surgery under navigation guidance. J Surg Oncol. 2009;100(3):227–32. BACKGROUND: Recently, the navigation system has been introduced to orthopedic oncology. It can apply MRI and/or CT images to intraoperative visualization. We performed navigation-assisted limb salvage surgeries on patients with a malignant bone tumor of the metaphysis of the long bone or the iliac bone while preserving the adjacent joint. METHODS: When preoperative chemotherapy was estimated to be effective by imaging studies and the residual remaining epiphysis was expected to be more than 1 cm long after tumor resection with 1-2 cm of surgical margin, joint-preserving surgery was performed under navi

gation guidance. We carried out CT and MRI data fusion to use MR images as an intraoperative guide. A deep frozen strut allograft was placed in the defect for the restoration of anatomical continuity. RESULTS: Resection margin measured on pathological examination was in accordance with that of the preoperative plan. The functional scores of all patients were satisfactory. There was no evidence of recurrence on the regional radiographs and CT on the chest until the last follow-up. CONCLUSION: Navigation-assisted surgery can be indicated for limb salvage and it can help to preserve the adjacent joint in selected cases.

2. Cho HS, et al. Computer-assisted sacral tumor resection. A case report. J Bone Joint Surg Am. 2008;90(7):1561–6.
3. Court C, et al. Surgical excision of bone sarcomas involving the sacroiliac joint. Clin Orthop Relat Res. 2006;451:189–94. Adequate (wide or marginal and uncontaminated) margins and reconstruction are difficult to achieve when performing an internal hemipelvectomy for bone sarcomas involving the sacroiliac joint. We evaluated whether adequate surgical margins could be achieved and if functional outcomes could be predicted based on the type of resection and reconstruction. Forty patients had resections of the sacroiliac joint. Vertical sacral osteotomies were through the sacral wing (n = 2), ipsilateral sacral foramina (n = 27), sacral midline (n = 9), or contralateral foramina (n = 2). Iliac resections were Type I, Type I-II with partial or total acetabular re-section, or Type I-II-III. Surgical margins were adequate in 28 of 38 patients (74%), two (7%) of whom experienced local recurrence, compared with seven of 10 (70%) patients with inadequate margins. Reconstruction consisted of restoring continuity between the spine and pelvis. Resection of the entire acetabulum and removal of the lumbosacral trunk were the two main determinants of function, as assessed using the Musculoskeletal Tumor Society score. There were no life-threatening or function-threatening complications. Internal hemipelvectomy with a limb salvage procedure can be achieved with adequate surgical margins in selected patients. Functional outcomes can be predicted based on the type of resection and reconstruction, which helps the surgeon plan the procedure and inform the patient.
4. Fehlberg S, et al. Computer-assisted pelvic tumor resection: fields of application, limits, and perspectives. Recent Results Cancer Res. 2009;179:169–82. The treatment of malignant tumors involving the pelvic area is a challenging problem in musculoskeletal oncology due to the complex pelvic anatomy and the often large tumor size at presentation. The use of navigation systems has effectively increased surgical precision aiming at optimal preservation of pelvic structures without compromising oncologic outcome by means of improved visibility of the surgical field, and enabling intraoperative display and 3D reproduction of preoperatively determined pelvic osteotomy and resection levels. In the following sections, current developments in computer-assisted pelvic surgery are reviewed and possible fields of application, as well as limitations of navigation systems, are discussed.
5. Fuchs B, et al. Osteosarcoma of the pelvis: outcome analysis of surgical treatment. Clin Orthop Relat Res. 2009;467(2):510–8. Risk factors to explain the poor survival of patients with osteosarcoma of the pelvis are poorly understood. Therefore, we attempted to identify factors affecting survival and development of local recurrence and metastasis. We retrospectively reviewed 43 patients who had high-grade pelvic tumors and were treated surgically. Twenty lesions were chondroblastic, 10 fibroblastic, 11 osteoblastic, and one each was giant cell-rich and small cell osteosarcomas. At a median of 3.5 years (range, 0.3-21 years) postoperatively, 13 patients were alive with no evidence of disease. The overall and disease-free 5-year survival rates were 38% and 29%, respectively, at 5 years. Anatomic location, tumor size, and margin predicted survival. Fifteen patients (35%) had local recurrence. The 5-year cumulative incidence of recurrence with death as a competing risk factor was 34%. Location in the ilium and size of the tumor predicted local recurrence. Twenty-one (49%) of 43 patients had metastases develop. The cumulative incidence of metastasis with death as a competing risk factor was 48% at 5 years. Six patients who presented with metastasis had a worse survival than patients who had no evidence of metastasis at presentation (2-year survival, 33% versus 76%). If distant metastasis is diagnosed subsequent to primary treatment, aggressive therapy may be justified. LEVEL OF EVIDENCE: Level II, prognostic study. See the Guidelines for Authors for a complete description of levels of evidence.

6. Kawai A, et al. Osteosarcoma of the pelvis. Oncologic results of 40 patients. Clin Orthop Relat Res. 1998;(348):196–207. The cases of 40 patients with osteosarcoma of the pelvis treated between 1977 and 1994 were reviewed. The location of the tumor was ilium in 30 patients, ischium in four, pubis in one, and sacrum in five. Most (58%) of the tumors were of the chondroblastic subtype. Thirty patients had surgical excision of the tumors: 10 with hemipelvectomies and 20 with limb sparing procedures. A wide margin was achieved in 16 of 30 (53%) patients, including 12 of 14 who had no sacral tumor involvement. Positive margins occurred at the sacrum in 11 patients, lumbar vertebra in one, perirectal space in one, and contralateral pubic body in one. Macroscopic tumor emboli within the regional large vessels were found in seven patients. The incidence of local recurrence was 32%: 13% in wide excisions, 38% in marginal excisions, and 80% in intralesional excisions. The 1- and 5-year overall patient survivals were 73% and 34%, respectively. Patients who had a surgical excision of the primary tumor had a significantly better survival than did those treated without surgery (5-year survival; 41% and 10%, respectively). Tumor size, surgical excision of the primary tumor, surgical margin, and type of surgical procedure were the prognostic factors for patients with Stage IIB tumors.
7. Pring ME, et al. Chondrosarcoma of the pelvis. A review of sixty-four cases. J Bone Joint Surg Am. 2001;83-A(11):1630–42. BACKGROUND: Treatment of pelvic chondrosarcoma is a difficult problem for the musculoskeletal oncologist. Poor rates of survival and high rates of local recurrence after surgical treatment have been reported in previous studies. The present study was designed to review the long-term oncologic and functional outcomes of surgical management in a large series of patients with pelvic chondrosarcoma who were treated at a single institution. METHODS: The cases of sixty-four patients with localized pelvic chondrosarcoma that had been surgically treated between 1975 and 1996 were reviewed retrospectively. The study was limited to patients who had received no previous treatment for chondrosarcoma. There were forty-one male and twenty-three female patients who had a mean age of forty-seven years (range, fifteen to eighty-eight years). The patients were followed for a minimum of three years or until death. The median duration of follow-up of the living patients was 140 months (range, thirty-nine to 295 months). RESULTS: Thirty-three of the sixty-four patients were first seen with grade-1 chondrosarcoma; twenty-three, with grade-2; one, with grade-3; and seven, with grade-4 (dedifferentiated chondrosarcoma). Thirteen patients had a hemipelvectomy to achieve local tumor control, whereas fifty-one patients underwent a limb-salvage procedure. Twelve patients (19%) had local recurrence, and eleven (17%) had distant metastases. At the time of the final follow-up, forty-four patients (69%) were alive without evidence of disease, thirteen (20%) had died of the disease, six (9%) had died of unrelated causes, and one (2%) was alive with disease. Less than a wide surgical margin correlated with local recurrence ($p = 0.014$). High-grade tumors correlated with poor overall survival ($p < 0.001$). All patients who had a limb-salvage procedure were able to walk at the time of the final follow-up, and they had a mean functional score of 77%, according to the system of the Musculoskeletal Tumor Society. CONCLUSIONS: Aggressive surgical resection of pelvic chondrosarcoma results in long-term survival of the majority of patients. There is a high correlation between tumor grade and overall or disease-free survival.
8. Sucato DJ, et al. Ewing's sarcoma of the pelvis. Long-term survival and functional outcome. Clin Orthop Relat Res. 2000;(373):193–201. Fifty patients with Ewing,s sarcoma of the pelvis were treated using a multidisciplinary approach; followup of surviving patients averaged 137 months (range, 40-276 months). The addition of surgical resection to the multidisciplinary treatment for all patients was associated with improved survival compared with survival of patients treated with chemotherapy and radiation therapy alone; the addition of surgery to the treatment regimen of 37 patients without metastases also was associated with improved survival. There were no significant differences between the surgical and nonsurgical groups in terms of tumor size, stage of disease, patient age, duration of symptoms before diagnosis, or anatomic site. Surgery was used more often in recently treated patients, but the year of diagnosis and treatment did not significantly affect overall survival, secondary to large confidence intervals. The Short Form-36 and the Musculoskeletal Tumor Society functional evaluation

instruments showed a superior level of function in the nonsurgical group, but this difference was not statistically significant. There have been many advances in the treatment of patients with Ewing's sarcoma during the past 3 decades, resulting in improved survival for patients with Ewing's sarcoma of the pelvis. The addition of surgery significantly improved survival and did not show a significant difference in functional outcome.

9. Wirbel RJ, et al. Surgical treatment of pelvic sarcomas: oncologic and functional outcome. Clin Orthop Relat Res. 2001;(390):190–205. The experiences in treating 93 consecutive patients (56 males, 37 females; mean age, 38.5 years; range, 4-69 years), including 76 patients with primary malignant bone tumors and 17 patients with soft tissue sarcomas involving the innominate bone, are reported. Oncologic and functional results were investigated in relation to the tumor stage, to the achieved surgical margin, and to the surgical procedure (hemipelvectomy, internal hemipelvectomy and endoprosthetic replacement, and continuity resection). The mean followup was 48 months (range, 8-222 months). The 5-year survival was 86% in patients with low-grade malignant bone tumors, 42% in patients with high-grade malignant bone tumors, and 25% in patients with high-grade soft tissue sarcomas. Survival was influenced by the grade of malignancy, the tumor stage, and the achieved surgical margins. Forty-six patients who survived were examined an average of 36 months after primary surgery. Excellent and good functional results were seen in 82% of patients who underwent continuity resection and in 55.5% of patients who underwent partial or total internal hemipelvectomy. All patients who survived hemipelvectomy had poor functional results. Surgical treatment of pelvic sarcomas is an extensive procedure with a considerable incidence of complications. It requires the knowledge of different techniques of resection and reconstruction of bone, joints, soft tissue, and intrapelvic organs.
10. Krettek C, et al. Computer aided tumor resection in the pelvis. Injury. 2004;35 Suppl 1:S-A79-83. Surgical treatment of malignant tumors within the pelvis is a complex problem due to the anatomy and biomechanics. There are standardized preoperative diagnostic tools like computed tomography (CT) or magnetic resonance imaging (MRI) that provide multidimensional information. However, this information cannot be transferred intraoperatively. Computer aided orthopedic surgery (CAOS) may be a solution for precise intraoperative accuracy for these indications. We report on two patients with tumors within the pelvis. In one patient, an infiltrating recurrent chordoma within the sacrum was resected with CAOS. The other patient presented with a periacetabular chondrosarcoma. Resection was done with navigation so precise that a custom-made hemipelvis prosthesis with a special coating fit. In both patients, a complete resection was achieved with tumor-free resection margins. Navigation may be helpful in tumor surgery within the pelvis.
11. Wong KC, et al. Image fusion for computer-assisted bone tumor surgery. Clin Orthop Relat Res. 2008;466(10):2533–41. The fusion of computed tomography and magnetic resonance images is a software-dependent processing technique that enables one to integrate and analyze preoperative images for planning complex musculoskeletal tumor resections. By integrating various imaging modalities into one imaging data set we may facilitate preoperative image analysis and planning of navigation computer-assisted bone tumor resection and reconstruction. We performed image fusion for computer-assisted tumor surgery in 13 consecutive patients, seven males and six females, with a mean age of 35.8 years (range, 6-80 years). Visual verification of fused images was accurate in all patients. The mean time for image fusion was 30.6 minutes (range, 8-80 minutes). After intraoperative registration, all tumor resections were performed as planned preoperatively under navigation image guidance. Resections achieved after navigation resection planning were validated by postoperative CT or resected specimens in seven patients. Histologic examination of all resected specimens showed tumor-free margins in patients with bone sarcoma. The fusion of computed tomography and magnetic resonance imaging has the potential to enhance computer-assisted bone tumor surgery. The fusion image, when combined with surgical navigation, helps surgeons reproduce a preoperative plan reliably and may offer substantial clinical benefits.
12. Schlondorff G. Computer-assisted surgery: historical remarks. Comput Aided Surg. 1998;3(4):150–2.

13. Stiehl JB, Heck DA. Computer-assisted surgery: basic concepts. Instr Course Lect. 2008;57:689–97. Computer-assisted surgery has been advocated as a significant enabling technology that will enhance the surgical technique of various orthopaedic procedures. The computer becomes a sophisticated measuring tool, determining the three-dimensional spatial orientation of fiducial points, which may be established by a variety of referencing methods. These fiducial points or arrays may define a bone, an instrument, or a prosthesis. Current referencing methods include using segmented computer tomograms; fluoroscopic images; ultrasound images; and imageless, direct anatomic point-picking methods. Tracking technologies use optical cameras and electromagnetic coils. Optical systems have high reliability with errors of less than 0.5 mm. Electromagnetic trackers have a similar capability, but are less reliable because of the distortion of the electromagnetic signal that may result from the complex operating room environment. Accuracy with current CT-referenced systems approximates 1 degrees or 1 mm. Other methods such as fluoroscopy or ultrasound are less precise because of difficulty related to the ability to consistently define a specific anatomic structure. Descriptive measures of outcome include standard deviation and quantification of error. Process capability indices or Six Sigma are suitable methods for comparing outcomes with computer-assisted surgery and can be generalized from various approaches.
14. Amiot LP, et al. Computer-assisted pedicle screw fixation. A feasibility study. Spine (Phila Pa 1976). 1995;20(10):1208–12. STUDY DESIGN: We evaluated a computer-assisted surgical tool for inserting pedicle screws. OBJECTIVES: This study reviewed the feasibility, usefulness, and accuracy of the proposed tool. SUMMARY OF BACKGROUND DATA: Reviews documented neurovascular damage caused by screw misplacement. Currently, screw hole position is assessed by radiologic means and curette palpation. METHODS: Three sheep vertebrae and one artificial object were reconstructed three-dimensionally from computed tomography scan slices. At surgery, the surgeon's movements were displayed relative to the three-dimensional vertebrae on a computer screen. The tool was used to detect pedicles and to verify the position of drilled holes. In our laboratory, we calculated the system's accuracy by taking measurements on the artificial object. RESULTS: All pedicles were identified with the computer. Five of the six drilled hole positions were correctly represented. An accuracy of 4.5 mm +/- 1.1 mm RMS (root of the mean squared) and 1.6 degrees +/- 1.2 degrees were calculated. CONCLUSIONS: Results suggested the proposed system could be useful for pedicle detection and assessing the intravertebral location of a drilled hole. The proposed system could be used for many different orthopedic procedures where structures are hidden from the surgeon's view.
15. Dessenne V, et al. Computer-assisted knee anterior cruciate ligament reconstruction: first clinical tests. J Image Guid Surg. 1995;1(1):59–64. Anterior cruciate ligament reconstruction is a delicate task. The procedure of choice is the patellar tendon bone autograft, but an anisometric position of this tendon often leads to failure. We allows positioning of the central part of the ligament graft at the least anisometric sites. The system uses a workstation and a three-dimensional optical localizer to create images that represent knee kinematics. The surgeon uses these images to guide the surgery. This technique has been validated on eight cadavers and 12 patients.
16. Amiot LP, et al. Comparative results between conventional and computer-assisted pedicle screw installation in the thoracic, lumbar, and sacral spine. Spine (Phila Pa 1976). 2000;25(5):606–14. STUDY DESIGN: A comparative study on the position of pedicle screws in patients treated surgically with and without computer assistance. OBJECTIVES: To evaluate the accuracy of computer-assisted pedicle screw installation, and to evaluate its clinical benefit as compared with conventional pedicle screw installation techniques. SUMMARY OF BACKGROUND DATA: In vitro and clinical studies have documented a significant rate of misplaced screws in the thoracolumbar area. Neurologic complications are recognized problems caused by screw misplacement. METHODS: Patients treated surgically with computer assistance were compared with a historical control group of patients treated surgically with conventional techniques in the same hospital and by the same surgical team. All screw positions were measured with a postoperative magnetic resonance tomography, and cortical effrac-

tions were categorized in 2-mm increments. Patients' charts also were reviewed to assess individual neurologic outcomes. RESULTS: The control cohort was composed of 100 patients, with 544 screws from T5 to S1. The computer-assisted cohort was composed of 50 patients, with 294 screws from T2 to S1. In the control cohort, 461 of 544 screws (85%) were found completely within their pedicles as compared with 278 of 294 screws (95%) correctly placed in the computer-assisted group ($P < 0.0001$). All 16 screws incorrectly placed with computer assistance were found 0.1 mm to 2 mm from the pedicle cortex. In the control cohort, 68 screws were found 0.1 mm to 2 mm, 10 screws 2.1 mm to 4 mm, and 5 screws more than 4 mm from the pedicle cortex. Seven patients in the control cohort were surgically retreated because of postoperative neurologic deficits, whereas no patients in the computer-assisted group were surgically retreated. CONCLUSIONS: Computer assistance can decrease the incidence of incorrectly positioned pedicle screws.

17. Castro WH, et al. Accuracy of pedicle screw placement in lumbar vertebrae. Spine (Phila Pa 1976). 1996;21(11):1320–4. STUDY DESIGN: The location of pedicle screws (n = 42) in four human specimens of the lumbar spine and in 30 patients (n = 131 screws) after lumbar spinal fusion was assessed using computed tomography. OBJECTIVES: To determine the accuracy of pedicle screw placement in lumbar vertebrae and the reproducibility and repeatability of the computed tomography examination. SUMMARY OF BACKGROUND DATA: Failures in the placement of transpedicular screws for lumbar fusion are reported. The evaluation of such screws using computed tomography examination has not been investigated. METHODS: After surgery, the specimens were dissected in transversal slices to observe macroscopically the location of the pedicle screw and to correlate these observations with the computed tomography images. All patients were examined by one observer. To determine the reproducibility and repeatability of the computed tomography examination, two observers studied computed tomography images of 12 patients (n = 58 screws) twice within 3 months. RESULTS: In the specimens, 10 screws were observed to penetrate the medial wall of the pedicle. This correlated fully with the images. In the patients' group, 40% of all screws penetrated the cortex of the vertebra. Of all screws, 29% penetrated the medial wall of the pedicle. From the computed tomography images, it appeared that a deviation of more than 6 mm medially was a high risk for nerve root damage. Three months after his first examination, Observer 1 documented a different position in three of 58 screws (kappa = 0.90). Observer 2 found a different position in eight screws (kappa = 0.65). The comparison between the reviews of the two observers showed a different opinion for the first evaluation, four disagreements (2-4 mm) and 17 disagreements (0-2 mm; kappa = 0.34), and for the second evaluation, four disagreements (2-4 mm) and 12 disagreements (0-2 mm; kappa = 0.43). CONCLUSIONS: Correct placement of transpedicular screws for spinal fusion seems to be more difficult than it looks. The computed tomography scanning is useful for differential diagnosis of postoperative radicular syndromes after lumbar transpedicular fixation.

18. Hufner T, et al. Computer-assisted fracture reduction of pelvic ring fractures: an in vitro study. Clin Orthop Relat Res. 2002;(399):231–9. A newly developed software module for computer-assisted surgery based on a commercially available navigation system allows simultaneous, independent registration of two fragments and real-time navigation of both fragments while reduction occurs. To evaluate the accuracy three fracture models were used: geometric foam blocks, a pelvic ring injury with disruption of the symphysis and the sacroiliac joint, and a pelvic ring fracture with symphysis disruption and a transforaminal sacral fracture. One examiner did visual and navigated reduction and in all experiments the end point was defined as anatomic reduction. Residual displacement was measured with a magnetic motion tracking device. The results revealed a significantly increased residual displacement with navigated reduction compared with visual control. The differences were low, averaging 1 mm for residual translation and 0.7 degrees for the residual rotation, respectively. Residual displacement was small in both set-ups and may not be clinically relevant. Additional development of the software prototype with integration of surface registration may lead to improved handling and facilitated multifragment tracking. Use in the clinical setting should be possible within a short time.

19. Langlotz F, et al. The first twelve cases of computer assisted periacetabular osteotomy. Comput Aided Surg. 1997;2(6):317–26. Image guided freehand navigation of surgical instruments has been applied to the Bernese periacetabular osteotomy, a complex surgical technique for the treatment of dysplastic hips. This navigation system has been introduced into the operating room and has so far been used for 12 patients. Image data from computed tomography (CT) scans are presented in various ways to support the preoperative plan and to provide optimized control of surgical action. Special attention has been paid to the implementation of a sophisticated surgeon-machine interface. This paper describes the features of this novel surgical navigation system and its introduction into the clinical environment.
20. Hufner T, et al. New indications for computer-assisted surgery: tumor resection in the pelvis. Clin Orthop Relat Res. 2004;(426):219–25. The resection of recurrent malignant pelvic tumors was supported by a commercially available navigation system in three patients. Preoperatively three-dimensional images from the pelvis were obtained by computed tomography or magnetic resonance imaging to identify the tumor extension. During surgery navigated tools oriented the surgeon to excise the tumor with adequate virtual margins. Navigation was helpful for tumor identification in one patient with a recurrent presacral mesenchymal chondrosarcoma. In the other two patients the tumor resection in the bone was done with three-dimensional observation of the osteotomies in the sacrum. In all three patients the histopathologic analysis confirmed that the neoplasms were excised accurately within their margins. We think that computer-assisted surgery is a potential method to increase the accuracy of tumor resections.
21. Cheong D, Letson GD. Computer-assisted navigation and musculoskeletal sarcoma surgery. Cancer Control. 2011;18(3):171–6. BACKGROUND: Despite advances in medical, surgical, and radiation oncology, deep-seated bone sarcomas that require large osseous resections continue to present resection and reconstructive challenges to musculoskeletal surgeons. METHODS: We describe our experience with computer navigation techniques combined with complex pelvic resections and limb-preserving surgeries. RESULTS: Computer-assisted navigation has shown promise in aiding in optimal preoperative planning and in providing more accurate and precise feedback during surgery. CONCLUSIONS: Computer-assisted navigation offers precise instrumentation, technology-oriented imaging systems, and powerful information processing, all of which can assist in decision making, preoperative planning, and surgical accuracy.
22. Jeys L, et al. Can computer navigation-assisted surgery reduce the risk of an intralesional margin and reduce the rate of local recurrence in patients with a tumour of the pelvis or sacrum? Bone Joint J. 2013;95-B(10):1417–24. We hypothesised that the use of computer navigation-assisted surgery for pelvic and sacral tumours would reduce the risk of an intralesional margin. We reviewed 31 patients (18 men and 13 women) with a mean age of 52.9 years (13.5 to 77.2) in whom computer navigation-assisted surgery had been carried out for a bone tumour of the pelvis or sacrum. There were 23 primary malignant bone tumours, four metastatic tumours and four locally advanced primary tumours of the rectum. The registration error when using computer navigation was < 1 mm in each case. There were no complications related to the navigation, which allowed the preservation of sacral nerve roots (n = 13), resection of otherwise inoperable disease (n = 4) and the avoidance of hindquarter amputation (n = 3). The intralesional resection rate for primary tumours of the pelvis and sacrum was 8.7% (n = 2): clear bone resection margins were achieved in all cases. At a mean follow-up of 13.1 months (3 to 34) three patients (13%) had developed a local recurrence. The mean time alive from diagnosis was 16.8 months (4 to 48). Computer navigation-assisted surgery is safe and has reduced our intralesional resection rate for primary tumours of the pelvis and sacrum. We recommend this technique as being worthy of further consideration for this group of patients.
23. Reijnders K, et al. Image guided surgery: new technology for surgery of soft tissue and bone sarcomas. Eur J Surg Oncol. 2007;33(3):390–8. AIM: Providing the surgical oncologist with a new means of performing safe and radical sarcoma surgery with the help of image guidance technology. METHOD: Two patients with pelvic sarcomas were operated upon with the help of an intra-operative navigation system. The technology of image guided surgery is described

in one patient with a retroperitoneal sarcoma invading the bony pelvis and another patient with a chondrosarcoma of the iliac crest. RESULTS: We show that this new procedure enables optimal radical surgical resection with minimal treatment related morbidity or loss of function. CONCLUSION: Image guided surgery is a new technical tool in sarcoma surgery.

24. So TY, et al. Computer-assisted navigation in bone tumor surgery: seamless workflow model and evolution of technique. Clin Orthop Relat Res. 2010;468(11):2985–91. BACKGROUND: Computer-assisted navigation was recently introduced to aid the resection of musculoskeletal tumors. However, it has not always been possible to directly navigate the osteotomy with real-time manipulation of available surgical tools. Registration techniques vary, although most existing systems use some form of surface matching. QUESTIONS/PURPOSES: We developed and evaluated a workflow model of computer-assisted bone tumor surgery and evaluated (1) the applicability of currently available software to different bones; (2) the accuracy of the navigated excision; and (3) the accuracy of a new registration technique of fluoro-CT matching. METHODS: Our workflow involved detailed preoperative planning with CT-MRI image fusion, three-dimensional mapping of the tumor, and planning of the resection plane. Using the workflow model, we reviewed 15 navigation procedures in 12 patients, including four with joint-saving resections and three with custom implant reconstructions. Intraoperatively, registration was performed with either paired points and surface matching (Group 1, n = 10) or a new technique of fluoro-CT image matching (Group 2, n = 5). All osteotomies were performed under direct computer navigation. Postoperatively, each case was evaluated for histologic margin and gross measurement of the achieved surgical margin. RESULTS: The margins were free from tumor in all resected specimens. In the Group 1 procedures, the correlation between preoperative planned margins and actual achieved margins was 0.631, whereas in Group 2 procedures (fluoro-CT matching), the correlation was 0.985. CONCLUSIONS: Our findings suggest computer-assisted navigation is accurate and useful for bone tumor surgery. The new registration technique using fluoro-CT matching may allow more accurate resection of margins.
25. Wong KC, et al. Precision tumour resection and reconstruction using image-guided computer navigation. J Bone Joint Surg Br. 2007;89(7):943–7. The use of a navigation system in musculoskeletal tumour surgery enables the integration of pre-operative CT and MRI images to generate a precise three-dimensional anatomical model of the site and the extent of the tumour. We carried out six consecutive resections of musculoskeletal tumour in five patients using an existing commercial computer navigation system. There were three women and two men with a mean age of 41 years (24 to 47). Reconstruction was performed using a tumour prosthesis in three lesions and a vascularised fibular graft in one. No reconstruction was needed in two cases. The mean follow-up was 6.9 months (3.5 to 10). The mean duration of surgery was 28 minutes (13 to 50). Examination of the resected specimens showed clear margins in all the tumour lesions and a resection that was exactly as planned.
26. Wong KC, et al. Computer assisted pelvic tumor resection and reconstruction with a custom-made prosthesis using an innovative adaptation and its validation. Comput Aided Surg. 2007;12(4):225–32. Computer aided musculoskeletal tumor surgery is a novel concept. Ideally, computer navigation enables the integration of preoperative information concerning tumor extent and regional anatomy to facilitate execution of a surgical resection. Accurate resection helps oncological clearance and facilitates precise fitting of a custom prosthesis. We adapted a commercially available computer navigation platform for spine, and used it to plan and execute pelvic bone resection and custom pelvic prosthetic reconstruction in a patient with a metastatic tumor affecting the acetabulum. The surgery was simulated and validated using a plaster bone model based on the patient's preoperative CT data, before performing the procedure on the patient.
27. Wu K, et al. Intraoperative navigation for minimally invasive resection of periarticular and pelvic tumors. Orthopedics. 2011;34(5):372. The surgical approach to benign, metastatic, and some low-grade malignant tumors is often difficult due to their typically precarious locations. This article presents a series of cases where intraoperative stealth navigation was used to treat periarticular tumors. The use of paired point imaging with image fusion has made approaching

tumors through an accurate and minimally invasive technique a viable option for the treatment of a subset of musculoskeletal tumors.
28. Young PS, et al. The evolving role of computer-assisted navigation in musculoskeletal oncology. Bone Joint J. 2015;97-B(2):258–64. We report our experience of using a computer navigation system to aid resection of malignant musculoskeletal tumours of the pelvis and limbs and, where appropriate, their subsequent reconstruction. We also highlight circumstances in which navigation should be used with caution. We resected a musculoskeletal tumour from 18 patients (15 male, three female, mean age of 30 years (13 to 75) using commercially available computer navigation software (Orthomap 3D) and assessed its impact on the accuracy of our surgery. Of nine pelvic tumours, three had a biological reconstruction with extracorporeal irradiation, four underwent endoprosthetic replacement (EPR) and two required no bony reconstruction. There were eight tumours of the bones of the limbs. Four diaphyseal tumours underwent biological reconstruction. Two patients with a sarcoma of the proximal femur and two with a sarcoma of the proximal humerus underwent extra-articular resection and, where appropriate, EPR. One soft-tissue sarcoma of the adductor compartment which involved the femur was resected and reconstructed using an EPR. Computer navigation was used to aid reconstruction in eight patients. Histological examination of the resected specimens revealed tumour-free margins in all patients. Post-operative radiographs and CT showed that the resection and reconstruction had been carried out as planned in all patients where navigation was used. In two patients, computer navigation had to be abandoned and the operation was completed under CT and radiological control. The use of computer navigation in musculoskeletal oncology allows accurate identification of the local anatomy and can define the extent of the tumour and proposed resection margins. Furthermore, it helps in reconstruction of limb length, rotation and overall alignment after resection of an appendicular tumour.
29. Ozaki T, et al. Osteosarcoma of the pelvis: experience of the Cooperative Osteosarcoma Study Group. J Clin Oncol. 2003;21(2):334–41. PURPOSE: To define patients and tumor characteristics as well as therapy results, patients with pelvic osteosarcoma who were registered in the Cooperative Osteosarcoma Study Group (COSS) were analyzed. PATIENTS AND METHODS: Sixty-seven patients with a high-grade pelvic osteosarcoma were eligible for this analysis. Fifteen patients had primary metastases. All patients received chemotherapy according to COSS protocols. Thirty-eight patients underwent limb-sparing surgery, 12 patients underwent hemipelvectomy, and 17 patients did not undergo definitive surgery. Eleven patients received irradiation to the primary tumor site: four postoperatively and seven as the only form of local therapy. RESULTS: Local failure occurred in 47 of all 67 patients (70%) and in 31 of 50 patients (62%) who underwent definitive surgery. Five-year overall survival (OS) and progression free survival rates were 27% and 19%, respectively. Large tumor size (P =.0137), primary metastases (P =.0001), and no or intralesional surgery (P <.0001) were poor prognostic factors. In 30 patients with no or intralesional surgery, 11 patients with radiotherapy had better OS than 19 patients without radiotherapy (P =.0033). Among the variables, primary metastasis, large tumor, no or intralesional surgery, no radiotherapy, existence of primary metastasis (relative risk [RR] = 3.456; P =.0009), surgical margin (intralesional or no surgical excision; RR = 5.619; P <.0001), and no radiotherapy (RR = 4.196; P =.0059) were independent poor prognostic factors. CONCLUSION: An operative approach with wide or marginal margins improves local control and OS. If the surgical margin is intralesional or excision is impossible, additional radiotherapy has a positive influence on prognosis.
30. Cartiaux O, et al. Surgical inaccuracy of tumor resection and reconstruction within the pelvis: an experimental study. Acta Orthop. 2008;79(5):695–702. BACKGROUND AND PURPOSE: Osseous pelvic tumors can be resected and reconstructed using massive bone allografts. Geometric accuracy of the conventional surgical procedure has not yet been documented. The aim of this experimental study was mainly to assess accuracy of tumoral resection with a 10-mm surgical margin, and also to evaluate the geometry of the host-graft reconstruction. METHODS: An experimental model on plastic pelvises was designed to simulate tumor resection and reconstruction. 4 experienced surgeons were asked to resect 3 different tumors and to reconstruct pelvises. 24 resections and host-graft junctions were available for evaluation.

Resection margins were measured. Several methods were created to evaluate geometric properties of the host-graft junction. RESULTS: The probability of a surgeon obtaining a 10-mm surgical margin with a 5-mm tolerance above or below, was 52% (95% CI: 37-67). Maximal gap, gap volume, and mean gap between host and graft was 3.3 (SD 1.9) mm, 2.7 (SD 2.1) cm3 and 3.2 (SD 2.1) mm, respectively. Correlation between these 3 reconstruction measures and the degree of contact at the host-graft junction was poor. INTERPRETATION: 4 experienced surgeons did not manage to consistently respect a fixed surgical margin under ideal working conditions. The complex 3-dimensional architecture of the pelvis would mainly explain this inaccuracy. Solutions to this might be to increase the surgical margin or to use computer- and robotic-assisted technologies in pelvic tumor resection. Furthermore, our attempt to evaluate geometry of the pelvic reconstruction using simple parameters was not satisfactory. We believe that there is a need to define new standards of evaluation.

31. Docquier PL, et al. Computer-assisted resection and reconstruction of pelvic tumor sarcoma. Sarcoma. 2010;2010:125162. Pelvic sarcoma is associated with a relatively poor prognosis, due to the difficulty in obtaining an adequate surgical margin given the complex pelvic anatomy. Magnetic resonance imaging and computerized tomography allow valuable surgical resection planning, but intraoperative localization remains hazardous. Surgical navigation systems could be of great benefit in surgical oncology, especially in difficult tumor location; however, no commercial surgical oncology software is currently available. A customized navigation software was developed and used to perform a synovial sarcoma resection and allograft reconstruction. The software permitted preoperative planning with defined target planes and intraoperative navigation with a free-hand saw blade. The allograft was cut according to the same planes. Histological examination revealed tumor-free resection margins. Allograft fitting to the pelvis of the patient was excellent and allowed stable osteosynthesis. We believe this to be the first case of combined computer-assisted tumor resection and reconstruction with an allograft.
32. Kojima T, et al. The usefulness and limits of magnetic resonance imaging in the differential diagnosis of pelvic tumors. Oncol Rep. 2001;8(4):867–9. Three cases of benign pelvic tumors are presented (2 leiomyomas and 1 fibroma). All three tumors were suspected of being malignant neoplasms because they were visualized as heterogeneous high signal intensity on T2-weighted images, and thus they were difficult to diagnose preoperatively. One of the leiomyomas was located in the retroperitoneum and had been misdiagnosed as an ovarian tumor. All three tumors exhibited secondary myxoid changes, these changes may have been responsible for the high signal intensity on the T2-weighted MR images. Since benign tumors sometimes mimic malignant tumors on MR images, exploratory laparotomy is essential to make a definitive diagnosis.
33. Berlemann U, et al. [Computer-assisted orthopedic surgery. From pedicle screw insertion to further applications]. Orthopade. 1997;26(5):463–9. Computer assisted orthopaedic surgery is a new but rapidly evolving field. Based on previous research and development in the area of stereotactic neuronavigation a few groups have adapted these technologies for the image interactive insertion of pedicle screws. The present paper summarizes past and current work in the field of computer assisted orthopaedic surgery and describes the state of the art of research and future innovations, particularly in in vivo applications.
34. Delp SL, et al. Computer assisted knee replacement. Clin Orthop Relat Res. 1998;(354):49–56. Accurate alignment of knee implants is essential for the success of total knee replacement. Although mechanical alignment guides have been designed to improve alignment accuracy, there are several fundamental limitations of this technology that will inhibit additional improvements. Various computer assisted techniques have been developed to examine the potential to install knee implants more accurately and consistently than can be done with mechanical guides. For example, computer integrated instrumentation incorporates highly accurate measurement devices to locate joint centers, track surgical tools, and align prosthetic components. Image guided knee replacement provides a three-dimensional preoperative plan that guides the placement of the cutting blocks and prosthetic components. Robot assisted knee replacement allows one to machine bones accurately without the use of stan-

dard cutting blocks. The rationale for the development of computer assisted knee replacement systems is presented, the operation of several different systems is described, the advantages and disadvantages of different approaches are discussed, and areas for future research are suggested.

35. Jaramaz B, et al. Computer assisted measurement of cup placement in total hip replacement. Clin Orthop Relat Res. 1998;(354):70–81. The introduction of image guided systems in total hip replacement surgery provides the ability to plan precisely the alignment of the acetabular cup before surgery, and to perform the surgery according to the preoperative plan. Preoperative planners (interactive computer programs for surgical planning) based on three-dimensional medical images allow planning of optimal placement of implant components based on simulated implant performance. Exact measurement of the cup position during surgery allows precise placement of the cup and accurate measurement of the final position of the cup relative to the pelvis. This measurement is used to evaluate the radiographic techniques for postoperative measurement of cup alignment. Malposition of the acetabular component increases the occurrence of impingement, reduces the safe range of motion, and increases the risk of dislocation and wear. Dislocation of the implant after total hip replacement remains a significant clinical problem. Not fully understanding the interaction between pelvic orientation and final acetabular cup alignment may be one of the main contributing factors in the continued significant incidence of dislocations after total hip replacement. In this study an attempt was made to link the preoperative planning, intraoperative placement, and postoperative measurement of cup placement in total hip replacement using computer assisted techniques.
36. Gautier E, et al. Accuracy of computer-guided screw fixation of the sacroiliac joint. Clin Orthop Relat Res. 2001;(393):310–7. Computer-assisted image guidance allows precise preoperative planning and intraoperative localization of surgical instruments. The technique recently was validated for the insertion of pedicle screws. In the laboratory, the precision of a surface-matching algorithm was evaluated for registration and accuracy and safety of screw placement into the vertebral bodies of S1 and S2 for fixation of the sacroiliac joint. Using six plastic pelves, 24 screw holes were made through the sacroiliac joint into the vertebral body of S1, and 12 holes were made through the sacroiliac joint into S2. The accuracy of the hole position was evaluated using a postoperative computed tomography examination. The safety factor was assessed by analysis of the remaining bone stock around the holes calculating a theoretical cylindrical volume being outside bone with increasing bore hole diameters. The registration was accurate with a mean error less than 1.4 mm in the posterior parts of the pelvis. The drilling followed precisely the preoperatively planned trajectories; perforation of the cortex of the sacrum was not observed. The safety factor of the S1 vertebral body is higher than that of S2 allowing larger diameter screw insertion into S1. This technique provides a safe and precise guide for transcutaneous or open insertion of iliosacral screws in cases of iliosacral dislocation or sacral fracture.
37. Hufner T, et al. Computer-assisted fracture reduction: novel method for analysis of accuracy. Comput Aided Surg. 2001;6(3):153–9. Anatomic reduction of displaced fractures is limited by the chosen surgical approach and intraoperative visualization. Preoperative Computed Tomography (CT) enhances the analysis of the fracture pattern and provides accurate spatial relationships. Computer Assisted Surgery (CAS) was introduced to increase the accuracy of specific surgical procedures. CAS systems can be used for implant placement or osteotomies in intact bone or reduced situations prior to obtaining the CT data, as differentiation into different datasets related to specific fragments is not yet possible. We present a model that allows "virtual" controlled reduction, providing computer assistance during the fracture reduction. Prior to clinical application, the accuracy of the process of virtual reduction must be proven in an experimental setting. An in vitro fracture model with two body fragments and a motion tracking system for three-dimensional (3D) control (accuracy 0.1 mm and 0.1 degrees) was used. Two methods were employed: direct visualization and reduction by the examiner, and "virtual" reduction, performed solely with the use of a computer image, in which the examiner lacks any direct visualization of the fragments. The results of this very simplified "fracture" model indicate that the overall difference between direct and virtual controlled reduction was

very small. A significant difference of 0.3 mm (0-1.8 mm) was seen for the residual displacement represented by the Euclidean distance ($p < 0.01$), whereas the difference in the residual angulation was not significant ($p > 0.05$). The methods tested revealed that virtual controlled reduction is nearly as accurate as direct visualization. Reduction control utilizing a motion tracker system reveals accurate 3D information in this simplified reduction setup, and is now used as a standard setup for analyzing realistic fracture models.

38. Zura RD, Kahler DM. A transverse acetabular nonunion treated with computer-assisted percutaneous internal fixation. A case report. J Bone Joint Surg Am. 2000;82(2):219–24.
39. Ritacco LE, et al. Accuracy of 3-D planning and navigation in bone tumor resection. Orthopedics. 2013;36(7):e942–50. Surgical precision in oncologic surgery is essential to achieve adequate margins in bone tumor resections. Three-dimensional preoperative planning and bone tumor resection by navigation have been introduced to orthopedic oncology in recent years. However, the accuracy of preoperative planning and navigation is unclear. The purpose of this study was to evaluate the accuracy of preoperative planning and the navigation system. A total of 28 patients were evaluated between May 2010 and February 2011. Tumor locations were the femur (n=17), pelvis (n=6), sacrum (n=2), tibia (n=2), and humerus (n=1). All resections were planned in a virtual scenario using computed tomography and magnetic resonance imaging fusion. A total of 61 planes or osteotomies were performed to resect the tumors. Postoperatively, computed tomography scans were obtained for all surgical specimens, and the specimens were 3-dimensionally reconstructed from the scans. Differences were determined by finding the distances between the osteotomies virtually programmed and those performed. The global mean of the quantitative comparisons between the osteotomies programmed and those obtained through the resected specimen was 2.52+/-2.32 mm for all patients. Differences between osteotomies virtually programmed and those achieved by navigation intraoperatively were minimal.
40. Ritacco LE, et al. Bone tumor resection: analysis about 3D preoperative planning and navigation method using a virtual specimen. Stud Health Technol Inform. 2013;192:1162. The use of three-dimensional preoperative planning and bone tumor resection guided by navigation has increased in the last ten years. However, no study to date, as far as we know, has directly provided evidence of accuracy of this method. The objective of this study was to describe a method capable of determining the accuracy of osteotomies performed for tumor resection planned and guided by navigation. We hypothesize that matching the 3D reconstructed surgical specimen is an acceptable method to determine the accuracy of virtual planning and navigation. A total of seven patients and 14 osteotomies were evaluated. After surgery, all surgical specimens were 3D reconstructed from CT images. The mean of quantitative comparisons between osteotomies planned and osteotomies obtained through the resected specimen was in a global mean of 1.56 millimeters (SD: 2.91) for all the cases. Based on our observations, a three-dimensional model obtained from the tumor surgical specimen is a useful tool to determine accuracy of 3D planning and surgical navigation.
41. Jones BC, et al. Synovial sarcoma: MR imaging findings in 34 patients. AJR Am J Roentgenol. 1993;161(4):827–30. OBJECTIVE: MR imaging is considered the procedure of choice for detecting and staging soft-tissue tumors. Its ability to show differences between benign and malignant soft-tissue tumors and its usefulness in suggesting a specific histologic diagnosis remain controversial. We studied the MR features of synovial sarcoma in 34 patients to determine if these tumors have specific MR findings that can be used to suggest the diagnosis. MATERIALS AND METHODS: MR imaging studies of 34 patients with synovial sarcoma were collected from two institutions and studied to determine the following characteristics of the tumor: size, shape, location, signal intensity and homogeneity, margin definition, presence of hemorrhage, and relationships to adjacent structures. These findings were then correlated with pathologic findings. RESULTS: The tumors tended to be deep, large (85% were > or = 5 cm in diameter), and located in the extremities with epicenters close to joints (63% within 7 cm of a joint). The lesions were usually inhomogeneous on T2-weighted images (82%) and clearly delineated from surrounding tissues (91%). Forty-four percent had high signal consistent with hemorrhage on both T1- and T2-weighted images. Fluid-fluid levels, best visualized

on T2-weighted images, were present in 18% of patients. Thirty-five percent of the lesions had areas that were hyper-, iso-, and hypointense relative to fat on T2-weighted images, constituting a triple signal intensity. The tumors frequently involved adjacent bone, with 71% invading, eroding, or touching bone. No association of pathologic subtypes with specific imaging findings was noted. CONCLUSION: Our results show a spectrum of MR imaging findings in synovial sarcoma. Nevertheless, the results suggest that synovial sarcoma should be considered when MR images show a relatively well-defined but inhomogeneous hemorrhagic lesion near a joint and in contact with bone. Fluid-fluid levels and areas hyper-, hypo-, and isointense relative to fat (triple signal) on T2-weighted sequences support the diagnosis.

42. Takao M, et al. Application of a CT-3D fluoroscopy matching navigation system to the pelvic and femoral regions. Comput Aided Surg. 2012;17(2):69–76. OBJECTIVE: The aim of this study was to find the proper location of the fluoroscopic imaging center in order to apply a CT-based 3D fluoroscopy matching navigation system in the pelvic and femoral regions. MATERIALS AND METHODS: To simulate surgeries around the hip joint, a dry human pelvis and femur were used. A total of 16 fiducial markers, each consisting of a metal ball 1.5 mm in diameter, were fixed to the pelvis and femur. For the pelvis, the pubic symphysis, the acetabular fossa, and a site on the ilium 3 cm above the acetabular roof were selected as fluoroscopic imaging centers. For the proximal femur, the base of the femoral neck, the femoral shaft at the level of the lesser trochanter, and the inferior border of the great trochanter were selected as fluoroscopic imaging centers. RESULTS: Target registration error (TRE) differed significantly among the selected fluoroscopic imaging centers. The best mean TRE for the pelvis was 0.8 mm (range: 0.2 to 1.6 mm) with the imaging center on the ilium (3 cm above the acetabular roof). The best mean TRE for the proximal femur was 1.1 mm (range: 0.2 to 2.0 mm) with the imaging center on the femoral shaft at the lesser trochanter level. CONCLUSION: Fluoroscopic imaging center location had a significant effect on the accuracy of the CT-based 3D fluoroscopy matching navigation system in the pelvic and femoral regions. The proper fluoroscopic imaging centers for CT-3D fluoroscopic matching were, for the pelvis, a site on the ilium 3 cm above the acetabular roof, and for the proximal femur, the femoral shaft at the level of the lesser trochanter.
43. Lionberger R. The attraction of electromagnetic computer-assisted navigation in orthopaedic surgery. In: Stiehl JB, Konermann W, Hacker R, editors. Navigation and MIS in orthopaedic surgery. Heidelberg: Springer; 2006. p. 44–53.
44. Frantz DD, et al. Accuracy assessment protocols for electromagnetic tracking systems. Phys Med Biol. 2003;48(14):2241–51. Electromagnetic tracking systems have found increasing use in medical applications during the last few years. As with most non-trivial spatial measurement systems, the complex determination of positions and orientations from their underlying raw sensor measurements results in complicated, non-uniform error distributions over the specified measurement volume. This makes it difficult to unambiguously determine accuracy and performance assessments that allow users to judge the suitability of these systems for their particular needs. Various assessment protocols generally emphasize different measurement aspects that typically arise in clinical use. This can easily lead to inconclusive or even contradictory conclusions. We examine some of the major issues involved and discuss three useful calibration protocols. The measurement accuracy of a system can be described in terms of its 'trueness' and its 'precision'. Often, the two are strongly coupled and cannot be easily determined independently. We present a method that allows the two to be disentangled, so that the resultant trueness properly represents the systematic, non-reducible part of the measurement error, and the resultant precision (or repeatability) represents only the statistical, reducible part. Although the discussion is given largely within the context of electromagnetic tracking systems, many of the results are applicable to measurement systems in general.
45. Khadem R, et al. Comparative tracking error analysis of five different optical tracking systems. Comput Aided Surg. 2000;5(2):98–107. OBJECTIVE: Effective utilization of an optical tracking system for image-based surgical guidance requires optimal placement of the dynamic reference frame (DRF) with respect to the tracking camera. Unlike other studies that measure the overall accuracy of a particular navigation system, this study investigates the precision of one

component of the navigation system: the optical tracking system (OTS). The precision of OTS measurements is quantified as jitter. By measuring jitter, one can better understand how system inaccuracies depend on the position of the DRF with respect to the camera. MATERIALS AND METHODS: Both FlashPointtrade mark (Image Guided Technologies, Inc., Boulder, Colorado) and Polaristrade mark (Northern Digital Inc., Ontario, Canada) optical tracking systems were tested in five different camera and DRF configurations. A linear testing apparatus with a software interface was designed to facilitate data collection. Jitter measurements were collected over a single quadrant within the camera viewing volume, as symmetry was assumed about the horizontal and vertical axes. RESULTS: Excluding the highest 5% of jitter, the FlashPoint cameras had an RMS jitter range of 0.028 +/- 0.012 mm for the 300 mm model, 0.051 +/- 0.038 mm for the 580 mm model, and 0.059 +/- 0.047 mm for the 1 m model. The Polaris camera had an RMS jitter range of 0.058 +/- 0.037 mm with an active DRF and 0.115 +/- 0.075 mm with a passive DRF. CONCLUSION: Both FlashPoint and Polaris have jitter less than 0.11 mm, although the error distributions differ significantly. Total jitter for all systems is dominated by the component measured in the axis directed away from the camera.

46. Milne AD, et al. Accuracy of an electromagnetic tracking device: a study of the optimal range and metal interference. J Biomech. 1996;29(6):791–3. The positional and rotational accuracy of a direct-current magnetic tracking device commonly used in biomechanical investigations was evaluated. The effect of different metals was also studied to determine the possibility of interference induced by experimental test fixtures or orthopaedic implants within the working field. Positional and rotational data were evaluated for accuracy and resolution by comparing the device output to known motions as derived from a calibrated grid board or materials testing machine. The effect of different metals was evaluated by placing cylindrical metal samples at set locations throughout the working field and comparing the device readings before and after introducing each metal sample. Positional testing revealed an optimal operational range with the transmitter and receiver separation between 22.5 and 64.0 cm. Within this range the mean positional error was found to be 1.8 percent of the step size, and resolution was determined to be 0.25 mm. The mean rotational error over a 1-20 degree range was found to be 1.6% of the rotational increment with a rotational resolution of 0.1 degrees. Of the metal alloys tested only mild steel produced significant interference, which was maximum when the sample was placed adjacent to the receiver. At this location the mild steel induced a positional difference of 5.26 cm and an angular difference of 9.75 degrees. The device was found to be insensitive to commonly used orthopaedic alloys. In this study, the electromagnetic tracking device was found to have positional and rotational errors of less than 2 percent, when utilized within its optimal operating range. This accuracy combined with its insensitivity to orthopaedic alloys should make it suitable for a variety of musculoskeletal research investigations.

47. Stiehl JB, et al. Accuracy of acetabular component positioning with a fluoroscopically referenced CAOS system. Comput Aided Surg. 2005;10(5–6):321–7. OBJECTIVE: This study evaluated the accuracy, repeatability, and reproducibility of a fluoroscopic referenced system used for guiding acetabular component positioning. METHODS: Calibration of the Medtronic StealthStation Treon Plus system was performed using a Weber gage block to assess linearity. Metrologic validation of repeatability and reproducibility was done using a cadaveric pelvis with an uncemented cup placed in the target position of 45 degrees inclination and 17.5 degrees anteversion. A baseline assessment was done with a National Institute of Standards and Technology (NIST) traceable coordinate measuring machine (CMM). RESULTS: Weber gage block analysis revealed a mean bias of 0.69 mm. For the cadaveric pelvis, the anterior pelvic plane was determined using the bilateral anterior superior iliac spines with the symphysis pubis as the inferior landmark. The mean CMM measurement was inclination of 46.023 degrees (SD=1.075; range: 43.318-46.844 degrees) and anteversion of 15.787 degrees (SD=0.411; range: 15.068-16.384 degrees). One surgeon performed a repeatability assessment (n=8), finding mean inclination of 42.8 degrees (SD=1.5; range: 39.5-44.5 degrees) and anteversion of 17.5 degrees (SD=3.0; range: 14.5-22.5 degrees). Three surgeons performed a reproducibility assessment (n=24), finding mean overall inclination of 48.5 degrees (SD=0.9;

range: 46-50 degrees) and anteversion of 17.8 degrees (SD=2.5; range: 13.5-23.5 degrees). All measurements were within a predefined acceptability range of+/-5 degrees. DISCUSSION: The accuracy and reproducibility of the fluoroscopic referencing method was found to be suitable for determination of cup position in the surgical setting. Anteversion measurements were more variable for the fluoroscopic method and this may be related to the difficulty for the surgeon in predictably picking the anatomical points from the fluoroscopic image.

48. Lembeck B, et al. Pelvic tilt makes acetabular cup navigation inaccurate. Acta Orthop. 2005;76(4):517–23. BACKGROUND: Modern navigation techniques allow precise positioning of the acetabular cup relative to the anterior pelvic plane. Variations in pelvic tilt will affect the resulting spatial orientation of the cup. METHODS: We measured pelvic tilt in 30 volunteers with an inclinometer combined with an ultrasonographic position measurement system. A mathematical algorithm was developed to calculate the resulting cup position measured on standard radiographs, depending on pelvic tilt. RESULTS: Average pelvic tilt at rest was -4 degrees in the lying position and -8 degrees in the standing position, and ranged from -27 degrees to +3 degrees. Pelvic reclination of 1 degree will lead to functional anteversion of the cup of approximately 0.7 degree. INTERPRETATION: Pelvic tilt makes navigation systems referring to the anterior plane inaccurate.
49. Thaler M, et al. Accuracy of an image-guided navigation system for pelvic surgery based on a multimodality registration object: a cadaver study. Am J Orthop (Belle Mead NJ). 2010;39(8):382–5. Accurate registration of external landmarks is often required for computer-aided surgery. In the study reported here, we investigated the influence of a new externally fixated multimodality registration object (MRO) on the accuracy of an image-guided navigation system in a human cadaver pelvis. With the MRO placed on the ipsilateral anterior superior iliac spine (ASIS), 14 of 17 target points showed a mean deviation (1.1 mm) that was significantly lower than that registered with the MRO on the contralateral ASIS (2.5 mm). In addition, the distance of target points from the MRO and the deviation of target points were highly correlated. This MRO provides a feasible means for achieving improved registration in computer-aided surgery of the pelvis.
50. Van Hellemondt G, et al. Computer-assisted pelvic surgery: an in vitro study of two registration protocols. Clin Orthop Relat Res. 2002;(405):287–93. An in vitro study was done to test the accuracy and functionality of computer-assisted surgery in pelvic orthopaedic surgery. The study was done on two fresh hips from one cadaver. In each hip, 10 titanium marker screws were inserted through standard pelvic osteotomy incisions. After a computed tomography scan was obtained the data were introduced into the navigation system. For the accuracy measurements the location of the center of the spherical heads of the marker screws was determined relative to a reference base attached to the pelvis using a special pointer that corresponded to the spherical head of the screws. A randomized trial was done with two surgeons to test the accuracy of two different anatomy-based registration protocols. The deviation between the virtual position of the marker screws in the pelvis, calculated by the computer after each anatomy based registration, and the real position were compared for each registration. Accuracy is not only related to the distance of the computed tomography slices and the necessary computed tomography field of view but also depends on the location of the point on the pelvis.
51. Sternheim A, et al. Navigated pelvic osteotomy and tumor resection: a study assessing the accuracy and reproducibility of resection planes in Sawbones and cadavers. J Bone Joint Surg Am. 2015;97(1):40–6. BACKGROUND: This Sawbones and cadaver study was performed to assess the accuracy and reproducibility of pelvic bone cuts made with use of a novel navigation system with a navigated osteotome and oscillating saw. METHODS: Using a novel navigation system and a three-dimensional planning tool, we navigated pelvic bone cuts that were representative of typical cuts made in pelvic tumor resections. The system includes a prototype mobile C-arm for intraoperative cone-beam computed tomography, real-time optical tracking (Polaris), and three-dimensional visualization software. Three-dimensional virtual radiographs were utilized in addition to triplanar (axial, sagittal, and coronal) navigation. In part one of the study, we navigated twenty-four sacral bone cuts in Sawbones models and validated our results in sixteen similar cuts in cadavers. In part two, we developed three Sawbones models of pelvic tumors based

on actual patient scenarios and compared three navigated resections with three non-navigated resections for each tumor model. Part three assessed the accuracy of the system with multiple users. RESULTS: There were ninety navigated cuts in Sawbones that were compared with fifty-four non-navigated cuts. In the navigated Sawbones cuts, the mean entry and exit cuts were 1.4 +/- 1 mm and 1.9 +/- 1.2 mm from the planned cuts, respectively. In comparison, the entry and exit cuts in Sawbones that were not navigated were 2.8 +/- 4.9 mm and 3.5 +/- 4.6 mm away from the planned osteotomy site. The navigated cuts were significantly more accurate (p </= 0.01). In the cadaver study, navigated entry and exit cuts were 1.5 +/- 0.9 mm and 2.1 +/- 1.5 mm from the planned cuts. The variation among three different users was 1 mm on both the entry and exit cuts. CONCLUSIONS: Navigation to guide pelvic bone cuts is accurate and feasible. Three-dimensional radiographs should be used for improved accuracy. Navigated cuts were significantly more accurate than non-navigated cuts were. A margin of 5 mm between the target tumor volume and the planned cut plane would result in a negative margin resection in more than 95% of the cuts. CLINICAL RELEVANCE: The accuracy of pelvic bone tumor resections and pelvic osteotomies can be improved with navigation to within 5 mm of the planned cut.

52. Cho HS, et al. Direct application of MR images to computer-assisted bone tumor surgery. J Orthop Sci. 2011;16(2):190–5. BACKGROUND: We describe a method for the direct application of MR images to navigation-assisted bone tumor surgery as an alternative to CT-MRI fusion. METHOD: Six patients with an orthopedic malignancy were employed for this method during navigation-assisted tumor resection. Tumor types included osteosarcoma (4), high-grade chondrosarcoma (1), and adamantinoma (1). Mean patient age was 25.3 years (range 18-52 years). Mean duration of follow-up was 25.8 months (range 18-32 months). Resorbable pin placement and rapid 3-dimensional spoiled gradient echo sequences made the direct application of MR images to computer-assisted bone tumor surgery without CT-MR image fusion possible. A paired-point registration technique was employed for patient-image registration in all patients. RESULTS: It took 20 min on average to set up the navigation (range 15-25 min). The mean registration error was 0.98 mm (range 0.4-1.7 mm). On histologic examination, distances from tumors to resection margins were in accord with preoperative plans. No patient had a local recurrence or distant metastasis at the last follow-up. CONCLUSION: Direct patient-to-MRI registration is a very useful method for bone tumor surgery, permitting the application of MR images to intraoperative visualization without any additional costs or exposure of the patient to radiation from the preoperative CT scan.

53. Pappas IP, et al. New method to assess the registration of CT-MR images of the head. Injury. 2004;35 Suppl 1:S-A105-112. Due to their complementary information content, both x-ray computed tomography (CT) and magnetic resonance (MR) imaging are employed in certain clinical cases to improve the understanding of pathology involved. o spatially relate the two datasets, image registration and image fusion are employed. However, registration errors, either global or local, are common and are nonuniform within the image volume. In this paper, we propose a new algorithm that assesses the quality of the registration locally within the CT-MR volume and provides visual, color-coded feedback to the user about the location and extent of good and bad correspondence between the two images. The proposed registration assessment algorithm is based on a correspondence analysis of bone structures in the CT and MR images. For that purpose, a custom segmentation algorithm for bone in MR images has been developed that is based on a stochastic threshold computation method. This segmentation method for MR images and the CT-MR registration assessment algorithm were validated on simulated MR datasets and real CT-MR image pairs of the head. Some partial-volume effects occur at the borders of the bone structures and at the bone interfaces with air, which cannot be separated from bone in the MR image. The presented assessment method of CT-MR image registration offers the user a new tool to evaluate the overall and local quality of the registration. With this information, the user does not have to blindly trust the fused CT-MR datasets but can easily identify areas of inaccurate correspondence. The application of the algorithm is so far limited to T1-weighted MR and CT images of the head area.

54. Amiot LP, Poulin F. Computed tomography-based navigation for hip, knee, and spine surgery. Clin Orthop Relat Res. 2004;(421):77–86. A review of CT-based orthopaedic navigation is

presented with a specific emphasis on arthroplasty for the hip and the knee. Fundamental issues about the laboratory and clinical validation of the applications are addressed. The ability to compute the position and orientation of an acetabular implant using a postoperative CT scan was investigated. Angle deviations relative to known positions were computed with an error of less than 1 degree. Then, the system accuracy for three-dimensional reconstruction and registration of two cadaveric pelvis specimens was measured with more than 350 registrations. We observed a maximal inclination error of 5 degrees in 99% of cases and a maximal anteversion error of 5 degrees in 97% of cases. The accuracy of the three-dimensional reconstruction and registration for knee arthroplasty also was measured and computed with an angular accuracy of 0.5 degrees in the AP plane and accuracy of 3 degrees in the lateral plane. A clinical study then was done in 109 cases where 96% of implants were installed with a hip-knee-ankle angle of 180 +/- 3 degrees . Computed tomography-based navigation for orthopaedic surgery provides greater accuracy and reproducibility than conventional surgery. As noted by learning curves, software improvements are needed to bring it into daily clinical routine.

55. Docquier PL, et al. Registration accuracy in computer-assisted pelvic surgery. Comput Aided Surg. 2009;14(1–3):37–44. INTRODUCTION: An in vitro study was performed to assess the global registration accuracy of a computer-assisted system in pelvic orthopaedic surgery. The system was applied to a putative tumor resection in a pelvic sawbone. METHODS: Twenty landmarks were created on the surface of the pelvis, and a virtual model of the sawbone was constructed based on surface extraction from computed tomography. The coordinates of the landmarks were defined in the CT-scan coordinate system, and registration of the sawbone with the virtual model was achieved using a surface-based matching algorithm. The landmarks were considered as control points, and deviations between their physical locations and their locations in the virtual model were calculated, thereby quantifying the global accuracy error. RESULTS: The location of the initialization points was unimportant. The dynamic reference base gave the best results when placed far from the working area. Accuracy was improved when the sampling area was increased, but was decreased by its excessive expansion. CONCLUSIONS: It is recommended that the DRB be located on the contralateral side of the pelvis. Extending the approach posteriorly and including the entire working area in the sampling surface area, if possible, will also help increase accuracy in computer-assisted pelvic surgery.

56. Mayr E, et al. The effect of fixation and location on the stability of the markers in navigated total hip arthroplasty: a cadaver study. J Bone Joint Surg Br. 2006;88(2):168–72. In navigated total hip arthroplasty, the pelvis and the femur are tracked by means of rigid bodies fixed directly to the bones. Exact tracking throughout the procedure requires that the connection between the marker and bone remains stable in terms of translation and rotation. We carried out a cadaver study to compare the intra-operative stability of markers consisting of an anchoring screw with a rotational stabiliser and of pairs of pins and wires of different diameters connected with clamps. These devices were tested at different locations in the femur. Three human cadavers were placed supine on an operating table, with a reference marker positioned in the area of the greater trochanter. K-wires (3.2 mm), Steinman pins (3 and 4 mm), Apex pins (3 and 4 mm), and a standard screw were used as fixation devices. They were positioned medially in the proximal third of the femur, ventrally in the middle third and laterally in the distal portion. In six different positions of the leg, the spatial positions were recorded with a navigation system. Compared with the standard single screw, with the exception of the 3 mm Apex pins, the two-pin systems were associated with less movement of the marker and could be inserted less invasively. With the knee flexed to 90 degrees and the dislocated hip rotated externally until the lower leg was parallel to the table (figure-four position), all the anchoring devices showed substantial deflection of 1.5 degrees to 2.5 degrees . The most secure area for anchoring markers was the lateral aspect of the femur.

57. Wiles AD, Thompson D, Frantz DD. Accuracy assessment and interpretation for optical tracking systems. Med Imaging. 2004;5367:1–12.

58. Oszwald M, et al. Accuracy of navigated surgery of the pelvis after surface matching with an a-mode ultrasound probe. J Orthop Res. 2008;26(6):860–4. Computer-aided surgery (CAS)

allows for real-time intraoperative feedback resulting in increased accuracy, while reducing intraoperative radiation. CAS is especially useful for the treatment of certain pelvic ring fractures, which necessitate the precise placement of screws. Flouroscopy-based CAS modules have been developed for many orthopedic applications. The integration of the isocentric flouroscope even enables navigation using intraoperatively acquired three-dimensional (3D) data, though the scan volume and imaging quality are limited. Complicated and comprehensive pathologies in regions like the pelvis can necessitate a CT-based navigation system because of its larger field of view. To be accurate, the patient's anatomy must be registered and matched with the virtual object (CT data). The actual precision within the region of interest depends on the area of the bone where surface matching is performed. Conventional surface matching with a solid pointer requires extensive soft tissue dissection. This contradicts the primary purpose of CAS as a minimally invasive alternative to conventional surgical techniques. We therefore integrated an a-mode ultrasound pointer into the process of surface matching for pelvic surgery and compared it to the conventional method. Accuracy measurements were made in two pelvic models: a foam model submerged in water and one with attached porcine muscle tissue. Three different tissue depths were selected based on CT scans of 30 human pelves. The ultrasound pointer allowed for registration of virtually any point on the pelvis. This method of surface matching could be successfully integrated into CAS of the pelvis.

59. Arand M, et al. [Sources of error and risks in CT based navigation]. Orthopade. 2002;31(4):378–84. Based on the experience of 4 cervical, 102 thoracic/lumbar pedicle screw and 14 transiliosacral screw implantations all problems and complications were collected. Problems noted within the data collection in the preoperative CT were an incomplete acquisition of the surgical target (n = 3), an exceeding of the processable scan slices (n = 1) and a non focused field of view. Transmission of the CT datas often were documented as incomplete (n = 16). Segmentation of the CT dataset turned out to be the significant problem with incorrect differentiation of the bone-soft tissue transition (n = 2), where as the choice of the matching points and the trajectories did not provoke any mistakes in the planning modus. The intraoperative matching of both corresponding datasets was insufficient (n = 7), while the assignment of the CT dataset to the correct vertebral was not a major problem (n = 1). Navigation was not possible (n = 2) due to an instability of the spinal process. All fiducial based matching procedures (pelvis) were carried out without any problems. During intraoperative navigation potential complications resulted from deformation of instruments (n = 1) and interaction of instruments and the data reference base (n = 2). Further, the CT-based navigation of fractured vertebrae or unstable iliosacral joints is not safe, because dislocations between acquisition of the dataset and operation will lead to misguidance.

60. Sakai Y, et al. Simultaneous registration with ct-fluoro matching for spinal navigation surgery. A case report. Nagoya J Med Sci. 2006;68(1–2):45–52. Computer-assisted surgery, which provides simultaneous, multiplanar images of bone structures, has become widely used. However, registration maneuvering remains time consuming. The objective of this paper is to document the usefulness of CT-fluoro matching for spinal navigation. A spinal navigation system (VECTORVISION compact; Brain LAB, Germany) and a digital imaging system (OEC9800; CATHEX, Tokyo, Japan) were used for CT-fluoro matching in cases of L4/5 and L5/S1 posterior lumbar interbody fusion. A reference array was attached to the L4 spinous process. Preoperative CT images and intraoperative fluoro-shots including L4, L5, and S1 were superimposed on the navigation monitor. Following insertion of L4 screws, a reference array remained to be attached to the L4 spinous process, after which a level definition and preregistration of L5 and S1 vertebrae were performed and the screwing procedure of L5 and S1 was completed without additional fluro-shots. Registration of three vertebrae was completed without paired-point or surface-matching procedures. The calculation time for the registration in a single vertebra was 30 sec. All pedicle screws were seen to be successfully inserted on postoperative CT images. We performed the navigation surgery by matching the preoperative CT images to the intraoperative fluoro-shots without manual registration. This technique may

prove useful in the future for anterior spinal surgery and percutaneous screwing without the need for total exposure of the bone surface.

61. Stockle U, et al. Image guidance in pelvic and acetabular surgery—expectations, success and limitations. Injury. 2007;38(4):450–62. During the last decade navigation techniques in pelvic and acetabular surgery have been described. Nowadays, available techniques include CT-based navigation, 2D C-arm navigation and 3D C-arm navigation. The main indication is the navigated percutaneous SI screw fixation, but acetabular screw fixations are also reported. In this article, based upon a literature review and our own clinical experiences, the indications for and limitations of navigated techniques in pelvic and acetabular surgery are described.
62. Bachler R, et al. Restricted surface matching—numerical optimization and technical evaluation. Comput Aided Surg. 2001;6(3):143–52. Accurate and reliable registration is one of the most important issues in computer-aided surgery, as small errors may have a large influence on the overall accuracy of the system. The restricted surface-matching algorithm (RSM), initially developed for periacetabular osteotomy surgery (PAO), has been improved to become numerically more stable and reliable. To assess the accuracy and sensitivity of registration, a framework is presented that evaluates two aspects of registration: the sensitivity and raw performance of the registration algorithm are tested in a stand-alone environment, and the integration into a CAS system is analyzed by evaluating the accuracy of the complete system. For the latter tests, spherical-headed titanium screws used as fiducial landmarks provide a reference transformation for the registration. This framework was used to analyze the performance of RSM for PAO surgery. The sensitivity analysis showed the algorithm to be insensitive to noise up to a magnitude of 3 mm. Both the sensitivity analysis and simulated surgical environment tests showed that an accuracy can be attained of better than 2 mm in the region of interest, and better than 4 mm far away from the region of interest. This is sufficient for safely assisting PAO surgeries.
63. Wong KC, Kumta SM. Computer-assisted tumor surgery in malignant bone tumors. Clin Orthop Relat Res. 2013;471(3):750–61. BACKGROUND: Small recent case series using CT-based navigation suggest such approaches may aid in surgical planning and improve accuracy of intended resections, but the accuracy and clinical use have not been confirmed. QUESTIONS/PURPOSES: We therefore evaluated (1) the accuracy; (2) recurrences; and (3) function in patients treated by computer-assisted tumor surgery (CATS). METHODS: From 2006 to 2009, we performed CATS in 20 patients with 21 malignant tumors. The mean age was 31 years (range, 6-80 years). CT and MR images for 18 cases were fused using the navigation software. Reconstructed two-dimensional/three-dimensional images were used to plan the bone resection. The achieved bone resection was compared with the planned one by assessing margins, dimensions at the level of bone resection, or fitting of CAD custom prostheses. Function was assessed with the Musculoskeletal Tumor Society (MSTS) score. The minimum followup was 31 months (mean, 39 months; range, 5-69 months). RESULTS: Histological examination of all resected specimens showed a clear tumor margin. The achieved bone resection matched the planned with a difference of </= 2 mm. The achieved positions of custom prostheses were comparable to the planned positions when merging postoperative with preoperative CT images in five cases. Three of the four patients with local recurrence had tumors at the sacral region. The mean MSTS score was 28 (range, 23-30). CONCLUSION: CATS with image fusion allows accurate execution of the intended bone resection. It may be beneficial to resection and reconstruction in pelvic, sacral tumors and more difficult joint-preserving intercalated tumor surgery. Comparative clinical studies with long-term followup are necessary to confirm its efficacy. LEVEL OF EVIDENCE: Level IV, therapeutic study. See Guidelines for Authors for a complete description of levels of evidence.
64. Wong KC, Kumta SM. Joint-preserving tumor resection and reconstruction using image-guided computer navigation. Clin Orthop Relat Res. 2013;471(3):762–73. BACKGROUND: Joint-preserving surgery is performed in select patients with bone sarcomas of extremities and allows patients to retain the native joint with better joint function. However, recurrences may relate to achieving adequate margins and there is frequently little room for error in tumors close to the joint surface. Further, the tumor margin on preoperative CT and/or MR images is difficult to transpose to the actual extent of tumor in the bone in the operating room.

QUESTIONS/PURPOSES: We therefore determined whether joint-preserving tumor surgery could be performed accurately under image-guided computer navigation and determined local recurrences, function, and complications. METHODS: We retrospectively studied eight patients with bone sarcoma of extremities treated surgically by navigation with fused CT-MR images. We assessed the accuracy of resection in six patients by comparing the cross sections at the resection plane with complementary prosthesis templates. Mean age was 17 years (range, 6-46 years). Minimum followup was 25 months (mean, 41 months; range, 25-60 months). RESULTS: The achieved resection was accurate, with a difference of 2 mm or less in any dimension compared to that planned in patients with custom prostheses. We noted no local recurrence at latest followup. The mean Musculoskeletal Tumor Society score was 29 (range, 28-30). There were no complications related to navigation planning and procedures. There was no failure of fixation at the remaining epiphysis. CONCLUSIONS: In selected patients, the computer-assisted approach facilitates precise planning and execution of joint-preserving tumor resection and reconstruction. Further followup assessment in a larger study population is required in these patients. LEVEL OF EVIDENCE: Level IV, therapeutic study. See Instructions for Authors for a complete description of levels of evidence.

65. Salehi SA, Ondra SL. Use of internal fiducial markers in frameless stereotactic navigational systems during spinal surgery: technical note. Neurosurgery. 2000;47(6):1460–2. OBJECTIVE: The use of frameless stereotaxy has expanded the spine surgeon's ability to perform surgical procedures with instrumentation in areas of narrow anatomic tolerance. In many circumstances, however, it is difficult to register the frameless stereotactic probe using known anatomic landmarks. This occurs typically because landmarks are indistinct, and congenital or surgical defects limit the availability of anatomic fiducials. We propose an accurate and efficient method for registering the frameless stereotactic probe for spinal surgery when a staged procedure is planned. METHODS: During the first stage of a planned two-stage procedure, a minimum of four cranial fiducial screws are implanted in the posterior element of each vertebra in which stereotactic registration is desired. Stage 1 is completed, and all suture closure is performed. A computed tomographic scan formatted for the frameless stereotactic unit is obtained postoperatively. In the second stage of surgery, registration is performed using cranial screws as internal fiducial markers. RESULTS: Registration is performed easily and quickly using cranial screws as internal fiducial markers. No more than four registration points are necessary to calibrate the system to accuracy within 1.5 mm. CONCLUSION: Implantation of fiducial markers during Stage 1 of a complex staged spinal surgery renders the frameless stereotactic navigational system registration extremely fast and accurate. We advocate the technique to enhance the use of frameless navigational systems for reliable and quick registration of the spine.

66. Hulen CA, et al. Oncologic and functional outcome following sacrectomy for sacral chordoma. J Bone Joint Surg Am. 2006;88(7):1532–9. BACKGROUND: Sacral chordoma is a rare, low to intermediate-grade tumor that poses substantial challenges in terms of timely diagnosis and adequate treatment. Few studies have examined the oncologic and functional outcomes of patients treated for sacral chordoma. METHODS: The clinical records of sixteen patients who had undergone sacrectomy for chordoma between 1985 and 2001 were evaluated retrospectively. All patients underwent resection by means of a sequential combined anterior and posterior approach. Patients were followed clinically at six-month intervals following recovery from the index surgical procedure. The disease onset, treatment, hospital stay, recurrence rates, survival, adjuvant therapy, functional outcome measures, and complications were evaluated. RESULTS: The average age at the time of diagnosis was sixty-one years. The mean tumor size was 15.2 cm in diameter, and all patients had a resection involving S1 or S2. The mean duration of follow-up was sixty-six months, and the tumor recurred in twelve of the sixteen patients. The mean time to metastasis was fifty months. Four patients were clinically disease-free at a mean follow-up of 94.5 months, while five patients died as a result of progressive local or metastatic disease at a mean follow-up of 31.4 months. Only one patient had normal bowel and bladder control postoperatively, and only three were able to walk without assistive devices. Eight patients had wound complications, and one patient had

a deep-vein thrombosis. With the numbers available, neither negative margins at the time of initial tumor resection nor adjuvant radiation therapy had a significant impact on survival or local recurrence. More cephalad levels of resection were associated with significantly worse bowel (p = 0.01) and bladder (p = 0.01) control. Complications were frequent and were more common with a larger tumor size at the time of presentation (p = 0.034). CONCLUSIONS: The treatment of sacral chordoma is an arduous clinical undertaking that requires a multidisciplinary approach and attention to detail from the outset. Despite aggressive well-planned surgical management and adherence to strict surveillance protocols, frequent recurrence and the late onset of metastatic disease are to be expected in a substantial proportion of patients, especially those with a very large chordoma or one at a more cephalad level. Adequate surgical treatment results in substantial functional impairment and numerous complications; however, it does offer the possibility of long-term disease-free survival. We advocate an attempt at complete resection, when there is still a possibility of cure, and aggressive treatment of local recurrences. LEVEL OF EVIDENCE: Therapeutic Level IV. See Instructions to Authors for a complete description of levels of evidence.

67. Kendoff D, et al. Navigated Iso-C3D-based percutaneous osteoid osteoma resection: a preliminary clinical report. Comput Aided Surg. 2005;10(3):157–63. Minimally invasive osteoid osteoma resection under computer tomography (CT) guidance has yielded good results and has become a viable alternative to open surgical procedures. Limited visualization of the actual drill position under CT guidance can frequently result in inadequate and malpositioned drilling, especially at lesions located in less accessible anatomic regions. With the conventional CT-guided drilling technique, sterility and general operative management poorly correlate with standard operating room conditions, and are at risk of intra- and postoperative complications. The new Iso-C(3D) imaging device provides intraoperative multiplanar reconstructions. Adequate image quality and implementation in navigation systems were described for numerous indications. On the basis of multiplanar reconstructions, minimally invasive navigated techniques under three-dimensional surgical tool control become possible, which is not the case under fluoroscopic or CT-based navigation. We report on our first three cases of navigated Iso-C(3D) osteoid osteoma resection. A minimally invasive resection of the nidus was possible under permanent multiplanar image control. No complications were encountered and all patients reported successful outcomes. Minimally invasive-based navigation offered an effective and reproducible surgical approach. Dependence on CT imaging for proper positioning and complications associated with use away from the operating room environment can be avoided.

68. Cartiaux O, et al. Computer-assisted planning and navigation improves cutting accuracy during simulated bone tumor surgery of the pelvis. Comput Aided Surg. 2013;18(1–2):19–26. BACKGROUND: Resection of bone tumors within the pelvis requires good cutting accuracy to achieve satisfactory safe margins. Manually controlled bone cutting can result in serious errors, especially due to the complex three-dimensional geometry, limited visibility, and restricted working space of the pelvic bone. This experimental study investigated cutting accuracy during navigated and non-navigated simulated bone tumor cutting in the pelvis. METHODS: A periacetabular tumor resection was simulated using a pelvic bone model. Twenty-three operators (10 senior and 13 junior surgeons) were asked to perform the tumor cutting, initially according to a freehand procedure and later with the aid of a navigation system. Before cutting, each operator used preoperative planning software to define four target planes around the tumor with a 10-mm desired safe margin. After cutting, the location and flatness of the cut planes were measured, as well as the achieved surgical margins and the time required for each cutting procedure. RESULTS: The location of the cut planes with respect to the target planes was significantly improved by using the navigated cutting procedure, averaging 2.8 mm as compared to 11.2 mm for the freehand cutting procedure (p < 0.001). There was no intralesional tumor cutting when using the navigation system. The maximum difference between the achieved margins and the 10-mm desired safe margin was 6.5 mm with the navigated cutting process (compared to 13 mm with the freehand cutting process). CONCLUSIONS: Cutting accuracy during simulated bone cuts of the pelvis can be significantly improved by using a freehand process assisted by a navigation system. When fully validated with comple-

mentary in vivo studies, the planning and navigation-guided technologies that have been developed for the present study may improve bone cutting accuracy during pelvic tumor resection by providing clinically acceptable margins.

69. Cartiaux O, et al. Computer-assisted and robot-assisted technologies to improve bone-cutting accuracy when integrated with a freehand process using an oscillating saw. J Bone Joint Surg Am. 2010;92(11):2076–82. BACKGROUND: In orthopaedic surgery, many interventions involve freehand bone cutting with an oscillating saw. Such freehand procedures can produce large cutting errors due to the complex hand-controlled positioning of the surgical tool. This study was performed to investigate the potential improvements in cutting accuracy when computer-assisted and robot-assisted technologies are applied to a freehand bone-cutting process when no jigs are available. METHODS: We designed an experiment based on a geometrical model of the cutting process with use of a simulated bone of rectangular geometry. The target planes were defined by three variables: a cut height (t) and two orientation angles (beta and gamma). A series of 156 cuts were performed by six operators employing three technologically different procedures: freehand, navigated freehand, and robot-assisted cutting. After cutting, we measured the error in the height t, the absolute error in the angles beta and gamma, the flatness, and the location of the cut plane with respect to the target plane. RESULTS: The location of the cut plane averaged 2.8 mm after use of the navigated freehand process compared with 5.2 mm after use of the freehand process ($p < 0.0001$). Further improvements were obtained with use of the robot-assisted process, which provided an average location of 1.7 mm ($p < 0.0001$). CONCLUSIONS: Significant improvements in cutting accuracy can be achieved when a navigation system or an industrial robot is integrated into a freehand bone-cutting process when no jigs are available. The procedure for navigated hand-controlled positioning of the oscillating saw appears to be easy to learn and use.
70. Arand M, et al. Computer-guidance in percutaneous screw stabilization of the iliosacral joint. Clin Orthop Relat Res. 2004;(422):201–7. Nine patients with instability and one patient with degeneration of the iliosacral joint were treated surgically. The posterior pelvic ring was stabilized with the assistance of an optoelectronic navigation system. Registration was ensured by using fiducial screws in the iliac crest or by collecting landmarks on the external fixator. Computed tomography scans taken postoperatively provided additional information regarding implant localization in all patients. Accurate placement of 21 of 22 implanted iliosacral screws was observed. Two of the 21 screws touched the wall of the second sacral foramen without perforating the canal. One screw perforated the anterior wall of the sacrum because the navigated guide wire was bent during implantation. The initial results indicate that computer-aided frameless navigation in surgery of the iliosacral joint can facilitate surgical performance during screw stabilization in selected patients. Two important issues must be considered in the clinical application of this technique: first, any relative migration of the iliac and sacral bone structures between computed tomography scans taken preoperatively and intraoperative navigation may result in an intolerable inaccuracy of computer guidance. Second, bending of the guide wire of the tracked power drive, which cannot be accommodated by the navigation system, will lead to misguidance; therefore, only navigated drill sleeves should be used.
71. Kawai A, et al. Prognostic factors for patients with sarcomas of the pelvic bones. Cancer. 1998;82(5):851–9. BACKGROUND: Treatment of malignant tumors of the pelvis represents one of the most difficult problems in musculoskeletal oncology. However, factors that influence the local and systemic control of the disease remain ill-defined. METHODS: One hundred and two patients with localized pelvic sarcomas who underwent a surgical excision of the tumors were analyzed. The tumor diagnosis was chondrosarcoma in 49 patients, osteosarcoma in 26 patients, Ewing's sarcoma in 20 patients, and other tumors in 7 patients. The tumor was located in the ilium in 65 patients, the pubis in 21 patients, the ischium in 8 patients, and the sacrum in 8 patients. Eighty-three patients underwent a limb-sparing surgery and 19 patients underwent hemipelvectomy. Prognostic factors for local recurrence, metastasis, and survival were analyzed. RESULTS: At last follow-up, 47 patients were disease free, 7 were alive with disease, and 48 had died. The 5-year survival rate was 55% (chondrosarcoma: 65%, osteosarcoma: 47%, and Ewing's sarcoma: 52%). Inadequate surgical margin emerged as the only

independent adverse prognostic factor for local recurrence. For distant metastasis, surgical stage remained as an independent prognostic factor. Patients who underwent a hemipelvectomy and those who had an inadequate surgical margin had significantly poorer survivals. CONCLUSIONS: Pelvic sarcomas remain diseases with a poor prognosis. Independent prognostic factors are few; an adequate surgical margin is critical to prevent local recurrence, and the surgical stage is related to the risk of distant metastasis. Surgical margins and hemipelvectomy were predictors of survival, but the patients who underwent hemipelvectomy also tended to have the largest, most advanced tumors. Hemipelvectomy should be considered when there is sacral involvement.

72. Cartiaux O, et al. Improved accuracy with 3D planning and patient-specific instruments during simulated pelvic bone tumor surgery. Ann Biomed Eng. 2014;42(1):205–13. In orthopaedic surgery, resection of pelvic bone tumors can be inaccurate due to complex geometry, limited visibility and restricted working space of the pelvis. The present study investigated accuracy of patient-specific instrumentation (PSI) for bone-cutting during simulated tumor surgery within the pelvis. A synthetic pelvic bone model was imaged using a CT-scanner. The set of images was reconstructed in 3D and resection of a simulated periacetabular tumor was defined with four target planes (ischium, pubis, anterior ilium, and posterior ilium) with a 10-mm desired safe margin. Patient-specific instruments for bone-cutting were designed and manufactured using rapid-prototyping technology. Twenty-four surgeons (10 senior and 14 junior) were asked to perform tumor resection. After cutting, ISO1101 location and flatness parameters, achieved surgical margins and the time were measured. With PSI, the location accuracy of the cut planes with respect to the target planes averaged 1 and 1.2 mm in the anterior and posterior ilium, 2 mm in the pubis and 3.7 mm in the ischium ($p < 0.0001$). Results in terms of the location of the cut planes and the achieved surgical margins did not reveal any significant difference between senior and junior surgeons ($p = 0.2214$ and 0.8449, respectively). The maximum differences between the achieved margins and the 10-mm desired safe margin were found in the pubis (3.1 and 5.1 mm for senior and junior surgeons respectively). Of the 24 simulated resection, there was no intralesional tumor cutting. This study demonstrates that using PSI technology during simulated bone cuts of the pelvis can provide good cutting accuracy. Compared to a previous report on computer assistance for pelvic bone cutting, PSI technology clearly demonstrates an equivalent value-added for bone cutting accuracy than navigation technology. When in vivo validated, PSI technology may improve pelvic bone tumor surgery by providing clinically acceptable margins.

73. Haider H, et al. Minimally invasive total knee arthroplasty surgery through navigated freehand bone cutting: winner of the 2005 "HAP" PAUL AWARD. J Arthroplast. 2007;22(4):535–42. Navigated freehand bone cutting (NFC) is introduced as a concept to eliminate alignment jigs and facilitate smaller arthroplasty incisions. We compare experimental cuts with this technique to conventional jigs. Using an in-house-built computer-aided orthopedic surgery system directly navigating a bone saw, users with different levels of surgical skills were timed performing full sets of distal femoral total knee arthroplasty cuts with jigs and with NFC. The cut surfaces were digitized to measure roughness and 3-dimensional translational/rotational errors. Navigated freehand cutting was 15% faster and produced 200% rougher surfaces than jigs, although its worst peaks/valleys were less than 1.2 mm. Implant fit/looseness, assessed by special navigated tools, was similar; but alignment was 400% better with NFC. Even at its infancy, NFC appears not to prohibitively compromise time and quality of cutting. Without requiring jigs, it has potential for radically less invasive total knee arthroplasty surgery.

74. Paul L, et al. Inaccuracy in selection of massive bone allograft using template comparison method. Cell Tissue Bank. 2008;9(2):83–90. The use of massive bone allografts is increasing year by year and selection method remains unchanged. Superposition of patient's radiograph over allograft image and comparison of distances is the gold standard. Experiment was led to test selection procedure of a major european tissue bank. Four observers were asked to select an allograft for 10 fictive recipients. Nine allografts were provided. To simulate a perfect allograft, recipient himself was inserted in the pool of allografts (trap graft). The 10 potential bone transplants were classified in four categories (from adequate to unacceptable). In addi-

tion, observers were asked to choose the three best grafts for a given recipient. Quadratic kappa measuring agreement on classification between two observers ranged between 0.74 (substantial) and 0.47 (moderate). Trap graft was quoted by observers as adequate four times (10%) and was cited eight times (20%) among the three best matching allografts. None of the observers discovered that recipient was among allograft panel. This study demonstrates that current selection method is inaccurate for hemipelvic allograft selection. New methods should be developed and tested to assist tissue banks in bone allograft selection.

75. Schmerber S, Chassat F. Accuracy evaluation of a CAS system: laboratory protocol and results with 6D localizers, and clinical experiences in otorhinolaryngology. Comput Aided Surg. 2001;6(1):1–13. OBJECTIVES: The objective of the study reported in this article was to evaluate (1) localizer inaccuracies, one of the major sources of errors in Computer-Assisted Surgery (CAS) systems, and (2) the final errors obtained using surface-based registration in ear, nose, and throat (ENT) surgery. These objectives were met through (1) a technical evaluation of the accuracy and usability of several optical localizers under laboratory test conditions, and (2) a clinical measure of the global errors obtained when using a CAS system including one of the standard localizer systems (Flashpoint 5000) in Functional Endoscopic Sinus Surgery (FESS). PATIENTS AND METHODS: The technical evaluation of localizers consisted of series of geometric tests on four commercial systems. Clinical evaluation included the development of a laboratory CAS system using a markerless, skin surface registration method. This was based on a standard optical digitizing system (Flashpoint 5000), which eliminates the need for the second CT scan, which is normally performed specifically to process the position of the fiducial markers. Global accuracy was then evaluated on 20 patients by subjective and visual comparison when placing a calibrated pointer on anatomical landmarks. RESULTS: The results of the technical study indicate that the four commercial systems tested have levels of inaccuracy deemed acceptable for most CAS applications, including ENT surgery. The clinical study obtained a registration and calibration accuracy of less than 1.5 mm in 89.2% (SD = 0.20 mm) of the cases studied. Our markerless skin surface points registration method is reliable, and allows patient head movements during the procedure. The accuracy tests performed show that this type of system can be used for ENT surgery with satisfaction. CONCLUSION: CAS systems enable the surgeon to have a more thorough understanding of the complicated anatomy of paranasal sinuses, and may be especially helpful in revision surgery when normal anatomic landmarks are lacking. Further studies are necessary in FESS to improve the CAS systems that are currently available, and to determine whether these systems can minimize the overall risk of complications.

76. Grimer RJ, et al. Hindquarter amputation: is it still needed and what are the outcomes? Bone Joint J. 2013;95-B(1):127–31. A total of 157 hindquarter amputations were carried out in our institution during the last 30 years. We have investigated the reasons why this procedure is still required and the outcome. This operation was used as treatment for 13% of all pelvic bone sarcomas. It was curative in 140 and palliative in 17, usually to relieve pain. There were 90 primary procedures (57%) with the remaining 67 following the failure of previous operations to control the disease locally. The indication for amputation in primary disease was for large tumours for which limb-salvage surgery was no longer feasible. The peri-operative mortality was 1.3% (n = 2) and major complications of wound healing or infection arose in 71 (45%) patients. The survival at five years after hindquarter amputation with the intent to cure was 45%, and at ten years 38%. Local recurrence occurred in 23 patients (15%). Phantom pain was a significant problem, and only 20% used their prosthesis regularly. Functional scores were a mean of 57%. With careful patient selection the oncological results and functional outcomes of hindquarter amputation justify its continued use.

77. Delloye C, et al. Pelvic reconstruction with a structural pelvic allograft after resection of a malignant bone tumor. J Bone Joint Surg Am. 2007;89(3):579–87. BACKGROUND: Reconstruction of the pelvic arch after resection of a malignant pelvic tumor remains a major surgical challenge because of the high rate of associated complications. The purpose of this investigation was to assess the functional outcome and complication rate following treatment with a bone allograft to reconstruct the pelvis. METHODS: Twenty-four consecutive patients

underwent excision of a malignant pelvic bone tumor and reconstruction with a pelvic bone allograft. The living patients were followed for a minimum of twenty-four months. There were nineteen primary malignant bone tumors, sixteen of which were high-grade sarcomas, and there were five isolated metastases. Patients were examined clinically and radiographically and were assessed functionally with the Musculoskeletal Tumor Society score. RESULTS: The mean age of the patients at the time of the index surgery was thirty-four years, and the mean duration of follow-up was forty-one months. Eighteen of the twenty-four resections involved the periacetabular area and were followed by reconstruction either with a hip prosthesis (thirteen) or with an osteochondral allograft alone (five). The six other resections involved the iliac bone. All patients received a massive bone allograft that had been sterilely procured without secondary irradiation. At the time of our last evaluation, eight patients were alive and free of disease. Seven patients had a local recurrence. Neurological deficits were present in six patients, and three had a deep infection. Nonunion of three of the sixteen allografts that could be evaluated was observed. Neither graft fracture nor lysis was observed. Eleven patients underwent surgical revision, with nine of these revisions related to the reconstruction. The average Musculoskeletal Tumor Society score at the time of the latest follow-up was 73% of the maximal possible score. The average score was 82% for the eleven patients with an age of less than twenty years at the time of the index procedure and 65% for the thirteen older patients. Ten patients walked without any assistive device, and five of them had normal function with no or only a slight limp. CONCLUSIONS: Pelvic reconstruction after a limb-sparing resection is associated with a high risk of surgical complications and usually should be reserved for patients with a primary bone sarcoma. A pelvic allograft can restore the anatomy and provide good functional results, especially in young patients. Nonunion was the most common allograft-related complication.

78. Carter TJ, et al. Application of soft tissue modelling to image-guided surgery. Med Eng Phys. 2005;27(10):893–909. The deformation of soft tissue compromises the accuracy of image-guided surgery based on preoperative images, and restricts its applicability to surgery on or near bony structures. One way to overcome these limitations is to combine biomechanical models with sparse intraoperative data, in order to realistically warp the preoperative image to match the surgical situation. We detail the process of biomechanical modelling in the context of image-guided surgery. We focus in particular on the finite element method, which is shown to be a promising approach, and review the constitutive relationships which have been suggested for representing tissue during surgery. Appropriate intraoperative measurements are required to constrain the deformation, and we discuss the potential of the modalities which have been applied to this task. This technology is on the verge of transition into clinical practice, where it promises to increase the guidance accuracy and facilitate less invasive interventions. We describe here how soft tissue modelling techniques have been applied to image-guided surgery applications.

79. Sugano N. Computer-assisted orthopaedic surgery and robotic surgery in total hip arthroplasty. Clin Orthop Surg. 2013;5(1):1–9. Various systems of computer-assisted orthopaedic surgery (CAOS) in total hip arthroplasty (THA) were reviewed. The first clinically applied system was an active robotic system (ROBODOC), which performed femoral implant cavity preparation as programmed preoperatively. Several reports on cementless THA with ROBODOC showed better stem alignment and less variance in limb-length inequality on radiographic evaluation, less incidence of pulmonary embolic events on transesophageal cardioechogram, and less stress shielding on the dual energy X-ray absorptiometry analysis than conventional manual methods. On the other hand, some studies raise issues with active systems, including a steep learning curve, muscle and nerve damage, and technical complications, such as a procedure stop due to a bone motion during cutting, requiring re-registration and registration failure. Semi-active robotic systems, such as Acrobot and Rio, were developed for ease of surgeon acceptance. The drill bit at the tip of the robotic arm is moved by a surgeon's hand, but it does not move outside of a milling path boundary, which is defined according to three-dimensional (3D) image-based preoperative planning. However, there are still few reports on THA with these semi-active systems. Thanks to the advancements in 3D sensor technology, navigation

systems were developed. Navigation is a passive system, which does not perform any actions on patients. It only provides information and guidance to the surgeon who still uses conventional tools to perform the surgery. There are three types of navigation: computed tomography (CT)-based navigation, imageless navigation, and fluoro-navigation. CT-based navigation is the most accurate, but the preoperative planning on CT images takes time that increases cost and radiation exposure. Imageless navigation does not use CT images, but its accuracy depends on the technique of landmark pointing, and it does not take into account the individual uniqueness of the anatomy. Fluoroscopic navigation is good for trauma and spine surgeries, but its benefits are limited in the hip and knee reconstruction surgeries. Several studies have shown that the cup alignment with navigation is more precise than that of the conventional mechanical instruments, and that it is useful for optimizing limb length, range of motion, and stability. Recently, patient specific templates, based on CT images, have attracted attention and some early reports on cup placement, and resurfacing showed improved accuracy of the procedures. These various CAOS systems have pros and cons. Nonetheless, CAOS is a useful tool to help surgeons perform accurately what surgeons want to do in order to better achieve their clinical objectives. Thus, it is important that the surgeon fully understands what he or she should be trying to achieve in THA for each patient.

80. Khan F, et al. Haptic robot-assisted surgery improves accuracy of wide resection of bone tumors: a pilot study. Clin Orthop Relat Res. 2013;471(3):851–9. BACKGROUND: Accurate reproduction of the preoperative plan at the time of surgery is critical for wide resection of primary bone tumors. Robotic technology can potentially help the surgeon reproduce a given preoperative plan, but yielding control of cutting instruments to a robot introduces potentially serious complications. We developed a novel passive ("haptics") robot-assisted resection technique for primary bone sarcomas that takes advantage of robotic accuracy while still leaving control of the cutting instrument in the hands of the surgeon. QUESTIONS/PURPOSES: We asked whether this technique would enable a preoperative resection plan to be reproduced more accurately than a standard manual technique. METHODS: A joint-sparing hemimetaphyseal resection was precisely outlined on the three-dimensionally reconstructed image of a representative Sawbones femur. The indicated resection was performed on 12 Sawbones specimens using the standard manual technique on six specimens and the haptic robotic technique on six specimens. Postresection images were quantitatively analyzed to determine the accuracy of the resections compared to the preoperative plan, which included measuring the maximum linear deviation of the cuts from the preoperative plan and the angular deviation of the resection planes from the target planes. RESULTS: Compared with the manual technique, the robotic technique resulted in a mean improvement of 7.8 mm of maximum linear deviation from the preoperative plan and 7.9 degrees improvement in pitch and 4.6 degrees improvement in roll for the angular deviation from the target planes. CONCLUSIONS: The haptic robot-assisted technique improved the accuracy of simulated wide resections of bone tumors compared with manual techniques. CLINICAL RELEVANCE: Haptic robot-assisted technology has the potential to enhance primary bone tumor resection. Further bench and clinical studies, including comparisons with recently introduced computer navigation technology, are warranted.

Sacral Biomechanics and Reconstruction 23

Matthew T. Houdek, Peter S. Rose, Steven L. Moran, Michael J. Yaszemski, and Franklin H. Sim

23.1 Introduction

En bloc resection is considered a mainstay of treatment for primary tumors of the sacrum. Based on the extent and location of the tumor, following en bloc resection spinopelvic continuity can be compromised, and as such reconstruction is necessary. However, en bloc resection often creates a difficult reconstructive challenge for orthopedic and plastic oncologic and reconstructive surgeons due to the combination of a segmental bony defect and the complex biomechanics of the sacrum. In addition to these significant mechanical issues, the surgical anatomy of the bony, vascular, and visceral pelvic structures contributes to a technically demanding reconstruction. The purpose of this chapter is to describe the biomechanical and technical challenges of reconstruction following sacral resection and the authors' suggestions to address those challenges.

M.T. Houdek, M.D. • P.S. Rose, M.D. • F.H. Sim, M.D. (✉)
Department of Orthopedic Surgery, Mayo Clinic, Rochester, MN, USA
e-mail: Houdek.Matthew@mayo.edu; Rose.Peter@mayo.edu; Sim.franklin@mayo.edu

S.L. Moran, M.D.
Division of Plastic and Reconstructive Surgery, Mayo Clinic, Rochester, MN, USA
e-mail: Moran.Steven@mayo.edu

M.J. Yaszemski, M.D. Ph.D.
Department of Orthopedic Surgery and Biomedical Engineering, Mayo Clinic, Rochester, MN, USA
e-mail: Yaszemski.Michael@mayo.edu

P. Ruggieri et al. (eds.), *Tumors of the Sacrum*,
DOI 10.1007/978-3-319-51202-0_23

23.2 Sacral Biomechanics

The sacrum is the only mechanical connection between the spine and pelvis/lower extremities. The sacroiliac (SI) joint is highly constrained and has to resist not only compression but also rotation, allowing for two degrees of motion and translation of only 0.7 mm [1, 2]. The constrained motion is due to the wedge shape of the sacrum between the iliac wings, which provides inherent stability similar to a "keystone" to prevent caudal migration, and the SI joint has an irregular and broad surface which interlocks the sacrum to the ilium. This allows the SI joint to not only resist compressive forces but also shear forces. In addition to the bony articulations, the SI joint is further stabilized by the intraosseous sacroiliac ligaments, the sacrotuberous ligaments, the sacrospinous ligaments, and the iliolumbar ligaments.

Following a sacrectomy, the biomechanical integrity of the SI joint can be compromised, and the need for reconstruction is largely based on the level of resection. It has previously been shown that the ability of the pelvis to resist axial loads is weakened by up to 50% with transverse resections of the sacral alae. However, this amount of weakening often does not prevent safe weight bearing [3, 4]. These early studies were expanded upon with a cadaveric model based on the effect of the level of resection. Hugate and colleagues showed that when a transverse partial sacrectomy was performed cranial to the S1 nerve root (Fig. 23.1a), then the residual

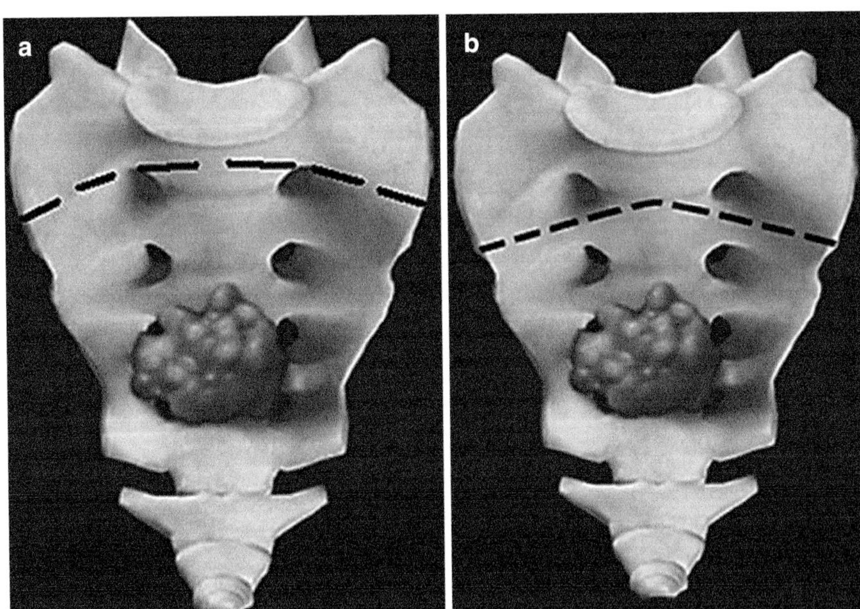

Fig. 23.1 Sacrectomies performed above the S1 neural foramen (**a**) were found to be unable to withstand postoperative mobilization compared to osteotomies performed below the S1 level (**b**). Due to these findings, reconstruction is recommended when an osteotomy is performed cranial to the S1 foramen

sacrum was at significant risk of a midline sagittal plane fracture during activities of daily living. Their recommendation was that reconstruction should be performed in this situation. However, if the transverse resection was distal to the S1 sacral segment (Fig. 23.1b), the authors felt that the sacrum would be able to withstand post-operative mobilization [5]. One criticism of this study was that the cadaveric specimens were from older patients, and sacrectomies are more often performed in younger patients. In order to address these issues, Yu and colleagues showed in a cadaveric model using "younger" pelvic specimens that resections involving S1 resulted in rotational instability and that further cephalad resection through half of the S1 body resulted in compressive instability [6]. Based on these findings, the authors recommended reconstruction when the osteotomy was at or above the S1–S2 vestigial disk level [6]. This has become the standard of practice at our institution, and we advocate for reconstruction if there is ablation of one of the SI joints or if there is a transverse osteotomy above the S1–S2 vestigial disk level. Clinically, the restoration of spinopelvic continuity has led to improved functional outcomes compared to patients where no reconstruction is performed [7, 8].

23.3 Spinopelvic Reconstruction

In order to restore spinal balance, and to reconstruct the spinopelvic instability that is generated by the sacrectomy, pedicle and iliac screw fixation with posterior rods and anterior support is currently our standard technique. Historically, the use of spinal instrumentation was associated with a high failure rate related to screw loosening and rod breakage, likely due to the use of posterior-only spinal reconstruction techniques without anterior column support at the resected sacral level. However, newer combined anterior and posterior reconstruction techniques have reduced failure rates [9, 10].

The ilium has two pathways of abundant cancellous bone: the upper (posterior superior iliac spine to the iliac crest) and lower segments (posterior superior spine to the anterior inferior iliac spine) which are ideal sites for anchoring iliac screws. It has been shown that if iliac screws are placed in both these paths, there is significant resistance to both compressive and torsional forces, especially with dual lower segment fixation [11]. In addition to improved iliac fixation techniques, changes have occurred in posterior rod instrumentation techniques, namely, the four-rod reconstruction technique. In an in vitro total sacrectomy model, Kelly and colleagues were able to demonstrate the superiority of a four-rod reconstruction technique compared to the traditional two-rod construct to provide significantly greater stability in flexion and extension [12]. Likewise, the addition of cross-links to the four-bar construct significantly increased the rotational stability of the construct [12]. In addition to a four-rod reconstruction with cross-linking, our preferred reconstruction technique includes an anterior column reconstruction of the sacral vertebral segment to augment the posterior reconstruction with anterior strut grafts (which are often preferably vascularized free fibulas), forming a "cathedral-shaped" reconstruction of the anterior spinal column at the sacral level [8].

23.3.1 Indications for Reconstruction

Reconstruction at our institution is performed when the SI joint has been disrupted, based on the Mayo Spino-Sacral-Pelvic Tumor Classification (Fig. 23.2), following either a total sacrectomy (Mayo Type IA), partial sacrectomy above the S1 foramen (Mayo Type IB), unilateral hemisacrectomy (Mayo Type II), amputative partial sacrectomy plus hemipelvectomy (Mayo Type III), or total sacrectomy and hemipelvectomy (Mayo Type IV). Reconstruction is not necessary for a lower sacrectomy which does not disrupt the SI joints (Mayo Type IC).

23.3.2 Cathedral Reconstruction

Staging of a total sacrectomy (Mayo Type 1A) has been shown to reduce patient morbidity and is currently our preferred technique [13]. We perform this procedure in three stages on three different surgical days. The anterior procedure, which we perform on day 1, includes the harvesting of a vertical rectus abdominis vascularized myocutaneous (VRAM) flap; the pelvic viscera mobilization; the sacral, spinal, and pelvic osteotomies as needed for a specific patient; the vascular mobilization; the nerve root sectioning as needed for a specific patient's tumor geometry; and the positioning of the VRAM flap in the pelvis over a Silastic sheet that identifies the plane of pelvic dissection. The second stage is the posterior approach and dissection, completion of osteotomies, tumor delivery and removal from the surgical field, and provisional VRAM flap inset followed by wound closure. The patient gets a spinopelvic CT scan on the way to the intensive care unit, which is used in the planning for the reconstruction which occurs as stage 3. The stage 3 reconstruction consists of bilateral bicortical pedicle screws in the two or three most distal remaining vertebrae and one or two iliac screws on each side. Docking sites for the two fibulae which constitute the anterior column sacral reconstruction are then created with a burr in the most caudal portion of the lowest remaining vertebra and in the ilia. The iliac docking sites may be prepared in the supra-acetabular region, in the ischial ramus, or in the ischial tuberosity area, depending on the locations that remain after specimen removal, as seen on the post-resection CT scan. The pelvic docking sites may be prepared during the anterior stage 1 operation, the posterior stage 2 tumor removal operation, or the stage 3 reconstruction operation, depending on the particular patient's tumor anatomy and which of the three operations present the optimum opportunity to prepare the docking sites. The ideal position of the docking sites in the ilium is at the intersection of the iliopectineal line and a straight line which intersects the center of the hip joint and the most caudal remaining vertebra (Fig. 23.3a). The position of these docking sites ultimately depends on the location and extent of the tumor removal in each patient and the bone areas that remain and are available for fibular strut graft docking.

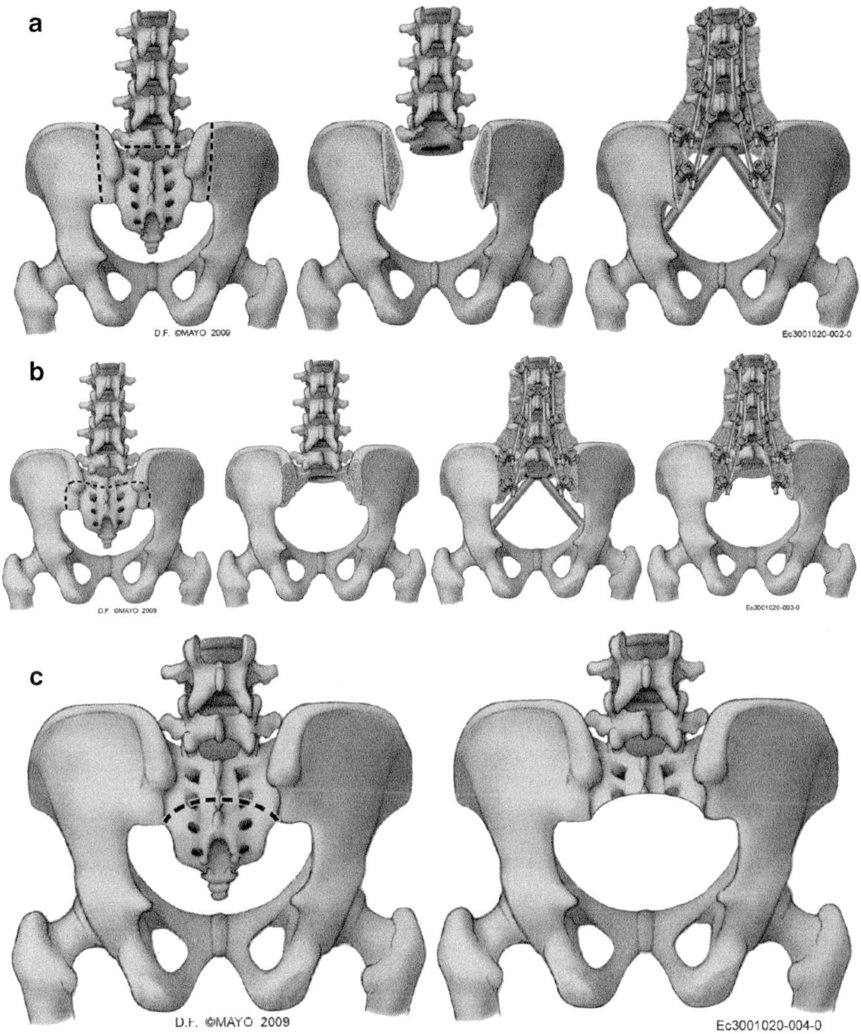

Fig. 23.2 The Mayo Spino-Sacral-Pelvic Tumor Classification assists in the planning of reconstruction based on the extent of resection and also if there is an amputative pelvic procedure. We perform a spinopelvic reconstruction for cases of Mayo Type IA (total sacrectomy, **a**), Type IB (subtotal sacrectomy above the S1 foramen, **b**), Type II (hemisacrectomy involving the ipsilateral sacroiliac joint, **d**), Type III (hemipelvectomy and hemisacrectomy, **e**), and Type IV (total sacrectomy and hemipelvectomy, **f**). Since the SI joints are not disrupted in a Type IC (subtotal sacrectomy below the S1 foramen, **c**), a reconstruction is not typically performed

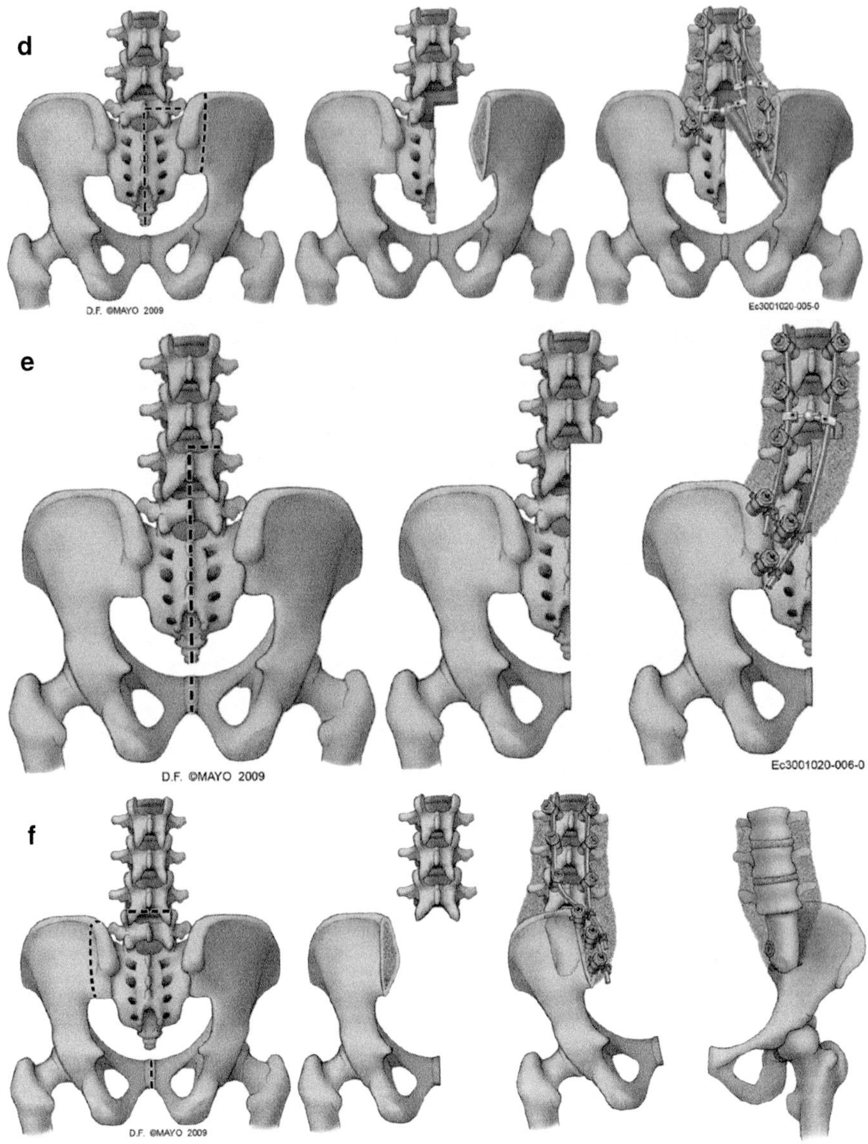

Fig. 23.2 (continued)

Fibular allografts or autografts are fashioned in order to be inserted into the docking sites, creating a "cathedral" appearance (Fig. 23.3b). We currently advocate the use of vascularized free fibulas instead of allografts in the setting of previous sacropelvic radiation. In such patients, healing of an allograft may likely be compromised. Following the docking of the fibulae to the most distal remaining vertebra, a bilateral four-rod posterior instrumentation reconstruction with cross-links is performed, and the instrumentation construct is compressed across the docking site (Fig. 23.3c).

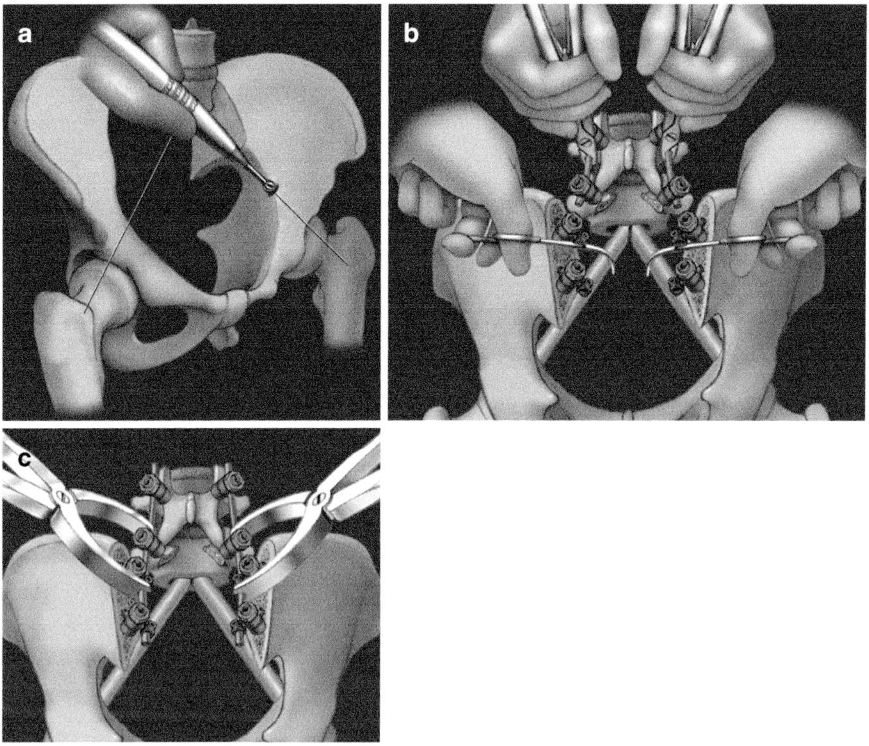

Fig. 23.3 During the anterior exposure of the tumor, receptacles for the strut grafts are made on the iliopectineal line at the crossing point from the center of the planned distal vertebrae and the center of the hip joint. Following tumor extirpation, bicortical pedicle screws are placed in the remaining lumbar vertebrae, and a docking site is made in the central portion of the most distal vertebrae. The fibular strut grafts are then placed into the docking sites of the ilium (**a**) and then inserted into the distal vertebrae in a "cathedral" fashion (**b**). Compression is then placed across the docking site, and the nuts of the pedicle screws are tightened (**c**)

The VRAM flap is then brought through the center of the cathedral (Fig. 23.4). The posterior abdominal wall is then reconstructed with a dermal replacement in order to prevent bowel and visceral herniation. It is important to leave a space in the caudal portion of the dermal replacement in order to allow for the VRAM pedicle. The VRAM flap is then sutured in place at the fascial, subdermal, and skin levels, and the patient is kept on a specialized pressure-equalizing bed mattress to allow for optimal flap healing.

23.3.3 Unilateral Reconstruction

In cases where only one SI joint has been resected, a unilateral cathedral technique can be performed (Fig. 23.5). This technique is used to recreate the biomechanical properties of the SI joint. Similar to a bilateral procedure, a compressive pedicle and iliac screw reconstruction is performed, augmented with either an allograft or autograft fibular strut.

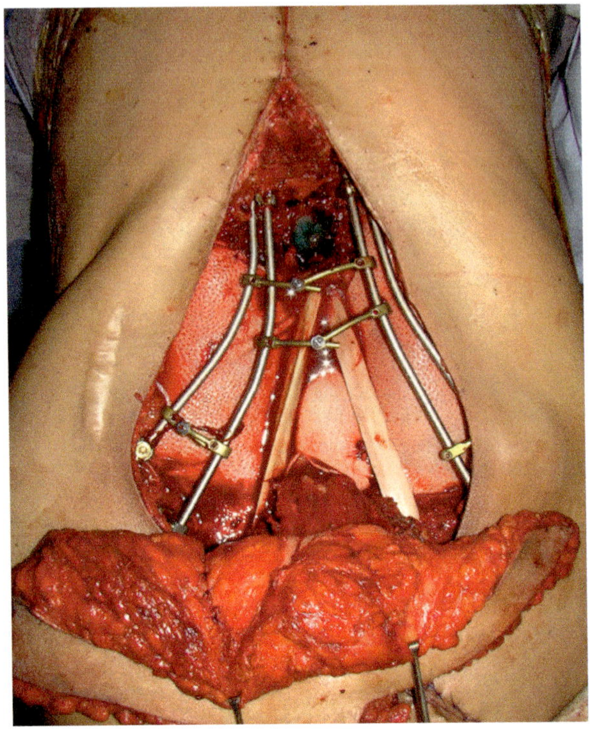

Fig. 23.4 Following reconstruction, a biologic matrix is used to reconstruct the posterior abdominal wall and placed between the abdominal contents and the hardware. An opening is created in the distal portion of the matrix in order to allow for the pedicle of the flap

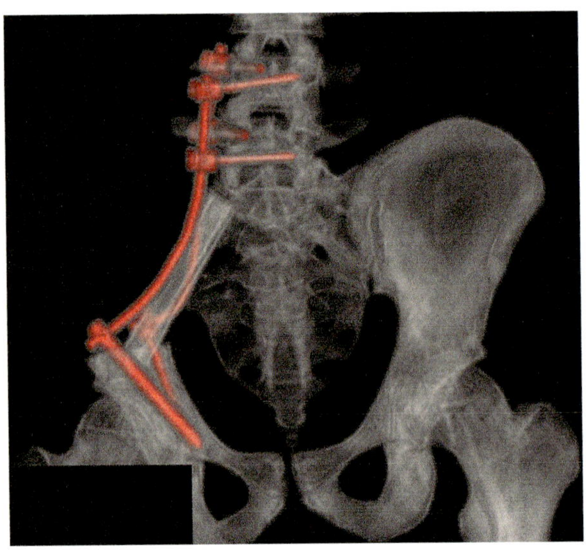

Fig. 23.5 Unilateral reconstruction and cathedral reconstruction using a fibular strut graft as well as pedicle and iliac screw fixation. Similar to the bilateral reconstruction, docking sites are created, and the fibula strut is placed in-between with compression across the docking sites

23.3.4 Amputative Sacrectomy

Combined sacrectomy and external hemipelvectomy procedures are rare, and there are few options to restore spinopelvic continuity. For a combined partial sacrectomy and external hemipelvectomy (Mayo Type III), spinopelvic continuity is maintained. However, this is not enough to support the forces transmitted during ambulation and sitting. We advocate for reconstruction whenever a spinal disk is entered as part of the tumor resection. Although there is no published biomechanical data that addresses this particular amputative resection, lumbar pedicle and iliac screw fixation appears to be a reasonable method from our perspective to restore spinopelvic stability following a Mayo Type III resection. Along with iliac fixation, the number of remaining vertebrae instrumented is based on individual patient characteristics, which include the extent of the tissues removed during tumor resection, patient weight, and patient bone quality. Two, three, or four vertebral levels are the usual range instrumented in patients following a Mayo Type III resection. Posterior rods and cross-links are used to connect the most proximal of the iliac screws and the lumbar pedicle screws (Fig. 23.6a). Likewise, the more caudal iliac screw is connected to the ipsilateral sacral pedicle screw and the contralateral lumbar pedicle screws. Compression is then placed through this construct, and morcellized bone graft is used in the ipsilateral posterolateral gutter. In addition, structural allograft bone is placed in each disk that is included in the instrumented levels of the arthrodesis (Fig. 23.6b). In the setting of previous radiation, a vascularized fibula can be used to enhance fixation.

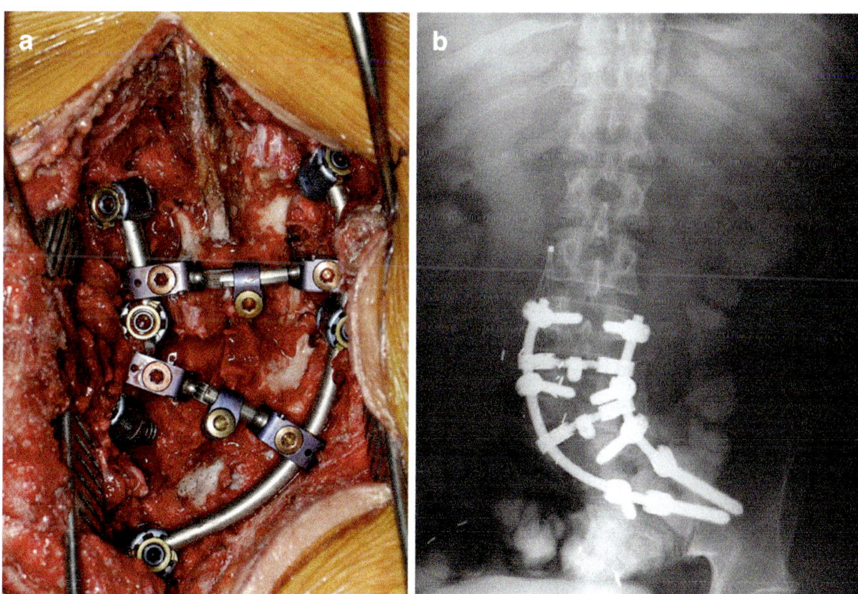

Fig. 23.6 Reconstruction following a Mayo Type III resection. The patient initially was left unreconstructed but developed severe pain related to instability of the lumbar vertebrae. As such, these vertebrae were reconstructed using pedicle and iliac screw fixation with crossbar linking of the remaining sacrum and pelvis (**a**). Following the procedure, there was solid fusion of the vertebrae to the pelvis, with a substantial reduction in pain (**b**)

In the setting of an amputative hemipelvectomy and total sacrectomy (Mayo Type IV, Fig. 23.7a), we use the amputated proximal femur for bone graft as long as there is no tumor located in this region. Similar to a Type III reconstruction, the remaining two, three, or four lumbar vertebrae are instrumented with bilateral pedicle screws, along with dual or triple iliac screw fixation in the remaining ilium. We then perform both an intertrochanteric osteotomy and a subtrochanteric osteotomy through the proximal femoral autograft to restore the anatomic distance between the spine and pelvis (Fig. 23.7b). The position of the subtrochanteric osteotomy is chosen to minimize either stretching or kinking of the vessels and nerves between the remaining lumbar spine and the remaining ilium. A docking site is created in the remaining ilium to allow for fixation of the cancellous bone of the amputated femur's intertrochanteric osteotomy to the remaining ilium and for fixation of the subtrochanteric osteotomy site of the amputated femur into the most caudal remaining vertebra (Fig. 23.7c). The angle of the intertrochanteric osteotomy is chosen so that the amputated femoral autograft aligns with the long axis of the patient's body.

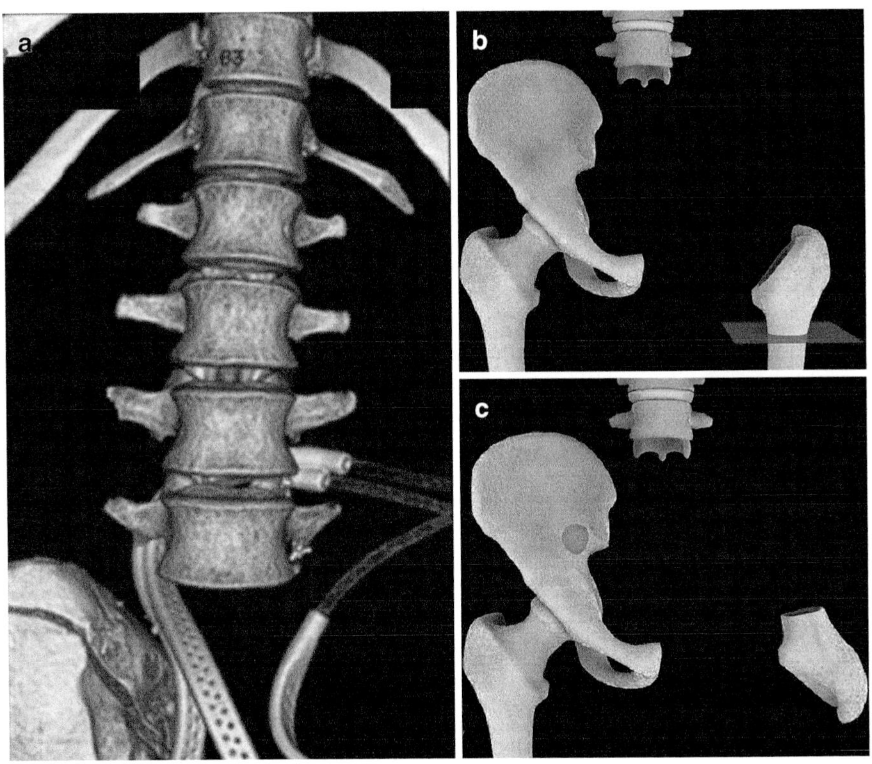

Fig. 23.7 Following a Mayo Type IV resection (**a**), the amputated proximal femur is used to restore the distance between the spine and pelvis. A subtrochanteric osteotomy is performed (**b**), and the proximal femur is "flipped," so the proximal femur's intertrochanteric osteotomy is in contact with the remaining ilium (**c**). The femur is then fixed to the ilium (**d**) along with multiple pedicle and iliac screws and posterior rods under compression (**e**)

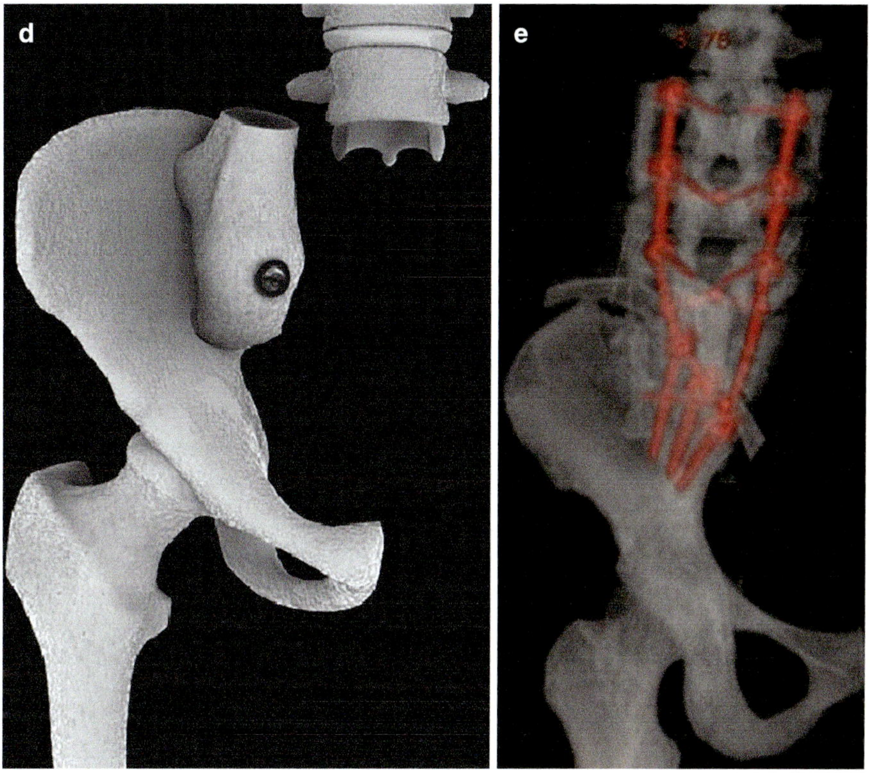

Fig. 23.7 (continued)

This reconstructive construct is held in place with a compression screw into the ilium (Fig. 23.7d) and via compression of the screw-rod instrumentation between the lumbar spine and the remaining ilium. An arthrodesis is performed between the remaining lumbar vertebrae and the remaining ilium.

Conclusion

Reconstruction following a sacrectomy is necessary to restore spinopelvic continuity and improve patient outcome. The use of the cathedral technique at our institution has resulted in an 89% success rate [8]. Currently, we advocate for the use of dual iliac screw fixation, double-bar constructs with cross-linking, and anterior column support for the defect that results from the sacral resection. A biomechanical analysis has shown decreased instrumentation failure when the anterior column is supported, when compared to posterior column only support [14]. Although it increases the surgical time, we feel that in patients who have a history of radiation to the pelvis, or who will receive chemotherapy following the reconstruction, the use of vascularized fibular autografts is a reasonable strategy to improve the reconstruction construct's stability and healing potential.

References

1. Egund N, et al. Movements in the sacroiliac joints demonstrated with roentgen stereophotogrammetry. Acta Radiol Diagn (Stockh). 1978;19(5):833–46.
2. Sturesson B, Selvik G, Uden A. Movements of the sacroiliac joints. A roentgen stereophotogrammetric analysis. Spine (Phila Pa 1976). 1989;14(2):162–5.
3. Gunterberg B. Effects of major resection of the sacrum. Clinical studies on urogenital and anorectal function and a biomechanical study on pelvic strength. Acta Orthop Scand Suppl. 1976;162:1–38.
4. Gunterberg B, Romanus B, Stener B. Pelvic strength after major amputation of the sacrum. An experimental study. Acta Orthop Scand. 1976;47(6):635–42.
5. Hugate Jr RR, et al. Mechanical effects of partial sacrectomy: when is reconstruction necessary? Clin Orthop Relat Res. 2006;450:82–8.
6. Yu B, et al. Biomechanical effects of transverse partial sacrectomy on the sacroiliac joints: an in vitro human cadaveric investigation of the borderline of sacroiliac joint instability. Spine. 2009;34(13):1370–5.
7. O'Connor MI, Sim FH. Salvage of the limb in the treatment of malignant pelvic tumors. J Bone Joint Surg Am. 1989;71(4):481–94.
8. Dickey ID, et al. Reconstruction after total sacrectomy: early experience with a new surgical technique. Clin Orthop Relat Res. 2005;438:42–50.
9. Tsuchiya K, et al. Minimum 5-year analysis of L5–S1 fusion using sacropelvic fixation (bilateral S1 and iliac screws) for spinal deformity. Spine. 2006;31(3):303–8.
10. Mindea SA, et al. Lumbosacropelvic junction reconstruction resulting in early ambulation for patients with lumbosacral neoplasms or osteomyelitis. Neurosurg Focus. 2003;15(2):E6.
11. Yu BS, et al. Biomechanical advantages of dual over single iliac screws in lumbo-iliac fixation construct. Eur Spine J. 2010;19(7):1121–8.
12. Kelly BP, et al. Biomechanical testing of a novel four-rod technique for lumbo-pelvic reconstruction. Spine. 2008;33(13):E400–6.
13. Brown MJ, et al. Sacral tumor resection: the effect of surgical staging on patient outcomes, resource management, and hospital cost. Spine (Phila Pa 1976). 2011;36(19):1570–8.
14. Bederman SS, et al. Surgical techniques for spinopelvic reconstruction following total sacrectomy: a systematic review. Eur Spine J. 2014;23(2):305–19.

Soft Tissue Reconstruction Following Sacrectomy

24

Matthew T. Houdek and Steven L. Moran

Primary sacral tumors are uncommon and fortunately the majority are low-grade malignancies; however, without negative surgical margins, these tumors have a high predilection for local recurrence [1]. Thus, the goal of surgery is complete tumor extirpation. In order to obtain a negative margin, large soft tissue defects are created. Unfortunately, these large resections are prone to infection and complications. The utilization of immediate soft tissue reconstruction with myocutaneous flaps has allowed the surgeon to bring well-vascularized tissue into the resection area, obliterate dead space, and preserve abdominal domain.

Local soft tissue flap reconstruction of these defects can be compromised by immobile radiated tissues and lack of local posterior soft tissue due to its removal with the tumor specimen. Historically, these wounds were left to close by secondary intention and often resulted in extensive scarring, as well as an unstable soft tissue envelope which leads to a prolonged hospital course due to the associated complications. Over the past 2 decades, myocutaneous flap reconstruction of these defects has lowered morbidity and also allowed for more aggressive surgical resection of the primary tumor. Over the past decade, we have found that there are two flaps that provide reliable soft tissue coverage for these complex defects. The purpose of this chapter is to provide an overview of the common indications and techniques for soft tissue reconstruction following sacrectomy and to review our reconstructive algorithm.

M.T. Houdek, M.D.
Department of Orthopedic Surgery, Mayo Clinic, Rochester, MN, USA
e-mail: Houdek.Matthew@mayo.edu

S.L. Moran, M.D. (✉)
Department of Orthopedic Surgery, Mayo Clinic, Rochester, MN, USA

Division of Plastic and Reconstructive Surgery, Mayo Clinic, Rochester, MN, USA
e-mail: Moran.Steven@mayo.edu

P. Ruggieri et al. (eds.), *Tumors of the Sacrum*,
DOI 10.1007/978-3-319-51202-0_24

24.1 Flap Planning

It is important to have a multidisciplinary team approach from the start of the case in order to mark out any colostomy or ileostomy sites to facilitate flap design. This is important because an inappropriately placed colostomy or ileostomy could potentially compromise abdominal flap elevation. In addition, prior to surgery, we advocate for the placement of ureteral stents that assist with identification of the ureters during tumor extirpation. Patient positioning for the case is dependent on the location of the tumor, if the tumor involves S2 or higher our preference is for a two-stage resection beginning with the patient supine for an anterior abdominal exploration followed by a posterior resection, which is performed with the patient in the prone position. Tumors which are located at S3 or lower may be removed through a pure posterior approach thus allowing the patient to be positioned prone on the operating room table. Prior to the start of the procedure, the plastic surgery team will mark the area for flap dissection based on the type of defect.

24.2 Sacral Reconstruction

Sacral resections have historically been associated with high postoperative morbidity due to the complex local anatomy and poor wound healing potential of these wounds. As previously mentioned, at our institution, distal sacral resections are typically performed through a posterior approach, while larger tumors, those spreading from the viscera (colon cancer) and cephalad to S3, require a combined anterior and posterior resection. Soft tissue reconstruction of these defects is either preformed with omental flaps, V–Y advancement flaps, or vertical rectus abdominis musculocutaneous (VRAM) depending on wound dimensions. These flaps obliterate the potential space left following tumor extirpation and allow for a tension-free closure of the wound. Depending on the size of the soft tissue defect, these flaps can be used in isolation or combined.

24.2.1 Omental Pedicled Flap

The omentum is easily accessible during the laparotomy used for exposure during the anterior approach. Since omentum can be scarred and adherent to abdominal organs, a previous history of abdominal surgery or abdominal infection may preclude the use of this flap.

The omentum flap may be based on either the right or left gastroepiploic artery. If the flap is based on the right gastroepiploic vessels, the short gastric vessels can be divided along the greater curvature of the stomach, allowing for mobilization of the omentum. The omentum can then be tucked into the residual soft tissue defect to obliterate the potential space left from tumor extirpation. While the flap is very good for obliterating dead space, it has little structural strength; thus, it is not an ideal flap when a significant portion of the abdominal wall or buttock area has been

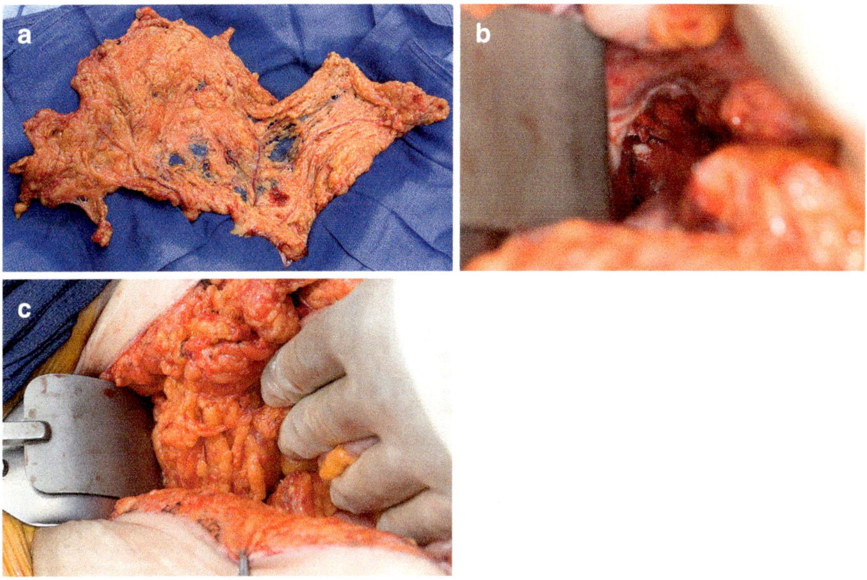

Fig. 24.1 During an anterior exposure, the omentum is easily accessible and significant mobilization can be acheived through the anterior laporotomy incision (**a**). Following removal of a tumor, there is often a large potential space (**b**). The omentum can be mobilized and "tucked" into this space obliterating the dead space (**c**)

excised. We prefer to use this flap for low-grade tumors where skin closure is not an issue. In these cases, the omentum can be tucked into the area of tumor extirpation and help to prevent the development of postoperative seroma and infection. Since the flap requires manipulation of the viscera, we recommend a gradual resumption of feeding until the bowel and stomach function return to baseline (Fig. 24.1).

24.2.2 V–Y Advancement Gluteal Flaps

The V–Y advancement flaps are performed as a composite flap (fasciocutaneous and myocutaneous). Due to the loss of gluteal strength following the procedure, the flap is safer from a functional standpoint to perform in paraplegic patients but can also be used in ambulatory patients if the flap is modified to not include the muscle. The flap is based on the superior and inferior gluteal vessels. The use of this flap is contraindicated if there is concern about the patency of the gluteal vessels (and this may be the cases if there has been substantial preoperative gluteal radiation or preoperative embolization of the internal iliac vessels). In most cases, the donor site may be closed primarily, but in cases of very large flaps, the donor site can be skin grafted or left to heal by secondary intention. We prefer to use this flap (Fig. 24.2) only for patients undergoing an entirely prone procedure (caudal to S3). The tissue available with this flap is limited, and it is often not possible to obliterate larger deep pelvic spaces with this flap.

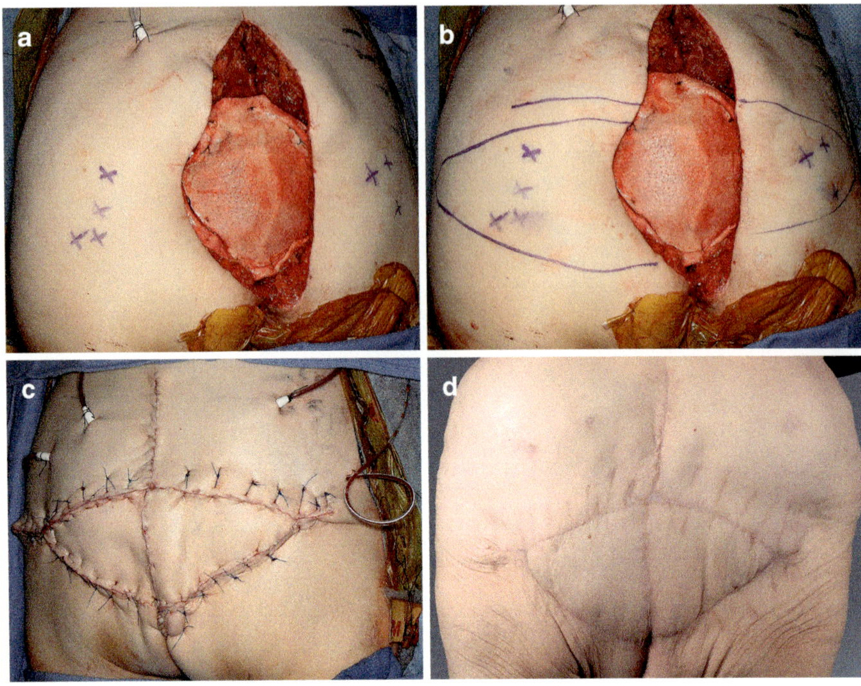

Fig. 24.2 For coverage of posterior-only sacrectomies, a V–Y advancement flap can be planned based on perforators from the gluteal vessels (**a**). Incisions are planned based on the location of the perforators (**b**), and the flaps can be elevated as either a fasciocutaneous or myocutaneous flap. The flaps are then mobilized to the midline (**c**). At 8-month postoperative, the flap has reliably healed (**d**)

24.2.3 Rectus Abdominis Musculocutaneous Flap

The rectus abdominis muscle can be elevated alone or as a composite flap with a skin paddle. The skin paddle can be elevated as a transverse rectus abdominis musculocutaneous (TRAM) or as a vertical rectus abdominis musculocutaneous (VRAM) flap, which can be either a distally based pedicle flap (inferior epigastric vessels) or microvascular free flap. We most commonly use a VRAM based on the deep inferior epigastric artery (DIEA). The DIEA arises above the inguinal ligament and lies superior to the peritoneum, but deep to the transversalis fascia. Once the pedicle enters the rectus sheath, it divides into the medial and lateral branches and located lateral to the muscle. The flap is elevated off the abdominal wall with both these perforators, with care taken to leave the flap attached the pubic ramus to prevent kinking of the pedicle.

The VRAM is the workhorse for reconstruction and can be used for a majority of soft tissue defects following sacrectomy. If there is a large skin defect, then we preferred to use a pedicled TRAM flap. Since these flaps are based on the inferior epigastric vessels, a detailed history of previous intra-abdominal surgery should be obtained in order to determine if the DIEA may have been previously divided (open appendectomy, inguinal hernia, colostomy, cesarean section, etc.). If there is a concern that the pedicle has been damaged, a duplex ultrasound or CTA should be performed to confirm patency.

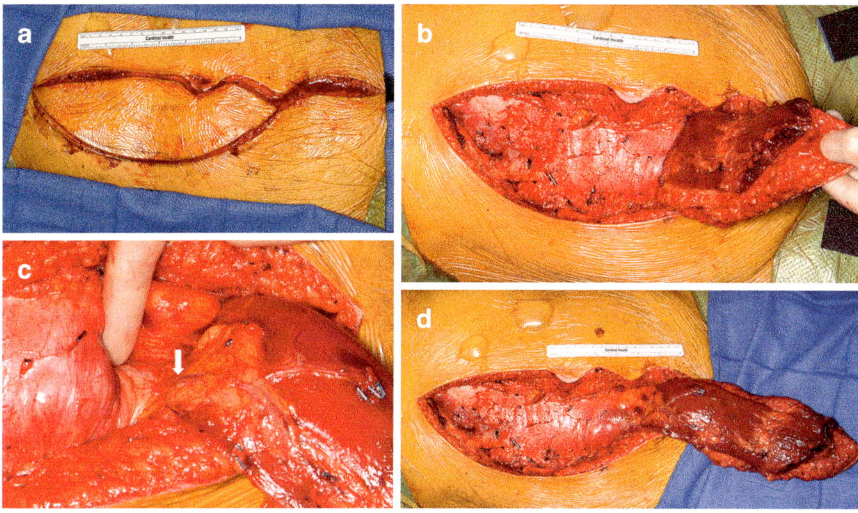

Fig. 24.3 The vertical rectus abdominis musculocutaneous (VRAM) flap is planned prior to the anterior exposure of the tumor (**a**) and is measured based on the anticipated amount of posterior skin resection. The rectus is elevated off the abdominal wall (**b**) with care taken not to kink the perforators of the deep inferior epigastric artery (**c**—*arrow*). Once mobilized (**d**), the anterior exposure of the tumor is undertaken and the flap is tucked into the abdomen

The VRAM flap should be elevated prior to abdominal exploration. A large skin paddle should be planned in order to close the posterior soft tissue defect (Fig. 24.3). The rectus sheath is opened near the midline and elevated off the rectus abdominis muscle in the areas that are away from the skin island. Care should be taken to avoid the pedicle which lies on the undersurface of the muscle. The flap is left attached to the pubis and a stich is placed to mark superior orientation of the skin paddle. The flap is placed in a plastic bag or wrapped in a laparotomy pad and placed over the anterior portion of the lumbar spine and sacrum for easy identification during the posterior approach. The flap is then left buried in the abdomen until the posterior portion of the procedure is performed.

If there is a large anterior fascial defect following flap harvest, the fascia can be reconstructed using a synthetic mesh or acellular dermal matrix. The repair of these defects should be tension-free preferably with an absorbable mesh such as Vicryl® (Ethicon Inc., Cincinnati, Ohio, USA) or a biologic mesh such as AlloDerm® (Lifecell Corporation, Branchburg, NJ, USA) or Surgisis® (Cook Surgical, Bloomington, IN, USA). Although both options are viable, the use of a biologic mesh is costly and patients can sustain an abdominal wall hernia or bulge in long-term follow-up.

During the posterior portion of the procedure, the VRAM flap is easily identified following resection of the sacrum (Fig. 24.4). Similar to the anterior reconstruction, a biologic mesh (AlloDerm®) is used to reconstruct the posterior abdominal wall. The pelvis and spine are stabilized, and the biologic mesh is then anchored to the pelvis deep to the surgical hardware to prevent herniation of the viscera. A small opening is left in the inferior portion of the mesh to allow for the pedicle of the VRAM flap to be passed through the defect. Following the reconstruction, the flap

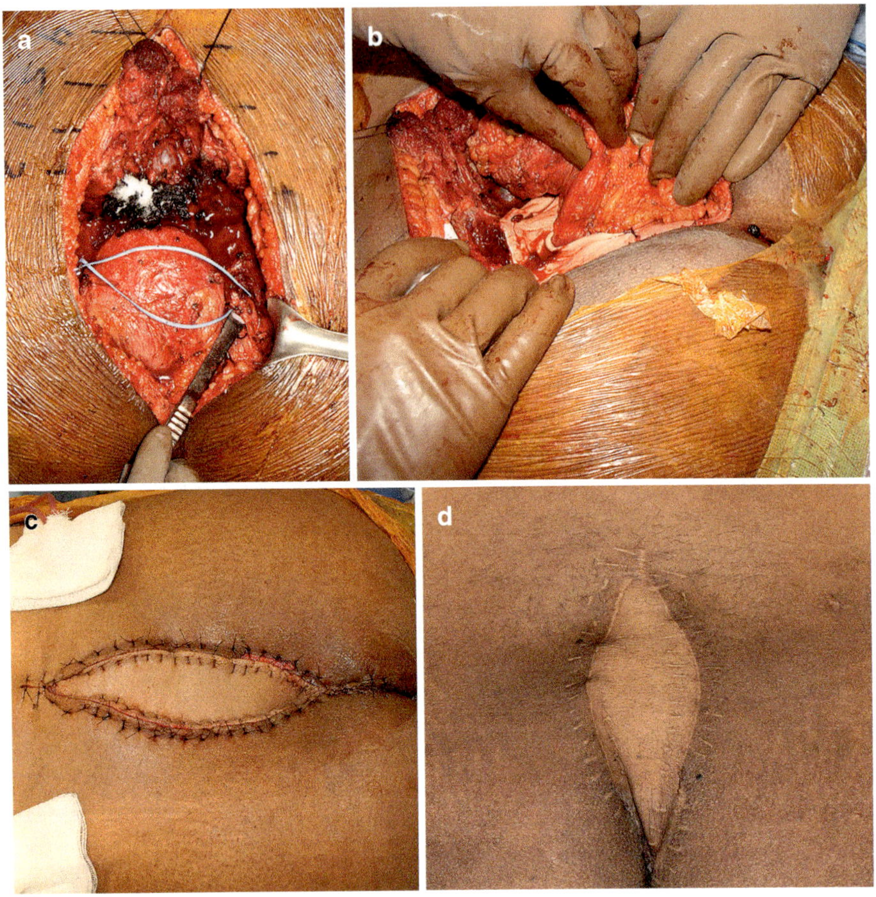

Fig. 24.4 Following a combined anterior and posterior approach to the sacrum, reconstructive surgeons are often faced with large posterior soft tissue defects (**a**). A biologic mesh is used to reconstruct the posterior abdominal wall, and the vertical rectus abdominis musculocutaneous (VRAM) is pulled through a small opening in the mesh (**b**). The flap is then inset into the posterior defect without tension (**c**). In this patient, the flap reliably healed (**d**)

should be inset without tension or kinking of the pedicle in order to prevent wound breakdown when the patients start to sit.

24.3 Postoperative Management

Patients are monitored in the ICU for at least the first postoperative night. Adequate fluid resuscitation improves flap perfusion; thus, blood pressure should be supported with fluids or blood products rather than vasopressors. We recommend for the use of a Clinitron® bed (Hill-Rom, Chicago, IL, USA) to avoid pressure injury to the flap, as many patients will be insensate over the ischial and sacral region. Physical and occupational therapy services are involved early, and when it is safe from surgical prospective, patients can begin ambulating and sitting.

Depending on the size of the defect, one or multiple drains can be placed to prevent hematoma or seroma formation. Large fluid accumulations can compromise the soft tissue reconstructions through direct pressure on the vascular pedicle or by the development of deep infection. In accordance with oncologic principles, the drains should exit the skin in line with and close to an incision in case it has to be resected at later date for tumor recurrence. Typically, drains are kept in place until the output decreases to less than 30 cc per day, but often are left in place longer in large or irradiated wound beds.

24.4 Complications

Wound complications are the most common postoperative complications following sacrectomy. In a series from our institution, authored by Maricevich and colleagues, we noted a 40% complication rate, with a majority of the complications related to skin dehiscence [2], even with the postoperative use of a Clinitron® bed. Since wound complications prevent adjuvant therapy (such as chemotherapy), uncomplicated wound healing is essential for optimum care and highlights the need for a multidisciplinary team including plastic surgeons to optimize wound healing. The high rate of complications following these complicated surgeries has been corroborated in other large series of partial and total sacrectomies [3, 4]. Despite a high rate of wound and abdominal complications, Maricevich and colleagues reported no flap loss following these procedures [2]. Wound complications were found to be associated with the surgical approach; patients reconstructed with a V–Y flap were at greatest risk of complications [2]. This is most likely due to the fact that the V–Y advancement flap lacks the bulk necessary to obliterate deeper spaces, elevating the risk for fluid accumulation. The study found that the use of acellular dermal matrix to reconstruct the posterior abdominal significantly reduces the risk of posterior bowel herniation and reduces the incidence of bowel obstruction and fistula formation [2].

Currently, at our institution, we use gluteal flaps for smaller defects following isolated posterior procedures. Even in the setting of smaller wound defects, any time there is a combined anterior and posterior approach, we advocate for the use of a VRAM flap. Although reconstruction is technically difficult following a sacrectomy, the use of the VRAM and biological matrix to reconstruct the posterior abdominal wall is our preferred technique to provide patients with the best outcomes.

References

1. Fuchs B, et al. Operative management of sacral chordoma. J Bone Joint Surg Am. 2005;87(10):2211–6.
2. Maricevich M, et al. Reconstruction following partial and total sacrectomy defects: an analysis of outcomes and complications. J Plast Reconstr Aesthet Surg. 2014;67(9):1257–66.
3. Miles WK, et al. Reconstruction of large sacral defects following total sacrectomy. Plast Reconstr Surg. 2000;105(7):2387–94.
4. Garvey PB, et al. Reconstructive strategies for partial sacrectomy defects based on surgical outcomes. Plast Reconstr Surg. 2011;127(1):190–9.

Embolization for Sacral Tumors

25

Andreas F. Mavrogenis, Vasilios Igoumenou, Andrea Angelini, Giuseppe Rossi, and Pietro Ruggieri

25.1 Introduction

Arterial embolization for tumors was first described in 1975 [1, 2]. Since then, embolization for sacral tumors either primary or metastatic has been used extensively as a useful primary, palliative, or adjuvant therapy [3–6]. Preoperative embolization of hypervascular metastatic lesions reduces intraoperative blood loss and improves the surgeon's ability for resection. Additionally, embolization may cause tumor growth arrest, pain alleviation, and shorter hospital stay [4–6]. The timing of preoperative embolization is important. Typically, best results are achieved when surgery is performed within 24–48 h after embolization [7, 8]. Serial embolization is safe and feasible; it can be performed in patients with persistent pain and/or imaging evidence of progressive disease. Serial embolization has been related with high rates of successful pain relief, tumor devascularization, tumor size reduction, and calcification of margins [9–11]. Serial embolization is typically performed in 4–6-week intervals until symptomatic improvement occurs, or the tumor's pathological vascularity disappears. Unless there is a clear indication for general anesthesia,

A.F. Mavrogenis, M.D., Ph.D. • V. Igoumenou, M.D.
First Department of Orthopaedics, National and Kapodistrian University of Athens, Athens, Greece
e-mail: afm@otenet.gr

A. Angelini, M.D., Ph.D. • P. Ruggieri, M.D., Ph.D. (✉)
Department of Orthopaedics and Orthopedic Oncology, University of Padova, Via N. Giustiniani, 3, Padova 35128, Italy
e-mail: andrea.angelini83@yahoo.it; pietro.ruggieri@unipd.it

G. Rossi, M.D.
Department of Interventional Radiology, Istituto Ortopedico Rizzoli, Bologna, Italy
e-mail: giuseppe.rossi@ior.it

P. Ruggieri et al. (eds.), *Tumors of the Sacrum*,
DOI 10.1007/978-3-319-51202-0_25

most procedures are performed under light conscious sedation. The optimal arterial approach is determined based on lesion location; most often is the common femoral artery using a Seldinger technique. Commonly, an arterial catheter is placed and standard 4 French or 5 French angiographic catheters are used for main arterial selection, and a 3 French microcatheter for subselectivity. A diagnostic angiography is performed from a major vessel, more commonly the aorta to delineate vascular supply to the tumor and to identify vessels of potential concern that may result in nontarget embolization. In general, microspheres of 100–700 μm are used because of their ease of delivery, range of available sizes, and lower potential for recanalization. Sponge gel, once the embolic agent of choice, has now fallen in disuse, because of its temporary nature and propensity for recanalization. Coils are avoided as an embolic agent for tumor vessels, because re-treatment may be necessary and blocking access sites should be avoided. Completion of the procedure is determined by complete occlusion of the tumor blush compared with the initial diagnostic angiography [12]. Complication rate is generally low [13]; reported complications include post-embolization syndrome (fever, pain, malaise), nerve palsy, subcutaneous or muscle necrosis, ischemic pain (usually transitory), infection, and tumor bleeding [14].

25.2 Embolization for Benign Tumors of the Sacrum

Osteoid osteomas, osteoblastomas, and hemangiomas have been reported to respond positively to embolization [15]. Preoperative embolization for hemangiomas provide for reduced blood loss intraoperatively [3]. Two well-known lesions, that may arise rarely in the sacrum but their management poses almost always a challenge for the surgeons, are aneurysmal bone cysts (Fig. 25.1) and giant cell tumors (Fig. 25.2). In these cases, surgery is often technically difficult and complicated by extensive hemorrhage and neurological compromise. Additionally, radiotherapy produces a limited benefit and is associated with a risk of postradiation sarcomas; moreover, radiation therapy should not be administered for benign tumors. Treatment is further complicated by the high rate of recurrence of these tumors. If however, these lesions are embolized prior to resection, a significant decrease in the preoperative blood loss is noted, facilitating surgery and offering better outcomes [15–18]. Embolization has also been used for palliation of pain related to unresectable aneurysmal bone cysts and giant cell tumors, where other modes of therapy have failed [15]. Embolization can also be the primary treatment option for these lesions as well [19, 20]. Current treatment of choice for spinal and sacral giant cell tumors is considered the sequel of preoperative arterial embolization, complete surgical removal, and postoperative denosumab; serial embolization, along with denosumab and radiation therapy, is also a treatment option for patients with unresectable tumors or at high risk for surgery [21]. Overall, the recurrence rate after embolization for aneurysmal bone cysts and giant cell tumors lesions is low, and when recurrence occurs it can be managed safely and usually successfully with repeat embolization.

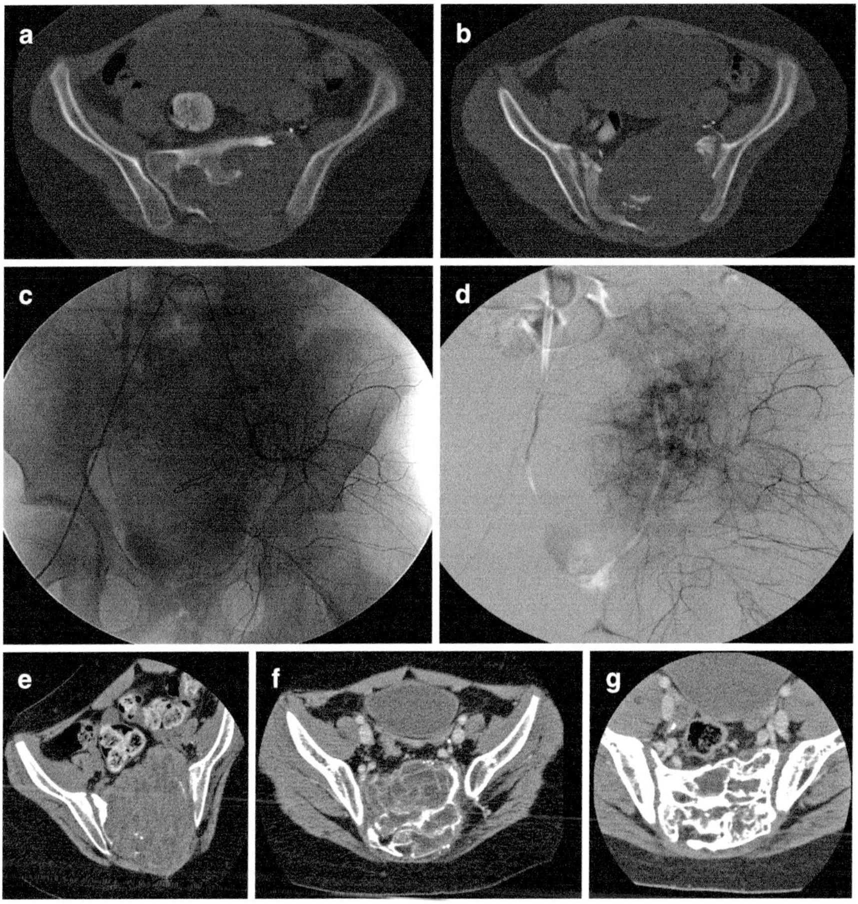

Fig. 25.1 An 11-year-old girl with external popliteal nerve deficit of 10 days duration. (**a**, **b**) Axial CT of the sacrum showed an osteolytic lesion involving the sacroiliac joint; biopsy showed aneurysmal bone cyst. (**c**, **d**) Digital subtraction angiography shows the high pathological vascularization originating from the pathologic feeding vessels of the tumor; NBCA embolization was done. (**e**) CT of the sacrum at 2-month follow-up because of persistent pain; a second NBCA embolization was done (**f**) CT of the sacrum at 3-month follow-up after the second embolization show partial ossification of the tumor. (**g**) CT at 1-year follow-up show almost complete ossification of the tumor; the patient is asymptomatic

Serial embolization is typically performed at 4–6-week intervals until symptomatic improvement occurs, or the tumor's vascularity disappears. Success of embolization is confirmed clinically by improvement of pain or with imaging using post-procedural angiography, MR imaging, or CT. Lesion ossification after embolization of aneurysmal bone cysts is considered a treatment success. Recurrence of symptoms should be evaluated with MR imaging, CT, or angiography. If there is an increase in tumor size or evidence of increased vascularity, then embolization should be repeated [15]. Puri et al. [22] consider serial embolization for benign

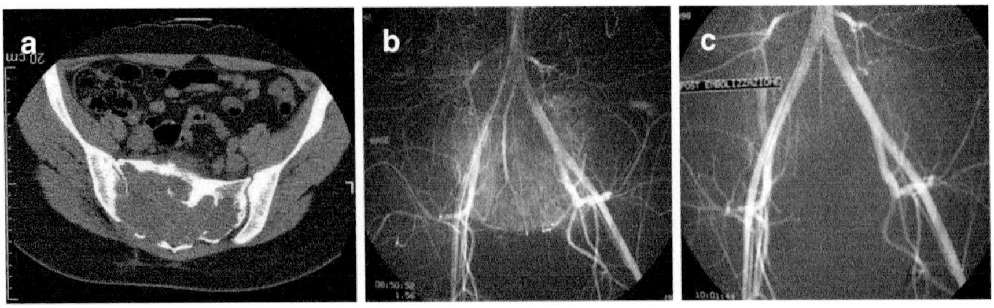

Fig. 25.2 (**a**) Axial CT of the pelvis of a 30-year-old man with a giant cell tumor of the sacrum. (**b**) Digital subtraction angiography shows the pathological tumor vascularization. (**c**) Digital subtraction angiography after NBCA embolization shows complete occlusion of the pathological tumor vessels

sacral tumors that extend above S3, in order to retain bladder and bowel control and minimize neurological dysfunction, in patients with preoperatively intact bladder and bowel function. In these cases, supplementary administration of parenteral bisphosphonates could be proved beneficial [22].

25.3 Embolization for Primary Tumors of the Sacrum

The complexity of the sacral neuroanatomy and its close relationship with vital organs adds additional challenges in the treatment of malignant tumors of the sacrum. Their management is governed by an interplay of complex factors, which includes their pathology, the extent of the disease, and presenting neurological symptoms [22]. Embolization has been used for such tumors as an adjunct to surgery, chemotherapy, and radiation therapy, or as palliative treatment [3]. Some tumors arising from the neural elements of the sacrum such as presacral schwannomas, neurofibromas, sacral meningiomas, malignant peripheral nerve sheath tumors, and intradural spinal tumors often are vascular and therefore responsive to embolization [22, 23]. In these cases, preoperative embolization is a useful adjunct to surgery to reduce blood loss during surgery and facilitate resection [22, 23]. In a recent study [23], the authors embolized preoperatively giant sacral neurogenic tumors, with a mean tumor size of 17.5 cm. All surgical procedures were performed through a single posterior approach, though most of the tumors were located above S3 level. The low recurrence and mortality rates, as well as the good functional outcome, were attributed to the preoperative embolization, which also facilitated surgeons' access to the tumor mass through a single posterior approach in all cases.

Chordomas are rare, slow-growing primary malignant bone tumors, thought to originate from embryonic remnants of the primitive notochord. They arise at the midline of the axial skeleton, most commonly at the sacrococcygeal (30–50%) region. Wide en bloc resection with tumor-free margins is considered the key to successful treatment. However, the special anatomic characteristics of the sacrococcygeal region, and the tumor's invasive nature, allow for a marginal or an intralesional tumor excision, rather than a wide one. Reducing the blood loss during the operation is a measure that could help the surgeon remove the tumor en bloc. In a recent study [24], the authors performed transcatheter arterial embolization of the main arteries that supplied the sacral chordomas. They reported significantly low intraoperative blood loss, and good functional outcomes with acceptable recurrence and mortality rates. These authors advocated that preoperative embolization can significantly decrease intraoperative blood loss, make the surgical field clear, possibly eliminate the need for using an anterior approach, and facilitate the maximal removal of the sacral chordoma [24].

25.4 Embolization for Metastases of the Sacrum

The spinal column is the most common site for metastatic bone disease, with an incidence of spinal metastases of about 20 times higher than that of primary spinal tumors [25]. If not all, most of the metastatic bone tumors are hypervascular; some are highly hypervascular due to angiogenetic factors, cytokines, and bone-resorbing factors being produced, which also contribute to bone failure. The hypervascularity of the metastatic tumors does not apply though universally. Tumors of typically high hypervascularity such as renal and thyroid, not rarely, have been found with low vascularization, whereas tumors considered non-hypervascular, such as lung and breast, have shown hypervascularity [26]. These observations emphasize the need of careful patient selection and a treatment strategy plan. Apart from the abovementioned spinal metastatic tumors, embolization has been also reported in metastases from melanomas, pheochromocytomas, and sarcomas, as well as from colon, prostate, uterus, ovarian, hepatobiliary, gastric, pancreatic, parotid, and lacrimal gland cancer and cancer of unknown origin [25, 26]. In general, embolization can serve as a palliative, as well as an adjuvant preoperative treatment in metastatic disease of the sacrum [20, 25]. It may successfully reduce intraoperative blood loss, improving surgeons' visibility and accessibility to the tumor, therefore, facilitating curettage, and reduce intraoperative morbidity and complications (Fig. 25.3). Preoperative embolization can also reduce the size, arrest tumor growth, alleviate pain, and shorten hospital stay [15].

There is lack of evidence in literature, however, regarding the outcomes of preoperative embolization in metastatic tumors of the sacrum [14, 15, 20, 25]. This could be attributed to the fact that surgical resection of a sacral metastasis consists a great risk accompanied with major complications and doubtful clinical benefits for the patient. Palliative embolization, on the other hand, has been reported as a satisfactory therapeutic alternative for these patients [14, 15, 20, 25]. Recently, Facchini et al. [25] reported good results in a large patient series with spinal metastases treated with *N*-2-Butyl-cyanoacrylate (NBCA) embolization. A fifth of patients had metastases of the sacrum, and good or moderate clinical response was noticed in 97% of the patients. Interestingly though, five patients, who showed no response,

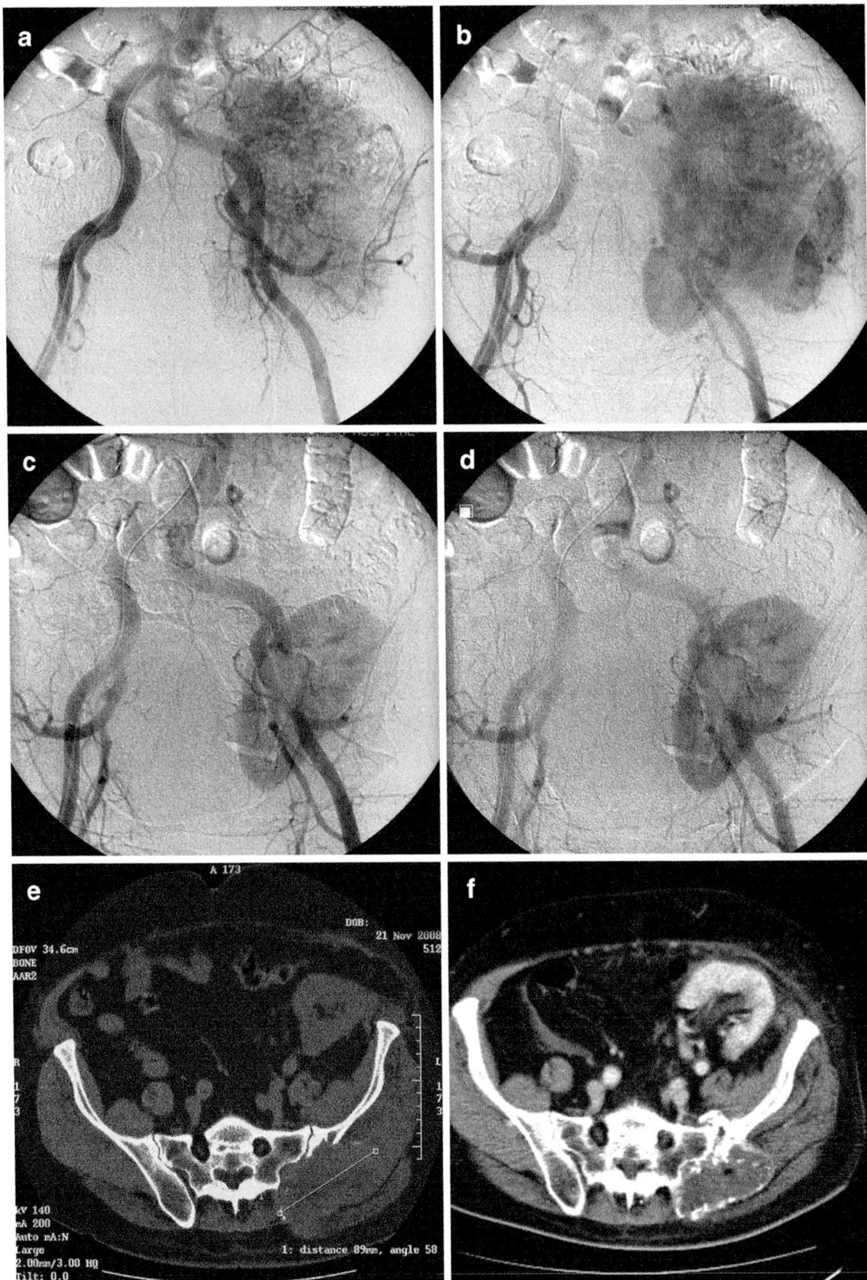

Fig. 25.3 A 63-year-old man with a painful sacroiliac metastasis from renal cancer originating at a transplanted kidney. (**a**, **b**) Digital subtraction angiography shows extensive tumor vascularization. (**c**, **d**) Digital subtraction angiography after NBCA embolization shows occlusion of the tumor vessels. (**e**) CT of the pelvis and sacrum at the time of embolization. (**f**) CT of the pelvis and sacrum at the 12-month follow-up show complete ossification of the metastatic lesion; the patient is asymptomatic

were patients with metastases of the sacrum. The mean duration of pain relief was 9.2 months, and for the patients who experienced recurrent intense pain similar to pre-embolization pain, the embolization was repeated one or two more times with significant pain relief and reduction in analgesics at the last follow-up. The authors concluded that embolization with NBCA should be considered for pain palliation of patients with metastases of the spine and sacrum, as it is a safe and effective procedure.

25.5 Palliative Embolization

The exact mechanism of pain relief following embolization is still unclear. In 1979, Chuang et al. [27] suggested that especially in hypervascular neoplasms the vascular occlusion decreases the size of the tumor and slows its progression. Subsequently, there is a decrease in the pressure of expansion or in the stretching of the periosteum, which contains the nerve fibers that are responsible for pain. This theory remains the only viable explanation of the pain relief mechanism of embolization [14]. The palliative properties of this technique can be extended in primary sacral sarcomas as well. In a recent study [28], selective embolization has been used for palliation of pain in patients with locally advanced sarcomas. In this cohort, patients with primary sacral sarcomas, recurrent or unresectable, responded satisfactory to this treatment with almost complete or moderate pain relief, along with a minimum 50% reduction of daily analgesic doses. Therefore, embolization should be recommended as a safe and effective local palliative treatment, providing optimum pain relief and improving the quality of the remaining life of these patients, by offering the least discomfort with the minimum possible complications [28].

In the question, which factors should be taken into consideration as predictors of the success of an embolization, the answer is the tumor's vascular properties before and after embolization (the tumor's vascularity, the completeness of the occlusion, and the availability of collateral circulation) along with the use of the appropriate embolic agent [25, 27, 28]. Therefore, selective and superselective embolization of the pathological tumor feeding vessels may provide for successful embolization.

Pain relief after embolization may be temporary; however, it occurs rapidly. Indeed, the pain-free period may averagely last 8–9 months; however the patients are relieved immediately, as soon as 12 h up to several days after the embolization procedure, usually within the first week from the procedure; this rapid response, of course, outmatches other methods, such as radiotherapy and chemotherapy [14, 25, 28, 29]. Tumors' size should not be considered when planning an embolization procedure, since it does not seem to affect the outcomes [25]. Therefore, embolization can be proved superior to thermal ablation and cryoablation as well, because sacral tumors are usually large, and ablations should be performed only in painful lesions of <3 cm of maximum diameter. Sacral tumors are also very close to neurovascular bundles; therefore, they cannot be adequately ablated, due to the risk of injuring those fine tissues [28].

25.6 Complications

Common embolization-related complications in most patients include nausea, emesis, low-grade fever, and pain, which usually last 3–7 days; this is known as post-embolization syndrome that has been reported in 18–86% of cases [14, 15]. The rates of major post-embolization complications are low ranging from 1 to 2%, or less [14, 29]. Ischemic neuropathy can result in motor and sensory deficits in the pelvis and lower extremities, and it is a potential complication of any pelvic embolization. During pelvic embolizations through the iliac artery and its major branches, ischemic neuropathies of the sciatic and femoral nerves may occur if neural vessels were occluded. To prevent these complications, the posterior branch of the internal iliac artery and the inferior gluteal artery must be spared at embolization. Complications related to the embolic agents have also been reported. Additionally, the neuraxis or the sacral plexus of nerves can be injured. Therefore, care must be taken to identify and avoid embolization of the neurovascular anatomy. Rectal ischemia can result from superior hemorrhoidal artery embolization. Any embolization of sacral tumors may result in injury to nontargeted tissue including muscle infarction, injury to the skin, or injury to the colon or other organs [14, 15].

25.7 Embolic Agents

Gelfoam, polyvinyl alcohol (PVA) particles, liquid (absolute alcohol), coils, tissue adhesives, ethanol, microfibrillar collagen, and autologous blood clot have been used as embolic agents [14]. Major considerations for choosing an embolic agent are speed and reliability of delivery, duration of occlusive effect, and preservation of normal tissue [14]. Operator's experience plays a key role in the embolization procedure and embolic agent selection. For distal location or lesions supplied by multiple feeding vessels, embosphere particles can be used. Their advantages include compressibility, allowing easy passage through a microcatheter with a luminal diameter smaller than that of the spheres and more uniform in size than poly-vinyl-alcohol (PVA), and the particle size does not change in liquids [30]. Coils are permanent embolic agents that come in a variety of shapes and sizes. In general, they are easy to see, control, and deploy. They are typically used for occlusion of larger vessels and cause complete occlusion equivalent to surgical ligation. In managing hypervascular bone tumors, however, there have been reports of being ineffective because the rich vascularization of these lesions can open collateral channels within hours after the procedure [31–33]. Stainless steel-fibered and platinum coils are usually reserved for single- and large-vessel occlusion. Prior to particulate or liquid embolization, coils may be placed to protect the distal vasculature from these agents [30]. For multiple lesions, distal location or lesions supplied by numerous collateral (accessory) blood pathways, particles can be used. However, injection of particles is not precise and may be difficult to deliver through small microcatheters or through tortuous anatomy. In addition, the particles themselves are not radiopaque, making fluoroscopic documentation of their site of occlusion impossible [20, 27]. Moreover, if particles are used, their size has to be adjusted to the diameter of potential collateral vessels and shunts because these entities are often present in hypervascular malignant bone tumors [9, 32, 33]. Gelatin sponge is a dissolvable material that is available in small, flat, rectangular blocks that can be cut with scissors into elongated rectangles and rolled into pledgets, which can then be injected by catheters or microcatheters. It is considered a temporary occluding agent, with the occluded vessel recanalizing in 2–4 weeks [28]. Once stasis or near stasis has been achieved with the sponge, many interventional radiologists use coil embolization for final and complete vessel occlusion [30].

Liquid embolic agents including absolute alcohol, NBCA, Ethibloc (Ethicon, Norderstedt, Germany), sodium tetradecyl sulfate, and Onyx (Micro therapeutics, Irvine, CA, USA) offer advantages of low viscosity for easy injection through small catheters or catheters with many bends through tortuous blood vessels [3, 20]. NBCA or "liquid glue" is a liquid embolic agent that spreads according to its polymerization time and the vascular flow. Although NBCA can pass through bent catheters, thus navigating tortuous blood vessels, it does not permeate all the way to the capillary level and therefore does not cause tissue death. Another distinct advantage of NBCA with Lipiodol, compared with particles, is its dense radiopacity [20, 28]. Thus, its exact site of occlusion can be observed and documented. Moreover, it can be used in patients with clotting pathologies. This characteristic decreases the risk of organ ischemia, which could cause tissue death in the organ [20, 27]. Bolus administration of small doses (0.1–0.2 mL) of sandwiched NBCA under fluoroscopic control, followed by arteriography provides for the efficacy and safety of the procedure. *N*-2-Butyl-cyanoacrylate, according to some investigators, is considered as the most appropriate embolic agent for controlled and permanent occlusion of the target vessels and subsequently completes tumor devascularization [13, 34]. Embolization is considered technically complete when there is stasis of intravascular contrast material and either complete elimination of the tumor's hypervascular staining, or 80% or greater elimination of the tumor pathological vasculature compared to the initial diagnostic angiogram [11]. If occlusion is not complete or more feeding vessels were observed, the procedure can be repeated in the same method.

Conclusions

Embolization should be considered as a primary, adjuvant, or palliative treatment for primary benign, malignant, and metastatic tumors of the sacrum. The procedure is effective and safe. The effect is immediate; if persistent of recurrent, embolization can be safely repeated. There have been also reports of inoperable tumors that became resectable after palliative embolization. However, life expectancy is not influenced by embolization therapy, and this is not surprising owing to the fact that embolization only targets a portion of the tumor burden aiming to improve the quality of life of musculoskeletal tumor patients. Pain relief on the other hand is usually temporary; however, the patient can be relieved almost immediately from pain, and it is a safe method that can be repeated more than once, until clinical response is met. Complications do occur. However, when embolization is planned carefully and the pathological vessels are occluded selectively and super-selectively, they occur rarely. Most complications are related to the post-embolization syndrome that usually resolves completely within several days or some weeks. Other major complications are uncommon. Nevertheless, strict adherence to the principles of arterial embolization is recommended for achieving simultaneously the most of the desired clinical response with the least adverse effects.

Conflict-of-Interest Statement No benefits have been or will be received from a commercial party related directly or indirectly to the subject matter of this article.

References

1. Feldman F, Casarella WJ, Dick HM, et al. Selective intra-arterial embolization of bone tumors. A useful adjunct in the management of selected lesions. Am J Roentgenol Radium Therapy, Nucl Med. 1975;123(1):130–9.
2. Hilal SK, Michelsen JW. Therapeutic percutaneous embolization for extra-axial vascular lesions of the head, neck, and spine. J Neurosurg. 1975;43(3):275–87.
3. Mavrogenis AF, Rossi G, Rimondi E, Papagelopoulos PJ, Ruggieri P. Embolization of bone tumors. Orthopedics. 2011;34:303–10.
4. Hess T, Kramann B, Schmidt E, Rupp S. Use of preoperative vascular embolisation in spinal metastasis resection. Arch Orthop Trauma Surg. 1997;116(5):279–82.
5. Prabhu VC, Bilsky MH, Jambhekar K, Panageas KS, Boland PJ, Lis E, Heier L, Nelson PK. Results of preoperative embolization for metastatic spinal neoplasms. J Neurosurg. 2003;98(2 Suppl):156–64.
6. Sundaresan N, Choi IS, Hughes JE, Sachdev VP, Berenstein A. Treatment of spinal metastases from kidney cancer by presurgical embolization and resection. J Neurosurg. 1990;73(4):548–54.
7. Gellad FE, Sadato N, Numaguchi Y, Levine AM. Vascular metastatic lesions of the spine: preoperative embolization. Radiology. 1990;176(3):683–6.
8. Chiras J, Cognard C, Rose M, Dessauge C, Martin N, Pierot L, Plouin PF. Percutaneous injection of an alcoholic embolizing emulsion as an alternative preoperative embolization for spine tumor. Am J Neuroradiol. 1993;14(5):1113–7.
9. Forauer AR, Kent E, Cwikiel W, Esper P, Redman B. Selective palliative transcatheter embolization of bony metastases from renal cell carcinoma. Acta Oncol. 2007;46(7):1012–8.
10. Hansch A, Neumann R, Pfeil A, Marintchev I, Pfleiderer S, Gajda M, Kaiser WA. Embolization of an unusual metastatic site of hepatocellular carcinoma in the humerus. World J Gastroenterol. 2009;15(18):2280–2.
11. Barton PP, Waneck RE, Karnel FJ, Ritschl P, Kramer J, Lechner GL. Embolization of bone metastases. J Vasc Interv Radiol. 1996;7(1):81–8.
12. Marciel AM, Van Zandt BL, Baxter AJ. Transcatheter arterial embolization for the palliation of painful bone lesions. Tech Vasc Interv Radiol. 2011;14(3):141–9.
13. Rossi G, Mavrogenis AF, Rimondi E, Braccaioli L, Calabro T, Ruggieri P. Selective embolization with N-butyl cyanoacrylate for metastatic bone disease. J Vasc Interv Radiol. 2011;22(4):462–70.
14. Mavrogenis AF, Angelini A, Vottis C, Pala E, Calabro T, Papagelopoulos PJ, Ruggieri P. Modern palliative treatments for metastatic bone disease: awareness of merits, demerits and guidance. Clin J Pain. 2016;32(4):337–50.
15. Gottfried ON, Schmidt MH, Stevens EA. Embolization of sacral tumors. Neurosurg Focus. 2003;15(2):E4.

16. Lackman RD, Khoury LD, Esmail A, et al. The treatment of sacral giant-cell tumours by serial arterial embolisation. J Bone Joint Surg Br. 2002;84:873–7.
17. Lin PP, Guzel VB, Moura MF, et al. Long-term follow-up of patients with giant cell tumor of the sacrum treated with selective arterial embolization. Cancer. 2002;95:1317–25.
18. Pogoda P, Linhart W, Priemel M, et al. Aneurysmal bone cysts of the sacrum. Clinical report and review of the literature. Arch Orthop Trauma Surg. 2003;123:247–51.
19. Henrichs MP, Beck L, Gosheger G, Streitbuerger A, Koehler M, Heindel W, Hardes J, Vieth V. Selective arterial embolisation of aneurysmal bone cysts of the sacrum: a promising alternative to surgery. Rofo. 2016;188(1):53–9.
20. Rossi G, Mavrogenis AF, Rimondi E, Ciccarese F, Tranfaglia C, Angelelli B, Fiorentini G, Bartalena T, Errani C, Ruggieri P, Mercuri M. Selective arterial embolisation for bone tumours: experience of 454 cases. Radiol Med. 2011;116(5):793–808.
21. Luksanapruksa P, Buchowski JM, Singhatanadgige W, Rose PC, Bumpass DB. Management of spinal giant cell tumors. Spine J. 2016;16(2):259–69.
22. Puri A, Agarwal MG, Shah M, Srinivas CH, Shukla PJ, Shrikhande SV, Jambhekar NA. Decision making in primary sacral tumors. Spine J. 2009;9(5):396–403.
23. Chen K, Zhou M, Yang H, Qian Z, Wang G, Wu G, Zhu X, Sun Z. Pre-operative embolization facilitating a posterior approach for the surgical resection of giant sacral neurogenic tumors. Oncol Lett. 2013;6(1):251–5.
24. Yang H, Zhu L, Ebraheim NA, Liu J, Shapiro A, Castillo S, Liu X, Tang T. Surgical treatment of sacral chordomas combined with transcatheter arterial embolization. J Spinal Disord Tech. 2010;23(1):47–52.
25. Facchini G, Di Tullio P, Battaglia M, Bartalena T, Tetta C, Errani C, Mavrogenis AF, Rossi G. Palliative embolization for metastases of the spine. Eur J Orthop Surg Traumatol. 2016;26(3):247–52.
26. Nair S, Gobin YP, Leng LZ, Marcus JD, Bilsky M, Laufer I, Patsalides A. Preoperative embolization of hypervascular thoracic, lumbar, and sacral spinal column tumors: technique and outcomes from a single center. Interv Neuroradiol. 2013;19(3):377–85.
27. Chuang VP, Wallace S, Swanson D, Zornoza J, Handel SF, Schwarten DA, Murray J. Arterial occlusion in the management of pain from metastatic renal carcinoma. Radiology. 1997;133(3 Pt 1):611–4.
28. Mavrogenis AF, Rossi G, Altimari G, Calabrò T, Angelini A, Palmerini E, Rimondi E, Ruggieri P. Palliative embolisation for advanced bone sarcomas. Radiol Med. 2013;118(8):1344–59.
29. Gottfried ON, Schloesser PE, Schmidt MH, Stevens EA. Embolization of metastatic spinal tumors. Neurosurg Clin N Am. 2004;15(4):391–9.
30. Owen RJ. Embolization of musculoskeletal tumors. Radiol Clin N Am. 2008;46:535–43.
31. Vaidya S, Tozer KR, Chen J. An overview of embolic agents. Semin Intervent Radiol. 2008;25(3):204–15.
32. Sun S, Lang EV. Bone metastases from renal cell carcinoma: preoperative embolization. J Vasc Interv Radiol. 1998;9:263–9.
33. Manke C, Bretschneider T, Lenhart M, et al. Spinal metastases from renal cell carcinoma: effect of preoperative particle embolization on intraoperative blood loss. AJNR Am J Neuroradiol. 2001;22:997–1003.
34. Rossi G, Mavrogenis AF, Casadei R, Bianchi G, Romagnoli C, Rimondi E, et al. Embolisation of bone metastases from renal cancer. Radiol Med. 2013;118(2):291–302.

Palliative Treatments for the Sacrum

26

Andreas F. Mavrogenis, Georgios N. Panagopoulos, Andrea Angelini, Giuseppe Rossi, Alberto Bazzocchi, and Pietro Ruggieri

26.1 Introduction

A wide array of tumors can occur in the sacrum. Benign tumors include giant cell tumors (60%), aneurysmal bone cysts (4%), and osteoblastomas [1]. Malignant tumors of the sacrum include chordomas (50%), hematopoietic malignancies (lymphoma and multiple myeloma, 18%), Ewing's sarcoma in children (8%), chondrosarcoma, and osteosarcoma [2]. However, the most common malignancy to occur in the sacrum is represented by metastatic tumors [3]. The most frequently implicated primary cancers include breast, lung, prostate, renal and thyroid, lymphoma, melanoma, and tumors of unknown origin follow, but are less common primary locations [4–9]. Spread is mainly by hematogenous dissemination, although direct extension in case of recurrent rectal tumors and drop metastases of intradural tumors have been also described [8, 9]. Sacral metastases are usually diagnosed in advanced stages, when they have already extended beyond bony margins and around sacral nerves and other surrounding structures [3, 10]. They generally grow insidiously causing ambiguous symptoms in the early stages, thus frequently resulting in a delayed diagnosis.

A.F. Mavrogenis, M.D., Ph.D. • G.N. Panagopoulos, M.D.
First Department of Orthopaedics, National and Kapodistrian University of Athens, Athens, Greece
e-mail: afm@otenet.gr

A. Angelini, M.D., Ph.D. • P. Ruggieri, M.D., Ph.D. (✉)
Department of Orthopedics and Orthopedic Oncology, University of Padova, Via N. Giustiniani, 3, Padova 35128, Italy
e-mail: andrea.angelini83@yahoo.it; pietro.ruggieri@unipd.it

G. Rossi, M.D. • A. Bazzocchi, M.D.
Diagnostic and Interventional Radiology, Istituto Ortopedico Rizzoli, Bologna, Italy
e-mail: giuseppe.rossi@ior.it; abazzo@inwind.it

P. Ruggieri et al. (eds.), *Tumors of the Sacrum*,
DOI 10.1007/978-3-319-51202-0_26

Patients may live with cancer for many years [11]. Their most common symptom is pain, which may be local, mechanical, or radicular in nature. This is typically followed by a progressive neurological deficit, eventually leading to bladder, bowel, and/or sexual dysfunction [12–14]. The treatment of sacral metastatic lesions is usually palliative, aiming primarily at pain control and preservation of neurological function [8, 9, 15–30]. The goal of palliative therapy is the prompt and cost-effective relief of symptoms, thus improving function and quality for the remainder of the patient's life, with as little treatment-related morbidity as possible. Palliative care is not restricted to terminally ill patients and is an important aspect of overall cancer management.

There is a paucity of studies dealing with the management of sacral metastases, since most papers refer to primary sacral tumors [8, 9, 15–30]. There is also no consensus or precise strategy algorithm as to which method is the most appropriate, making management highly individualized on a patient-to-patient basis, depending to an extent on institutional preferences. The modalities commonly employed include radiotherapy and stereotactic surgery, surgical debulking, sacroplasty, embolization, various ablation techniques, and electrochemotherapy.

26.2 Radiotherapy

Radiotherapy is frequently chosen as a first-line initial therapy for radiosensitive sacral metastases, in patients without evidence of spinal instability or acute neurological deterioration, where pain reduction and neurological improvement are attainable [31, 32]. In fact, palliative radiotherapy as a first-line intervention for spinal metastasis has been the mainstay of management since the late 1960s, after several authors compared radiotherapy with laminectomy, finding no significant difference in patient outcome [33–35]. It must be taken into account that radiosensitivity varies among primary cancer types. In general, prostate and lymphoid tumors are radiosensitive; breast cancer is 70% sensitive and 30% resistant, whereas gastrointestinal tumors, renal cell carcinomas, and melanomas are radioresistant [3]. Radiation doses of 30–50 Gy are indicated for palliation with minimal associated risk. Dose fractioning is controversial. Cummings et al. [36] reported no differences in survival, duration of symptomatic response, and progression-free survival in a heterogeneous group of patients who underwent 50–60 Gy radiotherapy compared with conventional fractions to less than 50 Gy or by a hyperfractionated regimen of 44 Gy delivered in 1-Gy fractions, four times daily for 14 days. To achieve higher doses, specialists at the Harvard Cyclotron Laboratory used a combined treatment of X-ray and proton-beam radiation therapy [37].

Conventional radiotherapy for spinal metastasis is delivered through simple portals to doses of 30–40 Gy in 2- to 3-Gy fractions. For isolated sacral lesions, an opposed anterior posterior field is typically used, encompassing one or two vertebral segments above and below the lesion. Alternatively, a three-field arrangement with two lateral portals and a single posterior field is used to spare anterior pelvic structures. A single posterior field arrangement is generally avoided for sacral lesions, particularly if lower energy beams are used, because the treatment depth will vary along the sacral hollow [38].

26.3 Stereotactic Radiosurgery

Stereotactic radiosurgery has been initially established as a safe and effective treatment modality for intracranial lesions. Precise tumor localization was achieved by fixation of stereotactic frames to the patient's skull [1]. Spinal stereotactic radiosurgery (SRS) is an emerging form of radiotherapy, which allows more precise radiation delivery and high-dose hypofractionation. SRS makes it possible to administer a tumoricidal radiation dose even for radioresistant tumors, with minimal exposure of the surrounding normal tissues. Current commercial spinal SRS systems include the CyberKnife® (Accuray Incorporated, Sunnyvale, California, USA) and Novalis® (BrainLAB, Heimstetten, Germany) [3]. These systems consist of a lightweight linear accelerator mounted on a robotic arm, also incorporating an X-ray imaging feedback system. Spatial accuracy can be achieved in a frameless manner, with real-time imaging tracking. The patients are fitted with a custom body mold for immobilization, and fiducial markers (self-retaining tacks or self-tapping screws) are implanted via stab incisions in the sacrum in an ambulatory setting [38]. Unlike conventional radiation therapy in which a full dose is delivered to both the vertebral body and the spinal cord or cauda equina, the CyberKnife® can deliver a high-dose single fraction to the target tissue while sparing most of the adjacent neural elements, thus significantly reducing the possibility of radiation-induced myelopathy or injury to the nerve roots. This is the main advantage of stereotactic radiosurgery for treatment of many spinal and sacral tumors [39]. Recently, in an attempt to obviate the need for invasive fiducial marker insertion, a new tracking algorithm for fiducial-free tracking of spine and sacral lesions has been introduced for the CyberKnife® system [40].

26.4 Surgery

Metastatic disease to the sacrum is mostly treated nonoperatively with radiation, chemotherapy, embolization, or other palliative modalities. However, there are circumstances in which these therapies fail and surgical intervention is warranted. Whether surgery can be beneficial for these patients is not clearly defined [9]. Care must be taken in the decision making process, as sacral resections are challenging operations with a high incidence of potential complications, in a patient with an already limited life expectancy and compromised general health status [41]. On the other hand, resective surgery in carefully selected patients with sacral metastases may result in a palliative benefit. If pain derives from overt mechanical instability, as a result of structural failure of the lumbosacropelvic junction, it is unlikely for nonsurgical measures to have substantial benefit [9]. In such cases, stabilization with a modified Galveston technique can offer symptom control and improvement of ambulatory function [42].

Primary tumor type is also a variable that must be taken into account. Breast and prostate cancer are generally quite responsive to nonsurgical therapies, making surgery a rarely necessary therapeutic option, whereas lung, gastrointestinal, renal cell cancer, and melanoma tend to respond poorly to medical treatment [9]. Histology and overall tumor burden should be considered as well. For example, removal of secondary lesions of renal cell carcinoma tends to be associated with an increase in overall survival. A minimal disease burden (single-site metastasis) may signify that there is a greater change for surgery to achieve definitive local control [9].

Once a decision for surgery is undertaken, its extent should take into account tumor location in the sacrum. The majority of sacral metastases involve the S1–S3, making en bloc resection too morbid a procedure to undertake for palliation. In such cases, aggressive intralesional resection is preferred. If the distal sacrum is involved, en bloc resection with preservation of the S1–S3 nerve roots may be feasible [15, 43, 44]. Wound healing is another potential issue of surgery. As soft tissue coverage in this territory may be challenging, plastic surgery feedback is frequently necessary [45].

26.5 Sacroplasty

Sacroplasty is gaining favor in cases of metastatic disease without instability or neurologic compromise and represents a minimally invasive alternative to open procedures [46]. Mostly described in the degenerative/osteoporotic literature, sacroplasty has also been examined as a palliative option for metastasis-related insufficiency fractures [47–50]. The technique of sacroplasty is similar to vertebroplasty. Preoperative evaluation consists in obtaining a CT and/or MR imaging scan. The procedure may be done under local or general anesthesia. Image guidance is usually achieved by single-plain fluoroscopy. However, as exclusive fluoroscopy guidance might cause difficulty in visualizing the sacral foramina, many authors advocate for the use of a CT-guided approach [25]. This better defines spatial relationships within the treatment field and aids in preventing iatrogenic injury. A combination of the CT and fluoroscopic guidance may be the best alternative at present, allowing for both precise needle placement and real-time visualization of cement delivery [51]. Needle entry points are dictated by the fracture plane and conformation; cement is then injected under direct fluoroscopic vision to ensure maximal bony penetration and to prevent extravasation [49]. Sacral cement augmentation is not without risk. Potential complications of sacroplasty include hemorrhage, infection, durotomy with cerebrospinal fluid leak, direct injury of nerve roots or the lumbosacral plexus, ectopic cement injection (into the sacroiliac joint), migration, and embolization. Although cement migration is generally inconsequential, it might occasionally cause nerve root compression and radiculopathy, requiring decompression [49].

26.6 Selective Arterial Embolization

Embolization of sacral tumors is a useful, minimally invasive, palliative adjuvant therapy that may also aid in surgical management. Preoperative embolization of hypervascular metastatic lesions reduces intraoperative blood loss and improves the surgeon's ability to subsequently perform surgical resection. Studies have shown that embolization may cause tumor growth arrest, pain alleviation, and shorter hospital stay [52–54]. The timing of preoperative embolization is also important. Typically, best results are achieved when surgery is performed within 24–48 h after embolization [55, 56]. Serial embolization can also be performed, if there is persistent pain and/or evidence of progressive disease on imaging. This has been shown to lead to tumor devascularization, tumor size reduction, calcification of margins, and consistent pain relief [57–59]. Serial embolization is typically performed in 4–6-week intervals until symptomatic improvement occurs or the tumor's vascularity disappears. Unless there is a clear indication for general anesthesia, most procedures are performed under light conscious sedation. Arterial approach is determined based on lesion location and most often is the common femoral artery using a Seldinger technique. Commonly, a sheath is placed and standard 4 French or 5 French angiographic catheters are used for main arterial selection, and a 3 French microcatheter for subselectivity. A diagnostic angiogram is performed from a major vessel to delineate vascular supply to the tumor and to identify vessels of potential concern that may result in nontarget embolization. Typically, microspheres of 100–700 μm are used because of their ease of delivery, range of available sizes, and lower potential for recanalization. Sponge gel, once the embolic agent of choice, has now fallen in disuse, because of its temporary nature and propensity for recanalization. Coils are avoided as an embolic agent for tumor vessels, because retreatment may be necessary and blocking access sites should be avoided. Completion of the procedure is determined by complete loss of tumor blush compared with the initial diagnostic angiogram [60]. Complication rate is generally low [61]. Risks of the procedure include nerve palsy, subcutaneous or muscle necrosis, post-embolization syndrome (fever, pain, malaise), ischemic pain (usually transitory), infection, and tumor bleeding [62].

26.7 Radiofrequency and Other Ablation Techniques

Over the past few decades, percutaneous ablation has emerged as an effective, minimally invasive, local treatment alternative to conventional methods, aiming to provide either palliation of painful bone lesions or local control of oligometastatic disease. Various image-guided ablation techniques have been applied to the treatment of bone metastases with varied levels of published evidence [63–67]. Thermal ablation methods include radiofrequency ablation (RFA), cryoablation, microwave ablation, laser ablation, and more recently MR imaging-guided focused ultrasound (MRgFUS) [63].

Radiofrequency ablation uses high-frequency alternating electrical current (200–1200 kHz) produced by the electrode. Many of the newer RFA devices utilize bipolar technology, eliminating the need for grounding pads, necessary in the past to avoid soft tissue burning. The alternating electrical current causes ionic agitation with subsequent frictional heat. The heat generated causes coagulative necrosis, with irreversible cell damage typically occurring between 60 and 100 °C [64, 65].

Some of the currently used RFA devices for bone include OsteoCool® RFA system (Baylis Medical, Burlington, Massachusetts), Dfine STAR® ablation system (Dfine, San Jose, California), and UniBlate® RFA system (Angiodynamics, Latham, NY). RFA cycles are typically 10–15 min long, depending on the size, shape, location, and intrinsic characteristics of the tumor. RFA also has a cauterizing effect that reduces the risk of bleeding. A limitation of RFA includes the inability to clearly visualize the treatment zone during ablation. The active tips of the RFA probes can be difficult to see on CT due to streak (beam-hardening) artifact. Frequently, multiple sequential, overlapping ablations are necessary to cover large lesions while carefully maintaining an adequate safety margin adjacent to critical structures. Post-procedural pain is also a concern [63].

Cryoablation techniques take advantage of the thermal properties of highly pressurized gases, typically argon or nitrous oxide. As the gas travels through the thermal probe to the tip, the gas expands at the applicator tip causing the temperature to rapidly drop. This is known as the Joule-Thomson effect, with temperatures of −80 °C to as low as −160 °C possible. A temperature between −20 and −40 °C is necessary and needs to persist 1 cm beyond the tumor periphery [66]. Some of the cryoprobes currently used for cryoablation are produced by Endocare® (Healthtronics/Endocare Incorporated, Irvine, California) and Galil Medical® (Galil Medical, Arden Hills, Minnesota). Cryoablation has the advantage of smaller ablation probes; it has the benefit of a clearly visible ablation zone (ice ball) during ablation, which can be seen on CT, MR imaging, or ultrasonography. It is also thought to have less post-procedural pain. More recently, newer probes offer post-ablation cauterization, in order to reduce the risk of post ablation bleeding.

MRgFUS is a noninvasive thermal ablation method that uses extracorporeal-focused ultrasound energy to heat and destroy tissues without the need for invasive placement of applicators. This technology takes advantage of the bone's high acoustic absorption of ultrasound energy to palliate pain, presumably through destruction of periosteal innervation [67]. Evidence regarding MRgFUS of bone metastases is limited but promising. Potential complications include skin burns and injury to heat-sensitive structures, such as nerves and bowel.

26.8 Chemotherapy

Modern medical palliative chemotherapy regimens for painful bone metastases mainly include bisphosphonates and denosumab. The usefulness of these two classes of drugs derives from their ability to regulate osteoclast activity, each targeting a different component of the activation pathway. Bisphosphonates are an important advance in supportive care of patients with bone metastases. They inhibit normal and pathological osteoclast-mediated bone resorption by direct inhibition of osteoclast activity by cellular mechanisms that affect osteoclast attachment, differentiation, and survival. They also reduce osteoclastic activity indirectly, through effects on osteoblasts. In 1995, intravenous pamidronate was approved to treat patients with multiple myeloma or metastatic breast cancer, based on evidence from randomized controlled trials that pamidronate decreases the risk of skeletal complications [62]. In 2002, intravenous zoledronic acid was approved to treat patients with multiple myeloma and bone metastases from any solid tumor including prostate cancer [68]. Denosumab is a human monoclonal antibody for the treatment of osteoporosis, induced bone loss, bone metastases, rheumatoid arthritis, multiple myeloma, and giant cell tumor of bone. It is designed to target RANKL (RANK ligand), a protein that acts as the primary signal to promote bone loss. Denosumab was approved by US Food and Drug Administration (FDA) for use in postmenopausal women with risk of osteoporosis in June 2010 (Prolia®) and for the prevention of skeletal-related events in patients with bone metastases from solid tumors in November 2010 (Xgeva®) making it the first RANKL inhibitor to be approved by the FDA [62]. Direct comparisons of denosumab and bisphosphonates appear to favor denosumab [69]. Potential drawbacks of both drug families notably include the risk for osteonecrosis of the jaw and for the development of atypical femoral fractures [70, 71].

26.9 Electrochemotherapy

Electrochemotherapy (ECT) is an anticancer therapeutic approach that enhances the effectiveness of a chemotherapeutic drug due to increased uptake of the drug by applying electric pulses to tumor tissue. Short intense electric pulses cause transient and reversible permeabilization of the cell membranes, therefore increasing intracellular access of otherwise nonpermeant or poorly permeant drugs [72]. Various chemotherapeutic drugs have been tested, but bleomycin and cisplatin were found to be the most suitable for clinical use in electrochemotherapy [73]. Currently, ECT is used in treatment of cutaneous and subcutaneous tumors of different histological types with response rate of 84.1% and long lasting complete responses rate of 59.5% [74]. ECT is now being used predominantly in Europe, where there are currently 16 countries with at least one clinical center offering it to its patients, especially Italy and Germany [75]. Even though, current focus of ECT is on skin nodules, efforts are being made to apply the procedure on deep-seated solid tumors and bone metastasis. Fini et al. demonstrated the effectiveness of the procedure in the treatment of bone metastases in rats [76]. Currently, a phase I–II clinical trial has been approved and is ongoing at the Istituto Ortopedico Rizzoli, Bologna, Italy, in order to assess safety and feasibility of ECT on bone metastases. Preliminary results on this technology are encouraging [77].

26.10 Pain Management

Appropriate and effective use of pain medication is another crucial aspect for the palliative management of painful bone lesions. Prudent use of opioid analgesics is paramount. Every opioid prescription must include a provision for breakthrough pain. Adjuvant pain medications may improve pain management and reduce potential opioid toxicity. Nonsteroidal anti-inflammatory drugs (NSAIDS) are most useful in a patient with moderate bone pain. They should not be used by frail elderly patients with renal failure or previous peptic ulcer disease. Steroids are the choice for treatment of short-term relief from bone pain, as they can be given parenterally and act within 24–48 h. A dose of 4–16 mg of dexamethasone is typically used in palliative pain management. Cannabinoids are also helpful against cancer pain [78, 79].

Conflict-of-Interest Statement No benefits have been or will be received from a commercial party related directly or indirectly to the subject matter of this article.

References

1. Mavrogenis AF, Patapis P, Kostopanagiotou G, Papagelopoulos PJ. Tumors of the sacrum. Orthopedics. 2009;32(5):342.
2. Unni KK, Dahlin DC. Dahlin's bone tumors: general aspects and data on 11,087 cases. 5th ed. Philadelphia: Lippincott-Raven; 1996.
3. Quraishi NA, Giannoulis KE, Edwards KL, Boszczyk BM. Management of metastatic sacral tumours. Eur Spine J. 2012;21(10):1984–93. doi:10.1007/s00586-012-2394-9.
4. Steinmetz MP, Mekhail A, Benzel EC. Management of metastatic tumors of the spine: strategies and operative indications. Neurosurg Focus. 2001;11(6):e2.
5. Raque Jr GH, Vitaz TW, Shields CB. Treatment of neoplastic diseases of the sacrum. J Surg Oncol. 2001;76(4):301–7.
6. Llauger J, Palmer J, Amores S, Bague S, Camins A. Primary tumors of the sacrum: diagnostic imaging. AJR Am J Roentgenol. 2000;174(2):417–24. doi:10.2214/ajr.174.2.1740417.
7. Diel J, Ortiz O, Losada RA, Price DB, Hayt MW, Katz DS. The sacrum: pathologic spectrum, multimodality imaging, and subspecialty approach. Radiographics. 2001;21(1):83–104. doi:10.1148/radiographics.21.1.g01ja0883.
8. Kollender Y, Meller I, Bickels J, Flusser G, Issakov J, Merimsky O, Marouani N, Nirkin A, Weinbroum AA. Role of adjuvant cryosurgery in intralesional treatment of sacral tumors. Cancer. 2003;97(11):2830–8. doi:10.1002/cncr.11383.
9. Feiz-Erfan I, Fox BD, Nader R, Suki D, Chakrabarti I, Mendel E, Gokaslan ZL, Rao G, Rhines LD. Surgical treatment of sacral metastases: indications and results. J Neurosurg Spine. 2012;17(4):285–91. doi:10.3171/2012.7.SPINE09351.
10. Feldenzer JA, McGauley JL, McGillicuddy JE. Sacral and presacral tumors: problems in diagnosis and management. Neurosurgery. 1989;25(6):884–91.
11. Janjan N, Lin E, Delclos M, Crane C, Rodriguez-Bigas M, Skibber J, Cleeland C. Palliative therapy. In: Ajani J, Curley S, Janjan N, Lynch P, editors. Gastrointestinal cancer. M. D. Anderson cancer care series. New York: Springer; 2005. p. 299–312.
12. Miralbell R, Louis DN, O'Keeffe D, Rosenberg AE, Suit HD. Metastatic ependymoma of the sacrum. Cancer. 1990;65(10):2353–5.
13. Payer M. Neurological manifestation of sacral tumors. Neurosurg Focus. 2003;15(2):E1. doi:10.3171/foc.2003.15.2.1.
14. Hall JH, Fleming JF. The "lumbar disc syndrome" produced by sacral metastases. Can J Surg. 1970;13(2):149–56.
15. Ozdemir MH, Gurkan I, Yildiz Y, Yilmaz C, Saglik Y. Surgical treatment of malignant tumours of the sacrum. Eur J Surg Oncol. 1999;25(1):44–9. doi:10.1053/ejso.1998.0598.
16. Turgut M, Gokpinar D, Barutca S, Erkus M. Lumbosacral metastatic extradural Merkel cell carcinoma causing nerve root compression—case report. Neurol Med Chir. 2002;42(2):78–80.
17. Lee YY, Wen-Wei Hsu R, Huang TJ, Hsueh S, Wang JY. Metastatic meningioma in the sacrum: a case report. Spine (Phila Pa 1976). 2002;27(4):E100–3.

18. Nader R, Rhines LD, Mendel E. Metastatic sacral tumors. Neurosurg Clin N Am. 2004; 15(4):453–7. doi:10.1016/j.nec.2004.04.009.
19. Menegaz RA, Resende AD, da Silva CS, Barcelos AC, Murta EF. Metastasis of choriocarcinoma to lumbar and sacral column. Eur J Obstet Gynecol Reprod Biol. 2004;113(1):110–3. doi:10.1016/j.ejogrb.2003.09.029.
20. Uemura A, Matsusako M, Numaguchi Y, Oka M, Kobayashi N, Niinami C, Kawasaki T, Suzuki K. Percutaneous sacroplasty for hemorrhagic metastases from hepatocellular carcinoma. AJNR Am J Neuroradiol. 2005;26(3):493–5.
21. Gerszten PC, Burton SA, Ozhasoglu C, Welch WC. Radiosurgery for spinal metastases: clinical experience in 500 cases from a single institution. Spine (Phila Pa 1976). 2007;32(2):193–9. doi:10.1097/01.brs.0000251863.76595.a2.
22. Akasu T, Yamaguchi T, Fujimoto Y, Ishiguro S, Yamamoto S, Fujita S, Moriya Y. Abdominal sacral resection for posterior pelvic recurrence of rectal carcinoma: analyses of prognostic factors and recurrence patterns. Ann Surg Oncol. 2007;14(1):74–83. doi:10.1245/s10434-006-9082-0.
23. Fujibayashi S, Neo M, Nakamura T. Palliative dual iliac screw fixation for lumbosacral metastasis. Technical note. J Neurosurg Spine. 2007;7(1):99–102. doi:10.3171/SPI-07/07/099.
24. Kakutani K, Doita M, Nishida K, Miyamoto H, Kurosaka M. Radiculopathy due to malignant melanoma in the sacrum with unknown primary site. Eur Spine J. 2008;17(Suppl 2):S271–4. doi:10.1007/s00586-007-0561-1.
25. Zhang J, Wu CG, Gu YF, Li MH. Percutaneous sacroplasty for sacral metastatic tumors under fluoroscopic guidance only. Korean J Radiol. 2008;9(6):572–6. doi:10.3348/kjr.2008.9.6.572.
26. Albareda J, Herrera M, Lopez Salva A, Garcia Donas J, Gonzalez R. Sacral metastasis in a patient with endometrial cancer: case report and review of the literature. Gynecol Oncol. 2008;111(3):583–8. doi:10.1016/j.ygyno.2008.04.005.
27. Toro A, Pulvirenti E, Manfre L, Di Carlo I. Sacroplasty in a patient with bone metastases from hepatocellular carcinoma. A case report. Tumori. 2010;96(1):172–4.
28. Dozois EJ, Privitera A, Holubar SD, Aldrete JF, Sim FH, Rose PS, Walsh MF, Bower TC, Leibovich BC, Nelson H, Larson DW. High sacrectomy for locally recurrent rectal cancer: can long-term survival be achieved? J Surg Oncol. 2011;103(2):105–9. doi:10.1002/jso.21774.
29. Nebreda C, Vallejo R, Aliaga L, Benyamin R. Percutaneous sacroplasty and sacroiliac joint cementation under fluoroscopic guidance for lower back pain related to sacral metastatic tumors with sacroiliac joint invasion. Pain Pract. 2011;11(6):564–9. doi:10.1111/j.1533-2500.2010.00439.x.
30. Moussazadeh N, Laufer I, Yamada Y, Bilsky MH. Separation surgery for spinal metastases: effect of spinal radiosurgery on surgical treatment goals. Cancer Control. 2014;21(2):168–74.
31. Maranzano E, Trippa F, Chirico L, Basagni ML, Rossi R. Management of metastatic spinal cord compression. Tumori. 2003;89(5):469–75.
32. Loblaw DA, Laperriere NJ. Emergency treatment of malignant extradural spinal cord compression: an evidence-based guideline. J Clin Oncol. 1998;16(4):1613–24.
33. Gilbert RW, Kim JH, Posner JB. Epidural spinal cord compression from metastatic tumor: diagnosis and treatment. Ann Neurol. 1978;3(1):40–51. doi:10.1002/ana.410030107.
34. Khan FR, Glicksman AS, Chu FC, Nickson JJ. Treatment by radiotherapy of spinal cord compression due to extradural metastases. Radiology. 1967;89(3):495–500. doi:10.1148/89.3.495.
35. Marshall LF, Langfitt TW. Combined therapy for metastatic extradural tumors of the spine. Cancer. 1977;40(5):2067–70.
36. Cummings BJ, Hodson DI, Bush RS. Chordoma: the results of megavoltage radiation therapy. Int J Radiat Oncol Biol Phys. 1983;9(5):633–42.
37. Hug EB, Fitzek MM, Liebsch NJ, Munzenrider JE. Locally challenging osteo- and chondrogenic tumors of the axial skeleton: results of combined proton and photon radiation therapy using three-dimensional treatment planning. Int J Radiat Oncol Biol Phys. 1995;31(3):467–76. doi:10.1016/0360-3016(94)00390-7.
38. Gibbs IC, Chang SD. Radiosurgery and radiotherapy for sacral tumors. Neurosurg Focus. 2003;15(2):E8.
39. Gerszten PC, Ozhasoglu C, Burton SA, Welch WC, Vogel WJ, Atkins BA, Kalnicki S. CyberKnife frameless single-fraction stereotactic radiosurgery for tumors of the sacrum. Neurosurg Focus. 2003;15(2):E7.

40. Muacevic A, Drexler C, Kufeld M, Romanelli P, Duerr HJ, Wowra B. Fiducial-free real-time image-guided robotic radiosurgery for tumors of the sacrum/pelvis. Radiother Oncol. 2009;93(1):37–44. doi:10.1016/j.radonc.2009.05.023.
41. Randall RL, Bruckner J, Lloyd C, Pohlman TH, Conrad 3rd EU. Sacral resection and reconstruction for tumors and tumor-like conditions. Orthopedics. 2005;28(3):307–13.
42. Jackson RJ, Gokaslan ZL. Spinal-pelvic fixation in patients with lumbosacral neoplasms. J Neurosurg. 2000;92(1 Suppl):61–70.
43. Salehi SA, McCafferty RR, Karahalios D, Ondra SL. Neural function preservation and early mobilization after resection of metastatic sacral tumors and lumbosacropelvic junction reconstruction. Report of three cases. J Neurosurg. 2002;97(1 Suppl):88–93.
44. Todd Jr LT, Yaszemski MJ, Currier BL, Fuchs B, Kim CW, Sim FH. Bowel and bladder function after major sacral resection. Clin Orthop Relat Res. 2002;397:36–9.
45. Miles WK, Chang DW, Kroll SS, Miller MJ, Langstein HN, Reece GP, Evans GR, Robb GL. Reconstruction of large sacral defects following total sacrectomy. Plast Reconstr Surg. 2000;105(7):2387–94.
46. Masala S, Konda D, Massari F, Simonetti G. Sacroplasty and iliac osteoplasty under combined CT and fluoroscopic guidance. Spine (Phila Pa 1976). 2006;31(18):E667–9. doi:10.1097/01.brs.0000231962.04739.ac.
47. Bayley E, Srinivas S, Boszczyk BM. Clinical outcomes of sacroplasty in sacral insufficiency fractures: a review of the literature. Eur Spine J. 2009;18(9):1266–71. doi:10.1007/s00586-009-1048-z.
48. Hirsch JA, Barr JD, Zoarski GH. Sacroplasty: beyond the beginning. J Neurointerven Surg. 2013;5(5):395. doi:10.1136/neurintsurg-2012-010434.
49. Moussazadeh N, Laufer I, Werner T, Krol G, Boland P, Bilsky MH, Lis E. Sacroplasty for cancer-associated insufficiency fractures. Neurosurgery. 2015;76(4):446–50; discussion 450. doi:10.1227/NEU.0000000000000658.
50. Whitlow CT, Mussat-Whitlow BJ, Mattern CW, Baker MD, Morris PP. Sacroplasty versus vertebroplasty: comparable clinical outcomes for the treatment of fracture-related pain. AJNR Am J Neuroradiol. 2007;28(7):1266–70. doi:10.3174/ajnr.A0561.
51. Pommersheim W, Huang-Hellinger F, Baker M, Morris P. Sacroplasty: a treatment for sacral insufficiency fractures. AJNR Am J Neuroradiol. 2003;24(5):1003–7.
52. Hess T, Kramann B, Schmidt E, Rupp S. Use of preoperative vascular embolisation in spinal metastasis resection. Arch Orthop Trauma Surg. 1997;116(5):279–82.
53. Prabhu VC, Bilsky MH, Jambhekar K, Panageas KS, Boland PJ, Lis E, Heier L, Nelson PK. Results of preoperative embolization for metastatic spinal neoplasms. J Neurosurg. 2003;98(2 Suppl):156–64.
54. Sundaresan N, Choi IS, Hughes JE, Sachdev VP, Berenstein A. Treatment of spinal metastases from kidney cancer by presurgical embolization and resection. J Neurosurg. 1990;73(4):548–54. doi:10.3171/jns.1990.73.4.0548.
55. Gellad FE, Sadato N, Numaguchi Y, Levine AM. Vascular metastatic lesions of the spine: preoperative embolization. Radiology. 1990;176(3):683–6. doi:10.1148/radiology.176.3.2389026.
56. Chiras J, Cognard C, Rose M, Dessauge C, Martin N, Pierot L, Plouin PF. Percutaneous injection of an alcoholic embolizing emulsion as an alternative preoperative embolization for spine tumor. AJNR Am J Neuroradiol. 1993;14(5):1113–7.
57. Forauer AR, Kent E, Cwikiel W, Esper P, Redman B. Selective palliative transcatheter embolization of bony metastases from renal cell carcinoma. Acta Oncol. 2007;46(7):1012–8. doi:10.1080/02841860701280725.
58. Hansch A, Neumann R, Pfeil A, Marintchev I, Pfleiderer S, Gajda M, Kaiser WA. Embolization of an unusual metastatic site of hepatocellular carcinoma in the humerus. World J Gastroenterol. 2009;15(18):2280–2.
59. Barton PP, Waneck RE, Karnel FJ, Ritschl P, Kramer J, Lechner GL. Embolization of bone metastases. J Vasc Interv Radiol. 1996;7(1):81–8.
60. Marciel AM, Van Zandt BL, Baxter AJ. Transcatheter arterial embolization for the palliation of painful bone lesions. Tech Vasc Interv Radiol. 2011;14(3):141–9. doi:10.1053/j.tvir.2011.02.006.

61. Rossi G, Mavrogenis AF, Rimondi E, Braccaioli L, Calabro T, Ruggieri P. Selective embolization with N-butyl cyanoacrylate for metastatic bone disease. J Vasc Interv Radiol. 2011; 22(4):462–70. doi:10.1016/j.jvir.2010.12.023.
62. Mavrogenis AF, Angelini A, Vottis C, Pala E, Calabro T, Papagelopoulos PJ, Ruggieri P. Modern palliative treatments for metastatic bone disease: awareness of merits, demerits and guidance. Clin J Pain. 2015;32(4):337–50. doi:10.1097/AJP.0000000000000255.
63. Kurup AN, Callstrom MR. Ablation of skeletal metastases: current status. J Vasc Interv Radiol. 2010;21(8 Suppl):S242–50. doi:10.1016/j.jvir.2010.05.001.
64. Kaufman JA, Lee MJ. Vascular and interventional radiology: the requisites. 1st ed. Philadelphia: Mosby; 2004.
65. Randall RL, SpringerLink (Online service). Metastatic bone disease: an integrated approach to patient care. New York: Springer; 2016.
66. Chu KF, Dupuy DE. Thermal ablation of tumours: biological mechanisms and advances in therapy. Nat Rev Cancer. 2014;14(3):199–208. doi:10.1038/nrc3672.
67. Mercadante S, Fulfaro F. Management of painful bone metastases. Curr Opin Oncol. 2007;19(4):308–14. doi:10.1097/CCO.0b013e3281214400.
68. Michaelson MD, Smith MR. Bisphosphonates for treatment and prevention of bone metastases. J Clin Oncol. 2005;23(32):8219–24. doi:10.1200/JCO.2005.02.9579.
69. Fizazi K, Carducci M, Smith M, Damiao R, Brown J, Karsh L, Milecki P, Shore N, Rader M, Wang H, Jiang Q, Tadros S, Dansey R, Goessl C. Denosumab versus zoledronic acid for treatment of bone metastases in men with castration-resistant prostate cancer: a randomised, double-blind study. Lancet. 2011;377(9768):813–22. doi:10.1016/S0140-6736(10)62344-6.
70. Puhaindran ME, Farooki A, Steensma MR, Hameed M, Healey JH, Boland PJ. Atypical subtrochanteric femoral fractures in patients with skeletal malignant involvement treated with intravenous bisphosphonates. J Bone Joint Surg Am. 2011;93(13):1235–42. doi:10.2106/JBJS.J.01199.
71. Thompson RN, Armstrong CL, Heyburn G. Bilateral atypical femoral fractures in a patient prescribed denosumab—a case report. Bone. 2014;61:44–7. doi:10.1016/j.bone.2013.12.027.
72. Gehl J. Electroporation: theory and methods, perspectives for drug delivery, gene therapy and research. Acta Physiol Scand. 2003;177(4):437–47. doi:10.1046/j.1365-201X.2003.01093.x.
73. Sersa G, Miklavcic D, Cemazar M, Rudolf Z, Pucihar G, Snoj M. Electrochemotherapy in treatment of tumours. Eur J Surg Oncol. 2008;34(2):232–40. doi:10.1016/j.ejso.2007.05.016.
74. Mali B, Jarm T, Snoj M, Sersa G, Miklavcic D. Antitumor effectiveness of electrochemotherapy: a systematic review and meta analysis. Eur J Surg Oncol. 2013;39(1):4–16. doi:10.1016/j.ejso.2012.08.016.
75. Miklavcic D, Sersa G, Brecelj E, Gehl J, Soden D, Bianchi G, Ruggieri P, Rossi CR, Campana LG, Jarm T. Electrochemotherapy: technological advancements for efficient electroporation-based treatment of internal tumors. Med Biol Eng Comput. 2012;50(12):1213–25. doi:10.1007/s11517-012-0991-8.
76. Fini M, Salamanna F, Parrilli A, Martini L, Cadossi M, Maglio M, Borsari V. Electrochemotherapy is effective in the treatment of rat bone metastases. Clin Exp Metastasis. 2013;30(8):1033–45. doi:10.1007/s10585-013-9601-x.
77. Bianchi G, Campanacci L, Fini M. Electrochemotherapy for the treatment of osteolytic bone metastasis: a phase I/II clinical trial. Paper presented at the EMSOS 2010 Annual Meeting, Birmingham, UK, 6–7 May, 2010.
78. Bonneau A. Management of bone metastases. Can Fam Physician. 2008;54(4):524–7.
79. MacDonald N. Palliative medicine: a case-based manual. 2nd ed. Oxford: Oxford University Press; 2005.

Radiation Therapy for Primary Malignant Sacral Tumors

27

Joseph H. Schwab and Francis J. Hornicek

27.1 Introduction

Radiation therapy continues to evolve and play an ever larger role in the management of primary tumors of the sacrum. Radiation therapy has become much more precise, and the principle advances in radiation have been in the sparing of normal tissues around tumors. Highly conformal photon radiation, carbon ion radiation, and proton radiation are all the so-called high precision radiation delivery methods. This relative sparing allows much higher doses to be delivered to the tumor rendering previously "radiation-resistant" tumors susceptible to radiation effects. Chondrosarcoma and chordoma have the reputation for being radiation resistant and both are commonly found in the sacrum. However, the literature continues to expand with reports of good local control with radiation as an adjuvant to surgery and, in some cases, as stand-alone treatment. However, the side effects of radiation increase as the dose increases. Even though there is relative sparing of normal tissue, there continues to be off-target effects and the true side effect profile for high precision radiation therapy is not known.

27.1.1 History

Radiation as method of treatment for cancer has been used since Roentgen first introduced X-rays as a diagnostic tool. Initially, radiation as a therapy was delivered in one treatment session similar to how it was used as a diagnostic tool. However,

J.H. Schwab, M.D., M.S. • F.J. Hornicek, M.D., Ph.D. (✉)
Section of Orthopaedic Oncology, Department of Orthopaedic Surgery, Massachusetts General Hospital, Boston, MA, USA
e-mail: JHSCHWAB@mgh.harvard.edu; fhornicek@mgh.harvard.edu

P. Ruggieri et al. (eds.), *Tumors of the Sacrum*,
DOI 10.1007/978-3-319-51202-0_27

short-term complications such as skin slough tempered the initial enthusiasm for radiation as a therapy. At that time, the most immediate outcomes were that of complications and the concept of radiation-resistant tumors was not yet discussed. In order to avoid short-term complications, radiation oncologists started delivering radiation in divided doses to help prevent local complications. The divided dose or fraction is allowed for the normal structures to recover from the off-target effects of radiation delivery. The downside of fractionating radiation is that the tumor cells are also allowed to recover. Radiation oncologists began developing other methods of protecting normal structures such as changing the angle which radiation entered the body. This allowed some of the off-target effects of radiation to be shared by other normal structures rather than delivering to the same structures as it had been done initially. Even with these changes the total dose of radiation was limited by the off-target affects seen in sensitive structures such as the lining of the alimentary track or the skin. For axial tumors, the spinal cord was a rate-limiting structure owing to the known toxicity manifested in the spinal cord after 50 Gy of radiation. Most studies using radiation for primary bone tumors did not exceed doses of 40 Gy, and this proved to be an ineffective dose for most primary malignant bone tumors, which is why radiation has the reputation for being an ineffective salvage in cases where surgery has failed or thought impractical to apply. The so-called radiation-resistant tumors are actually resistant only at the doses historically delivered since all cells are susceptible to radiation when high enough doses are used. The principle advance in radiation therapy has been minimizing the off-target effects on normal structures; thereby allowing the radiation oncologist to increase the doses of radiation used.

27.1.2 Photon Radiation

Photon radiation is the most common type of radiation used to treat cancer, and it is the same type of radiation used in diagnostic X-rays. Photon radiation is most commonly produced by a linear accelerator in which alternating electromagnetic waves are used to accelerate elections towards a target. Conventional radiation therapy using photons was introduced previously, and it is far and away the most common type of radiation used today to palliate cancer. Many advances have been made to conventional radiation that enable the more precise delivery of the electrons. One means by which precision has been improved is by the use of real-time three-dimensional imaging such as en suite computed tomography. This allows for highly accurate depictions of the target. The patient and the target (tumor) are necessarily held in position and motion is limited to the greatest degree possible by using various harnesses and positioners. Most modern radiation suites place patients on a table, which can be moved in six plains in order to maximize the effectiveness of having imaging capacity. These methods help to localize the target and hold the target into position. The beam of radiation is also rotated about a gantry, again to help minimize off-target effects of radiation.

The beam of radiation can be further modified in order to maximize on target and minimize off-target affects. The so-called intensity-modulated radiation therapy (IMRT) involves using smaller beams of radiation about the size of a number 2 pencil. The radiation oncologist can modulate the energy delivered in each beam to help protect normal structures. Computer software has greatly facilitated this method of treatment. In fact, IMRT uses what is known as reverse planning where the dose delivered to the tumor is planned first. The software then helps decide how to deliver the radiation while sparing normal structures by modulating the beams of radiation utilized. The net effect is to allow higher doses of radiation to be used because radiation deliver is much more precise with tolerances of 2–3 mm when the target can be fully immobilized [1].

27.1.3 Carbon Ion Radiation

Unlike photon radiation, carbon ion radiation relies on accelerating carbon to nearly 70% of the speed of light. The principle advantage of carbon ion therapy is that the amount of radiation delivered increases with depth into the patient and then drops off precipitously in what is known as a Bragg peak. This is in contrast to photon radiation in which higher entry doses are seen which gradually taper off until the radiation passes through the target. There is both a high entry dose and a relatively high exit dose with photon radiation, whereas there is a smaller entry dose and essentially no exit dose with carbon ion therapy. The location of the Bragg peak can be adjusted based on where its effect is most needed. The lack of an exit dose and a smaller entry dose allow the total dose to the target to be increased when compared to conventional photon radiation. The principle disadvantage of carbon ion therapy is that a specialized facility is required for its delivery. The costs of these facilities are high. Carbon ion facilities exist in Japan and several are in use or under development in Europe [1].

27.1.4 Proton Radiation

Proton radiation relies on the acceleration of protons and, similar to carbon ion, the radiation dose has a Bragg peak pattern rather than a gradual drop off with depth seen with conventional photon radiation. It is the Bragg peak that allows for higher doses of radiation to be used as there are no exit doses which limits the off-target affects of radiation. Similar to carbon ion facilities, proton accelerators are costly to build but there are now over 20 facilities in the United States either in use or in development [1].

27.2 Radiation in Primary Malignant Tumors of the Sacrum

Chondrosarcoma and chordoma are the most common primary malignant tumors of the sacrum and both of them are considered radiation resistant. However, most reports of radiation in these sacral tumors were from retrospective studies in which radiation was used as a means to control positive margins or after local failure. Furthermore, the dose of radiation seldom exceeded 50 Gy owing largely to the inability to deliver radiation in a more conformal manner [2–6].

27.2.1 Carbon Ion Radiation for Chordoma

Carbon ions have been used in Japan to treat chordomas in the sacrum, where some centers are treating sacral chordomas with carbon ions alone. A recent study outlined the oncologic results of patients with sacral and lower lumbar chordomas treated between 64 and 74 Gy with a median follow-up of 62 months. The authors describe grade 3 toxicity in the peripheral nerves in six cases and grade 4 toxicity seen in two cases with 97% of the patients remaining ambulatory at the end of the study. The 5 and 10 year local control rates were 77 and 52% with carbon ions alone [7]. This study compares favorably to a surgical series from Mayo Clinic, where the 5 and 10 year local control rates were 59 and 46%. However, when one reviews only those cases in which negative margins were obtained the local control rate was 100% [4]. A multicenter experience from Italy recently reported local control of 70% at 5 years, 54% at 10 years, and 44% at 15 years [8]. In that series of 99 chordomas, the benefits of a negative margin seemed to diminish over time with only 50% of the R0 resections remaining without local failure after 15 years [8]. A study from Germany reviewed 56 patients (41 primary and 15 recurrent) with sacral chordoma treated with carbon ion-based radiation with a median dose of 66 Gy. After median, 25 months of follow-up actuarial local control was 76% after 2 years and 53% after 3 years [9]. This is in contrast to another study of 23 patients treated with either proton or carbon ion with local control after 3 years of 94% reported [10]. The results of carbon-based radiation appear to demonstrate some variability from center to center with regard to local control. The same is true when one considers surgery. Baseline variation in tumor size, patient characteristics as well as the experience and technique of the radiation oncologists all likely play a role in this variability.

27.2.2 Proton Radiation for Chordoma

A recently updated phase 2 study of proton radiation in primary malignant tumors of the spine and sacrum included 29 chordomas [11]. The data included patients treated with surgery and proton radiation. The overall local control rate was 74% after 8 years. Twenty-nine chordomas and 14 chondrosarcomas were included as well as 7 other sarcomas. Patients who were treated for primary tumors did better than patients who were being treated for a recurrence. Local control for primary tumors was 85% [11]. In another series focusing on chordomas in the mobile spine, en bloc resection was seen as advantageous over intralesional resection with regard to local control (LC 72% vs. 55%) with a trend towards improved local control with negative margins. Patients who had primary tumors treated with neoadjuvant radiation and en bloc resection ($n = 28$) did not have a local recurrence [12].

Definitive high dose proton radiation has been reported with good results. The study initially included 24 patients treated with 77.4 Gy for chordomas in the sacrum and spine. After 56 months, the local control rate was 79.8%.

The authors found that a larger tumor volume correlated with worse survival [13]. A follow-up study including 40 patients followed for 50.3 months revealed an local control rate of 85% [14].

27.2.3 Photon Radiation for Chordoma

Less has been written about the use of conformal photon radiation in sacral chordoma. Single fraction and hypo-fractionated, highly conformal photon radiation has been used an adjuvant and as a stand-alone procedure. The largest experience is from Memorial Sloan Kettering Cancer Center where they presented 24 cases and followed for a median of 24 months with an local control rate of 95% [15].

27.3 Complications

The most common complications reported after surgery in combination with high dose radiation is a postoperative wound infection with rates between 20 and 60% reported in the literature [16]. Most centers now employ local soft tissue rotational flaps to help mitigate the risk of infection. Another complication that has not been written about as frequently is that of insufficiency fractures. In a report of 62 patients treated with en bloc sacrectomy combined with high dose proton-based radiation revealed an overall fracture rate of 47% and a 76% fracture rate in high sacrectomies. Most of the fractures occurred within the first 12 months of treatment [17]. Unlike most other insufficiency fractures that one might see secondary to osteoporosis, the fractures associated with high dose radiation do not heal normally and can present a vexing problem.

Skin breakdown and peripheral nerve dysfunction have both been reported although they are relatively rare. However, it is known that many of radiation's untoward effects occur years after treatment, and it is unclear how well we are surveying patients for these types of complications. For instance, how well are we detecting bowel, bladder, and sexual dysfunction in patients who have been treated with radiation alone? Yet, the treatment calls for radiating areas with sympathetic, parasympathetic, and somatic nerves interacting to control bowel, bladder, and sexual function. It is assumed that these functions are preserved when one avoids sacrectomy; however, it is unclear how the radiation truly impacts these functions.

Conclusion

The benefit of radiation is clearly seen with improved local control in recent publications. However, this must be balanced with the morbidity associated with radiation and radiation plus surgery. In addition to the increased risk of infection, we have seen high rates of fractures, which have proven to be particularly difficult to treat. Many of the patients suffering with these fractures have no evidence of disease but they have a poor quality of life. At first glance, it seems that definitive radiation ought to be considered for the higher sacrectomies given the risk of fracture and the known detrimental effect on physical function and increased pain [18]. However, it is also true that radiation alone works poorly when tumors are large like the ones which require high sacrectomy [13]. Radiation works well for small tumors like those that present in the distal sacrum. However, patient reported quality of life and pain scores reveal that patients who have had a distal sacrectomy have functional scores and pain levels comparable to the general population [18]. In other words, surgery works well with low morbidity for distal sacral tumors.

Radiation therapy continues to demonstrate utility in the management of malignant sacral tumors. Questions still remain as to the timing and dosage of radiation. Furthermore, the untoward effects of radiation have not been fully defined and need to be clarified.

Conflict-of-Interest Statement No benefits have been or will be received from a commercial party related directly or indirectly to the subject matter of this chapter.

References

1. Pennicooke B, Laufer I, Sahgal A, Varga PP, Gokaslan ZL, Bilsky MH, et al. Safety and local control of radiation therapy for chordoma of the spine and sacrum: a systematic review. Spine (Phila Pa 1976). 2016;41(Suppl 20):S186–92.
2. Angelini A, Pala E, Calabro T, Maraldi M, Ruggieri P. Prognostic factors in surgical resection of sacral chordoma. J Surg Oncol. 2015;112(4):344–51.
3. Bergh P, Kindblom LG, Gunterberg B, Remotti F, Ryd W, Meis-Kindblom JM. Prognostic factors in chordoma of the sacrum and mobile spine: a study of 39 patients. Cancer. 2000;88(9):2122–34.
4. Fuchs B, Dickey ID, Yaszemski MJ, Inwards CY, Sim FH. Operative management of sacral chordoma. J Bone Joint Surg Am. 2005;87(10):2211–6.
5. Kaiser TE, Pritchard DJ, Unni KK. Clinicopathologic study of sacrococcygeal chordoma. Cancer. 1984;53(11):2574–8.
6. Schwab JH, Healey JH, Rose P, Casas-Ganem J, Boland PJ. The surgical management of sacral chordomas. Spine (Phila Pa 1976). 2009;34(24):2700–4.
7. Imai R, Kamada T, Araki N, Working Group for Bone and Soft Tissue Sarcomas. Carbon ion radiation therapy for unresectable sacral chordoma: an analysis of 188 cases. Int J Radiat Oncol Biol Phys. 2016;95(1):322–7.
8. Radaelli S, Stacchiotti S, Ruggieri P, Donati D, Casali PG, Palmerini E, et al. Sacral chordoma: long-term outcome of a large series of patients surgically treated at two reference centers. Spine (Phila Pa 1976). 2016;41(12):1049–57.
9. Uhl M, Welzel T, Jensen A, Ellerbrock M, Haberer T, Jakel O, et al. Carbon ion beam treatment in patients with primary and recurrent sacrococcygeal chordoma. Strahlenther Onkol. 2015;191(7):597–603.
10. Mima M, Demizu Y, Jin D, Hashimoto N, Takagi M, Terashima K, et al. Particle therapy using carbon ions or protons as a definitive therapy for patients with primary sacral chordoma. Br J Radiol. 2014;87(1033):20130512.

11. DeLaney TF, Liebsch NJ, Pedlow FX, Adams J, Weyman EA, Yeap BY, et al. Long-term results of phase II study of high dose photon/proton radiotherapy in the management of spine chordomas, chondrosarcomas, and other sarcomas. J Surg Oncol. 2014;110(2):115–22.
12. Rotondo RL, Folkert W, Liebsch NJ, Chen YL, Pedlow FX, Schwab JH, et al. High-dose proton-based radiation therapy in the management of spine chordomas: outcomes and clinicopathological prognostic factors. J Neurosurg Spine. 2015;23(6):788–97.
13. Chen YL, Liebsch N, Kobayashi W, Goldberg S, Kirsch D, Calkins G, et al. Definitive high-dose photon/proton radiotherapy for unresected mobile spine and sacral chordomas. Spine (Phila Pa 1976). 2013;38(15):E930–6.
14. Kabolizadeh P, Chen YL, Liebsch N, Hornicek FJ, Schwab JH, Choy E, et al. Updated outcome and analysis of tumor response in mobile spine and sacral chordoma treated with definitive high-dose photon/proton radiation therapy. Int J Radiat Oncol Biol Phys. 2016;97: 254–62.
15. Yamada Y, Laufer I, Cox BW, Lovelock DM, Maki RG, Zatcky JM, et al. Preliminary results of high-dose single-fraction radiotherapy for the management of chordomas of the spine and sacrum. Neurosurgery. 2013;73(4):673–80. Discussion 680.
16. Ruggieri P, Angelini A, Pala E, Mercuri M. Infections in surgery of primary tumors of the sacrum. Spine (Phila Pa 1976). 2012;37(5):420–8.
17. Osler P, Bredella MA, Hess KA, Janssen SJ, Park CJ, Chen YL, et al. Sacral insufficiency fractures are common after high-dose radiation for sacral chordomas treated with or without surgery. Clin Orthop Relat Res. 2016;474(3):766–72.
18. Phukan R, Herzog T, Boland PJ, Healey J, Rose P, Sim FH, et al. How does the level of sacral resection for primary malignant bone tumors affect physical and mental health, pain, mobility, incontinence, and sexual function? Clin Orthop Relat Res. 2016;474(3):687–96.

Tumors of the Sacrum: The Role of Chemotherapy

28

Stefano Ferrari

28.1 Introduction

The use of chemotherapy has changed the natural history of sarcomas, and as most of the lesions arising in the sacrum are primary bone sarcomas, they can benefit from systemic treatment with antineoplastic agents.

Osteosarcoma, Ewing sarcoma, and the group of undifferentiated high-grade pleomorphic bone sarcomas are the tumors where the effectiveness of chemotherapy is most apparent. In the most recent years, also for tumors previously considered refractory to systemic chemotherapy such as giant-cell tumors, chondrosarcomas, and chordoma, new medical treatments are now available.

In the absence of evidence regarding a possible relation between chemosensitivity and skeletal location of the tumors, systemic treatment of sacral tumors follows the same criteria used for the treatment of primary bone sarcomas with other skeletal locations. As stated in the other chapters, the main challenge posed by sacral tumors is local treatment. Chemotherapy, apart from the effect against micrometastatic diseases, may also contribute to improve local control.

The different entities that can be diagnosed in the sacrum require specific systemic treatments comprising classic antineoplastic agents and more recent treatments with targeted therapies.

In this chapter, the role of chemotherapy will be described focusing on the main primary bone sarcomas.

S. Ferrari, M.D. (✉)
Department of Chemotherapy, Istituto Ortopedico Rizzoli, Bologna, Italy
e-mail: stefano.ferrari@ior.it

P. Ruggieri et al. (eds.), *Tumors of the Sacrum*,
DOI 10.1007/978-3-319-51202-0_28

28.2 Osteosarcoma

Osteosarcoma, together with Ewing sarcoma, is the first primary bone tumor where chemotherapy displayed its effectiveness in the early 1970s [1]. When patients received only surgery, survival rate was lower than 20% [1]. Today, it is widely accepted that the treatment of osteosarcoma requires a combined approach of surgery of the primary tumor and systemic chemotherapy with an expected probability of survival, in case of localized disease and extremity tumors, of around 75% [2]. Standard strategy of chemotherapy for osteosarcoma is based on primary chemotherapy, delayed surgery followed by adjuvant chemotherapy (neoadjuvant chemotherapy) [2].

Thanks to its preoperative use, it is possible to evaluate chemotherapy-induced tumor necrosis by histological examination of the resected surgical specimen [3]. The extent of tumor necrosis is a surrogate marker of chemosensitivity and is predictive of survival [4, 5]. Imaging techniques such as PET and dynamic magnetic resonance have been used to evaluate the pathological response to primary chemotherapy, but their significance is still under discussion [2].

New insights are coming from studies of pharmacogenetics in osteosarcoma. Germline genetic polymorphisms predictive of sensitivity to chemotherapy have been recently described [6–8]. Microarray technology has been recently investigated to predict chemotherapy response and a multigene predictive model was developed to classify good and poor responders to preoperative chemotherapy [8].

Most chemotherapy regimens adopted for osteogenic sarcoma are based on methotrexate (MTX), cisplatin (CDP), doxorubicin, and ifosfamide (IFO). It is well-known that when only CDP and adriamycin (ADM) are used, a probability of disease-free survival (DFS) around 45% can be expected [9].

Strategies of chemotherapy based on the use of the four active drugs lead to a probability of DFS around 60–65% [9]. It is a matter of discussion whether all patients require intensive and prolonged treatment based on all four active drugs [10, 11].

In a recent study, the Italian Sarcoma Group (ISG) demonstrated that IFO can be given postoperatively and only to patients with a poor pathological response to primary chemotherapy based on MTX, CDP, and ADM [12]. This approach allowed the same results with lower toxicity than a chemotherapy based on the four drugs delivered since the primary phase in all patients. A study of the Children's Cancer Group and Pediatric Oncology Group has evaluated whether the addition of ifosfamide and/or muramyl tripeptide-phosphatidylethanolamine (MTP-PE) to methotrexate, cisplatin, and doxorubicin could improve prognosis [13]. MTP-PE is a component of the bacterial cell wall conjugated to phosphatidylethanolamine and encapsulated in liposomes with immunostimulating activity. Overall, the probability of survival was higher in those patients treated with MTP-PE and a trend was reported in terms of event-free survival (EFS) [14]. Based on these data, EMA licensed the drug for commercial use in Europe.

The possible role of immunotherapy in osteosarcoma patients was investigated in a large randomized trial. EURAMOS 1 study [15] randomized patients with good pathological response to the MAP regimen to receive maintenance treatment with interferon. Unfortunately, the results recently reported did not show advantages for patients assigned to the interferon arm [15]. In the same study, the use of a differentiated and intensified treatment in patients with a poor pathological response to MAP failed to show an advantage in survival.

These data are sufficiently robust to support the MAP regimen as the standard treatment in patients with osteosarcoma.

28.3 Ewing Sarcoma

Ewing sarcoma (ES) shares with osteosarcoma similarities in the strategy of treatment.

Neoadjuvant chemotherapy with the aim of reducing tumor mass, increasing the likelihood of local control, and facilitating conservative surgical approaches is considered the standard in patients with Ewing sarcoma [16].

Vincristine, dactinomycin, adriamycin, cyclophosphamide, ifosfmide, and etoposide are the drugs that, in different combinations, are recommended for the neoadjuvant treatment of Ewing sarcoma [16].

Contrary to osteosarcoma, local control in ES can be achieved by surgery or radiotherapy, this tumor being highly sensitive to this last technique. Nevertheless, there is a body of evidence on the superiority of surgery versus radiotherapy in terms of local control rate and late effects. For this reason, the surgical treatment of patients with ES is now preferred and recommended whenever possible [2, 16].

As in osteosarcoma, when ES is surgically treated, the pathological evaluation of chemotherapy-induced tumor necrosis can identify patients having a different probability of survival [2, 16]. Previous studies reported a probability of EFS ranging from 63 to 81% in case of good response and ranging from 20 to 38% in case of poor response [17–19].

In the light of the predictive significance of chemotherapy-induced tumor necrosis, imaging techniques such as PET and dynamic magnetic resonance have been investigated in order to predict tumor response to primary chemotherapy. The results of these studies, most of them being retrospective, are at present not conclusive [20–23].

There is no agreement in the sarcoma community about the best strategy of chemotherapy in patients with Ewing sarcoma. Several data indicate that dose intensification is beneficial [1].

In a joint study carried out by Italian Sarcoma Group and Scandinavian Sarcoma Group, a dose-intensified treatment with high-dose busulfan and melphalan followed by peripheral blood stem cell rescue was used in patients with poor response to primary chemotherapy comprising vincristine, dactinomycin, adriamycin, cyclophosphamide, ifosfmide, and etoposide. The results showed that poor responder patients had the same probability of event-free survival as good responder patients [24]. The use of high-dose chemotherapy in patients with ES is still a matter of debate [1]. A study protocol [25] was activated some years ago to investigate the role of high-dose chemotherapy in ES. Interesting results, superior to those reported in literature, were obtained in the group of the so-called very high-risk patients (patients with multivisceral metastases with or without bone marrow infiltration) who could receive high-dose chemotherapy [26]. In the same study, patients with poor response to primary chemotherapy or with lung metastases only were randomized to receive intensified treatment with high-dose chemotherapy or a postlocal treatment regimen with chemotherapy at standard dose. Unfortunately, the results of this group of patients are not yet available.

A different way to dose intensification was that followed by the Children Oncology Group. In a randomized study [27], standard chemotherapy courses were delivered every 3 or 2 weeks with the support of G-CSFs. All patients received the same treatment regardless of the response to primary chemotherapy. Overall, the results of the study were comparable to those obtained in protocols with high-dose chemotherapy in poor responder patients. Interestingly, results of the study demonstrated that dose intensification obtained by an interval compression (every 2 weeks) is more effective than a standard approach based on chemotherapy courses given every 3 weeks. The study population consisted mainly of children and adolescents and only 15% of patients were older than 18 years and this makes the sample not entirely representative of the real population of patients with ES. Furthermore, the survival advantage was apparent in young and not in adult patients. Nevertheless, these data are an important contribution to the clinical practice suggesting that an interval compression of chemotherapy courses should be recommended at least in younger patients.

28.4 Chondrosarcoma

Chondrosarcoma is, after osteosarcoma, the second most common primary bone tumor. Chondrosarcomas are a diverse group of tumors that share the characteristic of chondroid matrix production, but show different histology, biological behavior, and chemosensitivity [28].

Conventional chondrosarcoma, the most frequent type of chondrosarcoma, is a slow-growing tumor whose aggressiveness and tendency to metastasize is strictly correlated to the grade of the tumor. There is wide agreement that it is resistant to the antineoplastic agents used for bone sarcomas. Surgery, whenever possible, is the main treatment. Grade 3 and, less frequently, grade 2 chondrosarcoma can give metastases, especially to the lungs, and also in this case surgery is the recommended approach. Nevertheless, there are clinical situations of unresectability where the use of chemotherapy is part of the clinical practice. A recent retrospective study reported that overall survival for patients with unresectable diseases is poor, with a 3-year overall survival (OS) of 12% (5-year survival of 2%). Patients with only local unresectable disease had a better prognosis than those with metastatic disease, with an overall survival of 26% after 3 years [29]. It is interesting to note that when the treatment received was analyzed, the authors found a survival benefit for metastatic patients who underwent chemotherapy. The efficacy of systemic treatment was apparent only in patients with metastatic disease and not in patients with locally advanced unresectable chondrosarcoma. As stated by the authors, "the general result of improved survival after chemotherapy is rather unexpected because the common opinion is that chondrosarcoma patients do not benefit from nonsurgical treatment." These data, although coming from a retrospective analysis, support the use of chemotherapy also in chondrosarcoma in the presence of unresectable metastatic disease. No data supporting a specific chemotherapy regimen can be suggested, doxorubicin, ifosfamide, and cisplatin being the most frequently used antineoplastic agents. Recently, a long-lasting response to gemcitabine has been reported in a patient with metastatic chondrosarcoma [30].

Several attempts have been made to explore alternative targets in chondrosarcomas. Based on the evidence that the platelet-derived growth factor receptor (PDGFR) is expressed and phosphorylated, a clinical study with imatinib was carried out, but failed to demonstrate any activity [31]. Some interest was posed on the evidence of the expression of aromatase and estrogen receptors in chondrosarcoma, but the use of drugs inhibiting estrogen signaling was not found beneficial [32]. Preclinical data have shown that the Hedgehog pathway plays an important role in tumor proliferation of chondrosarcoma [33] and a phase 2 study (ClinicalTrials.gov Identifier: NCT01310816) with the smoothened inhibitor IPI-926 has been recently carried out, but the results are at present not available.

Rare variants of chondrosarcoma are mesenchymal chondrosarcoma, dedifferentiated chondrosarcoma, and clear cell chondrosarcoma.

Mesenchymal chondrosarcoma arises in patients of younger age compared to conventional chondrosarcoma; it is characterized by a bimorphic histological pattern in which a relatively well-differentiated cartilage tissue is admixed with a highly undifferentiated small cell component [28]. Small cells can appear to be round, oval, or spindle-shaped, and this component often resembles a hemangiopericytoma or Ewing sarcoma. There is a tendency to metastasize. On the contrary to what reported for conventional chondrosarcoma, some retrospective studies have shown a superior survival for those patients who received chemotherapy [34–36]. On the basis of what has been reported in literature, it is not possible to identify a standard chemotherapy treatment; nevertheless, it is interesting to note that most patients were given a chemotherapy regimen including antineoplastic agents commonly used for Ewing sarcoma.

Dedifferentiated chondrosarcoma is characterized by the presence of a high-grade component with histologic features of classic osteosarcoma or high-grade undifferentiated pleomorphic sarcoma [28]. The clinical behavior of this rare variant is that of an aggressive sarcoma with a very high rate of metastases. The probability of survival in this group of patients is very low, but patients can benefit from chemotherapy [35]. The largest retrospective study reporting data on the role of systemic chemotherapy in dedifferentiated chondrosarcoma shows a survival advantage in patients without metastases at presentation [37]. Most chemotherapy regimens employed are based on drugs commonly used in osteosarcoma with dose and schedule age adapted, since dedifferentiated chondrosarcoma is more frequent in adult and elderly patients. A prospective study exploring the role of an osteosarcoma-like chemotherapy protocol in patients with dedifferentiated chondrosarcoma has been recently closed to enrollment and the final results will be published in the next year [38].

28.5 Giant-Cell Tumor of Bone

Giant-cell tumor of bone (GCTB) is a rare, osteolytic tumor that mainly occurs in young adults. GCTB is locally aggressive and metastases (mostly to the lung) can occur in up to 6% of patients. The majority of patients can be adequately treated by surgery, but in some, due to site and/or size of the tumor, surgery is not feasible. In case of unresectable GCTB, several options are part of the clinical practice, radiotherapy, and embolization over all, but the results are usually poor and they have a meaning of palliation and not a curative intent. Interferons, bisphosphonates, classic chemotherapy have been tried with unsatisfactory results [39].

GCTB has been investigated and high levels of RANK ligand (RANKL) expression and activated RANK-positive osteoclast-like giant cells were found to be characteristic markers of disease and pivotal elements in the biology of the tumor. Denosumab is a fully human monoclonal antibody that inhibits RANKL and licensed for preventing osteoporosis and skeletal-related events in bone metastases [40]. The specific mechanism of action of denosumab and the relevance of the role of the axis RANK–RANKL in GCTB being witnessed, the drug was tested in patients with advanced/unresectable GCTB or in patients who were the candidates to major surgery in an attempt to downgrade the tumor reducing its morbidity and invasiveness for a less aggressive surgical procedure [41]. The response rate was remarkable; denosumab treatment delayed the immediate need for surgery in many patients, and 90% of patients had either no surgery or underwent a less morbid surgical procedure than originally planned. Based on these data, denosumab was licensed for the use in unresectable GCTB or in case of advanced lesions with the aim of reducing surgical morbidity. The possible treatment effects of denosumab can be attributed to its actions against RANKL leading to deep morphological changes: an almost complete disappearance of the giant-cell component and neoplastic RANKL-positive stromal cells replaced by dense fibro-osseous tissue, new woven bone [42]. The safety profile of denosumab is good and hypocalcemia and ONJ, known risks associated with denosumab, were observed in a small proportion of patients. The drug is allowed only in skeletally mature patients, as the presently available safety data are insufficient for skeletally immature patients. The recommended schedule envisages a loading dose of 120 mg of denosumab given by subcutaneous injection on day 1-8-15 afterward every month. If the tumor is surgically removed, an additional 6 months of therapy are recommended [43].

Denosumab is a drug that has changed the history of GCTB, but several questions are still open:

- Questions about the effectiveness in preventing local recurrence of the 6-month period of therapy after surgery,
- In case of unresectable lesions, do we have to use the drugs indefinitely or it is possible to suspend treatment and resume it in case of disease progression?
- In case of prolonged treatment, is it possible to modify the schedule and deliver the drug with longer intervals?

To answer these questions further studies are required.

28.6 Chordoma

Chordoma is a rare bone tumor (annual incidence 0.1/100,000) that develops from persistent notochordal elements. Sacrum is the most frequent location followed by the skull base and mobile spine. Median age at the time of diagnosis is 60 years [44].

Chordoma is a low-grade tumor with local aggressiveness and with a metastatic potential (metastases can occur in about 30% of patients, usually late in the history of the tumor and after repeated local recurrences). Dedifferentiated cases are observed in 5% of patients [44].

Expression of the brachyury gene (a transcription factor involved in notochord differentiation) has been identified as a definitive diagnostic marker of *chordoma* and immunohistochemistry positivity for brachyury is recommended to confirm diagnosis. Dedifferentiated chordomas may lose brachyury expression [45].

Surgery is the main option of treatment, but sometimes, mainly due to the site of the tumor, functional neurological sequelae can be remarkable and not accepted by the patient. In case of surgery with adequate (R0) margins, the expected 5-year recurrence-free survival is around 50%. When surgery is not feasible or not accepted by the patient, definitive radiation therapy is a valid alternative [46, 47].

Activity and effectiveness of radiotherapy is related to the technique adopted. High-dose protons or carbon ions are very effective and should be considered when radiotherapy is chosen as local treatment [48].

No systemic treatments of proven efficacy are at present available. The antineoplastic agents used in sarcoma patients are not active in patients with chordoma, with the possible exception of high-grade dedifferentiated chordoma.

The activity of imatinib in patients with advanced chordoma has been recently reported both in terms of clinical benefit and progression-free survival (PFS). In 46 patients with advanced progressive disease, imatinib 800 mg/die achieved disease stabilization in 75% and a median PFS of 10 months. Interestingly, 10 (21%) patients remained progression-free >18 months. Based on these data in patients with advanced and progressive chordoma, the use of imatinib should be considered [49].

Since chordoma showed evidence of expression of vascular endothelial growth factor receptor, a study with an EGFR inhibitor (Lapatinib) was carried out. The median PFS was 8 months and the reported clinical benefit rate was 22% [50].

Results achieved in these studies indicate that there is the possibility, also in a tumor-like chordoma, that some kind of systemic chemotherapy may affect the clinical behavior of this disease, suggesting that further clinical investigations are justified and recommended.

References

1. Picci P. Classic osteosarcoma. In: Picci P, Manfrini M, Fabbri N, Gambarotti M, Vanel D, editors. Atlas of musculoskeletal tumors and tumorlike lesions. Cham: Springer; 2014. p. 147–52.
2. ESMO/European Sarcoma Network Working Group. Bone sarcomas: ESMO clinical practice guidelines for diagnosis, treatment and follow-up. Ann Oncol. 2014;25(Suppl 3):iii113–23.
3. Picci P, Bacci G, Campanacci M, et al. Histologic evaluation of necrosis induced by chemotherapy. Regional mapping of viable and nonviable tissue. Cancer. 1985;56:1515–21.
4. Bielack SS, Kempf-Bielack B, Delling G, et al. Prognostic factors in high-grade osteosarcoma of the extremities or trunk: an analysis of 1,702 patients treated on neoadjuvant cooperative osteosarcoma study group protocols. J Clin Oncol. 2002;20:776–90.
5. Bacci G, Longhi A, Versari M, et al. Prognostic factors for osteosarcoma of the extremity treated with neoadjuvant chemotherapy: 15-year experience in 789 patients treated at a single institution. Cancer. 2006;106:1154–61.
6. Kager L, Diakos C, Bielack S. Can pharmacogenomics help to improve therapy in patients with high-grade osteosarcoma? Expert Opin Drug Metab Toxicol. 2015;11:1025–8.
7. Windsor RE, Strauss SJ, Kallis C, Wood NE, Whelan JS. Germline genetic polymorphisms may influence chemotherapy response and disease outcome in osteosarcoma: a pilot study. Cancer. 2012;118:1856–67.
8. Hattinger CM, Fanelli M, Tavanti E, et al. Advances in emerging drugs for osteosarcoma. Expert Opin Emerg Drugs. 2015;20:495–514.
9. Anninga JK, Gelderblom H, Fiocco M, et al. Chemotherapeutic adjuvant treatment for osteosarcoma: where do we stand? Eur J Cancer. 2011;47:2431–45.
10. Ferrari S, Serra M. An update on chemotherapy for osteosarcoma. Expert Opin Pharmacother. 2015;29:1–10.
11. Isakoff MS, Bielack SS, Meltzer P, Gorlick R. Osteosarcoma: current treatment and a collaborative pathway to success. J Clin Oncol. 2015;33:3029–35.
12. Ferrari S, Ruggieri P, Cefalo G, et al. Neoadjuvant chemotherapy with methotrexate, cisplatin, and doxorubicin with or without ifosfamide in nonmetastatic osteosarcoma of the extremity: an Italian sarcoma group trial ISG/OS-1. J Clin Oncol. 2012;30:2112–8.
13. Meyers PA, Schwartz CL, Krailo MD, et al. Osteosarcoma: the addition of muramyl tripeptide to chemotherapy improves overall survival—a report from the Children's Oncology Group. J Clin Oncol. 2008;26:633–8.
14. Meyers PA, Chou AJ. Muramyl tripeptide-phosphatidyl ethanolamine encapsulated in liposomes (L-MTP-PE) in the treatment of osteosarcoma. Adv Exp Med Biol. 2014;804:307–21.
15. Bielack SS, Smeland S, Whelan JS, et al. Methotrexate, doxorubicin, and cisplatin (MAP) plus maintenance pegylated interferon Alfa-2b versus MAP alone in patients with resectable high-grade osteosarcoma and good histologic response to preoperative MAP: first results of the EURAMOS-1 good response randomized controlled trial. J Clin Oncol. 2015;33:2279–87.
16. Gaspar N, Hawkins DS, Dirksen U, et al. Ewing sarcoma: current management and future approaches through collaboration. J Clin Oncol. 2015;33:3036–46.
17. Oberlin O, Habrand JL, Zucker JM, et al. No benefit of ifosfamide in Ewing's sarcoma: a nonrandomized study of the French Society of Pediatric Oncology. J Clin Oncol. 1992;10: 1407–12.
18. Bacci G, Ferrari S, Bertoni F, et al. Prognostic factors in nonmetastatic Ewing's sarcoma of bone treated with adjuvant chemotherapy: analysis of 359 patients at the Istituto Ortopedico Rizzoli. J Clin Oncol. 2000;18:4–11.

19. Paulussen M, Ahrens S, Dunst J, et al. Localized Ewing tumor of bone: final results of the cooperative Ewing's Sarcoma Study CESS 86. J Clin Oncol. 2001;19:1818–29.
20. Raciborska A, Bilska K, Drabko K, et al. Response to chemotherapy estimates by FDG PET is an important prognostic factor in patients with Ewing sarcoma. Clin Transl Oncol. 2016;18:189–95.
21. Ulaner GA, Magnan H, Healey JH, et al. Is methylene diphosphonate bone scan necessary for initial staging of Ewing sarcoma if 18F-FDGPET/CT is performed? Am J Roentgenol. 2014;202:859–67.
22. Gaston LL, Di Bella C, Slavin J, Hicks RJ, Choong PF. 18F-FDG PET response to neoadjuvant chemotherapy for Ewing sarcoma and osteosarcoma are different. Skeletal Radiol. 2011;40:1007–15.
23. Denecke T, Hundsdörfer P, Misch D, et al. Assessment of histological response of paediatric bone sarcomas using FDG PET in comparison to morphological volume measurement and standardized MRI parameters. Eur J Nucl Med Mol Imaging. 2010;37:1842–53.
24. Ferrari S, Sundby Hall K, Luksch R, et al. Nonmetastatic Ewing family tumors: high-dose chemotherapy with stem cell rescue in poor responder patients. Results of the Italian Sarcoma Group/Scandinavian Sarcoma Group III protocol. Ann Oncol. 2011;22:1221–7.
25. EURO-EWING 99. http://www.controlled-trials.com/ISRCTN6143862.
26. Ladenstein R, Pötschger U, Le Deley MC, et al. Primary disseminated multifocal Ewing sarcoma: results of the Euro-EWING 99 trial. J Clin Oncol. 2010;28:3284–91.
27. Womer RB, West DC, Krailo MD, et al. Randomized controlled trial of interval-compressed chemotherapy for the treatment of localized Ewing sarcoma: a report from the Children's Oncology Group. Clin Oncol. 2012;30:4148–54.
28. Fabbri N, Donati D. Chondrosacomas. In: Picci P, Manfrini M, Fabbri N, Gambarotti M, Vanel D, editors. Atlas of musculoskeletal tumors and tumorlike lesions. Cham: Springer; 2014. p. 111–37.
29. van Maldegem AM, Gelderblom H, Palmerini E, et al. Outcome of advanced, unresectable conventional central chondrosarcoma. Cancer. 2014;120:3159–64.
30. Provenzano S, Hindi N, Morosi C, et al. Response of conventional chondrosarcoma to gemcitabine alone: a case report. Clin Sarcoma Res. 2015;5:9.
31. Grignani G, Palmerini E, Stacchiotti S, et al. A phase 2 trial of imatinib mesylate in patients with recurrent nonresectable chondrosarcomas expressing platelet-derived growth factor receptor-α or -β: an Italian Sarcoma Group study. Cancer. 2011;117:826–31.
32. Meijer D, Gelderblom H, Karperien M, et al. Expression of aromatase and estrogen receptor alpha in chondrosarcoma, but no beneficial effect of inhibiting estrogen signaling both in vitro and in vivo. Clin Sarcoma Res. 2011;1:5.
33. Campbell VT, Nadesan P, Ali SA, et al. Hedgehog pathway inhibition in chondrosarcoma using the smoothened inhibitor IPI-926 directly inhibits sarcoma cell growth. Mol Cancer Ther. 2014;13:1259–69.
34. Cesari M, Bertoni F, Bacchini P, et al. Mesenchymal chondrosarcoma. An analysis of patients treated at a single institution. Tumori. 2007;93:423–7.
35. Italiano A, Mir O, Cioffi A, et al. Advanced chondrosarcomas: role of chemotherapy and survival. Ann Oncol. 2013;24:2916–22.
36. Frezza AM, Cesari M, Baumhoer D, et al. Mesenchymal chondrosarcoma: prognostic factors and outcome in 113 patients. A European Musculoskeletal Oncology Society study. Eur J Cancer. 2015;51:374–81.
37. Grimer RJ, Gosheger G, Taminiau A, et al. Dedifferentiated chondrosarcoma: prognostic factors and outcome from a European group. Eur J Cancer. 2007;43:2060–5.
38. Ferrari S, Smeland S, Bielack S, Comandone A, Dileo P, Picci P, Sundby Hall K, Eriksson M, Honegger H, Reichardt P. A European treatment protocol for bone sarcoma in patients older than 40 years. J Clin Oncol. 2009;27(Suppl; abstr 10516):15s.
39. Manfrini M. Giant cell tumor of bone. In: Picci P, Manfrini M, Fabbri N, Gambarotti M, Vanel D, editors. Atlas of musculoskeletal tumors and tumorlike lesions. Cham: Springer; 2014. p. 91–5.

40. Singh AS, Chawla NS, Chawla SP. Giant-cell tumor of bone: treatment options and role of denosumab. Biologics. 2015;9:69–74.
41. Rutkowski P, Ferrari S, Grimer RJ, et al. Surgical downstaging in an open-label phase II trial of denosumab in patients with giant cell tumor of bone. Ann Surg Oncol. 2015;22:2860–8.
42. Girolami I, Mancini I, Simoni A, et al. Denosumab treated giant cell tumour of bone: a morphological, immunohistochemical and molecular analysis of a series. J Clin Pathol. 2016;69:240–7. doi:10.1136/jclinpath-2015-203248.
43. Chawla S, Henshaw R, Seeger L, et al. Safety and efficacy of denosumab for adults and skeletally mature adolescents with giant cell tumour of bone: interim analysis of an open-label, parallel-group, phase 2 study. Lancet Oncol. 2013;14:901–8.
44. Fabbri N, Ruggieri P. Chordoma. In: Picci P, Manfrini M, Fabbri N, Gambarotti M, Vanel D, editors. Atlas of musculoskeletal tumors and tumorlike lesions. Cham: Springer; 2014. p. 233–9.
45. Presneau N, Shalaby A, Ye H, et al. Role of the transcription factor T (brachyury) in the pathogenesis of sporadic chordoma: a genetic and functional-based study. J Pathol. 2011;223:327–35.
46. Stacchiotti S, Sommer J, Chordoma Global Consensus Group. Building a global consensus approach to chordoma: a position paper from the medical and patient community. Lancet Oncol. 2015;16:e71–83. doi:10.1016/S1470-2045(14)71190-8.
47. Angelini A, Pala E, Calabrò T, Maraldi M, Ruggieri P. Prognostic factors in surgical resection of sacral chordoma. J Surg Oncol. 2015;112:344–51.
48. Rotondo RL, Folkert W, Liebsch NJ, et al. High-dose proton-based radiation therapy in the management of spine chordomas: outcomes and clinicopathological prognostic factors. J Neurosurg Spine. 2015;23:788–97.
49. Stacchiotti S, Longhi A, Ferraresi V, et al. Phase II study of imatinib in advanced chordoma. J Clin Oncol. 2012;30:914–20.
50. Stacchiotti S, Tamborini E, Lo Vullo S, et al. Phase II study on lapatinib in advanced EGFR-positive chordoma. Ann Oncol. 2013;24:1931–6.

Printed by Printforce, the Netherlands